LASERS IN GENERAL SURGERY

LASERS IN GENERAL SURGERY

EDITED BY

STEPHEN N. JOFFE, M.D.

PROFESSOR OF SURGERY
DEPARTMENT OF SURGERY
UNIVERSITY OF CINCINNATI MEDICAL CENTER
CINCINNATI, OHIO

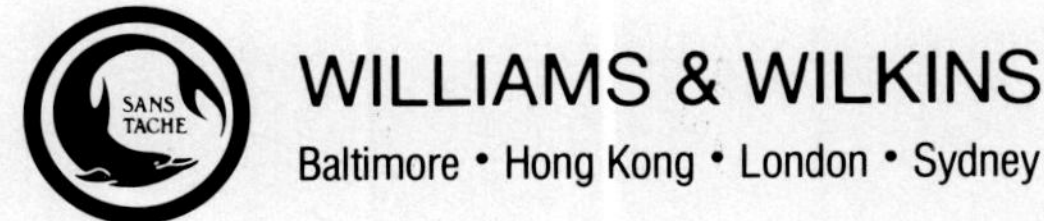

WILLIAMS & WILKINS
Baltimore • Hong Kong • London • Sydney

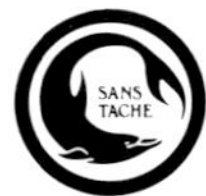

Editor: John N. Gardner
Associate Editor: Victoria M. Vaughn
Copy Editor: Shelley Potler
Design: Norman W. Och
Illustration Planning: Lorraine Wrzosek
Production: Barbara J. Felton

Williams & Wilkins
428 East Preston Street
Baltimore, Maryland 21202, USA

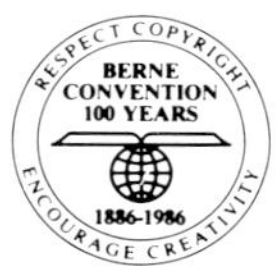

Accurate indications, adverse reactions, and dosage schedules for drugs are provided in this book, but it is possible that they may change. The reader is urged to review the package information data of the manufacturers of the medications mentioned.

Printed in the United States of America

Library of Congress Cataloging-in-Publication Data

Lasers in general surgery.

Includes index.
1. Lasers in surgery. I. Joffe, Stephen N. [DNLM:
1. Laser Surgery. WO 500 L3433]
RD73.L3L385 1989 617'.05 88-27986
ISBN 0-683-04460-5

The publishers have made every effort to trace the copyright holders for borrowed material. If they have inadvertently overlooked any, they will be pleased to make the necessary arrangements at the earliest opportunity.

89 90 91 92 93
1 2 3 4 5 6 7 8 9 10

DEDICATION

This book is dedicated to Theodore H. Maiman, Ph.D., a scientist who has combined the unique qualities of intellectual brilliance with compassion and humility. Since its invention by Dr. Maiman in 1960, the laser has found widespread applications in communications, industry, defense, and medicine. Lasers are the single most important advancement in surgery of the 20th century.

Patients, physicians, and the health care industry are all deeply indebted to Dr. Maiman. His wisdom, knowledge, foresight, and ingenuity have opened new vistas never before achievable.

PREFACE

It has been more than 28 years since the invention of the first ruby laser by Dr. Theodore H. Maiman.

Since that time, lasers have found numerous industrial, military, and medical uses. These versatile devices have evolved from the early short-pulsed lasers to the more sophisticated continuous-wave gas and solid-state lasers. Clinical application of lasers in general surgery, as well as basic and applied research, is still in evolution. Surgeons are just beginning to use the laser in a variety of surgical procedures. This textbook will illustrate operations, primarily in general surgery and related areas, in which the laser can be used.

The surgical specialties that have most readily adopted surgical lasers are ophthalmology, gynecology, and urology. Lasers have radically changed the ways in which many procedures can be done.

In gynecology, laser energy can be delivered through laparoscopes and hysteroscopes similar or identical to those already in use and by providing the ability to cut, vaporize, or coagulate tissue without the uncontrolled spreading effect of electrosurgery. Lasers render many existing procedures easier and more effective, and permit more conservative treatments of certain conditions. Laser endometrial ablation, for example, is replacing hysterectomy in many instances as an effective, yet less traumatic, treatment of chronic menorrhagia.

The situation is less clear in general surgery. The general surgeon encounters a wider variety of tissue types and operating conditions than most other surgical specialists, so that an instrument with narrowly defined capabilities would be useful in a correspondingly small number of cases. If a CO_2 laser will only cut, an argon or noncontact Nd:YAG will only coagulate, then in the absence of other procedural advantages it is difficult to justify—particularly in today's acutely cost-conscious hospital environment—using expensive equipment to do what simpler instruments will do almost or just as well. There would be no reason to encourage surgeons to give up familiar and proven methods in favor of complex technology that offers no specific advantages, except for being on the ''cutting edge'' and with ''state-of-the-art'' equipment.

The simple questions one ought to ask are: Can lasers perform more useful functions surgically than other currently available instruments? Can impossible procedures be rendered possible, or complex operations be simplified? Do lasers introduce less invasive surgical alternatives? Can lasers make surgery more effective, less painful and traumatic for the patient, or easier for the surgeon and operating room staff? Are there economic benefits, such as reduced length of hospital stay, that counterbalance the comparatively high purchase, maintenance, and utilization costs of most lasers?

Curiously enough, one of the laser's greatest handicaps in general surgery has been the unbridled zeal of its advocates. Some enthusiastic laser surgeons would introduce surgery more than may be reasonable. Certain steps, such as initial skin incisions, may be quicker and easier with an ordinary steel scalpel and electrocautery may give results indistinguishable from the laser technique, in which case the old familiar instruments may quite sensibly be selected due either to cost considerations or to the personal preference of the individual surgeon.

A great many general surgical procedures have been performed with lasers, including mastectomies, hemorrhoidectomies, cholecystectomies, solid organ surgery, and resections of the gastrointestinal tract. The literature on these procedures is sparse and often contradictory. Yet, credibly documented claims have been made that lasers can reduce bleeding, drainage, and postoperative pain. Because all lasers provide some hemostasis while cutting, there is less need for sutures, clips, or electrocautery. It is beyond question that in at least some procedures the laser technique allows shorter hospital stays and an earlier return of the patient to a normal routine.

Most general surgery laser procedures have been done with the CO_2 laser, which came into use about a decade ago, but the contact Nd:YAG, introduced in 1985, has taken over an increasingly larger number of applications and operative procedures.

Whereas the CO_2 laser delivers an intense, shallow thermal effect useful for cutting, and in the defocussed mode can provide superficial coagulation, the contact Nd:YAG can cut, coagulate, cut and coagulate, or vaporize tissue with a controlled depth of thermal penetration. The CO_2 beam is delivered through a cumbersome and sensitive articulated arm, and the delivery device must be used at some distance from the operative site. The contact Nd:YAG is delivered through a flexible optical fiber to a scalpel handpiece that can be used in contact with tissue. Fibers with handpieces are available in various lengths and configurations to suit particular procedures and personal techniques.

The contact Nd:YAG cuts as proficiently as the CO_2 laser, yet retains the coagulative properties of the Nd:YAG, a factor that contributes to its ability to seal blood vessels and lymphatics. Because one is working with a defined region of high-power density localized at the tip of the contact laser scalpel rather than with an open laser beam, there is no need for backstop devices to protect neighboring tissues or special anodized or ebonized instruments. The production of annoying and possibly noxious smoke is also greatly reduced.

The contact Nd:YAG laser preserves all of the surgical advantages of conventional noncontract lasers, yet adds tremendous procedural versatility and eliminates much of the mechanical complexity that has plagued surgical lasers thus far.

Laser surgery requires minimal training and practice in order to become skillful. The general surgeon easily acquires the ability to translate hand-eye-foot or hand-eye coordination to standard surgical procedures. Effective laser surgery may require a slightly different exposure or sequence of events in order to accomplish the task at hand. There is a learning curve, but once proficiency has been attained the benefits to patients are well worth the expended effort.

Lasers may be used in general surgery for cutting, vaporization, coagulation, and the newer areas of photodynamic therapy and interstitial hyperthermia. The histological effect on tissue closely resembles the scalpel and electrocautery when the laser is employed as a cutting instrument.

The primary objective of this textbook is to provide general surgeons and those working in related areas with current, substantive, and practical guidance in the comprehension and use of lasers in general surgery.

Stephen N. Joffe, M.D.
Cincinnati, Ohio

CONTRIBUTORS

Gregory T. Absten, M.A.
President
Advanced Laser Services Corporation
Columbus, Ohio

Vincent W. Ansanelli, M.D.
Breast Surgical Oncology
Plainview, New York

David B. Apfelberg, M.D.
Director, Comprehensive Laser Center
Palo Alto Medical Foundation
Palo Alto, California
Assistant Clinical Professor (Plastic Surgery)
Stanford University Medical Center
Stanford, California

B. L. Aronoff, M.D.
Director of Surgical Oncology and Laser Surgery
Baylor University Medical Center
Dallas, Texas

Peter-Wolf Ascher, M.D.
Professor of Neurosurgery
Department of Radiology
Karl-Franzens-University and Medical School
Graz, Austria

Jean-Luc Boulnois, Ph.D.
Scientific Manager
Quantel
Orsay, France

Jean-Marc Brunetaud, M.D.
Associate Professor of Medicine
University of Lille
Chief, Laser Center
University Hospital
Lille, France

Mary M. Cayton, B.S.N.
Cardiovascular Clinical Specialist
St. Luke's Hospital
Director of Laser Research Laboratory
Clement Zablocki Veterans Administration Medical Center
Milwaukee, Wisconsin

D. Cochelard, M.D.
Laser Center
Hopital C Huriez
Lille, France

A. Cortot, M.D.
Laser Center
Hopital C Huriez
Lille, France

Norio Daikuzono, M.Sc.
President, Surgical Laser Technologies (Japan) Ltd.
Tokyo, Japan

Christopher J. Daly, M.D.
Attending Staff
The Pittsburgh Laser Center
St. Francis Medical Center
Pittsburgh, Pennsylvania

Elizabeth C. Eddy, B.S.
Garden City, New York

Howard J. Eddy, Jr., M.D.
Attending Surgeon
Community Hospital at Glen Cove
Glen Cove, New York
St. John's Hospital and
Community Hospital of Western Suffolk
Smithtown, New York
Brookline Hospital
Brookline, Massachusetts
Hahnemann Hospital
Brighton, Massachusetts

Leon Goldman, M.D.
Laser Consultant
U.S. Naval Hospital
San Diego, California
Professor Emeritus, Dermatology
University of Cincinnati College of Medicine
Cincinnati, Ohio

John H. Graber, M.D.
Director, Leg Ulcer Clinic
Abbott Northwestern Hospital
Minneapolis, Minnesota

H. Raoul Herrera, M.D.
Chief of Plastic Surgery
Rochester General Hospital
Associate Clinical Professor
University of Rochester
Rochester, New York

David F. Hickok, M.D.
Clinical Associate Professor
University of Minnesota Medical School
Minneapolis, Minnesota

J. Raymond Hinshaw, M.D.
Professor of Surgery
University of Rochester School of Medicine and Dentistry
Chief of Surgery
Rochester General Hospital
Rochester, New York

Issei Ichimiya, M.D.
Department of Otolaryngology
Medical College of Oita
Oita, Japan

Kaichi Isono, M.D.
Second Department of Surgery
School of Medicine
Chiba University
Chiba, Japan

Stephen N. Joffe, M.D.
Professor of Surgery
University of Cincinnati Medical Center
President
Laser Centers of America
Cincinnati, Ohio

Teruo Kouzu, M.D.
Second Department of Surgery
School of Medicine
Chiba University
Chiba, Japan

Yuichi Kurono, M.D.
Department of Otolaryngology
Medical College of Oita
Oita, Japan

Johannes Lammer, M.D.
Associate Professor of Radiology
Department of Radiology
Karl-Franzens-University and Medical School
Graz, Austria

Raymond J. Lanzafame, M.D.
Assistant Professor of Surgery
University of Rochester
Director, Laser Center
Chairman
Laser Usage Committee
Rochester General Hospital
Rochester, New York

Jack M. Lomano, M.D.
Chairman of the Department of OB-GYN
Grant Medical Center
Director of Education and Development
Grant Laser Center
Clinical Assistant Professor
Obstetrics and Gynecology
Ohio State University
Columbus, Ohio

V. Maunoury, M.D.
Laser Center
Hopital C. Huriez
Lille, France

Adam Mester, M.D.
Assistant Professor
Laser Research Laboratory
Postgraduate Medical University
Department of Radiology
Semmelweis Medical School
Budapest, Hungary

Andrew F. Mester, M.D.
Research Associate
Department of Otorhinolaryngology and Human Communication, and Smell and Taste Center
University of Pennsylvania
Philadelphia, Pennsylvania

Mahmood Mirhoseini, M.D.
Assistant Clinical Professor of Cardiothoracic Surgery
Medical College of Wisconsin
Laser Laboratory
Clement Zablocki Veterans Administration Medical Center
Department of Cardiothoracic Surgery
St. Luke's Hospital
Milwaukee, Wisconsin

Goro Mogi, M.D.
Professor and Chairman
Department of Otolaryngology
Oita Medical College
Oita, Japan

Masaru Ohyama, M.D.
Professor and Chairman
Department of Otolaryngology
Faculty of Medicine
Kagoshima University
Kagoshima, Japan

J. C. Parris, M.D.
Laser Center
Hopital C Huriez
Lille, France

Ralph P. Pennino, M.D.
Clinical Assistant Professor of Surgery
University of Rochester School of Medicine and Dentistry
Attending in Surgery
Rochester General Hospital
Rochester, New York

Ernst Pilger
Department of Internal Medicine
Karl-Franzens-University and Medical School
Graz, Austria

O. Juhani Rämö, M.D.
II Department of Surgery
Helsinki University Central Hospital
Helsinki, Finland

M. Y. Sankar, M.D.
Assistant Professor of Surgery
University of Cincinnati Medical Center
Cincinnati, Ohio

Tom Schröder, M.D.
II Department of Surgery
Helsinki University Central Hospital
Helsinki, Finland

Leonard S. Schultz, M.D.
Chief, Department of Surgery, Abbott
Northwestern Hospital
Minneapolis, Minnesota
Surgical Staff, Fairview
Ridges Hospital
Burnsville, Minnesota

David H. Sliney, Ph.D.
Chief, Laser Branch
Laser Microwave Division
U.S. Army Environmental Hygiene Agency
Aberdeen Proving Ground, Maryland

Norman Sohn, M.D.
Clinical Assistant Professor of Surgery
New York Medical College
Valhalla, New York
Associate Surgeon
Lenox Hill Hospital
New York, New York

Raymond A. Sultan, M.D.
Head of the Laser Platform
Departmental Hospital Stell
Quest University
Paris, France

S. Suzuki, M.D.
Department of Internal Medicine
Tokai University School of Medicine
Kanazawa, Japan

Hisao Tajiri, M.D.
Department of Internal Medicine
National Cancer Center Hospital
Tokyo, Japan

CONTENTS

CHAPTER
1

Types of Surgical Lasers

Gregory T. Absten

To discuss the various types of surgical laser systems, this chapter will examine the principles of operation of different systems and advantages of various features found on many surgical lasers. Other than to mention their existence, ophthalmic laser systems will not be discussed. The information provided is based on available information.

When considering the acquisition of any laser system, three specific areas should be examined to determine which system to purchase. These are technology, training, and service.

TECHNOLOGY

The cliche is: *Buy only state-of-the-art.* There is considerable truth to this statement, but the question is: What is state-of-the-art? The truth is that most of the laser systems on the market will work well for their designed use. Most systems utilize the same basic technologies with minor variations and the addition of "ringers and bells." There are some exceptions such as the difference between flowing gas and sealed-tube carbon dioxide (CO_2) laser technologies, although each system still has some definite advantages.

Laser designs change quickly, but most involve changes in cosmetic appeal, convenience, and ease of use. When examing various lasers of the same wavelength, they all accomplish the same surgical tasks. Examine the ease of operation of the unit, its mobility, and ease of storage. In clinics, offices, or small operating rooms, the size of the unit may be an important consideration. How much noise does the system generate? What are the installation requirements and how much will those cost? What accessories are included in the package for the laser. Acessories can become a significant additional cost to a system.

Although one should seek up-to-date technology, obsolescence should not be a cause for anxiety in the selection of equipment. If the laser accomplishes the surgical task needed, it will continue to do so years in the future if properly maintained. Newer lasers simply become easier to use and more convenient. The attachments and delivery systems will be the focus of change and development. These can be added to the system at a later date, and most attachments are increasingly being made available from third parties to adapt to most systems.

Older laser systems do not become outdated and have to be discarded because of age and reliability. Older laser systems can be refurbished for a fraction of the cost of new laser systems. These refurbished systems become like new and, because of newer optical technologies, many are better refurbished than when originally new.

The hospital may want to evaluate systems in-house before their purchase. Most companies will make arrangements for a demonstration or evaluation in-house, but certain courtesies should be extended to the companies in return. Let the company know where you stand in the evaluation process, how many and which lasers are left to evaluate, and when they can expect a purchase order issued after the last evaluation. Be as expedient as possible in the evaluation process. It is not necessary to keep a unit for an entire month to evaluate its use. At most, a few days are sufficient if the hospital has organized the demonstration by making sure the physicians are aware of place and times, and assuring that all key individuals will be able to examine the unit. Do not arrange in-house trials or demonstrations if the staff is not yet properly educated on laser use; they must know which questions to ask and how to evaluate features. CO_2 lasers have been evaluated by pulling out a tape measure to assess the length of the articulated arm. The longest arm won the evaluation. If the staff is not knowledgeable on the basics of lasers, provide these presentations before an evaluation is conducted. Evaluations can sometimes be performed more satisfactorily by arranging on-site visits to other facilities with a key group from the hospital. This allows conversation with more experienced users of the system, and examination of the unit after it has been in use for a while.

TRAINING

Who can provide the most training support? Training is the single most important factor in the safe, frequent use of any laser system. Training is operationally important for the laser specialists, nurses, or technicians that operate the equipment and implement safety policies. It is important for physicians to learn the correct use and application of lasers, and it is important for management to learn to package laser resources.

Most manufacturers will provide some type of training with the purchase of the laser. Specific information should be obtained as to the type of training, the number of people who will be trained, the quality and time frame of the training, and the levels of training, such as nursing and physician courses.

Training is additionally available from third parties such as independent laser consultants. Hands-on physician training programs conducted in-house, as well as nursing training, can be provided by consultants. If the manufacturer has not detailed the costs of their education package included in the laser purchase, request that information. Considering quality, convenience, and money, decide whether it is better to acquire training from the manufacturer or consultant groups. Training should not be deleted from any laser purchase, even if the hospital is otherwise experienced in laser. A pushbutton inservice would be the minimum level of training.

SERVICE

What is the reputation of the manufacturer? Most companies will promise a response within 24 hours to a service request. Call other hospitals to learn what their experiences have been. Manufacturers will supply a list of users if requested, but these references obviously will be select.

As a condition of laser purchase, the manufacturer should be requested to supply a technical service manual with the unit. This should be a complete manual to include calibration and alignment procedures. It is good policy to maintain these types of manuals, and if the manufacturer should ever go out of business, the hospital will have the necessary information to maintain the unit.

Independent service providers are available to service most types of surgical laser units. Service contracts are frequently available from groups such as this at much lower costs than from the manufacturer inasmuch as the manufacturer must support sales efforts with service personnel. If the manufacturer does cease operations in the future, the laser can still be maintained by these groups. Most laser parts are readily accessible from the original component manufacturers.

TYPES OF LASERS

Lasers that currently have found the widest applications in medicine are those based on carbon dioxide (CO_2), argon, neodymium: yttrium aluminum garnet (Nd: YAG), krypton, and various dyes. In general surgery, the CO_2 and contact Nd:YAG lasers are the main ones used.

Carbon Dioxide (CO_2) Lasers

When the CO_2 gas mixture is energized and stimulated to emit light, there is a concomitant dissociation of the molecule into carbon monoxide and a free oxygen radical, unlike the argon or neodymium atoms, which do not break apart (Fig. 1.1). There is actually a more complicated chemistry involving a CO_2-helium-nitrogen laser gas, but this simplification suits the purpose of this discussion.

The resulting molecule is no longer able to produce the CO_2 laser light. This is complicated by the fact that electrodes in the laser tube emit contaminants that further degrade the gas mixture. Two basic configurations of CO_2 lasers have resulted for medical use.

Flowing Gas CO_2 Systems

A flowing gas system purges the tube of the contaminants and dissociated molecule by continuously replenishing the gas. Flowing gas systems are the oldest and most established technology for CO_2 lasers. They require cylinders of replacement gas, pressure regulators, and a vacuum pump to draw the gas through the system. All of this adds to the maintenance, noise, and expense of operating the laser.

Laser gas is relatively expensive, costing $75–105 per bottle. Lasers that are used infrequently

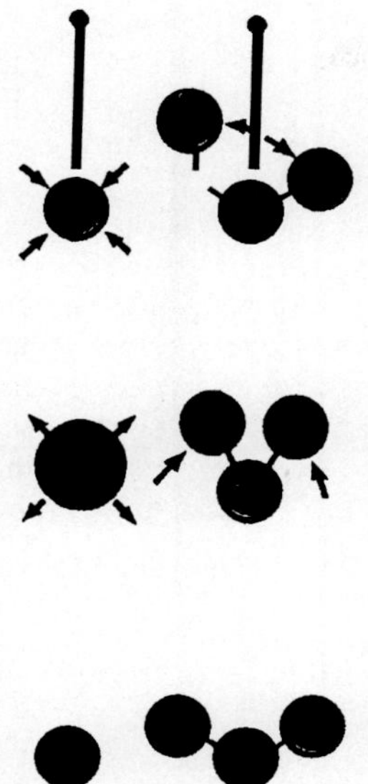

Figure 1.1. Dissociation of the CO_2 molecule.

will not incur large gas charges, however, heavily used lasers can consume several thousand dollars per year in gas.

Flowing gas systems do produce reliable, steady outputs and easily generate powers up to 100 W for medicine. At the low end of the power scale (1–5 W), the output is stable and reliable. Superpulse modes on the flowing gas systems are generally ''cleaner'' than the sealed tube variety.

Hi-Tech utilizes what is termed a micro-flow system on their lasers. This is used to reduce substantially the amount of gas the laser consumes.

Companies that produce fllowing gas systems include Cooper, Coherent, Hi-Tech, Nippon Infrared Industries Corporation (N.I.I.C.), and Sharplan. Some of these companies also produce sealed-tube lasers.

Prices range from approximately $18,000–32,000 for small office-type units of 15–25 W. Hospital-type units of 35–100 W range from $35,000–55,000 for 40- to 50-W units, up to approximately $115,000 for 100-W units. A rough guide of $1/W is sometimes used.

Sealed-Tube, Free Space CO_2 Lasers

These are a newer generation laser tube that eliminates the need for replacement laser gas mixture, regulators, and vacuum pumps. They can produce power levels comparable to flowing gas systems, of up to approximately 100 W. It simplifies operation and maintenance of a CO_2 laser.

This type of sealed-tube laser uses the same type of direct current (DC) excitation as do the fllowing gas systems. (each type still plugs into a standard AC outlet). Catalysts and inhibitors are added to the self-contained gas mixture to retard gas breakdown, and electrodes must be specially designed and treated to avoid emission of contaminants. The tubes will need to be recharged after several years as the power gradually falls from the high end of output.

Sealed-tube lasers appear to be the definite trend in the industry. Sealed systems of both varieties are generally simpler to operate, quieter, and require less routine maintenance than flowing gas systems.

Power output at the low end of the scale, less than 5 W, is not quite as stable as with flowing gas systems. Some of the higher powered sealed systems do not actually operate in a continuous wave (CW) mode at 1 or 2 W. Instead they oscillate on and off at a slightly higher power to provide an average power of the desired output. This is similar to a superpulse or chopped mode at the low end of the scale. Superpulsing a sealed-tube system, although quite satisfactory, is not technically as clean as with flowing gas systems.

Companies that handle this type of sealed-tube laser include Heraeus Lasersonics, Surgilase, California Laboratories, and Sharplan. Some of them also handle flowing gas systems.

Radiofrequency (RF) Waveguide CO_2 Lasers

These are the other type of sealed-tube laser, but instead of using direct current through electrodes in the tube, they utilize a RF that is transmitted transversely across the tube to excite the gas molecules. This eliminates electrode contamination. The ceramic bore of the tube is impregnated with catalysts and inhibitors to retard gas degradation. A waveguide structure of the laser head contains the RF. There is no interference with monitors or electrical equipment.Coherent, previously Xanar, has introduced the highest powered (55 W) RF waveguide laser in their XL 55, but other RF units typically produce lower power (25 W and less).

Companies that produce RF waveguide lasers include BioQuantum Technologies, Coherent (previously the Xanar line), and Pfizer. Coherent

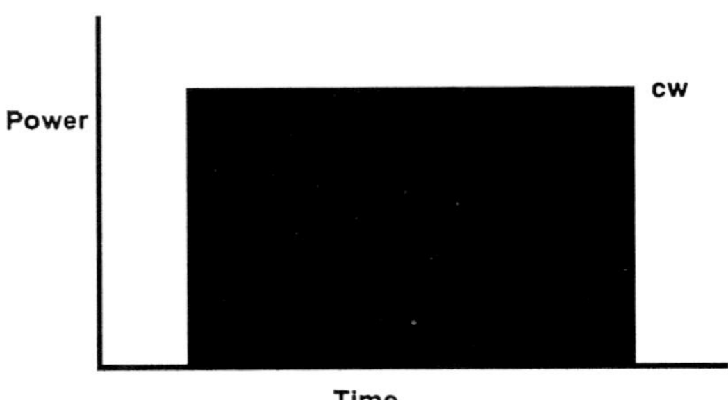

Figure 1.2. Continuous wave (CW) mode.

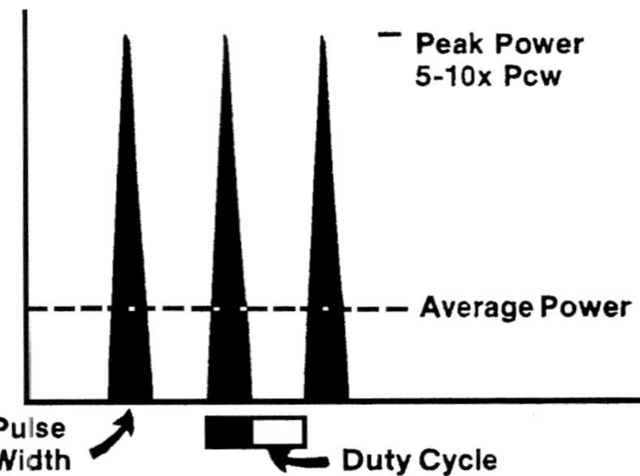

Figure 1.3. Superpulse parameters.

produces the only RF systems with articulated arms for general surgical use.

CO_2 Laser Modalities

The choices for the surgeon when requesting the operational mode of the CO_2 laser include CW, pulsed, repeat pulse, and superpulse. The surgeon manipulates the laser by controlling the mode, power, and spot size of the focused beam. In using the CO_2 laser as a general surgical instrument, to cut and vaporize tissues, particularly in a bloody field, an articulated arm is required and power capability of 50 W or higher is suggested. The higher the power available on a CO_2 laser the better, but 50–60 W will perform satisfactorily for all procedures.

In *CW* operation, the laser is emitted as a steady output for the entire time the beam is emitted. (Fig. 1.2). All CO_2 lasers have the CW capability. The Sharplan 1100 uses a chopped mode in place of the CW mode on this 100-W laser. The chopped mode cycles on and off at several hundred times per second—so fast that it appears continuous. Each pulse of the cycle jumps to a power approximately 1 and ½ times higher than that set on the laser. It averages out to give the set power. This is an engineering function to provide higher powers from a short tube than would otherwise be possible. The chopped mode appears a little "hotter" than a CW mode and is slightly cleaner for incision and vaporization.

A *pulsed* mode on a CO_2 laser provides one single pulse of a predetermined length, at whatever power is set. This provides a short burst of energy that reduces heat spread and provides more reaction time and control for the surgeon. This is merely a timer on the CW mode. It goes very slowly but with a high degree of precision. The surgeon will have to "pump" the foot pedal for each pulse.

Some lasers have preset options on the length of pulses. Four common settings are routinely provided between 0.05 and 0.5 sec. Some lasers provide continuous selection of pulse lengths from the microprocessor. A starting point of 0.1 sec is usually good on a pulse. If the effect is too much, the length is shortened to 0.05 sec. If it is not enough it is lengthened to 0.2 sec.

Repeat pulse is the same as a pulse except that the beam will automatically keep pulsing instead of the surgeon having to pump the foot pedal. Some lasers have preset rates at which the pulses are emitted—approximately 0.5 sec between each pulse. Others allow the user to vary the speed at which pulses are emitted. A variable rate is a very useful feature that retains the precision of pulsing and allows faster work than is gained by the slower preset rates.

Superpulse (Fig. 1.3) is a very useful feature for CO_2 lasers that provides a high degree of precision, but at slower speeds than in a CW mode. Superpulse has been vastly overstated by most of the manufacturers. It is called by various names including superpulse, megapulse, varipulse, enhanced, and spiked modes. They are all essentially the same even though there may be slight technical differences between manufacturers. Some combine the effects of superpulse and a chopped mode.

From the surgeon's view, superpulse is most useful in making cleaner incisions with a focused beam. It reduces the amount of charring created, but is less useful in vaporizing tissue with a

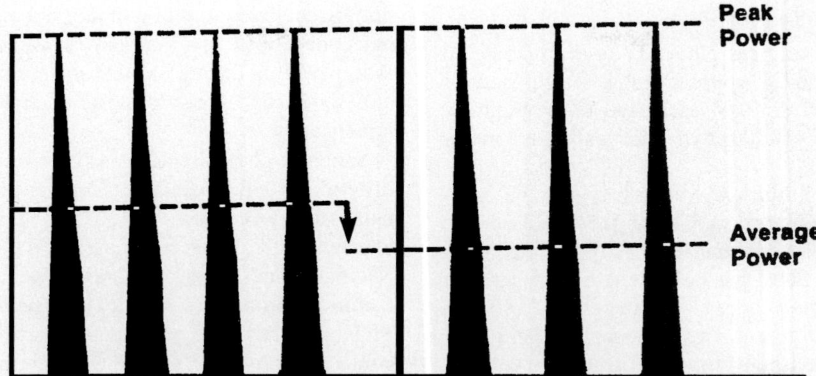

Figure 1.4. Superpulse average power changed by decreasing the frequency.

defocused beam. Superpulse is cleaner but offers less hemostasis than a CW mode.

Superpulse cycles on and off at several hundred times per second—like chopped mode—except that the power of each spiked pulse may go to 7–10 times the usual maximum output of the laser. In other words, an 80-W laser may produce a superpulse of 500 W at peak power.

Some lasers preset the power of this spike to maximum, then adjust the average power by changing pulse widths and frequency (i.e., Surgilase and N.I.I.C.) (Fig. 1.4). Other lasers preset the pulse widths and frequency, and adjust the average power by adjusting the power of the spike (i.e., Sharplan). Both types of systems will work well.

It is beyond the scope of this chapter to expand on the technical variations in superpulse and what they mean to the surgeon. Most of the differences are very subtle clinically. Superpulse does expand the precision capability of a CO_2 laser, but lasers that have only CW capability can perform any procedure that a superpulse laser can perform. It is a very useful feature, but not absolutely necessary to perform surgery.

CO_2 lasers do not have special installation requirements. They all have self-contained cooling systems and plug into standard 100 V outlets. Some of the higher powered lasers use two separate 110 V lines.

Neodymium: Yttrium-Aluminum-Garnet Lasers (Nd:YAG)

These units have higher power and cooling requirements than do CO_2 lasers. Most systems require power of approximately 208 volts, three phase electricity. They also require an external water hookup for cooling. This water is usually tapped from a nearby water line and returned to a drain in a sink.

Surgical Laser Technologies Inc (SLT) produced the first Nd:YAG laser with no requirement for external water cooling. It allows continuous operation at high power without shutting down. Unlike most Nd:YAG lasers, the flashlamps that drive the YAG crystal are not left at full power when the laser is in a ready mode. Instead, the lamps come up to full power only when the foot pedal is depressed. This, combined with the lower 60-W output, allows the unit to be operated with internal cooling, like a CO_2 laser. The SLT YAG also requires single phase power rather than the three-phase power of some other systems.

MBB has released a 40-W Nd:Yag laser that is also internally cooled. The 60-W Heraeus Nd:YAG laser operates from single phase electricity.

The lastest development in Nd:YAG laser technology is a 100 W CW system that requires no external water hookups and utilizes a single, standard 110 V wall outlet for power. This is accomplished through the use of a radically different internal power supply for the laser. The advantages of this configuration include greater mobility of the unit and elimination of installation costs. Living Technologies manufactures these units; more information is required regarding the reliability of these units. Laserscope, manufacturers of the KTP laser, produce one model that is a combination of Nd:YAG and KTP systems.

Nd:YAG Laser Modalities

All of the surgical Nd:YAG lasers operate in the CW mode as opposed to a Q-switched or mode-locked Nd:YAG laser used in ophthalmology to create small sparks and snap apart membranes.

The surgical Nd:YAG laser may also be operated in a timed pulse, similar to the CO_2 laser but for longer pulse lengths from 0.10 sec up to 10 sec or more. Setting a pulse length of 5 sec, for instance, actually is just a "safety limit" to turn off the laser in 5 sec. The surgeon can also terminate the pulse at any time before the 5-sec limit by lifting his foot from the pedal. On the next pulse, the timer would reset to give the full 5 sec.

In many instances it is useful to operate the laser in a true continuous mode so that the emission does not automatically stop every 10 sec or so. The surgeon controls the laser emission entirely with the foot pedal. Not all Nd:YAG lasers have this continuous capability with the foot pedal. Many require the use of a timer for all applications with an upper limit on pulse time from 10–26 sec. The use of contact sapphire probes, in particular, makes the continous mode useful.

Aiming Beams for the Nd:YAG Laser

A red helium neon laser is the standard aiming beam for most Nd:YAG lasers. This works quite well in most instances. However, there are times when using the laser in a noncontact manner that the aiming beam does not show up very well on the target. Heraeus has addressed this with multicolored aiming beams in their high-power laser, and variable intensity in their lower power 60-W laser.

Nd:YAG Laser Fibers and Probes

Some Nd:YAG laser manufacturers still offer reusable fibers, in addition to disposable ones. These systems must be cleaved, polished, and reassembled each time the tip burns out. Reusable fibers are relatively expensive, in the range of $1500, but may be used up, then restrung relatively inexpensively. Fiber polishing requires time and attention from the hospital staff. Most manufacturers now offer disposable fibers for their Nd:YAG lasers following the introduction initially by SLT, Inc.

When evaluting Nd:YAG lasers, the options in cooling the fiber should also be considered. Gas options include internal compressed air and external connections for nitrogen or carbon dioxide. Water cooling through a fiber is very useful in the closed spaces of gastrointestinal endoscopy and laparoscopy.

Sapphire probes significantly expand the versatility of any Nd:YAG laser. Contact probes, originally developed by SLT, Inc., are available through SLT, Heraeus Lasersonics, Surgilase, Sharplan, and Living Technologies. Each manufacturer's probes are slightly different. However, SLT, Inc. has several patents approved on their contact sapphire probes and they are the leaders in this technology and its applications to general surgery. In addition, SLT, Inc. was the first to obtain approval for their laser equipment and contact probes in general surgery.

Surgical Nd:YAG lasers are also available from Laser Industries, Ltd. (distributed by Sharplan), Medical Energy Inc., Surgilase, Surgical Laser Technologies (SLT), Trimedyne, and Living Technologies. MBB (Messerschmidt-Bolkow-Blohm) previously distributed lasers under the trade name Medilase and distributed in the U.S. through Endolase, Inc. Endolase is no longer in business. Service may be obtained through Advanced Laser Services Corporation. Discounted, new MBB YAG lasers, acquired from the Endolase bankruptcy, may be obtained through MedLaser, Inc.

Sixty-W Nd:YAG lasers are available in the cost range of $70,000–95,000; 100-W systems range from approximately $85,000–100,000. Attachments can run an additional $10,000 so this should be considered in the purchase.

Green Light Lasers—Argon and KTP

Both argon and KTP lasers produce green light, although of slightly different wavelengths. Their tissue effects are very similar if not identical. Both are fiberoptically delivered lasers. The only freestanding general use argon laser is made by HGM Laser. Similarly, Laserscope produces the only medical KTP laser system.

Laserscope utilizes fibers intended to be used only as bare fibers. When the fiber burns out a special cleaving device is provided to repair the tip quickly. The laser is controlled through a microprocessor. Power outputs are in the maximum range of 12–15 W. This laser uses a Nd:YAG laser at its heart and requires 208 V, three-phase electricity, and external water connections for cooling.

Laserscope also produces a combination Nd:YAG-KTP laser. With the push of a button, the physician may select between the green KTP or infrared Nd:YAG outputs.

HGM makes several models of argon lasers with power outputs of up to 15–20 W. Water cooling is required on all but the lowest power model, but only single phase 208 V electricity is required.

Trimedyne also makes an argon laser, but primarily designed for use with their "hot metal tips." The light from the fiber heats up the metal tip, which causes tissue vaporization from direct heat contact. Arterial recannulization in vascular surgery has been a main area of interest. These hot tips have also been used to vaporize esophageal tumors and to open the common bile duct. Trimedyne now uses primarily the Nd:YAG laser to power these hot tips.

Argon systems range from approximately $35,000–65,000 depending on output. The KTP is available for approximately $85,000. Consideration should be given to which attachments are included in these prices.

Dye Lasers

CW dye lasers, producing red light at 630 nm, are used for photodynamic therapy. California Laboratories produce a dye laser for this purpose. Gold vapor lasers eventually may be used for this application. Eventually solid-state semiconductor lasers may be used as this red light source.

The key to delivering the red light in photodynamic energy is the type of fiber used and accurate measurement of the output. Special fiber diffusers, probes, beam splitters, and power meters are available from Laserguide.

Pulsed dye lasers are generating considerable interest for selective dermatological application, and for fragmenting kidney (laser lithotripsy) and other stones. Candella Corporation is the only company now producing systems for lithotripsy and Candella, Coherent, California Laboratories, and MediTec make dermatological units.

The 504-nm, green light system is approved for laser lithotripsy. It is delivered fiberoptically through a very fine 0.2-mm fiber to cause fragmentation of stones. Biliary stone fragmentation is being examined with these units.

The 577–585 nm yellow light systems are used in highly selective dermatological use.

SMOKE EVACUATION EQUIPMENT

The vaporized plume from laser ablation is, at the very least, obnoxious. For this and for potential safety reasons the plume should be sucked away by a high-flow smoke evacuation system. Regular wall suction will usually not suffice. CO_2 lasers produce much more smoke than Nd:YAG lasers used with contact probes.

The majority of smoke evacuators in this country are produced by Stackhouse Associates or Lase, Inc. Surgimedics also produces a smoke evacuator and accessories that include some in-line filters for suction.

SUMMARY OF LASER COMPANIES

Some of the information that follows is provided by the respective companies. Other companies did not provide information. Details of product model numbers, power outputs, and completeness of product line should be verified with each company. The information listed below, although substantially true and correct, is not represented as complete or comprehensive.

Advanced Interventional Systems, Inc.
Irving, California
714–586–1342

This company is involved with cardiovascular applications of laser. They make a laser angioplasty catheter.

Advanced Laser Services Corporation
P.O. Box 99
Grove City, OH 43123
614–228–0252

This organization does not manufacture or sell any laser system and so can serve as an independent source for laser consulting and technical services.

Advanced Laser provides nursing training and introductory programs. Consulting is available for program development.

Advanced Laser Services serves as a comprehensive source for service contracts on most types of medical laser systems. Service engineers are well trained and experienced in the medical laser industry.

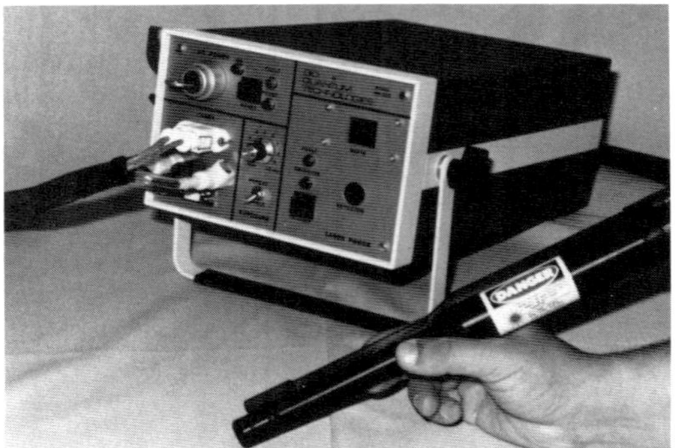

Figure 1.5. Model HH-550 advanced handheld CO_2 laser (Courtesy of BioQuantum Technologies).

Refurbishment of older laser systems is also provided. In most cases, these refurbished systems are better than the originally new laser inasmuch as optics technology has improved over the last few years.

BioQuantum Technologies
8275 El Rio, Suite 180
Houston, TX 77054
713–747–2654

Two models of CO_2 lasers are produced: the model HH-550 handheld 10-W system (Fig. 1.5) and the model 7600 microsurgical 5-W system (Fig. 1.6).

The model 7600 (Fig. 1.6) provides a higher degree of precision than obtained with conventional CO_2 microsurgical laser systems. Spot sizes down to 325 μ on a 300-mm lens are available. The model 7600 takes the approach of power density to microsurgery. Very small spots assure high power density. The joystick utilizes a finesse switch to dampen movement for work in critical procedurues. The digital readout is directly in front of the surgeon. It incorporates an integral digital laser power meter, manual and timed laser exposure control, finesse control, auto/lock tracking, sealed tube, and self-contained cooling.

The model 550 (Fig. 1.5) handheld system is a sealed-tube 10-W system producing power densities up to 30,000 W/cm_2.

California Laboratories, Inc.
2270-L Camino Vida Roble
Carlsbad, CA 92009-4894
619–931–1299

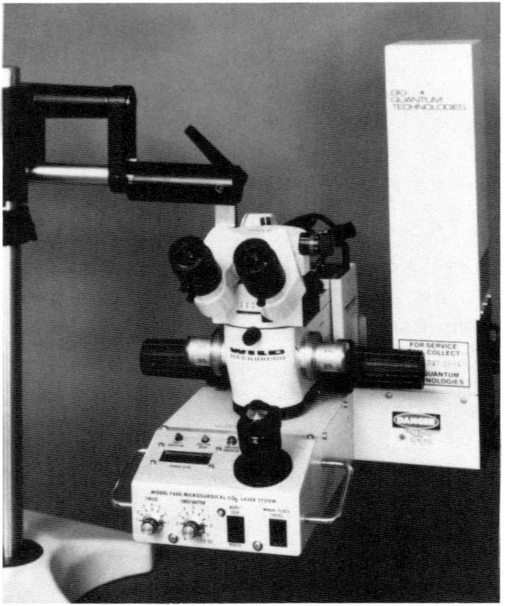

Figure 1.6. Model 7600 Microsurgical CO_2 Laser (Courtesy of BioQuantum Technologies).

California labs produces the Chrys laser, a 25 W sealed tube CO_2 laser system that weighs only 45 pounds and is transportable. Its small articulated arm is actually a waveguide delivery system rather than a true articulated arm, though it functions nicely in most situations.

California labs also makes two models of dye lasers, one for photodynamic therapy and one for dermatology.

Candela Laser Corporation
526 Boston Post Road
Wayland, MA 01778
508–358–7637
800–255–1287

Two models of pulsed dye lasers are produced. Model MDL-1 (Fig. 1.7) is the 504-nm Laser Lithotripter. A 250-μ fiber is used for transmission. Peak power per pulse is up to 40 kW with a delivered energy of up to 60 mJ.

The model SPTL-1 pulsed dye laser emits yellow light at 577 nm for selective thermolysis in dermatology. The pulse duration (300 μ) is longer than traditional flashlamp-pumped dye lasers so that the effects are deeper into the skin.

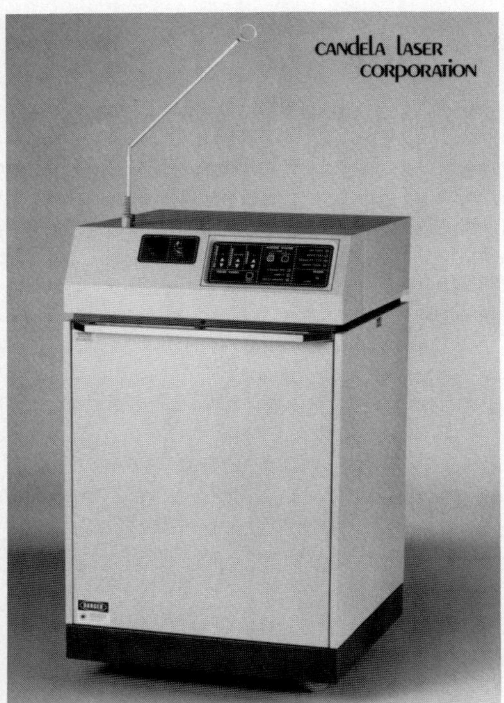

Figure 1.7. Candela Laser Lithotripter (Courtesy of Candela Laser Corporation).

Coherent Medical Group (includes Xanar)
3270 W. Bayshore Rd.
Palo Alto, CA 94303
800–525–2221

Coherent is one of the largest industrial laser companies in the world. Their historic involvement in medicine has been primarily in ophthalmic laser systems, producing argon, argon-krypton, argon-dye, and Q-switched Nd:YAG lasers, although they also produced a 40-W flowing gas CO_2 laser.

Coherent has acquired Xanar laser from Johnson & Johnson. This has significantly expanded their line into surgical systems.

Coherent makes a low-power (less than 20 W) RF waveguide sealed-tube CO_2 lasers: the Ambulase. They have introduced the XA5, a 55-W RF waveguide system that is microprocessor controlled.

Coherent offers a range of CO_2 lasers ranging from 20–55 W. All are sealed tube, RF excited. The Ambulase comes in a 20-W model with superpulse. The XA30/SP is a 30-W laser with superpulse, and the Excelase series (XL40 and XL55) is available in either 40 or 55 W with superpulse and milliwatt capability.

Coherent offers an Excelite Air-Fiber for use with their lasers for laparoscopy. This is not actually a CO_2 fiber. It is a hollow/ceramic metal waveguide that delivers the beam by hundreds of glancing reflections on the inside of the tube.

Heraeus LaserSonics (previously Cooper LaserSonics)
3420 Central Expressway
Santa Clara, CA 95051
408–720–1100
800–227–8372

Heraeus distributes an entire line of lasers including ophthalmic, CO_2, and Nd:YAG lasers.

Cooper previously had the Cavitron line of CO_2 lasers; it is no longer available. Cooper acquired Merrimack laser and now sells this line of flowing gas CO_2 lasers with powers up to 70 W. They also distribute the Illumina, a 40-W sealed-tube CO_2 laser.

Heraeus has a waveguide ''fiber'' available for their CO_2 lasers for use in laparoscopy called the Infraguide. As with the Coherent and Surgilase systems, this is a hollow waveguide and not actually a CO_2 laser fiber.

Molectron was the original manufacturer of Nd:YAG lasers for surgery in this country. Cooper acquired Molectron and sells this 100-W unit as the model 8000. Cooper has since developed two other models, i.e., Nd:YAG systems of 60 and 100 W. The 100-W model incorporates a choice of multicolor aiming beams. The 60-W model requires only single phase electricity and utilizes a multiple intensity aiming beam.

Dynatronics Research Corporation
270 W. Crossroad Square
Salt Lake City, UT 84115
801-485-4739

Dynatronics makes low-powered lasers used in the area of biostimulation. These are not surgical lasers.

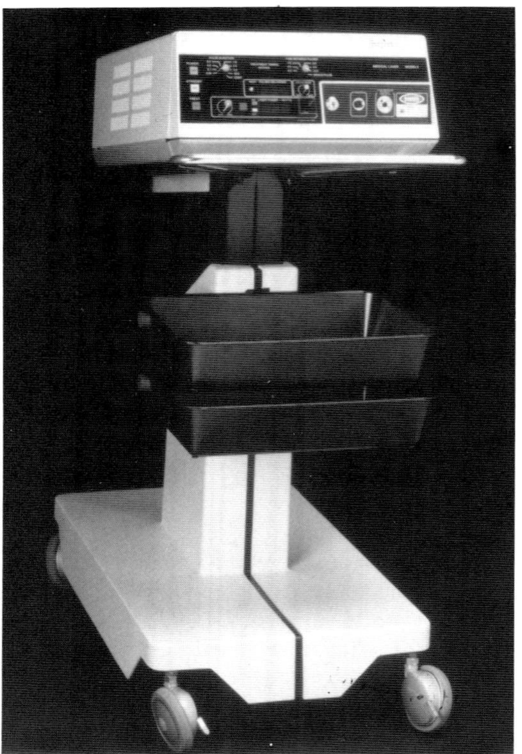

Figure 1.8. HGM model 5 Argon Laser (Courtesy of HGM).

GV Medical
3750 Annapolis Lane
Minneapolis, MN 55441
612-559-4000

GV Medical makes the Lastac argon laser angioplasty system. This sytem uses the straight argon beam, highly diverged with a small lens in the catheter system, and incorporated into a standard balloon dilatation catheter.

HGM, Inc.
3959 W. 1820 South
Salt Lake City, UT 84104–4996
801–972–0500

HGM manufactures four models of argon medical laser systems plus accessories. These are designed as portable units to be used by a variety of specialties including gynecology, otorhinolaryngology, neurosurgery, gastroenterology, dermatology, urology, and ophthalmology. Work is also underway in cardiovascular surgery.

The model 5 (Fig. 1.8) is a 3.5-W system requiring 208 V of single phase electricity. The unit is air cooled and requires no water hookup. The model PC (personal coagulator) is a 3.0-W system with similar installation requirements. The PC is designed as an office ophthalmic photocoagulator.

The model 8 system is a 6-W argon laser, with external water cooling and 208 V of single phase electricity. A krypton red version is available that would be useful in dermatology.

The model 20 system produces an output of 16 W. External water cooling is required and the 208 V now requires three phases. As a general surgery instrument, this higher powered unit would be more useful than the lower powered models.

The model 20 is also being used for laser angioplasty, using the argon laser to heat metal probes on the tip of a catheter. The laser utilizes a thermal feedback loop from the hot tip to maintain constant vaporization temperatures.

Accessories would include eye safety filters and shutters, collimated handpieces, disposable fibers, endoocular probes, and micromanipulators.

Hi-Tech, Medical Lasers, Inc.
1111 Chestnut St.
Burbank, CA 91506
213–849–5985
818–842–2199

Hi-Tech is the laser affiliate of Gyne-Tech, both privately owned by the same individual.

Hi-Tech manufactures several low-power CO_2 laser systems most often used in an office or clinic setting. These span the range from approximately 15–30 W. The units are available with articulated arms for use either freehand or coupled to a colposcope with a micromanipulator. These are flowing gas systems but incorporate what Hi-Tech refers to as micro-flow, which considerably decreases gas consumption.

The Hi-Tech lasers are amoung the least expensive office-type systems available.

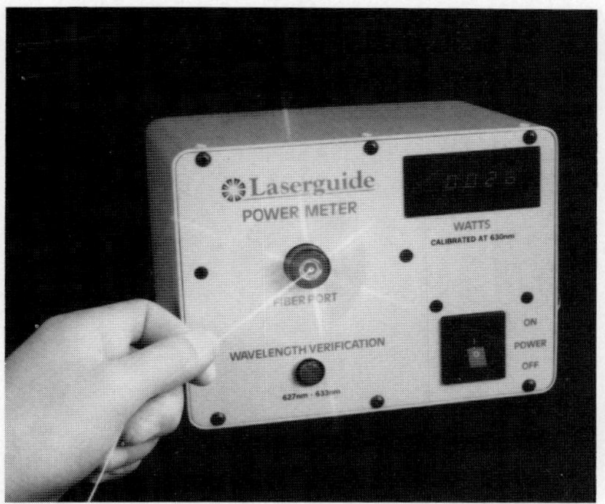

Figure 1.9. Laserguide Power Meter (Courtesy of Laserguide).

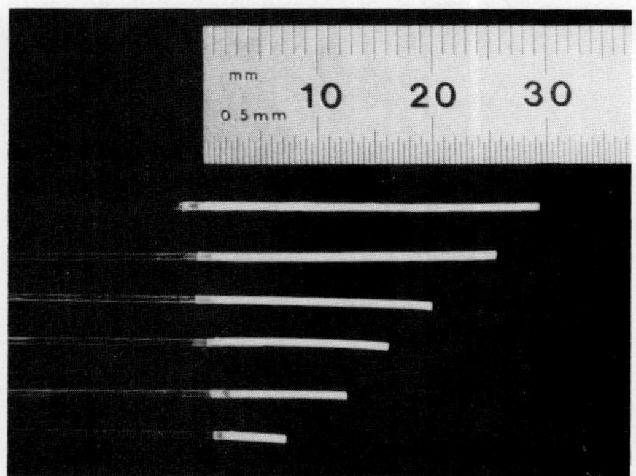

Figure 1.10. Cylindrical Diffusers (Courtesy of Laserguide).

Lase, Inc.
7209 E. Kemper Rd.
Cincinnati, OH 45249
513–489–6074

Lase manufactures smoke evacuators. These are the blue cart systems at the top end of the price range for smoke evacuators. Lase, Inc. is a subsidiary of U.S. Medical Corporation (a regional laser dealership), formerly the Paul Rogers Co. Lase also carries miscellaneous laser accessories such as safety signs.

Laserguide
51 Santa Felicia Dr.
Santa Barbara, CA 93117
805–968–6441

This company produces fibers and accessories for use in photodynamic therapy.

The power meter, model 2015 (Fig. 1.9) is an integrating sphere designed to display continuous output of single or bundled fibers. Output is read simultaneously in forward and radial emitting modes and displays the power of contact, diffusing, flat-cut, or microlens-tipped fibers.

The model 1220 remote fiber splitter allows one laser to be split to two or three fibers. Originally developed for photodynamic therapy, the splitter also works at other wavelengths by changing the internal optics.

The microlens and diffusing fiberoptics are designed to match the geometry of certain anatomical areas; e.g., the cylindrical diffusers (Fig. 1.10) are used in the trachea and esophagus and the spherical cavity diffusers are used in the bladder and nasopharyngeal areas.

Laser Industries, Ltd.
ATIDIM Science Based Industrial Park, Neve Sharet
P.O.B. 13135 Tel Aviv, Israel
Carried in the U.S. by:
Sharplan Lasers, Inc.
One Pearl Court
Allendale, NJ 07401
201–327–1666

Sharplan, a subsidiary of Laser Industries in Tel Aviv, carries a complete line of CO_2 lasers. They also produce a 100-W Nd:YAG system—the model 2100. Their entry into the ophthalmic markets is with an argon photocoagulator and Q-switched Nd:YAG system, although ophthalmics is not their primary market area.

The model 1100 is a 100-W flowing gas CO_2 laser system. This laser actually works in the chopped mode, providing peak spikes of about 150 W to give the 100-W average power. This model is popular for general surgical use because of the high-power output. It is also priced as a top of the line laser. The unit is microprocessor controlled.

The models 1060 and 1040 are 60-W and 40-W respectively, flowing gas systems.

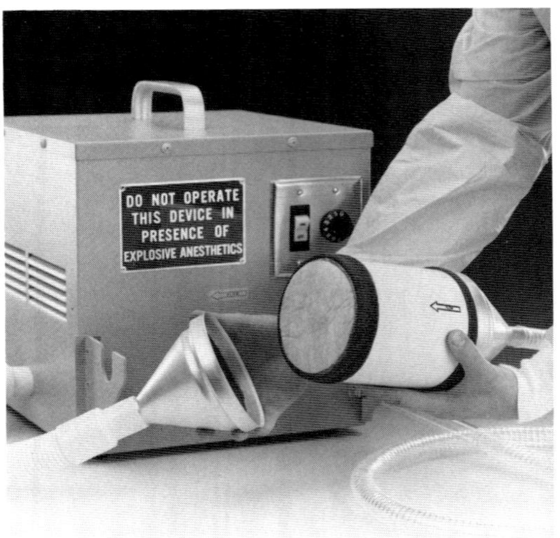

Figure 1.11. Stackhouse Biovac Smoke Evacuator (Courtesy of Stackhouse Associates).

Sharplan has many of the older models 733 and 743 lasers in place but have discontinued these lines. These are the orange and black colored 40-W and 80-W flowing gas CO_2 lasers.

Lasermatic OY
Lepolantie 21
00660 Helsinke, Finland

This company is introducing a combination CO_2-Nd:YAG laser into the U.S. marketplace.

Laserscope
3350 Scott Blvd., Bldg. 29
Santa Clara, CA 95054–3183
408–988–3466
800–356–7600

Laserscope produces the KTP laser. This laser is known by many different names including Omniplus (its trade name), frequency-doubled Nd:YAG, and green Nd:YAG. Laserscope prefers to use the term KTP, which is the crystal used to provide the green output.

This fiberoptic system is microprocessor controlled and produces a slightly greener beam of light than the argon laser. Applications are similar if not identical to argon laser use.

The KTP is a high-frequency pulsed system. This is fast enough so that, for all practical purposes, it operates as a CW mode laser. The unit produces power outputs of 12–15 W.

A variety of fibers and accessories are available.

Laserscope has introduced a combination Nd:YAG-KTP laser. The physician selects the desired output by the push of a button.

Living Technology, Inc.
440 Constance Drive
Warminster, PA 18974
215–674–3554
800–344–3554

Living Technology has developed a 100 W CW Nd:YAG laser unique in that it is both air cooled (no external water hookup) and requires only a standard 110v wall outlet to operate. The unit is left plugged into the wall while not in use which maintains a charge on its internal power supply.

Medical Energy, Inc.
8295 N. Military Trail
Suite B
Palm Beach Garden, FL 33410

This is a new entry into the CW Nd:YAG laser market. This company was formed after Endolase (the previous MBB distributor) dissolved, and some of the previous management from Endolase is now involved with this company.

This laser is to be released shortly.

Medilase, Inc.
2605 Fernbrook Lane
Minneapolis, MN 55447
612–559–8640

Medilase has developed a catheter system incorporating an aimable laser with an angioscope designed to perform intra-arterial endarterectomy.

MedLaser, Inc.
Tampa, Florida
813-971-4991

MedLaser was formed to purchase the liquidated CO_2 and Nd:YAG lasers from the Endolase bankruptcy. MBB 100 W CW Nd:YAG and LaFevre 100 W CO_2 lasers are available for lease or purchase at discounted prices.

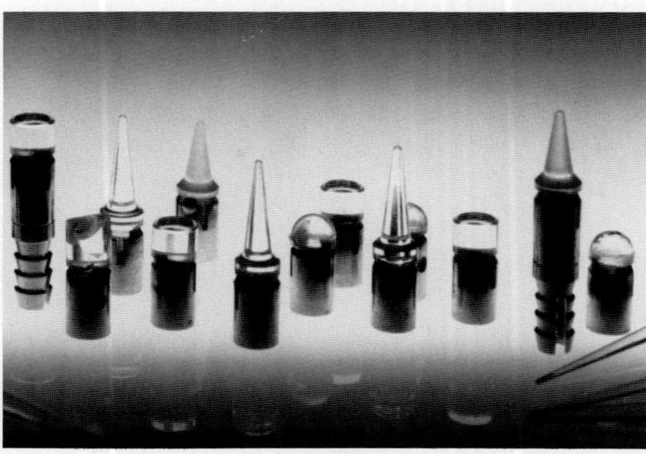

Figure 1.12. Sapphire Contact Probes (Courtesy of Surgical Laser Technologies).

Nippon Infrared Industries Co., Ltd. (N.I.I.C.)
460 Seaport Court
Redwood City, CA 94063
800–992–NIIC

N.I.I.C. markets their lasers directly in the U.S. They previously worked with both Heraeus (Cooper) LaserSonics and Xanar (now Coherent Medical Group) to supply this technology.

The Cooper-NIIC line was distributed as the models 250Z and 500Z lasers. These units have a very large installation base.

The XANAR-NIIC line was distributed as the Magnum line of CO_2 lasers. These included 40-W and 95-W systems.

N.I.I.C. now directly markets these lasers as the IR line, which includes a 40-W and 100-W CO_2 laser.

Pfizer Laser Systems
(Directed Energy, Inc.)
16700 Red Hill Ave.
Irvine, CA 92714
714–250–1757

These small, portable, handheld lasers are sealed-tube CO_2 lasers producing powers up to

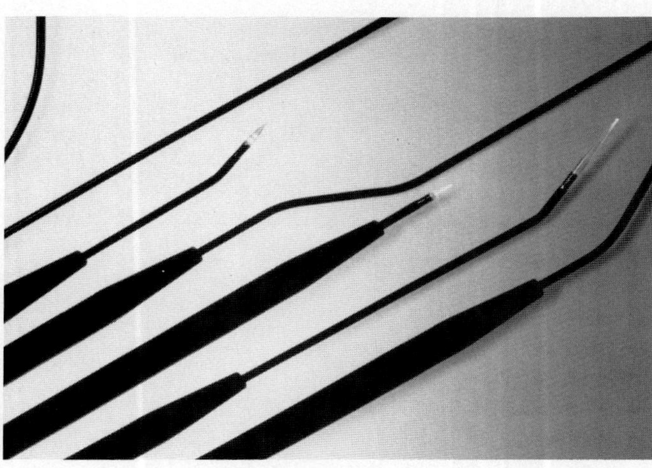

Figure 1.13. Surgical Handpieces with Contact Probes (Courtesy of Surgical Laser Technologies).

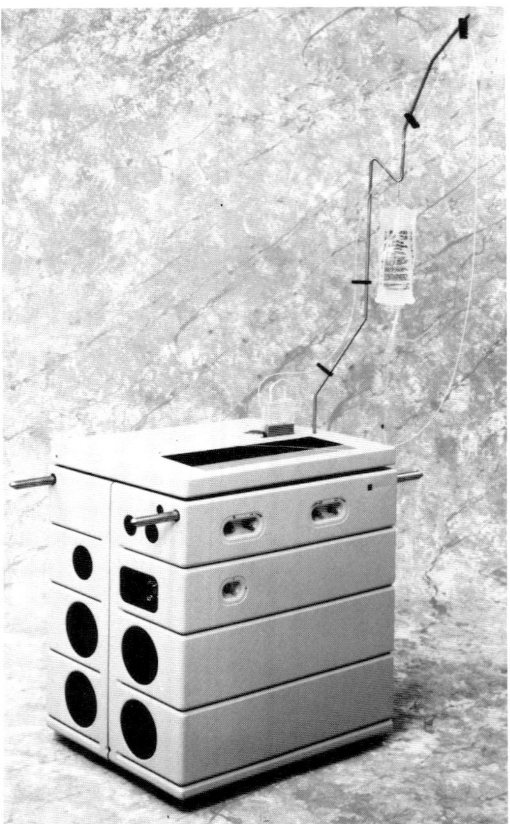

Figure 1.14. SLT Nd:YAG Laser (Courtesy of Surgical Laser Technologies).

approximately 20 W. No articulated arm or micromanipulator is used.

The units are popular for offices, particularly in podiatry, and are generating some interest in dentistry.

Spectranetics Corporation
80 Talamine Ct.
Colorado Springs, CO 80907

Spectranetics manufactures an excimer based laser system for laser angioplasty.

Stackhouse Assoc.
150 Sierra St.
El Segundo, CA 90245
213–322–6676

Stackhouse manufactures a full line of laser accessories and instruments. They do not manufacture or sell lasers. Accessories include laser safety glasses, ebonized surgical instruments (and a service to ebonize the hospital's existing instruments), backstops, laparoscopy smoke control valve sets, small in-line filters for wall suction, etc.

Stackhouse manufactures the most widely used smoke evacuation system—the Biovac (Fig. 1.11). This system quietly and efficiently vacuums and filters odor and particulate matter including fat, carbon, tissue cells, etc. The new Biovac:0.1 will filter all particulates, including microorganisms as small as 0.1 μ at 99.999% efficiency.

Summit Technology
150 Coolidge Ave.
Watertown, MA 02172
617–923–9633

Summit was the first company to design an excimer laser specificially for medical use. The 308 nm XeCl excimer is delivered through a fiberoptic and is used investigationally in laser recannulization of vessels.

The unit has the potential to change to other excimer wavelengths with a service call.

Surgical Laser Technologies (SLT)
1 Great Valley Pkwy.
Malvern, PA 19355
215–647–8277 or 1–800–772–5273

SLT developed the sapphire contact probe technology for use with the Nd:YAG laser. A complete line of probes are available for cutting, vaporization, coagulation, chiseling, photodynamic therapy, and laserthermia (Fig. 1.12). Probes are available as 1.8 or 2.2 mm diameters and come in various tip widths. Probes are available as either an endoprobe (an attachment to the fiber for endoscopy) or as handheld probes used on a surgical handpiece (Fig. 1.13).

The SLT CW Nd:Yag laser (Fig. 1.14) is a 60-W system specifically designed for stability with contact probes. It may be used as a conventional noncontact Nd:YAG laser or at lower powers with the probes. The unit is microprocessor controlled to provide 40 W of output power. Powers up to 60 W may be obtained by placing the unit in a manual override. Disposable fibers are used that

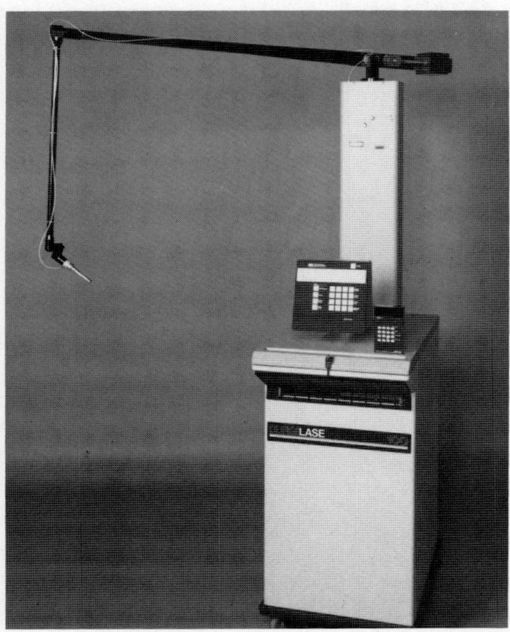

Figure 1.15. Surgilase Sealed Tube CO_2 Laser (Courtesy of Surgilase, Inc.).

may either be cooled with fluid or gas. A built-in pump and disposable cartridge allows fluid to be slowly dripped through the fiber for cooling. A built-in air compressor provides filtered room air, or CO_2 or nitrogen may be attached.

This Nd:YAG laser is air-cooled (internal heat exchanger) and requires 208 V of single phase electricity. The laser is extremely portable.

SLT also manufactures 25-W and 100-W Nd:YAG lasers. They are actively involved in the area of laser angioplasty with the use of their sapphire contact probes.

Surgilase, Inc.

I-95 Corporate Park
33 Plan Way
Warwick, RI 02886
401–732–6440

Surgilase was the first company to market the DC excited, free space, sealed-tube CO_2 lasers. These units are microprocessor controlled and come in 40-W, 55-W, and 100-W models (Fig. 1.15). Sealed technology increases reliability while reducing operating expense. Surgilase has announced the release of 15-W and 20-W lasers using the same technology and similar controls.

Articulated arms allow their use freehand, through the microscope or endoscopic couplers. Surgilase has available a waveguide delivery system for use in laparoscopy.

Surgilase also produces a 100 W CW Nd:YAG laser that is microprocessor controlled.

Trimedyne

1815 E Carnegie Ave.
Santa Ana, CA 92705
714–261–9041

Trimedyne originally utilized a surgical argon laser, primarily in conjunction with the hot metal tips. These metal tips at the end of the fiber are heated directly by the laser output. Tissue vaporization occurs as the hot tip touches the tissue. The Trimedyne system is FDA-approved for recanalization of vessels.

Trimedyne distributes a CW Nd:YAG laser that is now primarily used for this purpose.

Metal tips are available in a variety of configurations that allow for ''windows'' to emit some of the laser energy directly onto tissue. Some tips may be slipped over guidewires for steering.

Xanar (now Coherent Medical Group)

2868 Janitell Rd
Colorado Springs, CO 80906

See Coherent Medical Group

CHAPTER

2

Laser Safety in General Surgery

David H. Sliney

The introduction of lasers into general surgery has raised a number of laser safety issues. The safety guidelines introduced earlier for more dangerous lasers found in industrial and research applications (1) are often difficult to interpret and apply in the clinical setting. Both the potential hazards and applicable safety measures differ with the wavelength and type of laser. The output wavelength and power determines which of four hazard classes applies to any specific laser (1, 2). Virtually all surgical lasers, because of their requirement to cut or coagulate tissue, fall into Class 4, which is the most dangerous class. Stringent safety measures are needed with this class of laser in the research laboratory. However, because of the focused beam in the surgical application, the extent of the hazard is minimized and the risk of injury to eyes or skin of the bystanders and surgeon is limited. Nevertheless, certain precautions are still necessary.

Laser hazards depend upon the type of laser, the environment, and the personnel involved with the laser operation (the operator, ancillary personnel, and patient). The laser hazard is roughly defined by the hazard classification (Classes 1–4), whereas the other factors must be analyzed in each situation. A basic understanding of laser biological effects and hazards is necessary to assess laser hazards in the operating room intelligently. Once the hazards are understood, the safety measures become obvious.

BIOLOGICAL EFFECTS

General knowledge of the biological effects of lasers is a prerequisite to a solid understanding of the potential hazards associated with laser use. In addition, a general understanding of the hazards from exposure to ultraviolet, visible, and infrared radiation from conventional light sources is required to place laser hazards in perspective. The critical organ of interest is the eye. The nature of laser tissue interactions must be understood by the surgeon for optimal surgical use of the laser (3) and for the protection of the patient and assisting staff from laser hazards. At least five separate types of hazard from lasers and other optical sources to the eye and the skin have been identified.

1. Ultraviolet photochemical injury to the skin (erythema and carcinogenic effects), and to the cornea (photokeratitis) and lens (cataract) of the eye (200–400 nm) (2, 4);
2. Thermal injury to the retina of the eye (400–1400 nm);
3. Blue-light photochemical injury to the retina of the eye (principally 400–550 nm) (2,4);
4. Near-infrared thermal hazards to the lens (approximately 800–3000 nm);
5. Thermal injury (burns) of the skin (approximately 400 nm–1 mm) and to the cornea of the eye (approximately 1400 nm to 1 mm).

POTENTIAL HAZARDS

The principal hazard to personnel in the vicinity of an operating laser results from specular (mirror-like) reflections. Concern about such reflections led some to suggest the use of a safety measure commonly employed in industry, the door interlock. The application of this measure could produce additional risks in an operating theater, where a critically important laser procedure could be halted by the entry of a staff member. This has led to the development of modified safety rules for medical lasers.

A number of steps can be taken to minimize the potential hazards to both the patient and surgical staff. An example of a safety procedure that could be used with many CO_2 surgical lasers is presented in Table 2.1.

Table 2.1. Carbon Dioxide Surgical Laser Safety Checklist

1. Check beam alignment and output power.
2. Avoid surgical drapes, or saturate with water or saline.
3. Saturate swabs and gauze pads with water or saline.
4. Use quartz (not glass) guards behind tissue where applicable.
5. Tape the sterile stockingette to the articulated arm to prevent slippage.
6. Use clear plastic goggles or the operating microscope.
7. Use an effective fume evacuator.
8. Cap articulated arm (if not shuttered) when not connected to handpiece or operating microscope.
9. Use only a shielded pedal switch.
10. Always place laser in standby mode when delivery optics are moved away from surgical target.
11. Use saline to protect adjacent structures (e.g., bowel).
12. Assure proper identification of target site before laser emission.
13. Use intravenous or local rather than inhalation anesthesia.
14. Plug bowel to avoid ignition of rectal methane when surgical site is near.
15. Training is paramount. The surgeon, anesthesiologist, and operating room nurses must all be aware of laser hazards. The surgeon should understand basic laser physics and tissue interaction.

The most common type of laser currently employed in surgical applications is the CO_2 laser. Because CO_2 laser wavelength of 10.6 μm is in the far-infrared spectral region—and invisible—the presence of hazardous secondary beams could go unnoticed. This added hazard, resulting from an infrared laser beam's lack of visibility, is also common to other infrared lasers such as the neodymium:YAG (Nd:YAG) laser. Improper attention to safety with the use of Nd:YAG lasers has resulted in a number of serious retinal injuries (2, 5). The use of Nd:YAG lasers must be approached with even greater caution than the CO_2 laser. By contrast, the argon laser and the second-harmonic Nd:YAG laser (sometimes referred to as the KTP emit radiation in the blue-green spectrum with highly visible beams. In some ways, the argon lasers pose less of a potential hazard. Most of the current surgical lasers, such as the CO_2, Nd:YAG, or argon lasers are continuous wave (CW), or nearly so; even superpulse is quasi-CW compared to single-pulsed laser photodisruptors or some experimental excimer ablative lasers (6, 7). The biological effects and potential hazards from high-peak power pulsed lasers are quite different from those of CW lasers. This is particularly true of lasers operating in the retinal hazard region of the visible (400–760 nm) and near-infrared spectrum (IR-A: 760–1400 nm). The severity of retinal lesions from a visible or near-infrared (IR-A) CW laser is normally considered to be far less than that of a Q-switched or mode-locked laser. Another major factor that influences the potential hazard is the degree of beam collimation. Almost all surgical lasers are focused, thereby limiting the hazardous area, referred to as the "nominal hazardous zone" in ANSI Z-136.1 (1). An exception is the highly collimated beam from many of the argon laser photocoagulators, which may still be concentrated and hazardous at quite some distance from the instrument.

The potential optical radiation hazard to both the surgeon and onlookers during the clinical use of most types of lasers results primarily from either accidental misdirection of the primary beam or from its specular (mirror-like) reflections. Figure 2.1 shows the types of reflected beams that can be encountered when using a collimated laser beam and the focused laser beam. These reflections occur when incident light from the beam strikes a flat specular surface, characteristic of many metallic surgical instruments.

Many surgical instruments now have black anodized or sand-blasted, roughened surfaces to reduce (but not eliminate) potentially hazadous reflections. The surface roughening measures are generally more effective in reducing reflections than those that blacken (ebonize) the instrument surface. This difference is due to the diffusion of the beam on the roughened surface. Furthermore, any metal surface will absorb much of the energy emitted at the 10.6 μm CO_2 wavelength. It should be emphasized that both the surface finish and the reflectance observed in the visible spectrum do not indicate those qualities in the invisible far-infrared spectrum. In fact, a roughened surface at shorter visible or IR-A wavelengths will always be more specular at far-infrared wavelengths (e.g., the CO_2 laser wavelength). This results

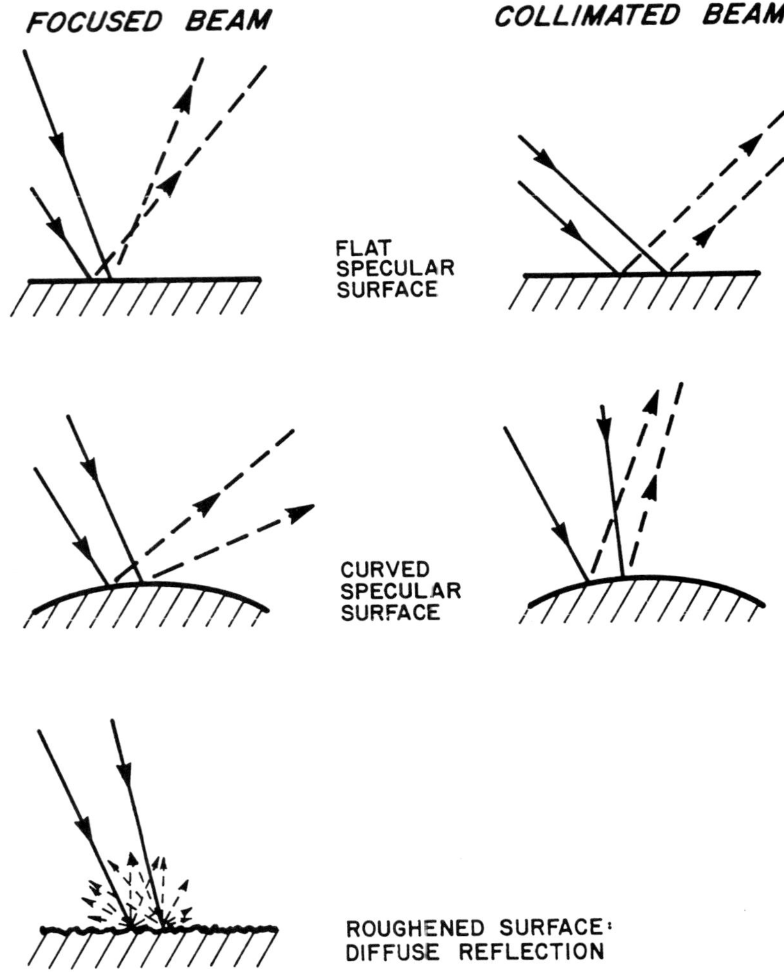

Figure 2.1. Examples of reflections of laser radiation from specular (mirror-like surfaces) e.g., metallic instrument surfaces.

from the fact that the relative size of the microscopic structure of the surface relative to the incident wavelength determines whether the beam is reflected as a specular or diffuse reflection (see Fig. 2.3). In any case, a specularly reflected beam with only 1% of the initial beam's power can still be hazardous. Hence, the rougher the surface of an instrument likely to intercept the beam, the safer the reflection. For example, even a 1% reflection of a 40 W laser beam is 400 mW!

It is indeed somewhat surprising that there have been few reported cases of eye injuries to resident physicians and others observing Nd:YAG laser surgery without eye protectors. Figure 2.2 shows the zones where hazardous reflected laser beams may be encountered when using a neurosurgical CO_2 laser. Hazardous specular reflections from a focused laser beam from a surgical instrument or other polished surface are limited in extent because of the focused beam shown in Figure 2.1.

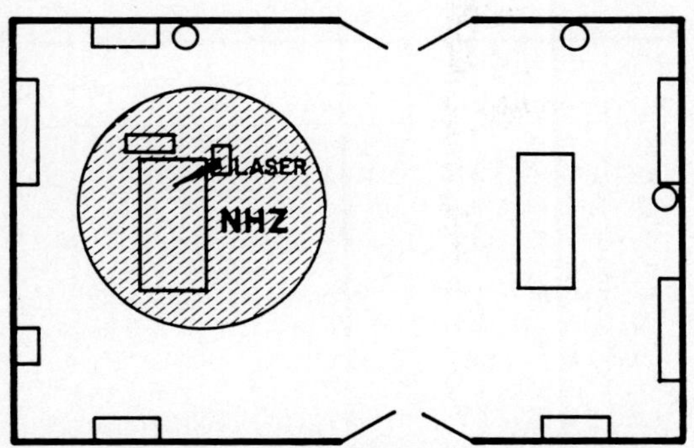

Figure 2.2. Reflected beam paths from flat metal surfaces and the potentially hazardous zones.

Most surgical lasers have a visible alignment beam. Infrared lasers most often make use of a low-power coaxial He-Ne (632.8) red laser. It is desirable, when feasible, for this alignment beam to be 1 mW or less, because the maximum CW, visible laser beam power that can safely enter the eye within the aversion response (i.e., within the blink reflex, etc. of 0.25 sec is 1 mW.

OCCUPATIONAL EXPOSURE LIMITS (ELs)

Relevant ELs for lasers of interest in this chapter are given in Table 2.2. The ELs in Table 2.1 are calculated or measured by the cornea. If the laser beam is less than 7 mm in diameter, it is assumed that the entire beam could enter the dark-adapted pupil. The maximal safe power of energy in the beam can then be expressed. It is the above EL multiplied by the area of a 7-mm pupil, i.e., 0.4 cm^2. This 1-mW value has a special significance in laser safety because it is a dividing line between two laser safety hazard classifications: Class 2 and Class 3 (1).

LASER HAZARD CLASSIFICATION

As mentioned, any CW visible laser (400–700 nm) that has an output of power less than 1.0 mW is termed a Class 2 (low-risk) laser. Exposure could be considered as more or less equivalent in risk to staring at the sun, at a tungsten-halogen spotlight, or at other bright light source. It should be noted that such exposures are capable of causing a photic maculopathy (central retinal injury) only if the individual forced themself to overcome the natural aversion response to bright light. An aiming beam or alignment laser operating at a total power of above 1.0 mW would fall into hazard Class 3, and could be hazardous even if viewed momentarily within the aversion response latency period. Only lasers that are totally enclosed, or

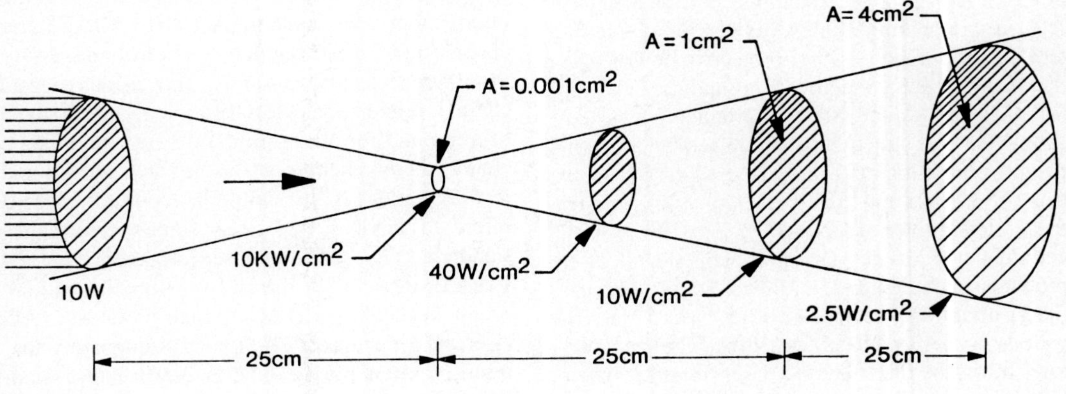

Figure 2.3. Beam irradiance of a focused laser beam as a function of distance from a laser. Note the rapid decrease of beam irradiance beyond the focal point.

Table 2.2. Selected Occupational Exposure Limits (ELs) for Surgical Lasers[a]

Laser	Wavelength (nm)	Exposure Limit			
		Eye		Skin	
Argon ion laser	488, 514.5 nm	3.2 mW/cm^2	for 0.1 sec	6.2 W/cm^2	for 0.1 sec
		2.5 mW/cm^2	for 0.25 sec	3.1 W/cm^2	for 0.25 sec
Helium-neon laser	632.8 nm	1.8 mW/cm^2	for 1.0 sec	1.1 W/cm^2	for 1.0 sec
		1.0 mW/cm^2	for 10 sec	0.2 W/cm^2	for >10 sec
Krypton ion laser	568, 647 nm				
Nd: YAG laser	1064 nm	16 mW/cm^2	for 0.1 sec	31 W/cm^2	for 0.1 sec
		9.0 mW/cm^2	for 1.0 sec	5.5 W/cm^2	for 1.0 sec
		5.1 mW/cm^2	for 10 sec	0.98 W/cm^2	for >10 sec
Carbon dioxide laser	10.6 μm	3.1 W/cm^2	for 0.1 sec	3.1 W/cm^2	for 0.1 sec
		0.56 W/cm^2	for 1.0 sec	0.56 W/cm^2	for 1.0 sec
		0.10 W/cm^2	for > 10 sec	0.10 W/cm^2	for >10 sec

[a]Source: ANSI Standard Z-136.1-1986 (1). Note: to convert ELs in mW/cm^2 to mJ/cm^2, multiply by exposure time t in seconds; e.g., the helium-neon or argon EL at 0.1 sec is 0.32 mJ/cm^2.

that emit extremely low-output powers, would be categorized as Class 1 and safe to view. Any CW laser with a output power of above 0.5W (500 mW) would fall into Class 4. Class 4 lasers are capable of posing hazards to skin and eyes, as well as risks of fire, if not properly used. The purpose of assigning hazard classes to laser products is to simplify the determination of adequate safety measures i.e., Class 3a measures are more stringent than Class 2 measures and Class 4 measures are more stringent than Class 3b measures. Virtually all surgical leasers are Class 4.

LASER SYSTEM SAFETY

System safety refers to the design and manufacture of a laser product. Examples of system safety features are: warning lights, built-in protective filters for the surgeon's eyes, protective covers over the foot switch, electrical grounding, and so forth. In the United States, certain laser system safety features are mandated by federal governmental regulations (9) under the Radiation Control for Health and Safety Act of 1968. Under these regulations (specifically, 21 CFR 1040), certain performance standards apply to all laser products marketed in the United States; whereas others apply only to specific laser hazard classifications or to specialized laser uses. The manufacturer must certify that the laser product meets these requirements and must file documents, which detail this certification, with the Center for Devices and Radiological Health (CDRH) of the Food and Drug Administration (FDA) in Rockville, MD.

The details of the FDA laser product performance standards can be quite complex, and shall not be covered here. However, the surgical staff may be assured that reasonable system safeguards have been designed into the construction of all commercially available lasers. This may not be true of some prototype or experimental laser devices, but final product lines should be in compliance with the standards. The FDA performance standards vary with hazard classification (denoted by Roman numerals I–IV). This laser hazard classification scheme (Classes I, II, III, and IV) should not be confused with the medical device classification scheme of Classes I, II, and III, which appear in the regulations (21 CFR 510, 519, 520, 807, etc.) that are used by FDA-CDRH to enforce the Medical Device Amendments to the Food, Drug and Cosmetic Act (10). These latter classes refer to the regulatory controls necessary to assure reasonable safety and effectiveness. Class I refers to the low-risk devices that have been around for a long time (e.g., an ophthalmic chair) where general controls are well known and few regulations if any should be required. Class II refers to devices that need some performance standards (e.g., an argon laser retinal coagulator). Class III devices are new instruments that require premarket approval (PMA), such as, a Nd:YAG laser photodisruptor. The laser system safety features required by the CDRH performance standards that are applicable to Nd:YAG photodisruptors are: (a) an interlocked or secured protective housing; (b) a remote connector that can be used to interlock an entrance door; (c) a key operated switch; (d) an emission indicator, such as a pilot light; (e) a beam attenduator, such as a mechanical shutter; (f) specified warning labels;

(g) protective viewing optics, for example by a filter or shutter system; and (h) operator controls positioned to limit the chance of exposure. In addition to these general requirements, all medical laser products must comply with three other requirements: (a) a means to measure output to within ±20%; (b) a measurement calibration schedule; and (c) a "laser aperture" label. In some instances, a self-monitoring fixed laser output is accepted as fulfilling the first medical requirement. Each manufacturer can obtain variances from the above standards, if alternative and effective controls are provided.

The protective filter in any viewing optical system such as an operating microscope is of key interest to the surgeon. Because the CO_2 laser wavelength and all far-infrared laser wavelengths beyond 4000 nm (4 μm) are not transmitted through glass (i.e., the infrared optical fiber problem), any optical microscope will filter out any potentially harmful reflections. In some medical laser instruments, such as ophthalmic photocoagulators or Nd:YAG pulsed laser photodisruptors, the laser system includes the viewing optics (e.g., the slit-lamp microscope) and the FDA requires the filter to be incorporated in the instrument. When the laser is used with any operating microscope, the user must be very careful to assure that a safety filter is in a quickly accessible mode when laser use is completed or is not required during part of a procedure. This precludes accidental firing and reduces the chance of a hazardous beam from an unsecured handpiece from being fired (out of distances exceeding 2 m). An interlock at the handpiece or at the connector to the delivery microscope could preclude unintentional firing of the laser beam except when properly connected, thereby assuring a focused (and less dangerous) laser beam. Indeed, the draft ANSI laser safety standard for health care facilities requires this feature (11).

SAFE SURGICAL SETTING

A surgical laser should be situated in a closed room with a controlled entrance. Conventional transparent glass or plastic windows filter out CO_2 laser radiation, but will transmit Nd:YAG or argon laser light. Windows for the room where a Nd:YAG or argon surgical laser is operated should be nonexistent or covered with a light-tight opaque screen. In this regard, many plastic "opaque" curtains actually transmit the 1064-nm Nd:YAG wavelength. Where feasible, the beam should be directed downward to limit the likelihood of a reflected beam or a misdirected beam intercepting the surgeon or an individual standing nearby. Although a strict interpretation of the earlier versions of the ANSI Z136.1 (1986) laser safety standard (1) would indicate that a door interlock should be installed to preclude laser operation when the door is ajar, it was determined that this was unwarranted for most medical applications because the direct beam of most surgical lasers is focused. This limits the extent of the potentially hazardous area to about 1 m in the direct beam or to either side of the surgeon. Furthermore, shutting off the laser beam during the surgical procedure may be more hazardous than the one-in-a-million chance of the beam being directed at the door at the moment of entry. A warning sign and/or light above the door is frequently employed to indicate when the laser is in use. A removable sign would also suffice. Figure 2.3 shows the effect of focusing the laser beam upon beam irradiance and hazard.

BUCK ROGER'S SYNDROME

The high technology, almost magical, aura of the new laser surgical tools may lead the laser surgeon into conflict with what this author refers to as the "Buck Roger's Syndrome." If laser safety training is inadequate, some members of the surgical or hospital staff may have fears. Proper training is essential to combat needless worries based upon an inadequate understanding of the laser's capabilities, hazards, and limits.

In this regard, it is worth considering the concerns that have emerged from time to time regarding the potential hazards of the laser to pregnant women. Any assertion that lasers could pose a hazard to the fetus is, of course, entirely without any scientific basis, and represents a profound misunderstanding about the clear differences between the biological effects of laser radiation and ionizing radiation, i.e., x-rays and gamma rays. Only ionizing radiation is capable of penetrating the uterus and possibly affecting the fetus. It is not a total surprise that this misunderstanding has occurred because ionizing radiation is often loosely referred to as "radiation." Therefore, when research scientists, nurses, and physicians quite correctly refer to laser radiation as "radiation," some confusion may develop. Some laser marketing people have requested that the scientific community use terms such as "laser light," which is, strictly speaking, only relevant to visible radiation (400–760 nm) or to "laser beams." However, there is simply no rationale for or likelihood that the scientific community would dilute the precision and accuracy of its technical language to ameliorate confusion among the uninformed. Improvements in the educational programs for the operating room staff are far more desirable and would be more more effective. It should be emphasized that light and infrared laser radiation do not deeply penetrate the body and that there is no mechanism for laser radiation to affect—either positively or negatively—the pregnancy.

It should also be realized that any nontechnical visitor to the laser surgical room will have difficulty comprehending such a high-technology device. The human propensity for making erroneous associations and overgeneralizing must be taken into consideration. If the laser was in use during the visit, the event will be strongly registered in the visitor's memory. If any visual change or impairment is noted sometime later, perhaps years, the individual may mistakenly associate it with the visit. Regardless of how unreasonable this may seem to one skilled in scientific logic, it has occurred many times in industrial laser facilities.

The most effective means of combating the Buck Roger's syndrome in visitors and staff is a strong educational program and an insistence upon following conservative safety measures. For example, the use of laser eye protectors may not be scientifically essential in all cases. However, it provides an important psychological assurance to less technically oriented persons, and it may help avoid needless liability controversies in the future.

INSTRUMENT SERVICING

There have been several severe eye injuries resulting from servicemen's inattention to safety measures. Because the laser beam is collimated before the final element of most delivery systems, i.e., before a focusing objective lens, the direct beam or a reflection from a flat surface (see Fig. 2.1) can be exceedingly dangerous and travel great distances before the irradiance falls to a safe level. In all instances, the service technician must wear eye protectors and onlookers should be barred from the closed room during servicing.

The burn marks on the walls in a CO_2 surgical laser facility confirm the observation that unterminated collimate beams are not unusual during alignment by service technicians. Unlike the CO_2 laser that can only burn the skin or unprotected cornea, the CW argon or Nd:YAG laser can coagulate the retina upon accidental exposure. Such retinal hazards are greatest when the collimated beam is focused by the relaxed normal eye or when a diverging beam originating from a focal spot is imaged to a point on the retina when the eye is focused on that same laser beam focal spot. These two instances, if they are to occur at all, are most likely to occur during servicing. Each accident to a serviceman occurred when the individual was not convinced of the need for eye protectors. When the beam is invisible, it is difficult to remember the dangers associated with its high irradiance and to remain aware that secondary beam reflections may be readily overlooked.

Over the past 20 years, at least eight and perhaps up to a dozen laser servicemen, technicians, and researchers have been electrocuted when failing to follow appropriate safety measures when working on high voltage laser power supplies. The voltages and currents found in most surgical laser power supplies can be lethal, and must be dealt with properly. Only experienced technicians should attempt servicing surgical lasers, and any high-voltage circuits (specifically capacitors) should be discharged before repair (2).

OBSERVERS

Surgical assistants and other members of the operating room team are typically present along with the surgeon during the laser operation. In some instances, a patient's relative or other nonmedical observer may be present during laser surgery. However, because of the potential presence of dangerous reflected beams, laser eye protectors should be made available, although it is frequently true that the zone of potentially hazardous reflections may be normally limited to the immediate vicinity of the laser as shown in Figure 2.2. This indicates that an observer standing only 1 m to the side of the laser need not be at risk. However, it be a good medical and legal practice to have these observers wear appropriate eye protectors. The eye protectors should have an optical density sufficient to reduce the laser beam irradiance or power to EL or less. The eye protectors normally have an attenuation factor of at least 4.0

at the appropriate laser wavelength. One should always be attuned to the need to provide more protection than what is normally required as a way of precluding unwarranted fears among visitors.

The use of a video monitoring system to permit visitors to observe the laser operation is not only safe, but is probably superior to most other modes of observation. If secondary observation stations in an operating microscope are used by a resident, or visiting surgeon, great care must be taken to ensure that all necessary protective filters are installed in the observer's viewing path. It should be noted that special filters are not required if a CO_2 laser is operated.

EYE PROTECTORS

Protective clothing is not a practical control procedure where Class 4 lasers are used. Industrial lasers that require protective clothing are usually operated remotely or are baffled and enclosed. These safeguards frequently make eye protectors unnecessary in industrial laser operations. However, the nature of laser surgical applications has made the use of eye protectors an important measure. Absorbing glasses and organic dye-impregnated plastics are normally employed as the attenuating protective filter materials. Filters used for protection against visible laser wavelengths are usually colored, but filters that absorb energy in the infrared bands are not necessarily colored. Infrared protective filters, as used with a CO_2 laser, can provide protection with high visual transmission and no color distortion. The following parameters are useful in specifying eye protectors: wavelength or range of wavelengths of protection, optical density at these wavelengths, visual exceeding and damage threshold. While clear plastic goggles will burn if placed near the focal point of the surgical laser, they provide adequate protection from reflections.

Laser eye protection devices should be comfortable to wear for the duration of the laser operation, and side shields are required only if oblique exposure to the eye is likely. Each type of protector design has its advantages and disadvantages regarding comfort, fit, and durability. The coverall goggle, with a flat glass plate as the absorbing material, may be worn over prescription spectacles but provides no peripheral vision and is often heavy. This type may be most suitable for visitors, who are observing for a short period. The soft plastic wrap-around styles are lightweight but less durable, and are subject to scratching. Tightly fitting goggles can be uncomfortable and are more subject to fogging. The spectacle type of laser eye protector with or without prescription lenses is the most popular type among people who must wear protectors for long periods. Side shields may be obtained for some of the spectacle types if desired. Ordinary spectacles can adequately serve as laser eye protectors for the CO_2 laser wavelength.

DELAYED EFFECTS AND FUTURE CONSIDERATIONS

At the present time, there is no indication of delayed effects from CO_2 or Nd:YAG laser exposure. Extensive medical surveillance of laser research workers has failed to reveal any ocular anomalies or even the presence of retinal lesions unknown to the individual worker (2). Monitoring of laser retinal injury accident victims (2, 5) has not revealed any delayed effects. The potential exposure levels to the skin from scattered radiant energy from this type of laser application would be so substantially below threshold that no delayed biological effects would be expected (12-16). The surgical laser user can be assured that an almost worldwide consensus currently exists (17) regarding the appropriate laser safety measures for precluding injury from acute or chronic exposure effects.

REFERENCES

1. American National Standards Institute. *Safety Use of Lasers*, ANSI Standard Z-136.1. New York: ANSI, 1430 Broadway, 1986.
2. Sliney DH, Wolbarsht ML. Safety with Lasers and Other Optical Sources, A Comprehensive Handbook. New York: Plenum Publishing Corp, 1980.
3. Sliney DH. Laser-tissue interactions. Clin Chest Med 1985; 6:203.
4. Sliney DH. Biohazards of ultraviolet, visible and infrared radiation. J Occup Med 1983; 25:203.
5. Boldrey EE, Little HL, Flocks M, Vassiliadis A. Retinal injury due to industrial laser burns. Ophthalmology 1981; 88:101-107.
6. Mainster MM, Sliney DH, Belcher CD III, Buzney SM. Laser photodisruptors, damage mechanisms, instrument design and safety. Ophthalmology 1983; 90:973-991.
7. Wolbarsht ML. Ablative laser surgery: CO-2 or HF. IEEE J Quant Electr 1984; QE-20(12):1427-1432.
8. Sliney DH, Mainster MA. Potential laser hazard to the clinician during photocoagulation. Am J Ophthalmol 1987; 103:758-760.

9. Center for Devices and Radiological Health. Federal Performance Standards for Laser Products, *21 CFR 1040*, (under the Radiation Control for Health and Safety Act), Rockville: CDRH-FDA 1987.
10. Center for Devices and Radiological Health. *Food and Drugs*. Title 21, *Code of Federal Regulations*, Parts 510, 519, 520, 807, (Medical Device Amendments to the Food, Drug and Cosmetic Act), Rockville: CDRH-FDA, 1987.
11. American National Standards Institute (ANSI). Safe Use of Lasers in Health Care Facilities, Draft Standard Z-136.3-1988, American National Standards Institute, Laser Institute of America, Toledo, OH, 1987.
12. ACGIH. TLV's, Threshold Limit Values and Biological Exposure Indices for 1987-1988, American Conference of Governmental Industrial Hygienists, Cincinnati, OH, 1987.
13. World Health Organization [WHO]. Environmental Health Criteria No. 23, Lasers and Optical Radiation, joint publication of the United Nations Environmental Program, the International Radiation Protection Association and the World Health Organization, Geneva, 1982.
14. ACGIH. Documentation for the Threshold Limit Values, 5th Ed, American Conference of Governmental Industrial Hygienists, Cincinnati, OH, 1987.
15. Forbes PD, Davies PD. Factors that influence photocarcinogenesis. In: Parrish JA, Kripke ML, Morison WL, Eds. Chapter 7, Photoimmunology, New York: Plenum Publishing Corp., 1982.
16. Hillenkamp F. Laser interactions with biological tissue. In: Hillenkamp F, Sacchi CA, Arrechi T, Eds. Lasers in Biology and Medicine, New York: Plenum Press, 1980.
17. International Electrotechnical Commission (IEC). Radiation Safety of Laser Products, Equipment Classification, and User's Guide, Document WS 825, IEC, Geneva, 1984.

CHAPTER
3

Breast Surgery with the Laser

Raymond J. Lanzafame, H. Raoul Herrera, Ralph P. Pennino, J. Raymond Hinshaw

The art of surgery is the melding of a variety of techniques and instrumentats to accomplish the task at hand. There are a number of benign and malignant processes of the breast that require surgical therapy. Breast cancer is an increasingly common problem affecting 1 of 9 women. The optimal surgical management of carcinoma of the breast remains controversial yet paramount at the present time. This chapter will present techniques for the use of lasers in surgery of the breast. The reader is referred to general surgical and laser surgical atlases for specific details of technique. The rationale for the use of the laser and its advantages will be discussed.

CHOICE OF LASER AND LASER PARAMETERS

The choice of wavelength and the basic parameters necessary for successful laser surgery must be determined. The CO_2 laser generates coherent radiation at a wavelength of 10.6 μ. This energy, which may be focused through a lens, interacts with tissue by superheating and vaporizing cellular water. It is suitable for use as a scalpel. When defocused, the energy vaporizes tissue fluid over a broader area and can also seal small blood vessels and lymphatics, and "sterilize" a wound. Because this energy is all absorbed by water at the point of incision, very little energy is transmitted to adjacent tissue. The zone of irreversible tissue damage is 100–300 μ and this degree of injury most closely resembles the histological effect of the scalpel.

The CO_2 laser has a number of advantages as a surgical instrument that makes it useful for breast surgery. It is an accurate cutting instrument, which permits access to confined spaces. It can effectively ablate lesions or coagulate vessels (up to 1 mm) and seal lymphatics, reducing intraoperative blood loss and postoperative edema. The 1500°C temperature of the beam effectively destroys cells and cell nuclei in the beam path and there is no contamination of surrounding tissue as can occur with traditional surgical instruments. Experimental evidence indicates that laser surgery results in fewer postoperative infections and a lower incidence of local tumor recurrence. The latter property is extremely useful in the case of breast cancer where the rate of local tumer recurrence varies from 3–35% depending upon the type of procedure chosen and the choice of postsurgical adjunctive therapies, such as radiation and chemotherapy.

Recent work with the contact tips for the Nd:YAG laser suggests that it too may have a place in breast and soft tissue surgery. However, a few cautions are in order. The 1.06 μ wavelength of the Nd:YAG laser is most intensely absorbed by protein. This laser has been most useful as a photocoagulator of tissue due to its deep tissue penetration and destruction (up to 2–6 mm). The contact probes appear to reduce the zone of injury to a tolerable 1–2 mm, comparable to electrosurgery (0.3–1.0 mm). The contact probe gives the surgeon some degree of tactile feedback, which he or she does not have when using the CO_2 laser, and it may further reduce operative blood loss. However, the Nd:YAG laser is unsuitable for skin incisions due to the relatively extensive lateral tissue damage and it is as yet unknown whether it, too, is capable of reducing local tumor recurrence as does the CO_2 laser. Studies are being conducted in this laboratory to answer these questions.

Therefore, at present, the CO_2 laser appears to be the instrument of choice for breast surgery. The basic parameters for the use of the CO_2 laser in breast surgery are listed in Table 3.1. This information is presented as a guide for the user and

Table 3.1. Parameters for the Use of the CO_2 Laser for Surgery of the Breast

Laser: CO_2
Mode: TEMoo
Handpiece: 125 mm
Operating mode: Continuous wave
Skin incision: 25 W, spot size: 0.2 mm (focused)
Breast dissection/raising of flaps: 40–80 W (0.2–1.0 mm)
Dissection from clavipectoral fascia: 30–40 W (1 mm)
Axillary dissection:[a] 40–60 W (1 mm)
Wound "sterilization":[b] 30–40 W (1.0–1.5 cm SPOT SIZE)

[a]Optional, requires Kocher bronchocele sound or similar instrument for safe dissection.
[b]The tissue is gently heated just to the point of dessication without blanching or charring of the wound.

is not meant to be unalterable. The surgeon must be completely familiar with the specific instrument he or she is using and must use power densities that are safe and comfortable. Again, a few cautions are in order. It is advisable to use a TEMoo laser as this will produce the smallest and most controllable spot size. Lasers that have maximum outputs below 40 W are still useful for breast surgery, particularly when used with a 50-mm handpiece that produces a spot size of 0.09 mm and is, therefore, capable of achieving high energy densities. The surgeon must then deal with the bulkier and often times shorter 50-mm lens that may, at times, be difficult to maneuver in tight quarters. The breast fat that tends to liquify and pool in the wound must be suctioned or swabed to permit efficient incision, to reduce wound cautery due to superheated oil, and to prevent flash fires in the surgical site. It is advisable to begin dissection laterally and work medially. This allows the liquified fat to flow away from the point of incision. Reflective instruments and retractors should be used with utmost caution and should be wrapped with moistened sponges to prevent accidental reflection of the beam. This latter statement is not intended to be unyielding. Surgeons have learned to use electrosurgery with metallic instruments safely and the same can be true with lasers. However, only nonreflective instruments must be used as backstops.

CLINICAL APPLICATIONS

Breast Biopsy

The CO_2 laser is quite useful for breast biopsy and for excision of benign and malignant masses. These operations are often performed as ambulatory procedures and they may be performed under either local or general anesthesia. Infiltration of the wound with 0.25% bupivacaine with epinephrine is preferred when local anesthesia is used. The epinephrine will enhance the hemostatic effect of the laser. Skin incision is accomplished at 25 W with constant tension and retraction of the wound maintained. Local flaps are raised at 40–60 W and the lesion is grasped and excised completely. Hemostasis is secured with laser and conventional techniques as needed. Wound "sterilization" is accomplished in the case of a malignant lesion by using the beam defocused to a 1.0 to 1.5-cm spot size at 30–40 W to heat the tissue to the point of surface dessication. Great care must be taken to avoid blanching or charring of the tissue and to prevent inadvertant damage to the skin edges. If desired, the breast tissue is approximated with absorbable suture material, although many surgeons prefer to omit this layer and to reapproximate the skin only. Drains are unnecessary. There has been no difficulty with interpretation by a pathologist of laser specimens, nor has there been any documented change in the ability to obtain accurate estrogen receptor information on these specimens. Similarly, there has been no clinically apparent difference in the rate of wound healing when the laser is used for making skin incisions.

Breast Abscess

The laser is particularly useful for the treatment of chronic breast abscessess and sinuses. The infected segment is excised en-bloc at 60 W and hemostasis is secured. The wound is irrigated copiously with saline to reduce further any bacterial innoculum and the wound is then sterilized as described above. Wound closure is accomplished over a closed-suction Silastic drain. Appropriate perioperative antibiotics are used. The laser facilitates the resection of all the infected tissue and minimizes the possibility of recontamination and reinfection of the wound.

Segmentectomy with Axillary Dissection

The CO_2 laser facilitates segmentectomy and axillary dissection in the appropriately selected patient. The dissection of the primary tumor and an adequate margin of uninvolved tissue is accomplished as described above. Histological confirmation of tumor-free margins is obtained, the wound is irrigated with sterile water, blotted, and then sterilized with the defocused beam. Drainage of this wound is unnecessary. Careful attention to wound closure and the restoration of breast contour is imperative. Local flaps may be undermined by using the laser at 40–60 W and the subcutaneous tissue is reapproximated with absorbable suture material. It should again be noted that many surgeons prefer not to attempt reapproximation of the breast tissue and reapproximate the skin only. This wound is covered with a small OP-Site or similar dressing and the axillary dissection is begun through a separate axillary incision. The axillary dissection may be accomplished using conventional surgical instruments or with the laser. When using the CO_2 laser for this purpose, an ebonized Kocher bronchocele sound is used to assist in the dissection of discrete bundles of tissue and to provide a backstop for the laser, permitting safe dissection without causing injury to the axillary vein or the long thoracic and thoracodorsal nerves. The laser is used at approximately 40 W for this portion of the dissection and the large vessels coursing through the specimen are ligated with absorbable suture material. The wound is closed over a closed-suction Silastic drain. Ansanelli has confirmed the observation that these wounds have less postoperative drainage and that the drainage has a lower hematocrit than is usually noted after conventional dissections. The reader is referred to the chapter on axillary dissection (Chapter 4) for further details. The reader should also note that axillary dissection is also easily accomplished with the contact probe and the Nd:YAG laser. Preliminary data suggest that the contact tip may be used safely in the vicinity of veins and nerves with little threat of iatrogenic trauma if used alongside or tangentially, not directly over, these structures.

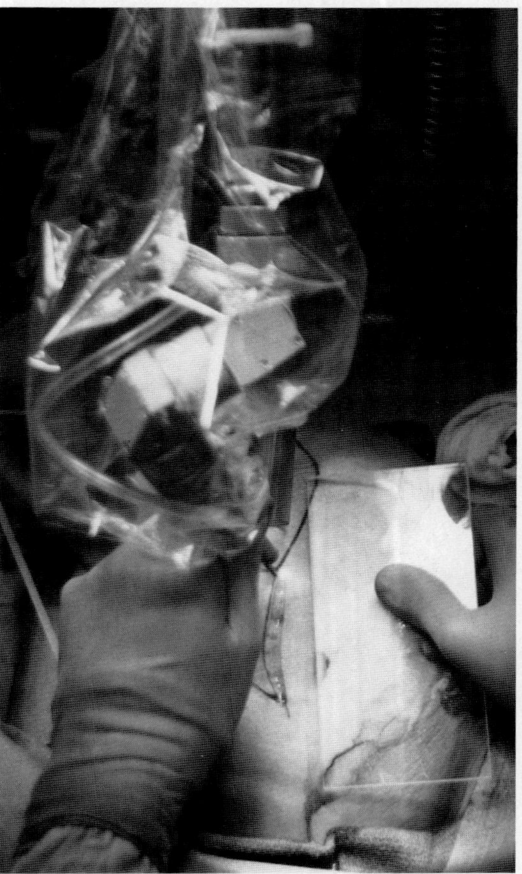

Figure 3.1. Skin incision in modified radical mastectomy is made at 25 W with the handpiece in focus. Note that the tissue is incised from a lateral to medial direction.

Modified Radical Mastectomy

Skillful performance of modified radical mastectomy is enhanced by the use of the CO_2 laser. The instrument is particularly useful for salvage mastectomy after radiotherapy because it easily dissects through tissue planes that are distorted and otherwise difficult to separate in the irradiated breast.

A transverse incision is preferred for mastectomy to produce a more favorable cosmetic result or to permit immediate or subsequent reconstructive surgery. As is noted in Table 3.1, the skin incision is made at 25 W in continuous wave form and in a lateral to medial direction (Fig. 3.1). Skin flaps of standard 5-mm to 1-cm

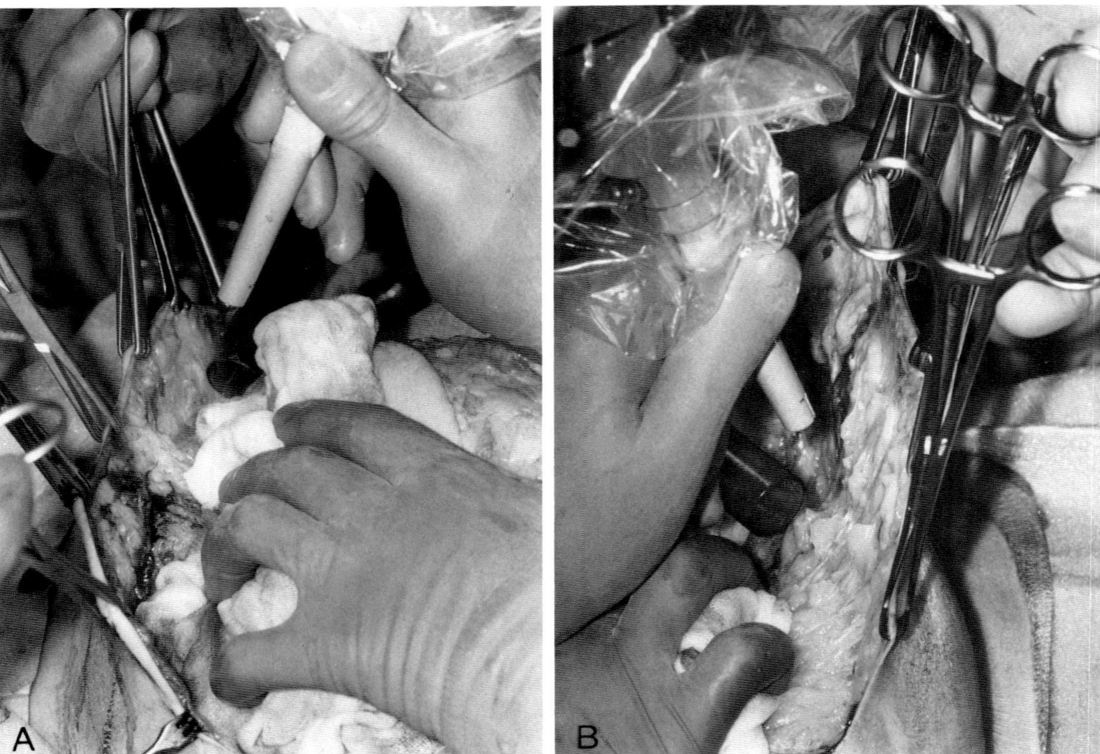

Figure 3.2A, The upper flap is raised using the laser at 60-80 W. The flap is held perpendicular to the chest wall and the laser is held parallel to the flap. **B,** The lower flap is raised in a similar fashion.

thickness are raised with the laser set at 60 to 80 W and the beam defocused to a 1-mm spot size so as to enhance hemostasis. The assistant must suction or swab away the liquefied fat and the flaps should be retracted perpendicular to the chest wall and maintained under constant traction. The surgeon should hold the laser handpiece parallel to the flap so as to avoid inadvertent injury to the flap. The lower flap is raised in a similar fashion (Fig. 3.2). Bleeders are easily controlled with electocautery or defocused laser energy. The breast is dissected from the clavipectoral fascia in a superomedial to an infralateral direction. The laser is used at 30–40 W. Subpectoral perforators should be coagulated with defocused laser energy before their division (Fig. 3.3). It is sometimes preferable to begin this peel with electrosurgery. The axillary envelope is incised and the axillary dissection may be accomplished with the laser and the Kocher bronchocele sound as is shown in Figure 3.4. The Nd:YAG contact tip, scalpel, or electrocautery may be used at the discretion of the surgeon. The wound is flushed with sterile water and sterilized once the specimen has been removed. Two suction drains are placed and the wound is closed in a single layer as is shown in Figure 3.5.

Immediate reconstruction of the breast is possible, particularly with the use of a mammary prostesis or tissue expander. A subpectoral flap is created (Fig 3.6) and the tissue expander is placed in a subpectoral plane between the pectoralis major and upper two insertions of the serratus anterior (Fig. 3.7). The pectoralis is reapproximated with absorbable suture material. A subcuticular wound closure is preferable in such cases. Many workers have performed mastectomy with immediate reconstruction. Tissue expanders have been shown to be a simple and safe procedure in properly selected patients. It permits breast reconstruction with contiguous tissues of similar color, texture,

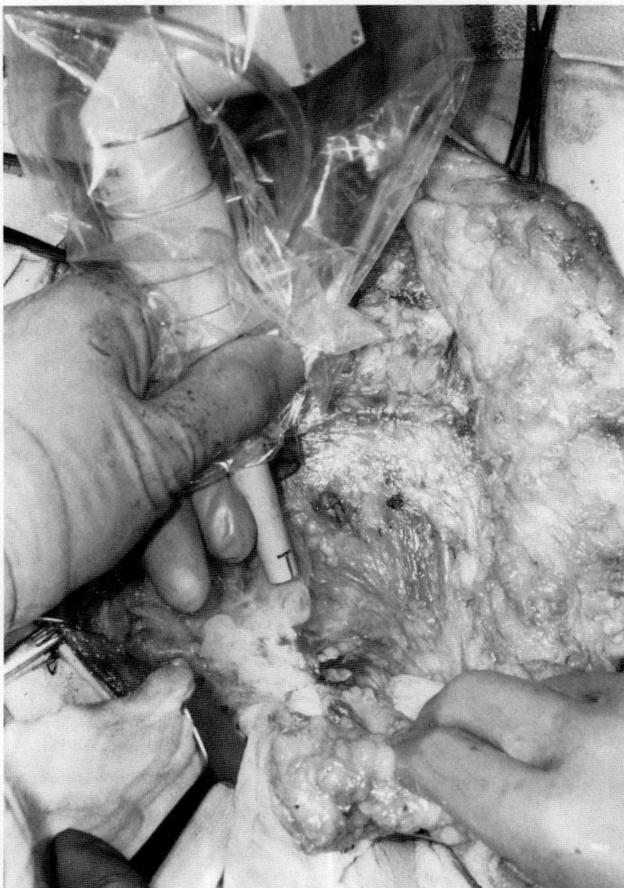

Figure 3.3. The breast is dissected from the clavipectoral fasia in a superomedial to inferolateral direction. The laser is set at 30–40 W and perforating vessels are coagulated before their division.

sensory appreciation, and with no donor site defects. There has been no evidence that immediate reconstruction affects the course of the primary tumor in properly selected patients. The laser should obviate concern about seeding of the wound and implant space by tumor cells and bacteria, and the reduced postoperative drainage should serve to make this operation more cost-effective by reducing hospital stay.

SUMMARY

The CO_2 laser represents a significant advance in the surgical repertoire of the breast surgeon. It is useful for the treatment of benign and malignant disorders of the breast. The nontouch, sterile nature of CO_2 laser permits the safe excision of infected lesions and tumors with a lowered risk of surgical contamination of the wound and experimental evidence of a reduced incidence of local tumor recurrence after laser excisions. Both intraoperative and postoperative wound drainage is reduced and there is no risk of destroying the pathological specimen or interfering with estrogen receptor analysis.

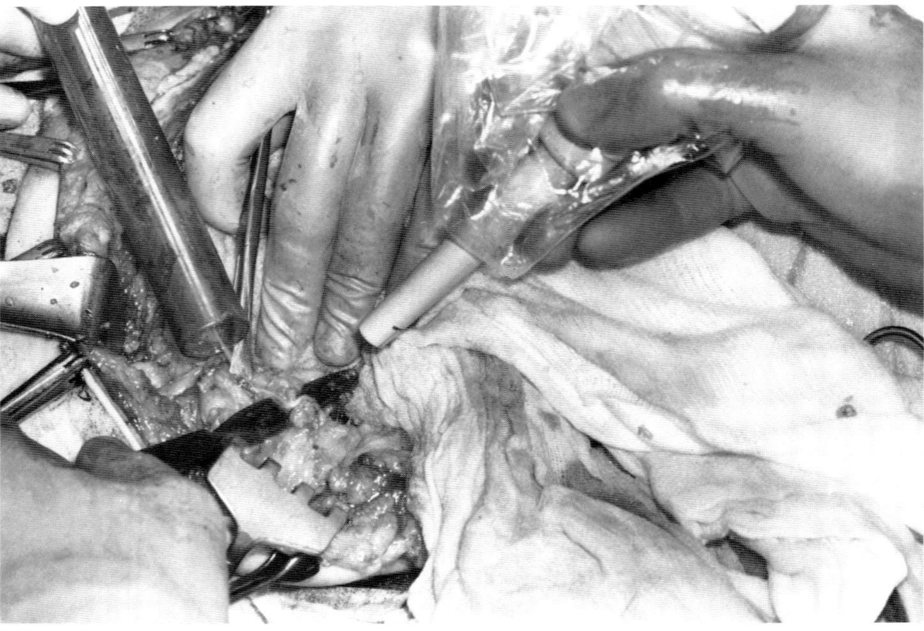

Figure 3.4. The axillary dissection is facilitated through the use of a Kocher bronchocele sound as both a dissecting instrument and laser backstop. The laser is set at 40 W for this portion of the procedure.

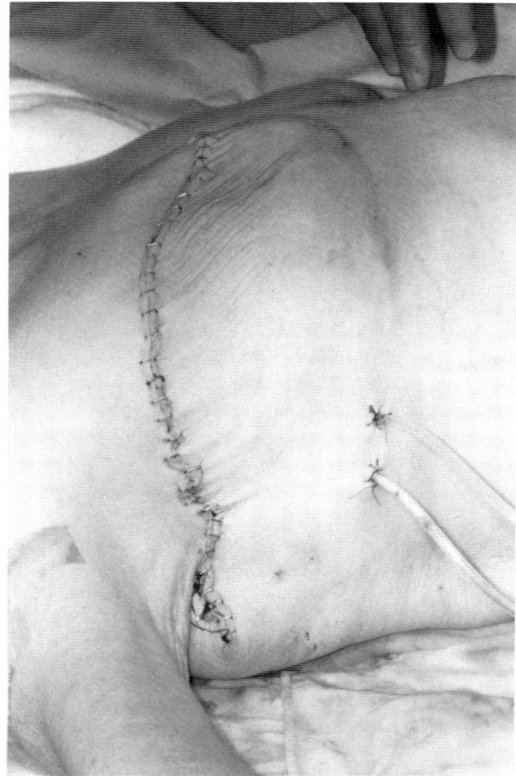

Figure 3.5. Silastic suction drains are placed and the wound is closed with staples.

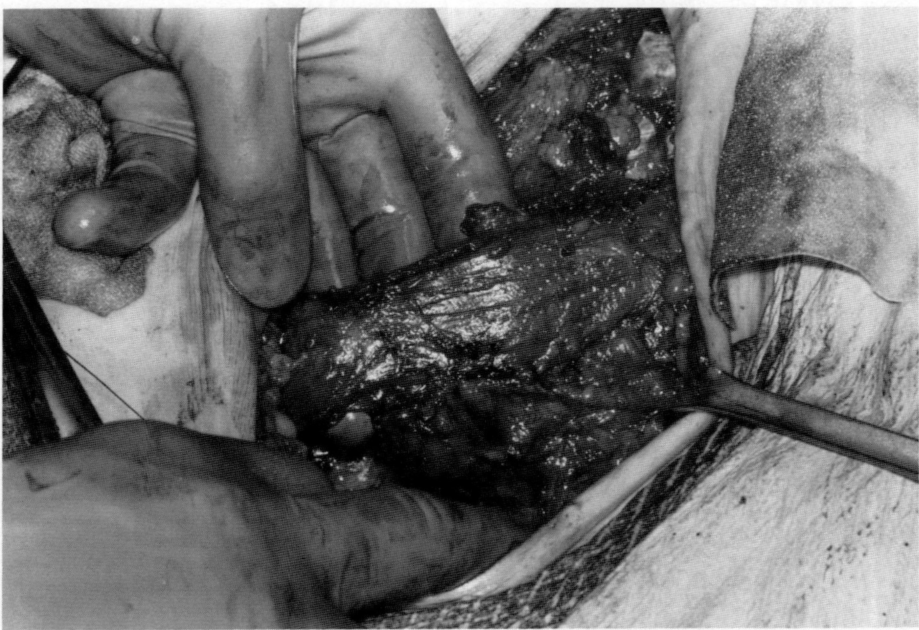

Figure 3.6. In the case of immediate reconstruction, a subpectoral flap is fashioned between the pectoralis major and serratus anterior.

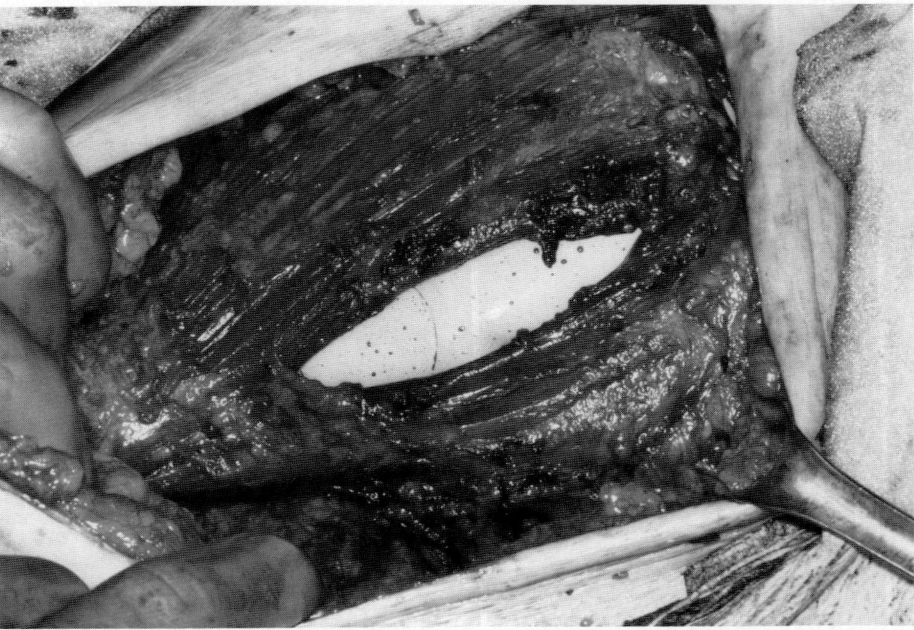

Figure 3.7. The mammary prosthesis is inserted into the subpectoral pocket. The pectoralis major will be reapproximated with absorbable suture material.

SUGGESTED READINGS

Surgical and Laser Atlases

Chassin JL. Operative Strategy in General Surgery, 2 Vol. New York: Springer-Verlag, 1980.

Cooper P. The Craft of Surgery, 2nd Ed. 3 Vol., Boston: Little Brown, 1971.

Lanzafame RJ, Hinshaw JR. Atlas of CO_2 Laser Surgical Techniques, St. Louis: Ishiyaku EuroAmerica, Inc., 1987.

Madden JL. Atlas of Technics in Surgery, 2nd Ed. 2 Vol. New York: Appleton-Century-Crofts, 1964.

Rob C, Smith R. Operative Surgery, 2nd Ed. 14 vol. Philadelphia: JB Lippincott Co., 1969.

Zollinger RM, Zollinger RM Jr. Atlas of Surgical Operations, 5th Ed. New York: Macmillan Publishing Co., 1983.

General Laser Information, Wound Healing

Andrews AH, Polanyi TG. Microscopic and Endoscopic Surgery with the CO_2 Laser. Boston: Wright Publishing Co., 1982.

Ben-Bassat M, Ben-Bassat M, Kaplan I. Electron microscopic studies of soft tissue incision by means of CO_2 laser. Laser Surg 1976; 1:95-100.

Brackett KA, Sankar MY, Joffe SN. Effects of Nd:YAG laser photoradiation on intra-abdominal tissues: A histological study of tissue damage versus power density applied. Lasers Surg Med 1986, 6:123-130.

Dixon JA. Lasers in Surgery. In: Ravitch MM, Ed. Current Problems in Surgery, Volume XXI, Number 9. Chicago, Year Book Medical Publishers, Sept. 1984.

Filder JP, Bendick PJ, Glover JL, et al. Effects of CO_2 laser on wound healing and infection. Lasers Surg Med 1983; 3:109.

Fidler JP, Law E, MacMillan BG. Comparison of carbon dioxide laser excision of burns with other thermal knives. Ann NY Acad Sci 1976; 267:254-262.

Fuller TA. Fundamentals of Lasers in Surgery and Medicine. In: Dixon JA, Ed. Surgical applications of lasers. Chicago: Year Book Medical Publishers, pp. 11-27, 1983.

Halldorsson TH, Langerholz J. Thermodynamic analysis of laser irradiation of biological tissues. Appl Optics 1978; 17:39-50.

Hishimoto K, et al. Carbon dioxide laser general surgery: Experience with 150 cases. In: Atsumi K, Nimsakul N. Eds. Laser Tokyo '81. Tokyo: Inter-Group, 1981.

Hishimoto K, Rockwell RJ Jr, Epstein RA, et al. Laser wound healing compared with other surgical modalities. Burns 1974; 1:13-22.

Kaplan I, Giler S. CO_2 Laser Surgery. Berlin: Springer-Verlag, 1984.

Lanzafame RJ, Naim JO, Rogers DW, Hinshaw JR. A comparison of continuous wave, chop wave and super pulse laser wounds. Lasers Surg Med (Abstr.) 1987; 7:69.

Lanzafame RJ, Pennino RP, Herrera HR, Hinshaw JR. Inexpensive retractors for laser surgery. Surg Gynecol Obstet 1985; 161:392-393.

Levine M, Ger R, Stellar S, et al. Use of the carbon dioxide laser for the debridement of third degree burns. An Surg 1974; 179:246-252.

Levine MS, Salisburg RE, Peterson HD, et al. Clinical evaluation of the carbon dioxide laser for burn wound excisions: A comparison of the laser, scalpel and electrocautery. J Trauma 1975; 15:800-807.

Madden JE, Edlich FR, Custer JR, et al. Studies in the management of contaminated wound: IV. Resistance to infection of surgical wounds made by knife, electrosurgery and laser. Am J Surg 1970; 119:222-224.

Pennino RP, Lanzafame RJ, Herrera HR, Hinshaw JR. Applications of CO_2 laser in general surgery. Contemp. Surg 1986; 28:13-21.

Slutzki S, Shafiri R, Bornstein LA. Use of the carbon dioxide laser for large excision with minimal blood loss. Plast Reconstr Surg 1977; 60:250-255.

Takiguchi S, et al. CO_2 laser surgery and hemorrhagic tendencies. In Laser Tokyo '81. Atsumi K, Nimsakul N, Eds. Tokyo: Inter-Group, 1981.

Unger M. Laser Surgery. In: Clinics in Chest Medicine. Philadelphia: WB Saunders, 1985.

Wound Sterilization; Infected and Purulent Wounds

Chegin VM, Brekhov EI, Skobelkin OK, Smolianinov MV, Eliseenko VI. Carbon dioxide laser in the complex treatment of suppurative diseases and wounds of the soft tissues. Khirurgiia (Mosk) 1983; Mar 3:29-32.

Chegin VM, Skobelkin OK, Brekhov EI. Laser surgery for soft tissue purulent diseases. Lasers Surg Med 1984; 4:279-82.

Giler S, Ben-Bassat M, Taube E, Kaplan I. The surgery of pilonidal sinus with the CO_2 laser. Laser Surg 1980; 3:201-203.

Glantz G, Korn A. The use of the CO_2 laser knife in the treatment of decubitus ulcers. Kaplan I, Ed. Laser Surgery, Volume I-II. Tel-Aviv. OT-PAZ, 1977.

Hinshaw JR, Herrera HR, Lanzafame RJ, Pennino RP. The use of the carbon dioxide laser permits primary closure of contaminated and purulent lesions and wounds. Lasers Surg Med 1987; 6:581-583.

Mullarky MA, et al. The efficacy of the CO_2 laser in the sterilization of skin seeded with bacteria: Survival at the skin surface and in the plume emissions. Laryngoscope 1985; 95:186.

Ovadia J, Levavi H, Edelstein T. Treatment of pruritus valve by means of CO_2 laser. Acta Obstet Gynecol Scand 1984; 63:265-7.

Serra Renom JM, Sanado L. Applications of the CO_2 laser scalpel in surgery. Rev Med Univ Navarra 1983; 27:45-49.

Skobelkin OK, Brekhov EI, Shablovski OR, Trizno TN. Treatment of purulent-inflammatory diseases of the soft tissues using carbon dioxide lasers in ambulatory care. Klin Chir 1984; 1:1-4 Jan.

Stellar S. The carbon dioxide surgical laser in neurological surgery, decubitus ulcers, and burns. Lasers Surg Med 1980; 1:15-33.

Breast Surgery with Lasers

Ansanelli VW. The CO_2 laser in cancer surgery of the breast. A comparative clinical study. Lasers Surg Med 1986; 6:470-472.

Ansanelli VW. The CO_2 laser in axillary dissection of breast cancer. Lasers Surg Med 1987; 7:87.

Giler S, Ben-Bassat M, Taube E, Kaplan I. The use of the CO_2 laser in palliative surgery for cancer. Proeedings of

4th Congress of the International Society for Laser Surgery 1981; 23:12-15.

Gollop TR, Hauschild D, Filho EA, et al. Use of CO_2 laser in mastectomy for breast carcinoma. Rev Paul Med 1980; 95:101-103.

Hira N, Steger AC, Moore KC. The use of the Nd:YAG laser in breast cancer surgery. Lasers Surg Med 1987; 7:87.

Kaplan I, Ger R. Partial mastectomy and mamoplasty performed with CO_2 laser—a comparative report. Br J Plast Surg 1973; 26:189-190.

Kott I, Reiss R, Giler S, Kaplan I. The CO_2 laser in mastectomy: A comparative study. Proceedings of 4th Congress of the International Society for Laser Surgery. 1981; 24:1-2.

Kott I, Reiss R, Giler S, et al. The CO_2 laser in mastectomy: A comparative study. In: Atsumi K, Nimsakul N, Eds. Laser Tokyo '81. Tokyo: Inter-Group, 1981.

Lanzafame RJ, Rogers DW, Naim JO, DeFranco C, Ochej H, Hinshaw JR. Reduction of local tumer recurrence by primary excision with the CO_2 laser. (Abstr.) Lasers Surg Med 1985; 5:142.

Lanzafame RJ, Rogers DW, Naim JO, DeFranco C, Ochej H, Hinshaw JR. Reduction of local tumor recurrence by excision with the CO_2 laser. Lasers Surg Med 1986; 6:103-105.

Lanzafame RJ, Rogers DW, Naim JO, DeFranco C, Ochej H, Hinshaw JR. Reduction of local tumor recurrence by excision with the CO_2 laser. Lasers Surg Med 1986; 6:439-441.

Lanzafame RJ. Breast surgery with the CO_2 laser. Laser Pract Rep 1986; 2:3S-4S.

Lanzafame RJ, Hinshaw JR, Eds. Atlas of CO_2 Laser Surgical Techniques. St. Louis, Ishiyaku EuroAmerica, Inc., 1987.

Lanzafame RJ, McCormack CJ, Rogers DW, Naim JO, Hinshaw JR. Effects of laser sterilization on local recurrence in experimental mammary tumor. Surg Forum 1986; 37:480-481.

Lanzafame RJ, McCormack CJ, Rogers DW, Naim JO, Herrera HR, Hinshaw JR. Mechanisms of carbon dioxide laser reduction of tumer recurrence in experimental mammary tumor. Lasers Surg Med (Abstr.) 1987; 7:87.

Lanzafame RJ, McCormack CJ, Rogers DW, Naim JO, Hinshaw JR. The effect of laser sterilization on local recurrence in experimental mammary tumors. Current Reports in Surgery (Abstr.) 1987; 3:21.

Pennino RP, Lanzafame RJ, Herrera HR, Hinshaw JR. Principles and techniques of free-hand CO_2 laser surgery. (Abstr.) Lasers Surg Med 6:197, 1986.

Pennino RP, Lanzafame RJ, Hinshaw JR. Roundtable: Lasers in general surgery. Surg Pract News 1986; 7:9-11.

Breast Cancer

Bonadonna G. Introduction: Breast cancer. Sem Oncol 13(4):383, 1986.

Bonadonna G, Valagussa P. Current status of adjuvant chemotherapy for breast cancer. Sem Oncol 1987; 14:8-22.

Carbone PP, Tormey DC. The clinical investigator and the evolution of the treatment of primary breast cancer. Sem Oncol 1986; 13:415-424.

Feig SA. The role of new imaging modalities in staging and follow-up of breast cancer. Sem Oncol 1986; 13:402-414.

Fisher B, Wolmark N. Conservative surgery: The American experience. Sem Oncol 1986; 13:425-433.

Goldie JH. Scientific basis for adjuvant and primary (neoadjuvant) chemotherapy. Sem Oncol 1987; 14:1-7.

Jones RC, Ed. Selected Readings in General Surgery. Overview of Papers on Breast Cancer. 1985; 12:1-32.

Jotti GS, Petit JY, Contesso G. Minimal breast cancer: A clinically meaningful term? Sem Oncol 1986; 13:384-392.

Pritchard KI. Current status of adjuvant endocrine therapy for resectable breast cancer. Sem Oncol 1987; 14:23-33.

Recht A, Connolly JL, Schnitt SJ, et al. Conservative surgery and radiation therapy for early breast cancer: Results, controversies, and unsolved problems. Sem Oncol 1986; 13:434-449.

Thor A, Weeks MO, Schlom J. Monoclonal antibodies and breast cancer. Sem Oncol 1986; 13:393-401.

Breast Reconstruction

Argenta L. Reconstruction of the breast by tissue expansion. Clin Plast Surg 1984; 11:257-264.

Argenta LC, Marks MW, Grabb WC. Selective use of serial expansions in breast reconstruction. Ann Plast Surg 1983; 11:188-202.

Asplund O. Capsular contracture in silicone gel and saline filled breast implants after reconstruction. Plast Reconstr Surg 1984; 73:270-275.

Georgiade GS: Immediate reconstruction of the breast following modified radical mastectomy for cancer of the breast. Clin Plast Surg 1984; 11:383-388.

Gruber RP, Kahn RA, Lash H, Morton M, Apfelberg D, Laub D. Breast reconstruction following mastectomy: A comparison of submusclar and subcutaneous techniques. Plast Reconstr Surg 1981; 67:312-317.

Guthrie RH. Breast reconstruction after radical mastectomy. Plast Reconstr Surg 1976; 57:14-22.

Guthrie RH, Cucin RL. Breast reconstruction after mastectomy: Problems in position, size and shape. Plast Reconstr Surg 1980; 65:595-602.

Radovan C. Breast reconstruction following mastectomy using temporary expander. Plast Reconstr Surg 1982; 69:195-206.

Synderman RK, Guthrie RH. Reconstruction of the female breast following radical mastectomy. Plast Reconstr Surg 1971; 47:565-567.

Versaci AD, Balkovich ME. Tissue expansion. In: Habel M, Ed. Advances in Plastic and Reconstructive Surgery, Vol. 1, Chicago: Yearbook Medical Publishers, pp 95-145, 1984.

CHAPTER

4

Radical Axillary Lymph Node Dissection with CO_2 Laser

Vincent W. Ansanelli

The decision to use adjuvant chemotherapy for breast carcinoma is usually based on the finding of mestastasis to the axillary nodes discovered on pathological examination. Radical axillary dissection provides information essential to this purpose and, in addition, offers some measure of prognosis.

In reviewing the literature, there is a paucity of information regarding the use of the CO_2 lasers in the performance of a radical axillary dissection as part of the surgical treatment for breast carcinoma. This is significant and indicates investigation is needed. Therefore, in an attempt to facilitate surgical dissection and to further minimize postoperative morbidity, the author has utilized the CO_2 laser in the majority of axillary dissections. The technique is described herein. Part of an incontinuity axillary dissection was used as with a modified radical mastectomy or via a separate incision as performed with segmentectomy (quadrantectomy [1] or lumpectomy [2]) and axillary dissection. Dissection included, at a minimum, levels I and II (3), level III being removed when readily accessible. Separate Jackson-Pratt drainage tubes were utilized to remove fluid from the chest wall and axilla. All tubes were removed and the patient was discharged when drainage measured less than 60 ml/day. All procedures are staged. Definitive surgery is usually preceded by excisional biopsy and full discussion of options with patient.

All surgery described is performed with the CO_2 laser Tem00, 125-mm handpiece, continuous wave (CW) of 25–60 W, with power densities ranging between 65,800 and 157,936 W/cm^2.

It is assumed in this presentation that the operating surgeon has fulfilled the basic requirement of laser usage.

1. Certification
2. Clinical preceptorship
3. Safety standards

Also of importance is a trained ancillary staff familiar with laser protocol. The operative time and ease of dissections with the laser depend on the surgeon's level of expertise, each surgeon develops his or her own comfort zone of laser usage.

OPERATIVE TECHNIQUE

1. *Anatomy of the axilla* with knowledge of axillary lymph node levels (Fig. 4.1) is necessary.
2. *Position of patient* (Fig. 4.2). The patient is placed in a supine position and a small pad is placed beneath the scapular to elevate the affected side approximately 20°. The arm is draped free and kept within the operative field. Exposure of the 2nd and 3rd portion of the axillary vein is often enhanced by adducting the arm across the chest wall.
3. *Skin Marking* (Fig. 4.2). In performing a separate incision for axillary dissection a sterile pen is used to mark the line of incision. The incisional line can either be made in a curved linear fashion across the axillar or in an oblique vertical fashion running from the apex to the axilla approximately at the level of the 5th rib inferior.
4. *Skin Incision and Flap Elevation* (Fig. 4.3). Skin incision is performed with the CO_2 laser set at a power of 25 W, penetrating into the subcutaneous fat.

   Power is now raised to 40–60 W and dissection was continued down to the inferior portion of the axillary fat pad. Anterior and

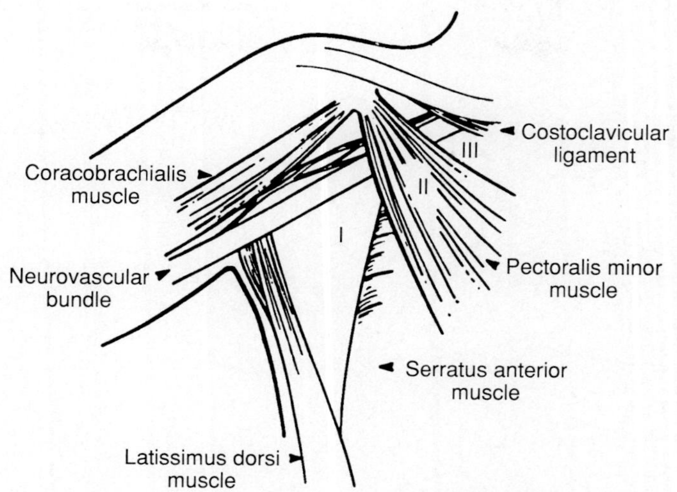

Figure 4.1. Axilla with lymph node levels (Pectoralis major muscle removed).

posterior flaps are elevated in order to identify the anterior border of the latissimus dorsi muscle and the lateral border of the pectoralis major muscle.

5. *Development of the boundaries of dissection.* Upon identification of the exposed border of the latissimus dorsi muscle, insertion of the index finger along this border and bluntly moving superiorly toward the humerous would point the index finger to the contents of the axillary sheath. The anterior aspect of the dissection, along the lateral border of the pectoralis major muscle is carried superiorly

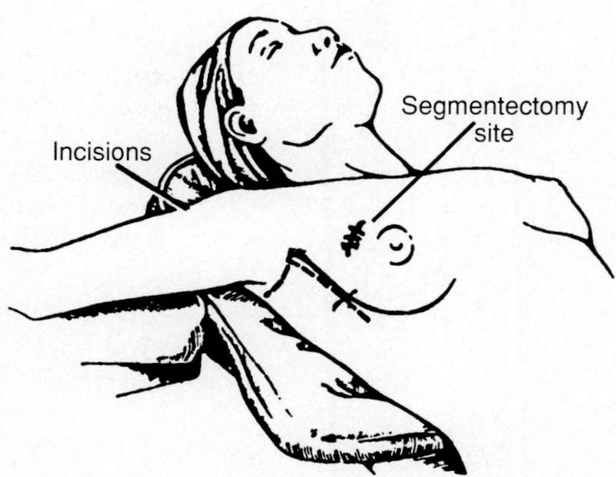

Figure 4.2. Position of patient. Skin marking.

with the laser set at 40–60 W. The clavi pectoral is now exposed.

By sharp technique, an incision is made parallel to and inferior to the axillary vein.

6. *Dissection along the axillary vein* (Fig. 4.4). After exposure of the axillary vein, dissection parallel to the vein is begun at its midpoint and proceeds anteriorly, beneath the pectoralis minor muscle to a point just inferior to the take off of the thoracoacromial trunk.

The apex of the dissection is tagged with silk. All of the fibroadipose tissue is removed from the ventral and inferior surface of the axillary vein with the bronchoseal sound. The laser is set at 25 W.

All axillary vein tributaries are secured by clamp, using the catgut technique. No attempts are made to dissect superior to the vein. This portion of the dissection is facilitated by placing the draped arm in a position of adduction across the chest wall with the hand touching the opposite shoulder. This offers complete relaxation to the pectoralis muscles and to the axillary contents. There is usually no need to transsect the pectoralis minor muscle.

7. *Anteromedial dissection* (Fig. 4.5). Protecting the axillary vein with a moist lap pad, the anteromedial aspect of the dissection proceeds by cutting the lateral portion of the

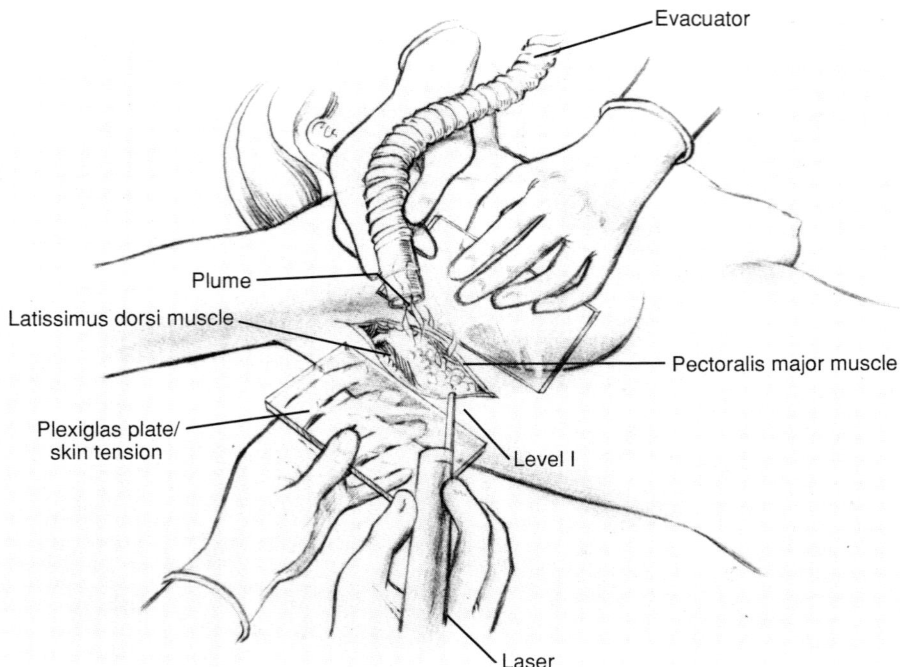

Figure 4.3. Skin incision and flap elevation. Evacuator suctions off vaporized tissue (plume).

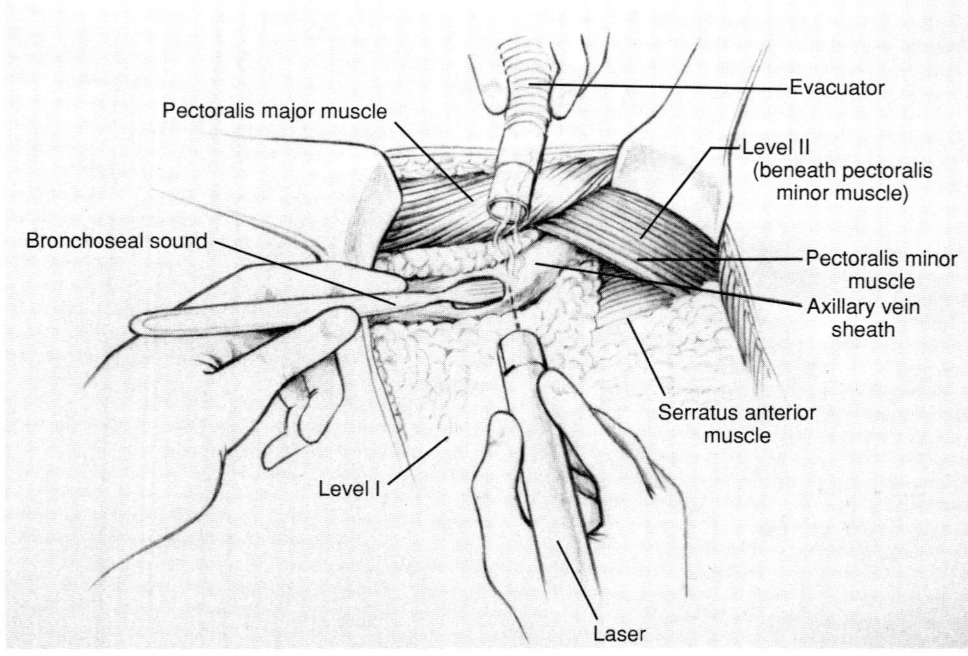

Figure 4.4. Dissection along the axillary vein.

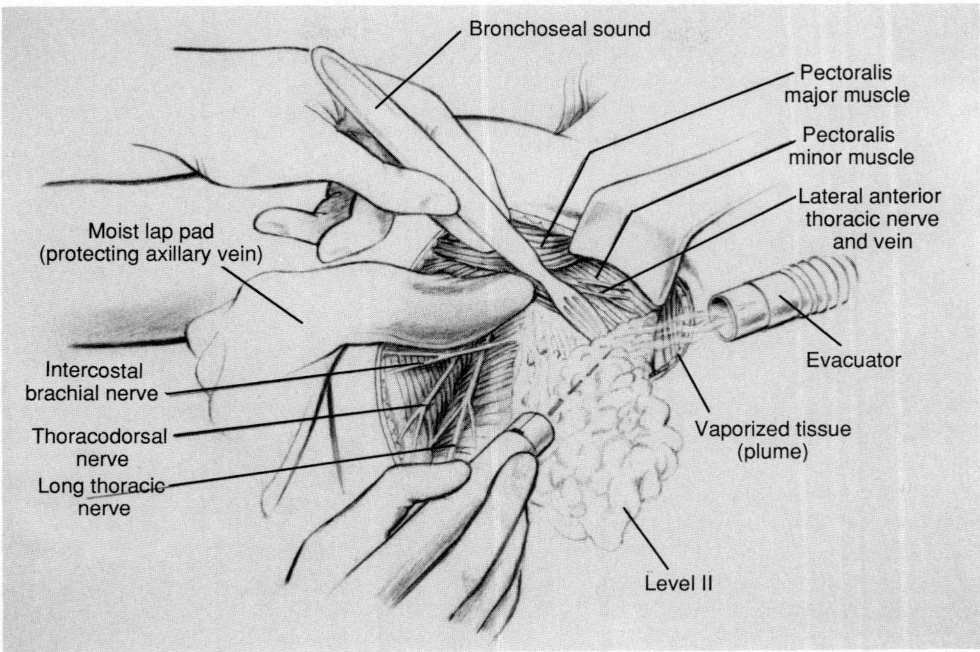

Figure 4.5. Anteromedial dissection (Rotter's node area).

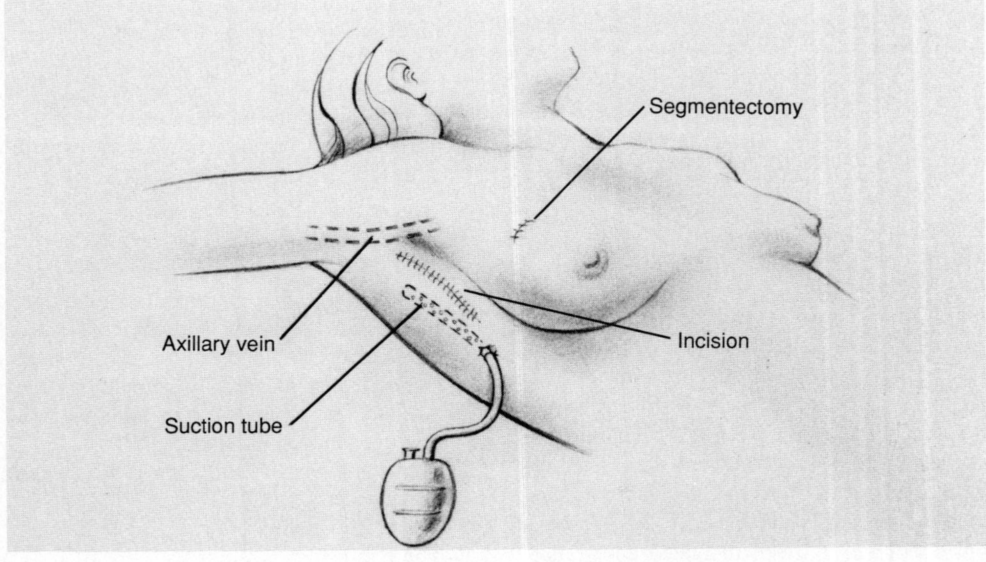

Figure 4.6. Wound dressing and drainage.

pectoralis major fascia in its length; dividing the medial anterior thoracic neurovascular trunk and simultaneously removing the interpectoral fatty areolar tissue (Rotter's node area), with the laser set at 40 W. Care is taken to preserve the lateral anterior thoracic neurovascular bundle. Blood vessel layers in the area are secured by conventional techniques.

8. *Intercostal-brachial nerve, long thoracic nerve, and thoracodorsal nerve.* The intercostal-brachial nerve is identified emerging from the 2nd intercostal space. It is usually located 1–2 cm anterior to the long thoracic nerve. Both of the intercostal-brachial nerve and the thoracic nerve are preserved. By blunt and sharp technique, the intercostal-brachial nerve is skeletonized as it crosses the base of the axilla until it enters the arm at a point where the latissimus dorsi border meets the axillary vein. With the aid of the bronchoseal sound and the laser set at 25 W, the distal portion of the axillary vein is now cleared of its fatty areolar tissue. The dissection stays superficial to the fascia of the anterior serratus muscle therefore protecting the long thoracic nerve. Dissection is carried inferiorly and laterally with the laser set at 25–40 W, preserving the thoracodorsal neurovascular trunk.
9. *Wound drainage and dressings* (Fig. 4.6). After removal of the specimen, a No. 10 Jackson-Pratt sump is inserted into the axilla and exteriorized via a small stab wound, at a point just inferior to the incision. This is fixed to the skin with a 2–0 silk suture. Closure of the wound is with staples and the wound is covered with a 1-inch gauze strip and collodion dressing.
10. *Postoperative management.* The sump tube is removed when drainage is less than 60 ml/day. This usually occurs within 24–48 hours (4) of surgery. Then the patient is discharged. Arm motion is not restricted except for abduction within the first 48 hours. Skin staples are left in situ between 8 and 10 days with good wound healing. Adjunctive radiotherapy is started approximately 2 weeks postoperatively. When indicated chemotherapy is usually started earlier.

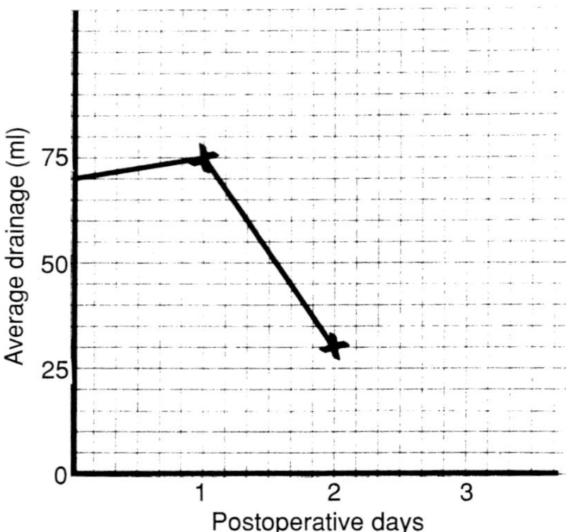

Figure 4.7. Postoperative drainage.

OBSERVATIONS

Sixty-seven patients with primary breast carcinoma (5) underwent a radical axillary dissection with the CO_2 laser. Selection was prospective, nonrandomized, and sequential. The following observations are noted.

Operative

1. Similar to training in conventional surgery, in equivocal anatomical situations, the operative time is inversely proportionate to the surgeon's level of expertise.
2. The surgical field is drier allowing for clearer identification of vial structures.
3. No operative complications were experienced with this modality.

Postoperative morbidity (Figs. 4.7 and 4.8).

1. Axillary drainage is dramatically reduced in volume and duration. This reduction involves lymphatic and bloody fluid. Patients are discharged without drains within 24–48 hours.
2. All patients require little or no analagesia and require minimal nursing care.
3. Arm function is excellent with no swelling or dysesthesias.
4. There are no infections.
5. There transient seromas were handled by simple fine needle aspiration.

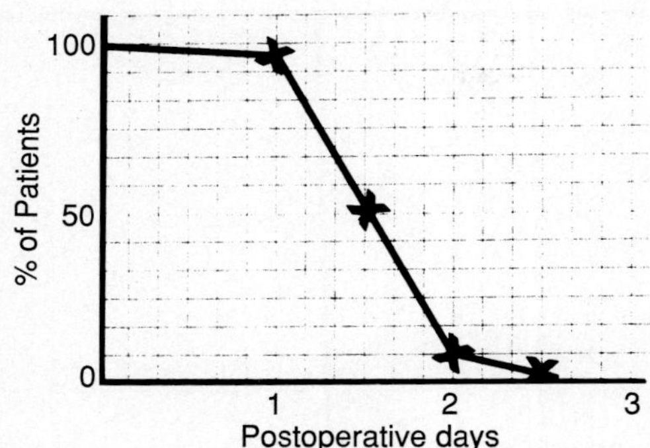

Figure 4.8. Postoperative hospitalization.

6. Since surgical experience has been relatively atraumatic, these patients are better prepared to adjust to adjunctive therapy that may be indicted.

Cost-effectiveness

In the United States, over 100,000 women per year will contract breast carcinoma. The majority of these patients will require major surgery including axillary dissection. One can easily comprehend the financial ramifications inherent in reduced postoperative morbidity and hospitalization.

REFERENCES

1. Veronesi U, Saccozzi R, Del Vecchio M, et al. Comparing radical mastectomy with quadrantectomy, axillary dissection and radiation therapy in patients with small cancers of the breast. N Engl J Med 1981; 305:6-11.
2. Fisher B, Bauer M, Margolese R, et al. Five year results from the NSABP trial comparing total mastectomy to segmental mastectomy, with and without radiation, in the treatment of breast cancer. N Engl J Med 1985; 312:665-673.
3. Rosen PP, Lesser ML, Kinne DW, et al. Discontinuous or ''skip'' metastases in breast carinoma. Am Surg 1983; 197:276-283.
4. Ansanelli V. CO_2 laser in cancer surgery of the breast. A comparative study, Laser Surg Med 1986; 6:470-472.
5. Ansanelli V. Use of CO_2 laser in radical axillary dissection for breast cancer. Presented at the 1987 Annual Meeting of the American Society for Laser Medicine and Surgery; 7th Congress of the International Society for Laser Surgery and Medicine. Munich, 1987.

CHAPTER

5

Laser Cholecystectomy

Christopher J. Daly

Laser technology has been commonly available in the operating rooms of most hospitals for 5–10 years. Traditionally, it has been only for "special" procedures and, therefore, was a tool unfamiliar both to the operating surgeon and to the remainder of the operating team. With the opening of the Laser Center at the St. Francis Medical Center in January of 1987, it became apparent that frequent—preferably daily—use of the laser would be essential to the smooth running of the Center.

Biliary tract operations are frequently performed and it was this author's belief at the outset that the application of laser technology would be advantageous for the patient. A MEDLINE search performed at that time revealed no articles in the literature regarding the use of lasers of any type for the performance of major biliary tract operations.

Therefore the performance of all biliary tract procedures with the laser was begun. The first cholecystectomy was performed using the CO_2 laser. The remainder were performed using the neodymium YAG (Nd:YAG) laser with the sapphire laser scalpel developed by Surgical Laser Technology laboratories. Patient selection, techniques employed, and the results in the first 25 patients, will be described. It should be stressed that there is a significant learning curve for the surgeon in beginning to use this equipment; this study represents the beginning of the learning curve.

PATIENT SELECTION

As the great majority of biliary tract operative procedures are performed electively, only patients admitted to the hospital for elective surgery were selected for this report. All patients had a diagnosis of chronic calculous cholecystitis documented preoperatively either by ultrasound or oral cholecystogram. A discussion was held in the office with each patient regarding the use of the laser during the course of their operation. It was stressed that the operation was not greatly different from that done with more traditional techniques. No special "laser operative permits" were obtained, but the routine hospital operative permission was utilized. The fact that the laser would be used was written in, e.g., permission for cholecystectomy utilizing the laser. All patients had complete blood count (CBC), urinalysis, SMA-12, and chest x-ray performed before surgery. Those over the age of 40 years had an electrocardiogram performed also. The majority of patients were admitted through the hospital's Short Stay Unit directly to the operating room on the morning of surgery, but 2 patients were admitted 1 day preoperatively because they dwelt a long distance from the hospital.

OPERATIVE TECHNIQUE

After the suitable induction of general endotracheal anesthesia, the abdomen was prepared and draped. In all patients a right subcostal incision was used (Fig. 5.1). The incision was marked with a scalpel and the remainder of all sharp dissection was performed utilizing the laser. In the majority of cases (24 of 25), the Nd:YAG contact laser was used. The 0.4-mm sapphire scalpel tip was used most commonly during the period of time when these operations were performed. The contact sapphire laser scalpel and Nd:YAG laser were obtained from Surgical Laser Technologies, Inc. (Malvern, PA). However, the 0.2-mm sapphire scalpel tip has been found to be more effective and is now the current choice. The laser was used in the continuous wave mode. In the beginning 8–10 W of power were used but, with more experience, the power was increased to approximately 15 W. It was found that dissection of the subcutaneous fat required about 15 W of power

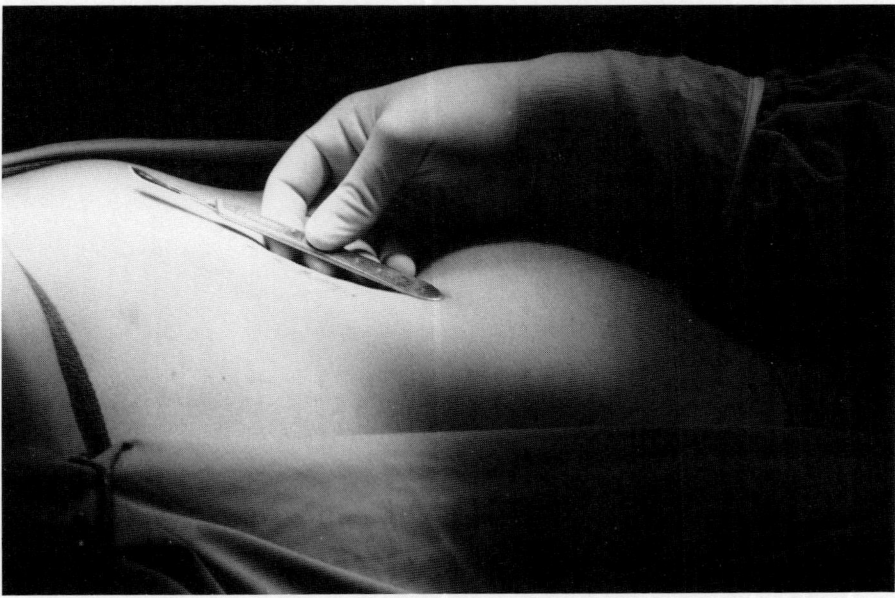

Figure 5.1. Right subcostal incision.

for smooth progress. Dissection was carried to the anterior rectus sheath which was cleansed utilizing the laser.

The anterior rectus sheath was then opened and the rectus muscle was bluntly dissected and elevated over an Army-Navy retractor (Fig. 5.2). The muscle was divided with the laser scalpel. It should be pointed out that traction and countertraction are extremely important when dissecting with the sapphire scalpel tips. This keeps the already divided tissue away from the sides of the tip where it will be heated and suffer thermal damage. Therefore, the only contact of the scalpel tip should be at its point directly on the tissue being incised.

Hemostasis for the majority of vessels encountered was performed utilizing the heat of the side of one scalpel tip. The larger vessels, particularly those under the rectus muscle, required electrocautery.

The posterior rectus sheath and peritoneum were then opened, again with the laser scalpel (Fig. 5.3). In contrast to the CO_2 laser, the contact tip technology allows the surgeon to open the peritoneum easily without fear of damaging the underlying viscera. Figure 5.3 shows the ability to utilize the laser close to one's own finger without fear of burning through the operating glove. Also noted in this figure is the plastic Yankauer suction tip. This was connected to the Stackhouse plume evacuator and proved to be an efficient, effective, and simple method of removing the laser plume from the operative field.

Exploration of the abdomen was carried out through this incision. The gallbladder was grasped with a Kelly clamp at its fundus and the pericholecystic adhesions, if any, were divided using the laser scalpel. The dissection was carried down until Calot's triangle was identified.

Moist laparotomy pads were then positioned to protect the viscera and to provide retraction on the common bile duct and duodenum. A Deaver retractor was placed medial to the gallbladder over the liver to expose the triangle of Calot. The gallbladder was placed on traction and the peritoneal reflection over the cystic duct and cystic artery was opened with the laser. In most cases, the cystic artery and cystic duct could be identified at this stage of the operation. The cystic duct was looped with a single chromic tie so as to prevent manipulation of stones downward during the course of dissection. The cystic artery was doubly clipped and divided when encountered. This was done adjacent to the gallbladder. When either

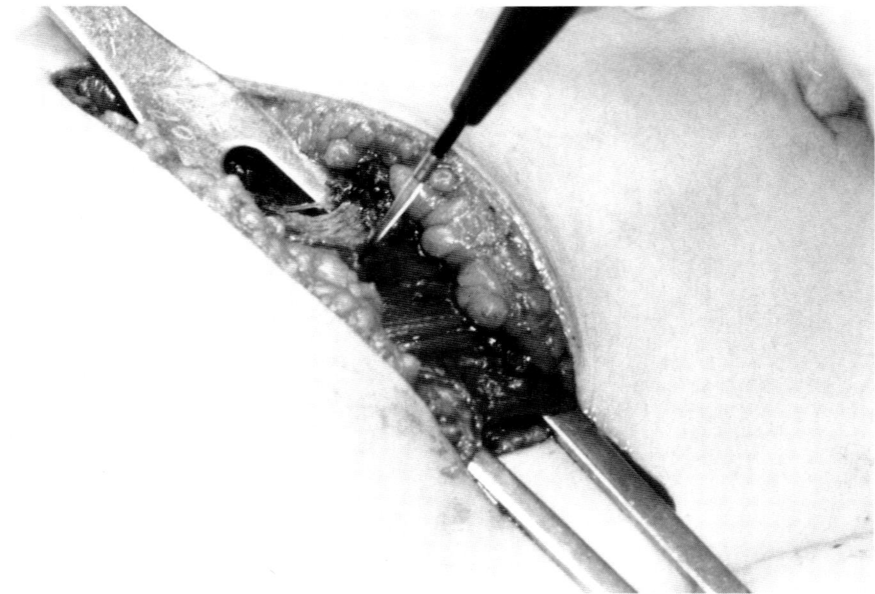

Figure 5.2. Dissection of anterior rectus sheath.

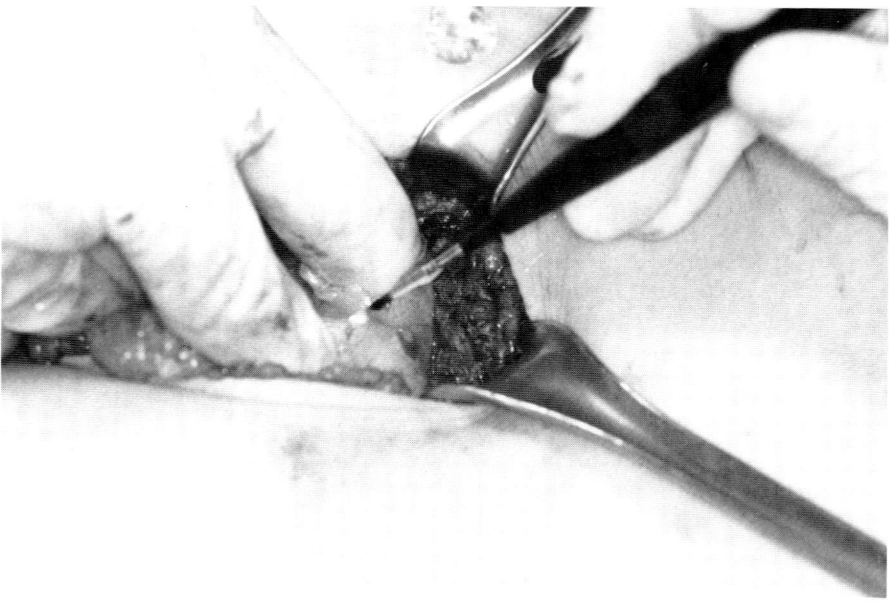

Figure 5.3. Dissection of posterior rectus sheath and peritoneum.

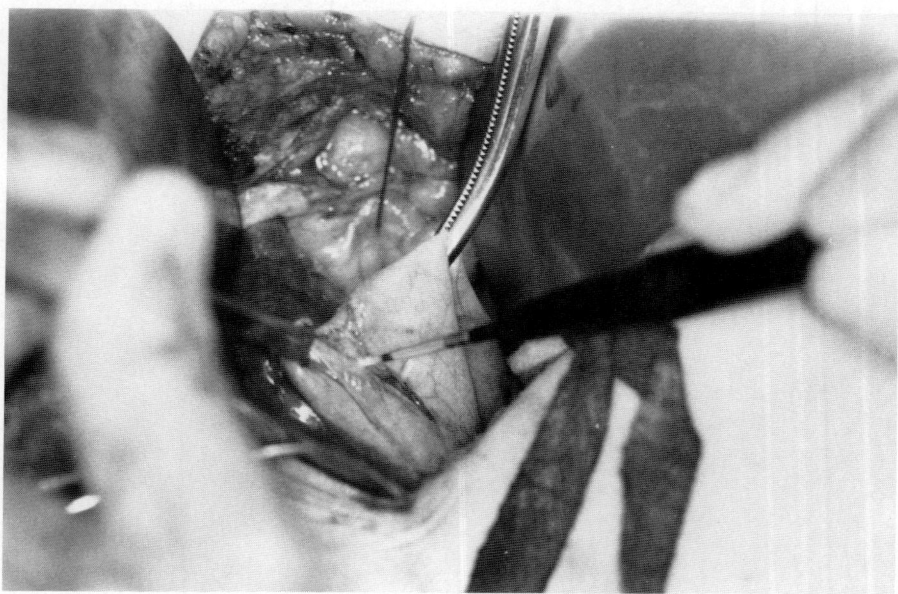

Figure 5.4. Opening the peritoneal reflection.

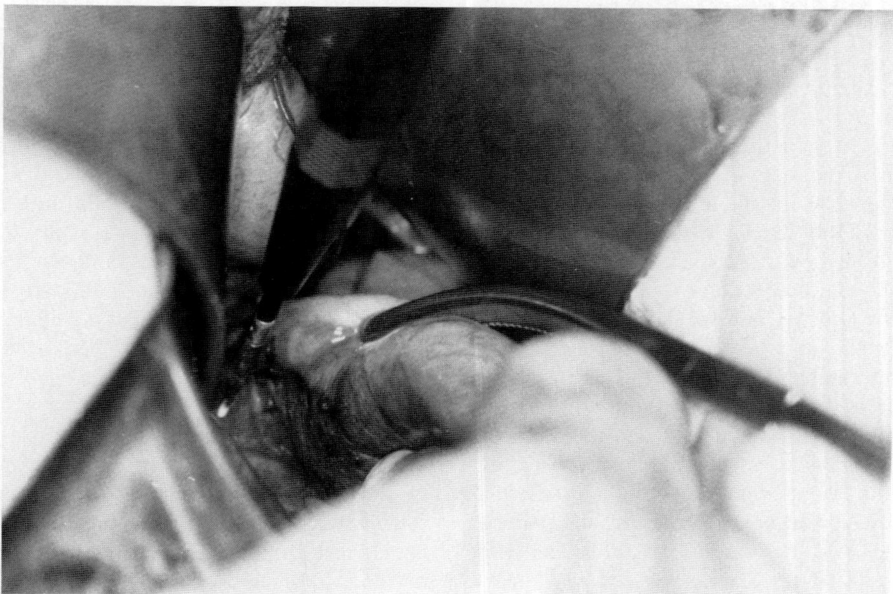

Figure 5.5. The cystic artery is doubly clipped.

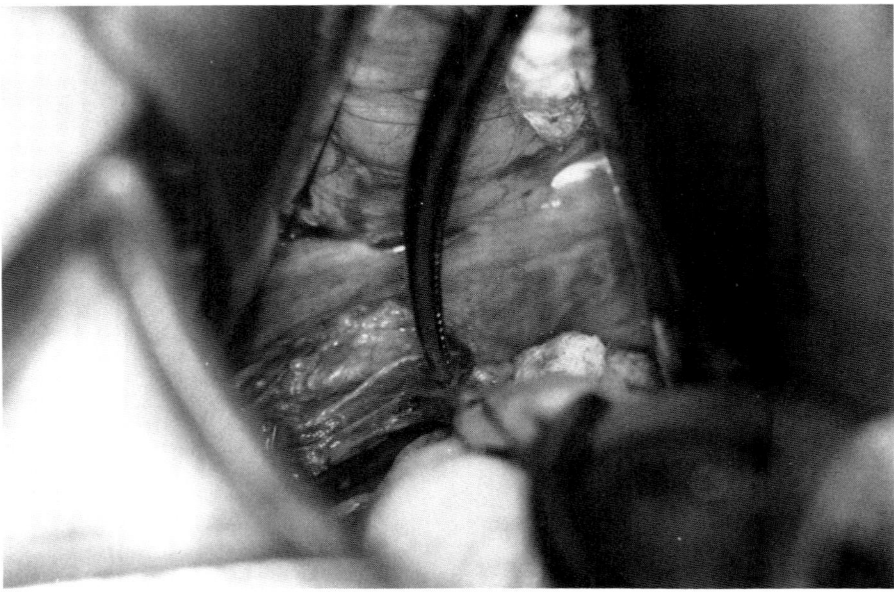

Figure 5.6. The cystic duct-common bile duct function.

could not be identified, in cases where acute inflammation made dissection difficult, the gallbladder was removed from the fundus downward without engaging in extensive dissection in this area.

Attention is again directed to the fundus of the gallbladder. The peritoneal reflection attaching the gallbladder to its bed in the liver was opened (Fig. 5.4) with the laser. The gallbladder was dissected from its bed in the liver with the laser and blunt dissection. Dissection was carried down until the cystic artery could be absolutely identified and the cystic artery was then doubly clipped close to the gallbladder and divided (Fig. 5.5). Dissection was then carried down until the cystic duct-common bile junction could be identified (Fig. 5.6). Care was taken to ensure that the common bile duct was not injured, that the cystic duct was doubly clipped with large clips, and that the gallbladder was removed. The gallbladder was then opened and inspected. Cultures were taken where appropriate. Cystic duct cholangiography was not routinely employed.

The operative site was then thoroughly irrigated. The bed of the gallbladder was inspected and bleeding points treated by removing the scalpel tip from its handle and applying the Nd:YAG laser as a bare fiber to cauterize these bleeding points. This was generally used at 40 W of power staying a distance of approximately 1–2 cm from the edge of the liver. It is important to keep the laser moving over the liver bed. This will keep the coagulation on one surface and prevent deep injury due to the ''popcorn'' effect.

Irrigation was performed again after bleeding had been secured. No attempt was made to close peritoneal reflection as it was completely excised. Neither Penrose nor suction drains are routinely used in this practice for elective gallbladder surgery unless a bile leak is discovered. No patient needed a nasogastic tube.

The would was then closed in layers with running suture technique utilizing heavy absorbable suture (0 Maxon). The subcutaneous tissue was irrigated with saline and checked for hemostasis. No subcutaneous sutures were used. The skin was approximated with intradermal sutures of fine absorbable suture material (Fig. 5.7). This was reinforced with SteriStrips and a suitable dressing was applied.

In the postoperative course, the patients were allowed and encouraged to ambulate on the evening of surgery. They were started on clear fluids the morning after surgery and progressed to a regular diet as tolerated. The great majority of patients were

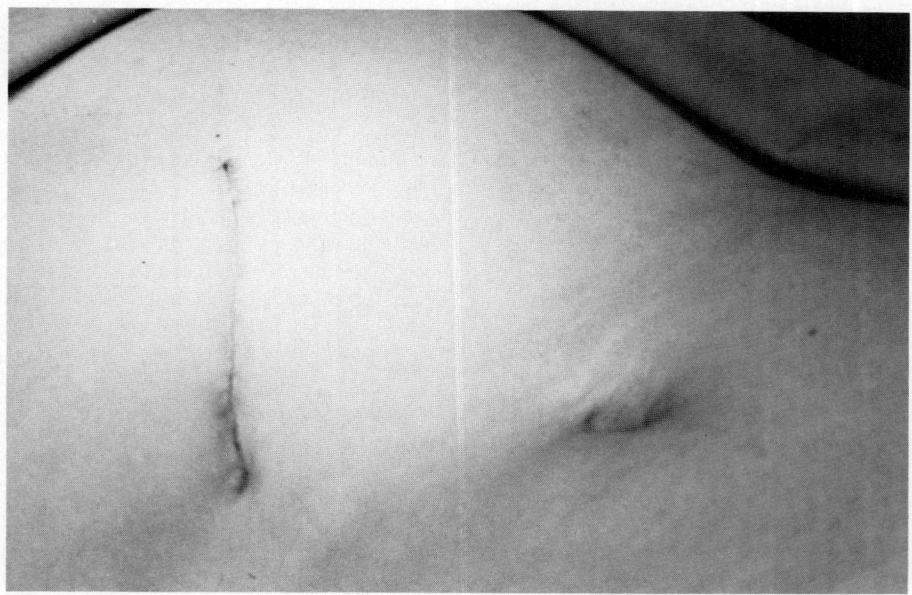

Figure 5.7. Intradermal sutures were used.

able to progress to a regular diet by 36 hours postoperatively and were discharged on the 2nd morning after their operation. Six patients were unable to take in nourishment until the 2nd day and they were kept until the 3rd postoperative day.

Intramuscular morphine sulfate has been the drug of choice for postcholecystectomy discomfort. In the group of patients under study, the average patient received 4.8 injections. No patient was discharged home on a prescription analgesic and none requested any. All patients were seen 7 to 10 days postoperatively in the office and for a second visit approximately 6 weeks postoperatively.

RESULTS

Twenty-five consecutive patients who underwent elective cholecystectomy for chronic calculous cholecystitis were studied from 1/8/87 through 9/9/87. They represented all elective admissions for this diagnosis on this service. There were 22 females and 3 males in the study. The average age was 42 years with a range of 24–76 years. Four patients were over 60 years old. Twenty-three patients were admitted on the day of surgery and 2 patients were admitted 1 day before because of the distance from their home to the hospital.

A review of the anesthetic records showed that the operating time for the procedures ranged from 40–75 min with an average of 59 min. The longer times represent cases performed earlier in the learning curve and also those patients who were found on later pathologic review to have acute cholecystitis. The dissection in these cases was more difficult than usual. It is this author's impression that the use of the laser adds a small

Table 5.1. Hospital Stays of Elective Cholecystectomy Patients

Patients	Age (yr)	Operating Time (min)	LOS[a] (days)	DRG 197 ALOS[b] (days)	DRG 198 ALOS[b] (days)	Cost to Hospital
25 (22 F/3 M)	24–76 (average = 42)	40–75 (average = 59)	2–5 (average = 2.56)	11.5	10.1	$1246–2496 AVG. $1871

[a]LOS—length of stay after SLT contact laser cholecystectomy.
[b]ALOS—Average length of stay.

amount of time to the performance of the operation initially, but that this addition becomes less marked with greater proficiency.

Complications were minimal. Twenty-two patients had no postoperative complications. Two patients developed slightly elevated temperatures. One of these patients, who was quite obese, required aspiration of a small seroma from the subcutaneous space. She represents the longest hospitalization at 5 days. One other patient was noted to have a small wound separation at the lateral edge of the wound on her first postoperative visit which cleared within several days and healed without any further incident.

The average hospital stay for the entire group (Table 5.1) was 2.56 days with a range of 2–5 days. The average cost to the hospital for the care of these patients was $1871 with a range of $1246–2496. This was particularly impressive considering that the average length of stay under DRG 197—total cholecystectomy without common duct exploration for the patient age over 69 years—is 11.5 days and that for DRG 198—total cholecystectomy without common duct exploration for the patient age 69 years or less—is 10.1 days.[a]

Although this group in no way represents a prospective clinical trial, this author believes that the results define obvious benefits to the patient and to the hospital resulting from the use of laser technology in the performance of biliary tract surgery. The use of the contact laser brings a degree of safety to intraabdominal laser surgery that is not present with the CO_2 laser. With that comes a degree of ''surgical comfort'' not previously available in laser surgery. This represents a significant advance in the treatment of one of the most common conditions requiring major surgery in the United States today.

[a] Diagnostic Related Groups, 3rd revision, Health Systems International, New Haven, CT, 1986, p 208.

CHAPTER

6

Percutaneous Treatment of Gallstones

Teruo Kouzu, Kaichi Isono

In recent years, endoscopic treatment for bile duct stones has become widespread. Endoscopic sphincterotomy (EST) has been used for common bile duct stones, while percutaneous lithotomy has been chosen for intrahepatic stones and gallbladder stones. The authors have mainly used percutaneous lithotomy for recurrent or residual intrahepatic stones (1).

Lithotripsy under cholangioscopy has improved so that it has become commonly used to indicate percutaneous treatment for bile duct stones. Depending upon the individual case, percutaneous treatment rather than surgical operations would be chosen to remove intrahepatic stones. However, in cases of gallstones, surgical operation becomes the first choice because it is only a minor surgical invasion of patients. Therefore, percutaneous treatment is confined to those cases where surgical operation is not indicated. In this chapter, the authors report a method of percutaneous treatment of gallstone using the laser.

METHOD

In preparation for percutaneous treatment, the accurate position and size of stones must be determined using echocardiography, endoscopic retrograde cholangiopancreatography (ERCP), and computed tomography (CT). To begin percutaneous treatment for gallstones, the gallbladder must be punctured using the ultrasonic probe (GCE-406M, 4 MHz by Toshiba). The probe is inserted in the intercostal region at the right ventrolateral side, and a PTCD needle (Chiba needle, no. 22 gauge) is inserted in the gallbladder (Figs. 6.1 and 6.2). During puncture, the needle should be manipulated toward the gallbladder neck as far as possible, so as to pass through the liver bed and into the gallbladder, thereby creating a dilated fistula with minimal complications.

After the position of the needle in the gallbladder is confirmed by fluoroscopy, a lead wire and a drainage catheter are inserted into the gallbladder. An enlarged tract (18–20 Fr) usually can be obtained using a dilator after two or three attempts. Then a cutaneous tract is formed ventrolaterally from the liver body to the surface (usually in 10–14 days). The cholangioscope is inserted into the gallbladder through the sinus tract.

The CHF-P cholangioscope (Olympus, 5.8-mm outside diameter, 2.6-mm biopsy channel diameter) or CHF-P10(4.9-mm outside diameter, 2.0-mm biopsy channel diameter), is used, depending on the size of the sinus tract. Small stones are removed from the gallbladder using the CHF-P. The instruments for lithotripsy are shown in Figure 6.3. The alligator forceps (**A**) are used for grasping stones, the basket catheter (**B**) is used for removing stones, and the Fogarty catheter (**C**) is used for swaying stones and turning stone surfaces toward the laser during irradiation. The brush instrument (**D**) removes mucus on the stone surface and sandy stones. If stones are larger than the diameter of the sinus tract, a laser beam is applied, removing it in small pieces.

The method of lithotripsy by laser for gallstones is shown in Figure 6.4. First, the Nd:YAG laser is applied, which makes stone friable. Next, instruments for lithotripsy are used to break the stones into small pieces and to extract them through the sinus tract using the basket catheter. During irradiation, part of the crumbled fragments may pass through the cystic duct and pile into the distal end of the common bile duct. At this point EST is not employed immediately; rather, the authors await dilation of the end of common bile duct caused by the obstruction of accumulated small stones. It is easier to remove stones by EST at that time. During percutaneous

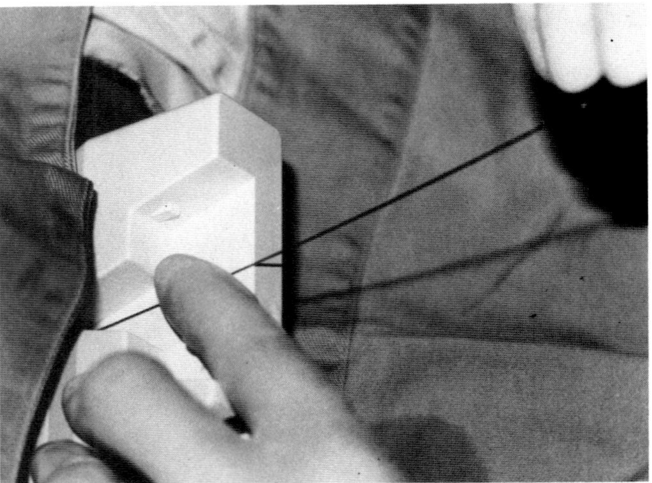

Figure 6.1. The echo-guided puncture of the gallbladder.

lithotomy, EST is used only for gallstones but not for intrahepatic stones. This is because of an unfortunate experience wherein a patient with intrahepatic stones died from hepatic abscess after EST. The continuous wave (CW) of the Nd:YAG laser has been used for lithotripsy.

Investigations were carried out on the fiber tip that lead the laser beam (Fig. 6.5). Figure 6.5**A**

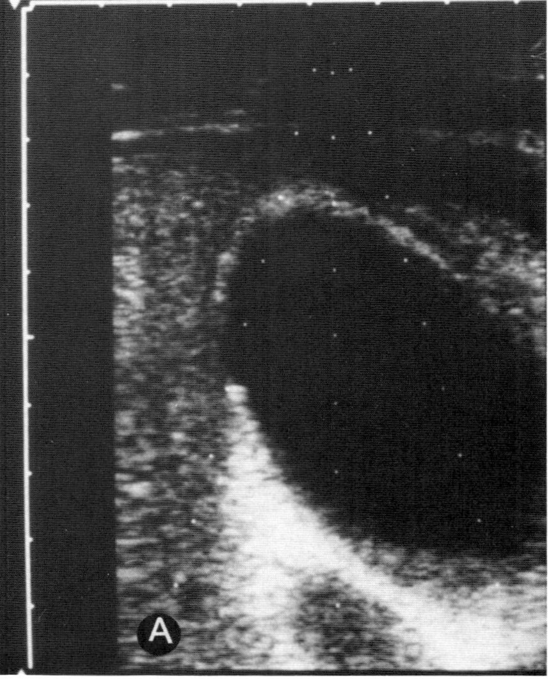

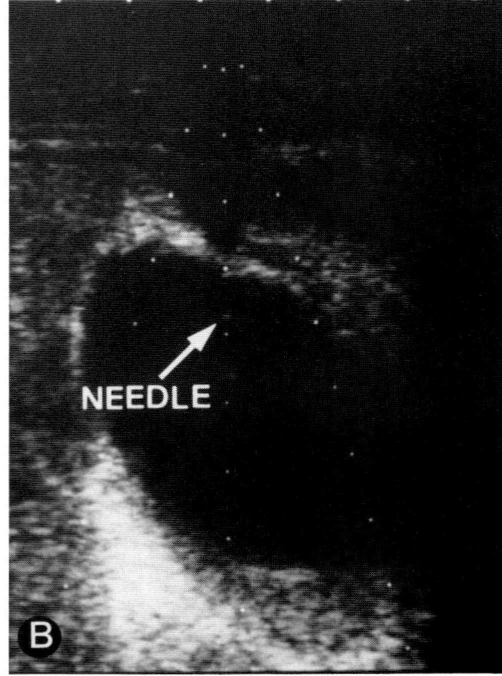

Figure 6.2. A Chiba needle is used to puncture the gallbladder. **A**, Before puncture. **B**, The *arrow* indicates the Chiba needle in the gallbladder.

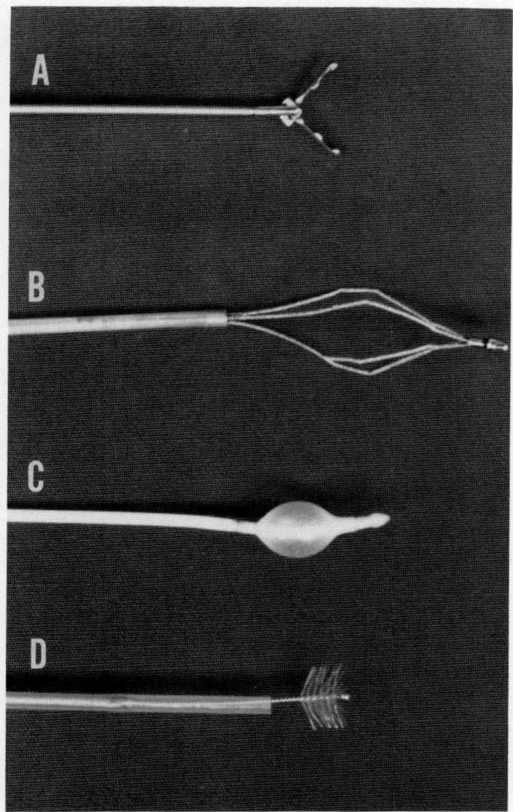

Figure 6.3. The instruments used for cholangioscopic lithotomy. A, The alligater forceps. B, The basket catheter. C, The Fogarty catheter. D, The brush.

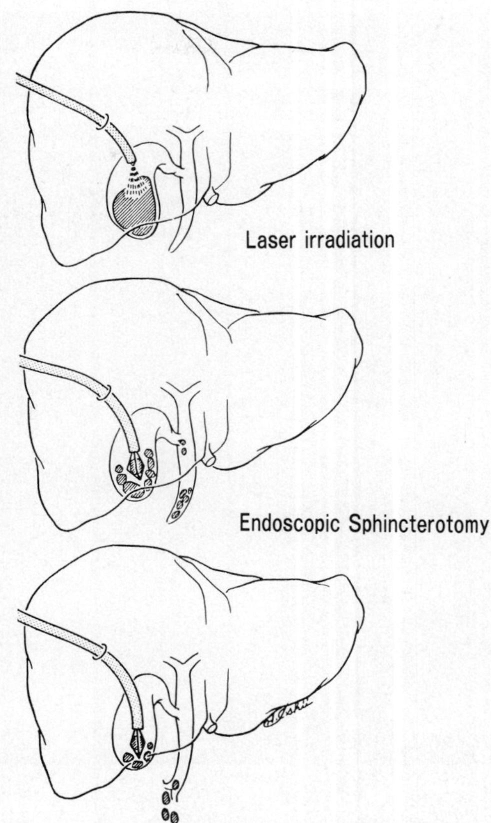

Figure 6.4. The method of lithotripsy for gallstones.

shows an ordinary fiber tip used for the treatment of digestive diseases. It has a weakness, however; that is, a metal nozzle for the gas jet surrounds the fiber tip making it impossible to view the irradiation directly in front of bending cholangioscopy. In Figure 6.5**B**, a metal nozzle is removed and a metal coil is inserted around the inner fiber. It is devised so that it may irradiate a laser beam from the center of the outer Teflon tube. It is used for the noncontact laser method even now. In Figure 6.5**C**, a laser beam of this fiber is adjusted to make a focal point 2–3 mm from the fiber tip by polishing. But this was not durable in clinical use. Figure 6.5**D** shows two fibers (a joint development by SLT-Japan and the authors) attached to new ceramic rods on the fiber tip and used for contact irradiation. In developing this fiber tip, the shape and durability of the rod we considered in relation to the drilling effect on the stones. A detachable ''bullet'' was manufactured as shown in the figure.

For lithotripsy of gallstones using noncontact irradiation, an output of 70–80 W of power is needed to crush a stone. In contact irradiation, however, sufficient results are obtained with an output of 15–20 W of power not only for bilirubinate stones but also for cholesterol stones.

RESULTS

From 1974 through January 1987, cholangioscopic lithotomy was performed in 109 cases. Of them, there were 28 cases of lithotripsy by laser for impacted large stones. The gallbladder lithotomy was performed in six patients (Table 6.1). All patients had an uneventful course without any complications. The success rate of complete cholangioscopic lithotomy using the Nd:YAG laser was 91.5% (61 of 67 cases). Using ordinary for-

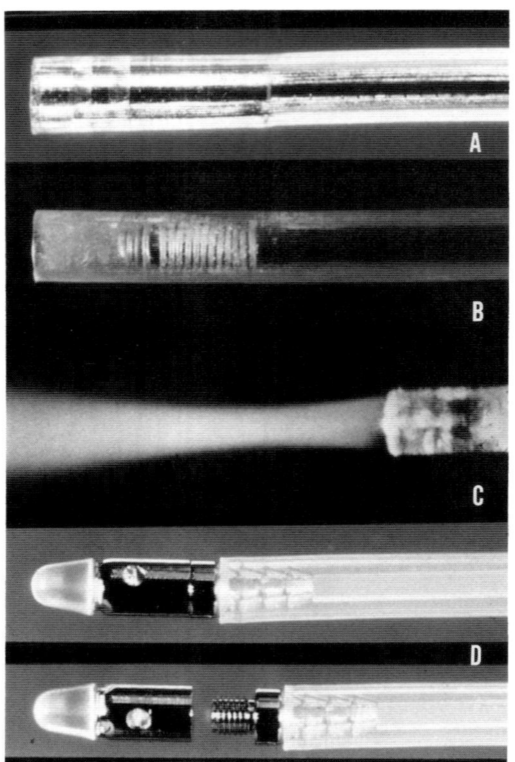

Figure 6.5. **A-D**, Various kinds of fiber tips leading the laser beam were investigated regarding the drilling effect on the stone surface.

ceps techniques, the success rate for complete lithotomy was only 66% (31 of 47 cases) (2).

Technique of Percutaneous Treatment

Case 1

A 59-year-old female patient was admitted to the hospital because of pain in the right hypochondrium. She was diagnosed as having cholecystolithiasis. She had previously undergone five abdominal operations and a mastectomy. Because of the previous multiple surgeries and frequent attacks of severe myocardial ischemia, cholangioscopic lithotomy treatment was chosen for her. Because a larger impacted stone was seen in the gallbladder, percutaneous transhepatic gallbladder drainage (PTGBD) was first carried out for reducing intracystic pressure (Fig. 6.6**A**). The sinus tract was then dilated one week later (Fig. 6.6**B**). The stone was a white cholesterol stone, 3 cm in diameter. Using the noncontact irradiation of the Nd:YAG laser, the stone was fragmented from the surface. Although some fragments passed through the cystic duct and piled up in the distal end of the common bile duct, most of them were extracted from the gallbladder after fragmented by laser irradiation (Fig. 6.7**A**). After lithotomy in the gallbladder was finished. EST was added to the procedure. Complete lithotomy was achieved after a total of seven percutaneous lithotomy treatments and one EST (Fig. 6.7**B**). Figure 6.8 shows the removed stones. It is possible to crush and extract large cholesterol stones easily using the laser. The endoscopic findings of the gallbladder during lithotomy are shown in Figure 6.9. Figure 6.9**A** shows a large stone before irradiation; **B** shows the patient cystic duct after lithotomy, and **C** shows a retroflex endoscopic finding in the gallbladder. Complete lithotomy is confirmed by endoscopy and fluoroscopy.

Case 2

A 58-year-old female patient was hospitalized with colic in the right hypochondrium. After a diagnosis of liver cirrhosis with bleeding esophageal varices, she underwent transabdominal esophageal mucosal transection for esophageal varices 2 years before this admission. A cholecystectomy was attempted but not completed because of severe adhesion and massive bleeding due to the well-developed collateral circulation. There-

Table 6.1. Patients Undergoing Percutaneous Treatment for Gallstones

Patient no.	Age (yr)	Sex	Reasons for Percutaneous Treatment	Lithotripsy Method	Follow-up Period
1	59	F	Polysurgery and heart attack	Nd:YAG laser	4 years[a]
2	58	F	Massive bleeding during surgery	Nd:YAG laser	4 years
3	84	M	Shock during surgery	Nd:YAG laser	4 years
4	66	F	Severe adhesion	Nd:YAG laser	8 months
5	77	F	Heart failure	Nd:YAG laser	3 years, 2 months
6	41	F	Severe adhesion	Ordinary forceps	4 years, 1 month

[a]Recurrence.

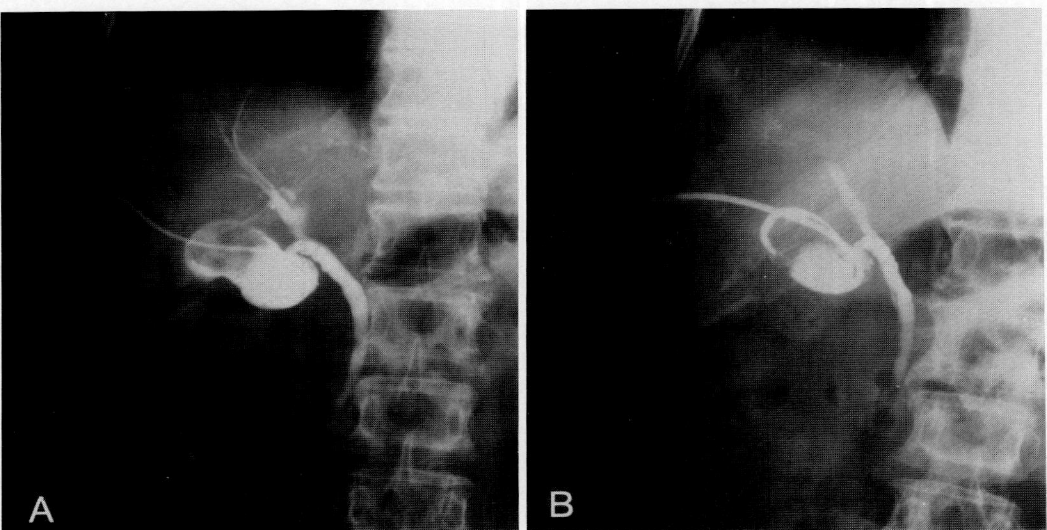

Figure 6.6. Case 1. A 59-year-old female patient. **A**, Percutaneous transhepatic gallbladder drainage (PTGBD). **B**, Dilation of the the sinus tract.

fore, percutaneous treatment was chosen. Cholesterol stones of varying sizes occupied the gallbladder, and an impacted stone was seen in the cystic duct (Fig. 6.10**A**). The patient underwent percutaneous lithotomy four times using the contact method of laser irradiation with the ceramic

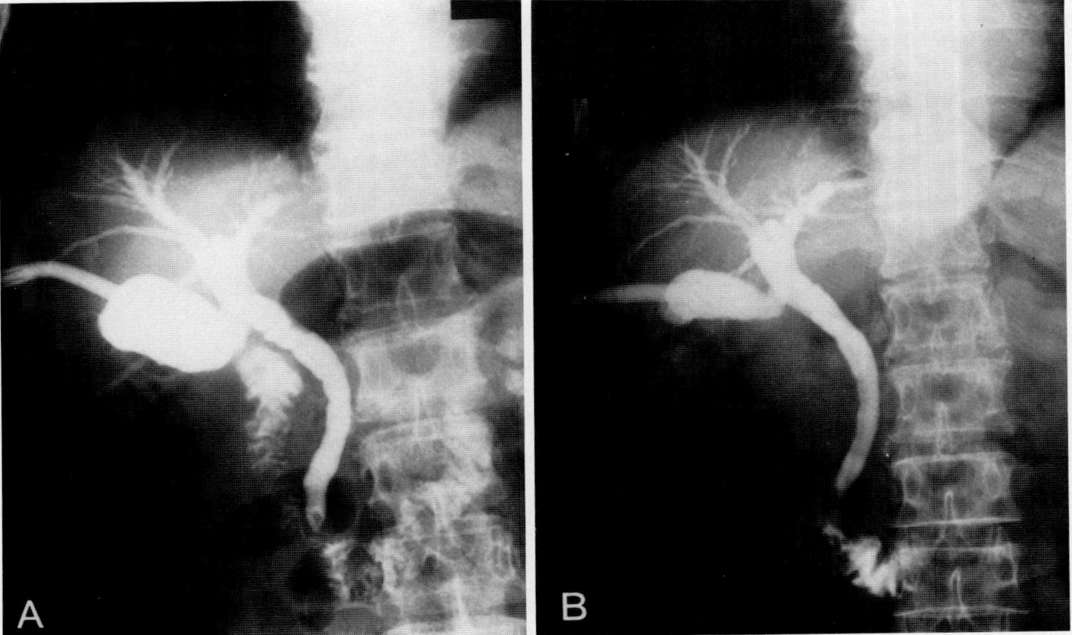

Figure 6.7. **A**, After the lithotripsy of the gallbladder, small pieces of the fragmented stones are piled up in the distal end of common bile duct. **B**, After EST, there is no stone shadow in the bile duct.

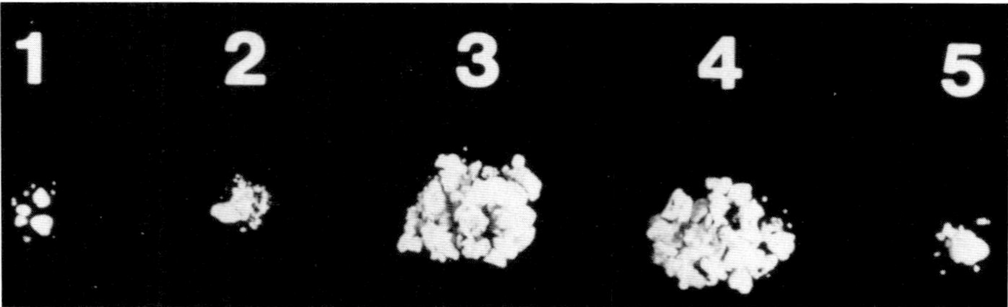

Figure 6.8. The stones removed from the gallbladder.

rods (Fig. 6.10**B**). Cholangioscopy was performed to direct the stone into the common bile duct. The small stone could be dislodged into the fundus of the gallbladder for removal by flash infusion with saline solution under direct observation (Fig. 6.11**A** and **B**). Besides these 2 patients with gallstones, there were three other cholecystolithiatic patients undergoing percutaneous treatment by laser, all of whom had severe concomitant diseases that made surgical operation impossible. However, percutaneous treatments are able to succeed without any complication (Table 6.1).

DISCUSSION

This report is mainly concerned with the treatment of gallstones, excluding the treatment of intrahepatic and common bile duct stones. At present, cholecystectomy is considered to be the safest and the most cost-effective treatment for gallstones. However, for risky and difficult patients who have severe disorders percutaneous treatment is chosen. Cholangioscopic lithotomy for bile duct stones has been performed actively since 1974. The most important benefit of this method is the fragmentation technique for removal of bile duct stones.

Presently, there are four fragmentation methods. Ultrasonic fragmentation (3), which crushes stones using vibration and sound waves of piezoelectric crystal, is one method. However, the probe is rigid so approaching routes are limited. Another method is electrohydraulic lithotripsy. Evaporization of water caused by the spark at two tips of electrode brings forth shock waves to crush stones. There are some reports about this efficient method (4). Except for direct touch, the bile duct wall is never damaged and the internal pressure rising within the bile duct is small. Recently, a new clinical method for lithotomy was reported. This method uses extracorporeal shock waves.

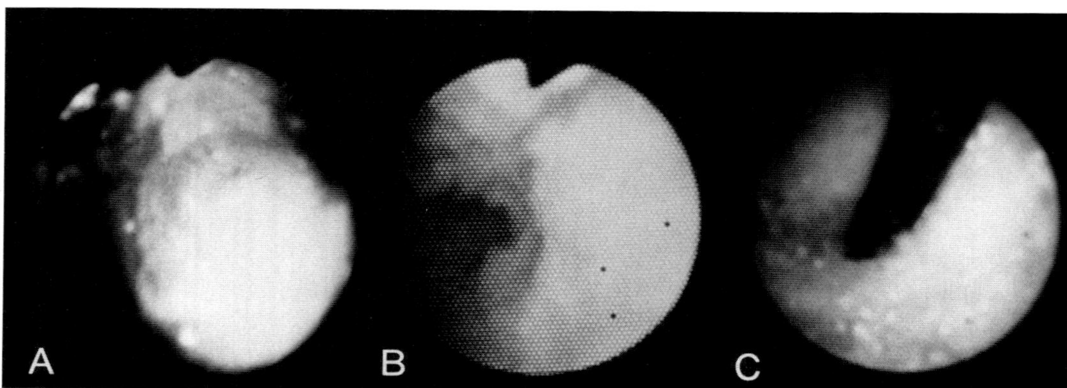

Figure 6.9. The endoscopic findings of the gallbladder. **A**, All large stone in the gallbladder before laser irradiation. **B**, The cystic duct after lithotomy. **C**, A retroflex endoscopic finding in the gallbladder.

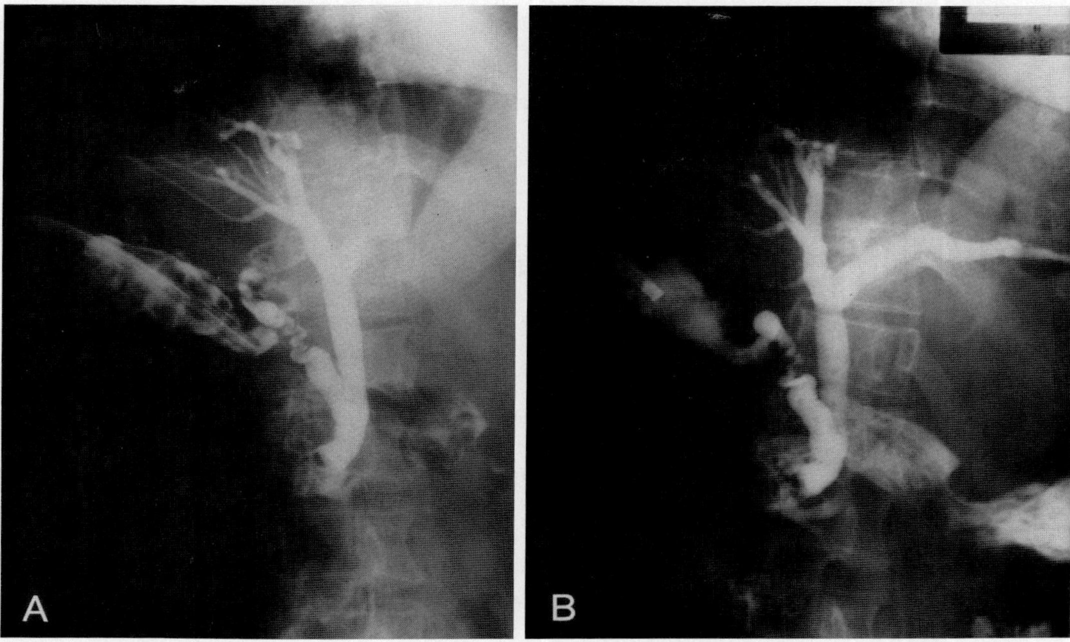

Figure 6.10. Case 2. A 58-year-old female patient. **A**, Before lithotomy. **B**, After lithotomy.

Patients with gallstones or common bile duct stones are immersed in the water bath and shock waves are directed toward the body (5). The trial of this technique has begun recently and its has a few underlying problems, e.g., there is possibility of lung injury, and the apparatus is expensive. Meanwhile, when the noncontact irradiation of the Nd:YAG laser was used, the stone component shifted the results of lithotomy. However, the ceramic rods of the contact type are often used providing same results in calcium bilirubinate stones and cholesterol stones. Moreover, the contact

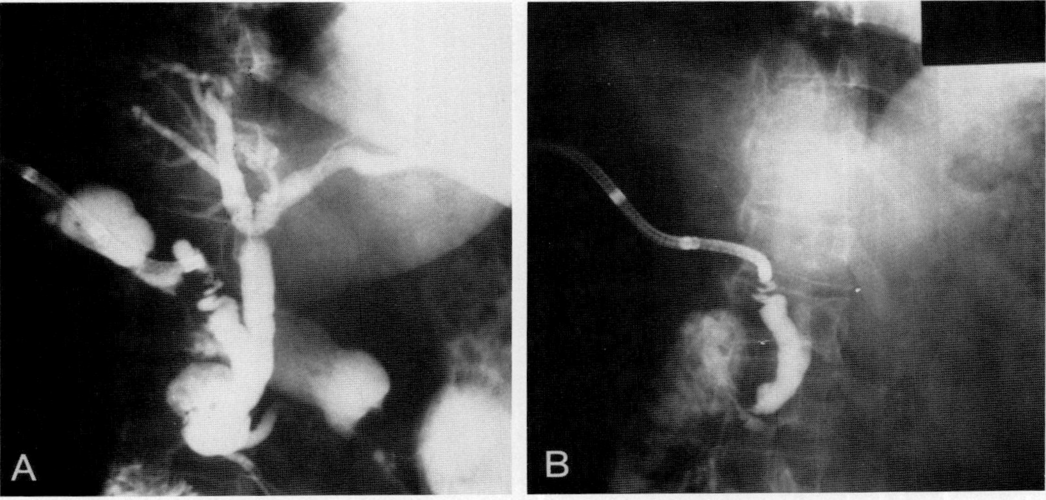

Figure 6.11. **A** and **B**, Study of the cystic duct of the previous case.

type takes only one-fourth or one-fifth power to crush stones compared to the noncontact type. The Nd:YAG laser uses continuous wave. Injury to the bile duct and the gallbladder wall by heat effect is cause for worry at times. Such is not a problem with cholangioscopic lithotomy because it is always performed under infusion of distilled water (1). Recently, the use of Nd:YAG laser with Q-switch has begun for lithotomy (6). Although percutaneous treatment can remove the stone completely, the possibility of stone formation is still left. Therefore, adequate care and follow-up are necessary to find recurrent stones. It is promising that this treatment method can be used repetitively.

REFERENCES

1. Kouzu T, Sato H. Endoscopic laser treatment of intrahepatic stones. Intrahepatic Calculi, ARL Inc., 1984, pp 321-332.
2. Kouzu T, Yamazaki Y. Cholangioscopic surgery using Nd:YAG laser. Reported from the Third International Nd:YAG Laser Symposium, PPS, 1986, pp 234-238.
3. Koch H, Stotle M, Wolf V. Endoscopic lithotripsy in the common bile duct. Endoscopy 1977; 9:95-98.
4. Reiter HJ. Electric treatment of bladder stones. Endoscopy 1968; 1:13-15.
5. Sauerbruch T, Delius M, Baumgartner G, et al. Fragmentation of gallstones by extracorporeal shock waves. N Engl J Med 1986; 314:818-822.
6. Ell C, Wondrazek F, Frank F. Laser induced shock wave lithotripsy of gallstones. Endoscopy 1986; 18:95-96.

CHAPTER
7

Advanced Intraabdominal Tumors

Leonard S. Schultz, David F. Hickok, John N. Graber

In no other field are the opportunites greater than in general surgery to apply lasers innovatively. To date, most work has been of a research nature; whereas clinical reports have been minimal. To their credit, surgeons in other fields (1 to 4) have helped develop the promise of lasers in clinical medicine by using them to make procedures simpler and less painful for patients. Such results are not yet apparent in abdominal surgical patients; nevertheless, efforts have revealed that lasers offer surgeons a wider range of therapeutic alternatives that may lead to less suffering by expanding the definition of operability. For example, follow-up of cancer patients exposed to laser techniques has indicated that a reasonable percentage can expect relief of complicating symptoms after hospital discharge (5, 6). Before the introduction of laser methods, complications such as gastrointestinal or ureteral obstruction usually represented terminal phases of the illness. Thus, the promise of lasers in abdominal surgery may not only be simplified techniques, but also enhanced treatment modalities for the seriously ill. This chapter will detail how carbon dioxide (CO_2) and neodymium: yttrium-aluminum-garnet (Nd:YAG) lasers can be used to achieve new solutions to old problems. Further therapeutic innovations will be left to the reader.

CARBON DIOXIDE LASER

While dermatologists have capitalized on the laser's ability to vaporize tissue with low power, general surgeons must think of using higher power densities for their needs.

The main use for the CO_2 laser, in terms of abdominal surgery, is for incision and tumor ablation. Although the limitations of this laser, even in experienced hands, may lead to greater use of the modified Nd:YAG laser, it is best for the novice to start with CO_2 because of its versatility and the need to use its full range of power to achieve successful clinical results. Once familiar with the machine and its capabilities through the use of the laboratory and minor skin surgeries, its use for skin incisions should be explored.

Incisions

A standard midline incision is used in the patient who is under general anesthesia. It is advised that no long-acting local anesthesia be used until the conclusion of the operation because the fluid will retard the effectiveness of the laser. The wattage is set at 30–35 W with the shutter open (''continuous'' mode), and the incision is made at a steady pace from xiphoid toward the umbilicus. Before using the foot pedal to switch on the laser, it is suggested that the surgeon inform the assistants not to touch his or her arm, that everyone has protective eyewear including the patient (who is covered with lenses or moist gauze sponges), that the machine be on the side of the table opposite the surgeon, and that the smoke evacuation system be readily available.

With the assistant holding the evacuation tubing close to the intended line of incision, the helium-neon (He-Ne) aiming beam is set at the focal point (smallest spot size) and lasing is begun. Once through the skin, experience has taught that the subcutaneous layer is best lased with a minimally defocused beam, which is achieved by pulling the laser slightly away from the skin. The widened diameter of the He-Ne aiming beam will alert the surgeon to this new position, which allows for some hemostasis as well as incising ability.

Should any vessels of reasonable size be encountered, now or later in the operation, it is best to defocus the beam and lase at the same wattage (35 W) over the visible length of the vessel and then bring the laser down to its focal point to cut the vessel. In this manner, minimal use of electrocautery will be needed. The fascial layer is incised in the same manner until the peritoneum is encountered. Once visible, it is best, (except in the most experienced hands where lower power at selected pulse durations are used) to cut an opening in the peritoneum with standard instruments. If desired, one can then place a moistened laparotomy pad over the abdominal viscera that underlies the rest of the incision, which can then be completed with the laser at reduced power (15–20 W).

Intraabdominal Use

Once the celiotomy is completed, adhesions can be lased at 10–15 W at whatever pulse duration the operator is comfortable. Continuous power will soon be utilized as the operator gains experience with the technique. In fact, there is nothing within the abdomen that cannot be lased with the CO_2 laser. It will soon be apparent, however, that certain drawbacks are inherent with its use.

The first disadvantage is the need for walling off susceptible tissue with moist packs to prevent inadvertent injury; this is both time-consuming and cumbersome. Another drawback is that larger blood vessels must still be handled with standard techniques of cautery and clamps. Further dissection of tumor tissue or highly vascular organs, such as the liver, results in unacceptable oozing because the hemostatic effect, even when the laser is defocused, is limited. Nevertheless, the primary advantage of precision, coupled with some hemostatic ability, has found the CO_2 laser to be very useful for removing adhesions and tumor nodules (7).

Please note the use of the term "nodules" and not "masses." This deserves some explanation. Nodules means small lesions such as tumor implants, whereas masses refers to reasonable size tumors, either malignant or benign. Although the authors believe it is best always to use the laser as a dissective tool rather than as a method of vaporization to limit blood loss and inordinate increases in opreative time, this is not always possible. While dissection of nodules or masses can be done at lower power (30–35 W), vaporization necessitates higher wattages in the range of 70–90 W, which then demonstrates the next two drawbacks of this laser.

The first shortcoming is the lateral absorption of heat by adjacent tissue, which can be extraordinary. While fat or muscle can survive this increased temperature by eventual scarring, vital adjacent structures cannot. Saline cannot be used in the field to cool such structures. This would cancel the effectiveness of the laser because it does not penetrate a water medium. Therefore, only lower power can be used and thus the increase in operating time.

The second problem is that if higher wattages can be used to vaporize the target tissue, a considerable smoke plume will be generated that cannot be adequately removed with present smoke evacuation devices. The exposure of these noxious fumes to operating personnel will be readily apparent and, at times, can be completely intolerable.

In general, however, for excision or vaporization of small nodules or tumors of 1 to 2 cm in widest diameter, the CO_2 laser is adequate and its use can be safely recommended.

Case History 1: Right Hemiabdominal Tumor

In the initial phases of the authors' clinical experiences, only CO_2 was available for use. Experience was gained with many abdominal wall incisions and relatively minor laser intraabdominal procedures, such as lysis of adhesions, mobilization of the right and left colon along the line of Toldt, and vaporization of tumor nodules. An 88-year-old white male patient then presented with a right abdominal tumor with extension into the groin. Initial biopsy indicated a highly undifferentiated carcinoma of undetermined primary origin. His presenting complaint was marked pain in the right lower extremity secondary to iliac vessel compression (Fig. 7.1) causing edema and hypoxemia to the extremity. A description of his clinical course follows to demonstrate the advantages and limitations of the CO_2 laser.

The right lower quadrant mass extended from the right hemi-pelvis to the inferior vena cava and right kidney, and completely encased the iliac vessels. The CO_2 laser was set at 90 W of power and was used in a continuous mode with resultant vaporization of the tumor. Despite some venous oozing, the use of the defocused beam provided adequate hemostasis but the length of the procedure was more than an elderly gentleman of 88 years should endure. For this reason, the CUSA (Cavitron ultrasonic aspirator) "ultrasonic scalpel" was substituted for the laser. This instrument did allow for more rapid removal of the residual tumor and proved safe for the iliac vessel dissections. Postoperatively, the patient was relieved of his right lower extremity swelling

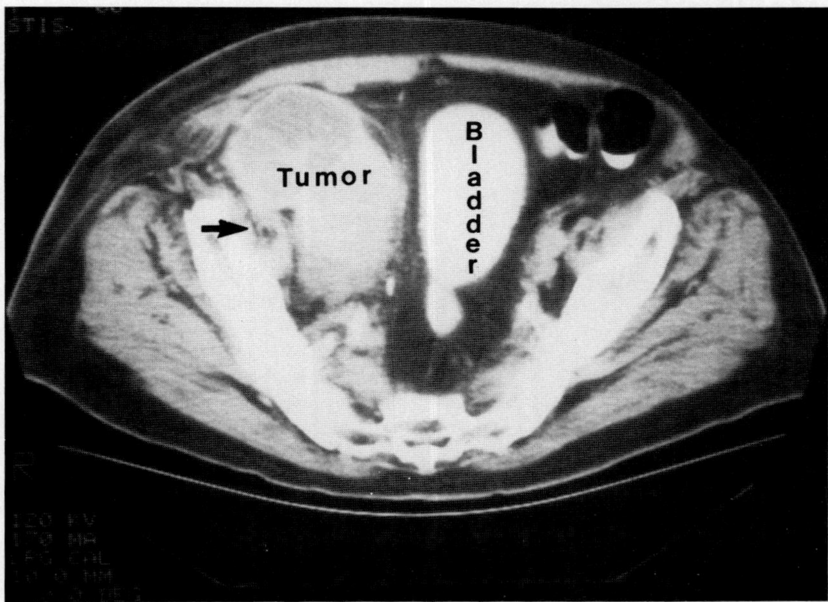

Figure 7.1. Case history 1. CAT scan indicating iliac vessel compression (*arrow*) by tumor in the right hemipelvis. (Reproduced with permission of Alan R. Liss, Inc. Publ., New York.) Reproduced with permission from Schultz LS, Hickok DF, Graber JN, Stephens WE, Eds. Laser Medicine and Surgery News. New York: Alan R. Liss, Inc., 1987.

and pain within 1 week. The final pathology report indicated lymphoma and he was subsequently started on a course of radiotherapy.

Several conclusions were drawn from this case. *(a)* Large tumor masses can be both dissected and vaporized with a CO_2 laser. *(b)* Dissection results in some blood loss, which was greater than the authors would prefer, while extensive vaporization was slow. Further, a significant lateral heat absorption was recognized and a noxious smoke plume was endured throughout the lasing period. *(c)* Vaporization of large tumor masses causes an unacceptable increase in operative time but is satisfactory for small lesions. *(d)* The CO_2 laser should be considered as only one of a group of tools available to the modern general surgeon.

These conclusions were reinforced by subsequent procedures and led the authors to pursue a search for another laser that would better fit the requirements of precision, enhanced hemostasis, and reduced operative time.

Nd:YAG LASERS

Publications by Joffe and coworkers (8, 9) and demands by members of this hospital's laser committee for a Nd:YAG laser fortuitously coincided, so that the general surgical service became the most active user of the device soon after its purchase. Since laser blades were not yet available, the free beam use of the device constituted initial experiences. Using the Nd:YAG laser in much the same way as a CO_2 laser for intraabdominal work, it became apparent that operative times were reduced because of better hemostasis without sacrifice of precision. These qualities also allowed extension of laser use to liver resection. Nevertheless, the increased depth of penetration, high wattage requirements, and production of smoke plume remained as drawbacks and limited more widespread use, such as with skin incisions. To prevent additional costs, rather than use the CO_2 laser, incisions were made with scalpel and cautery techniques. Local anesthesia was used for these standard procedures. Once entry into the abdomen was achieved, the advantages of the Nd:YAG laser became apparent.

Case History 2: Colon Tumors Metastatic to the Liver

MK was a 61-year-old white male patient admitted in October 1985 for upper abdominal tenderness.

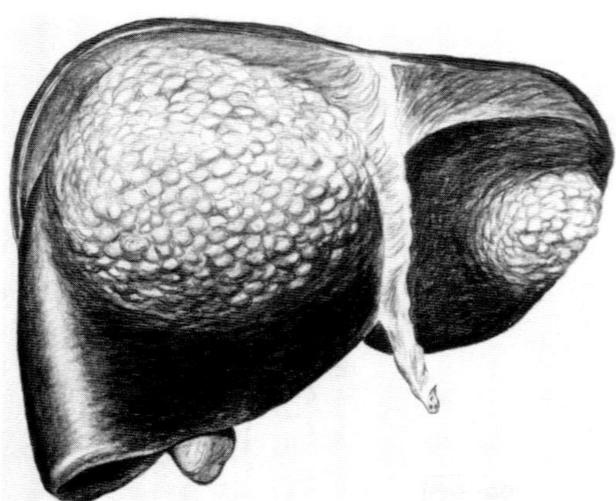

Figure 7.2. Case history 2. Artist's conception of the liver before resection. Note extension to the diaphragm.

This proved to be metastatic colon carcinoma with initial colectomy (Fig. 7.2). He presented on a prior chemotherapy program and was initially evaluated for placement of a hepatic artery infusion catheter with a continuous flow subcutaneous pump. A nonanatomic dissection was carried out because it was evident that the tumor mass representing two specific areas would require an extended right hepatic lobectomy as well as a significant wedge resection of the lateral segment of the left lobe, which the authors felt would not allow significant residual liver tissue for survival. The ultrasonic scalpel allowed for the nonanatomic resections as seen in Figure 7.3.

Of significance to this discussion was resection of the smaller tumor nodule in the lateral segment of the residual left lobe using a Nd:YAG laser at 80 W of power with continuous mode. This resection was carried out using both the focused and defocused beams to a liver depth that did not exceed 3 cm in any direction. When dissection with the laser deeper than this level was attempted, significant oozing was seen and it was concluded that the free beam Nd:YAG laser at the stated wattage was sufficient for heat sealing of liver tissue so long as one did not exceed approximately 3 cm in depth from the surface of the liver. Postoperatively, the patient did well except for a right upper quadrant fluid collection that was drained percutaneously. There was no leakage from the partial resection of the left lateral lobe done with the Nd:YAG laser.

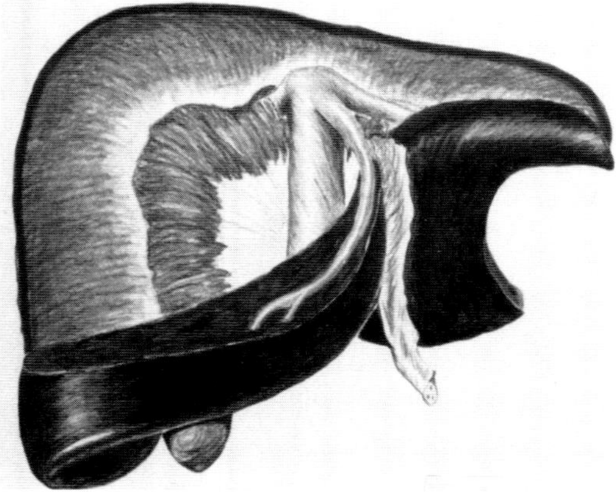

Figure 7.3. Case History 2. Artist's conception of the liver after completion of the hepatic resection.

As previously noted in the literature (10), and confirmed by this case, it was learned that the free beam Nd:YAG laser could be used for limited peripheral liver resection with a resultant dry margin of resection free of vascular or biliary leakage. Additional use of this technique on centrally located tumor nodules indicated the reality of hemostatic vaporization achieved at 70–80 W starting at the central part of the mass and working peripherally (7).

Still to be considered was the problem of lateral heat absorption, which was not of clinical significance with hepatic surgery. The next case history indicates how that problem of excessive heat buildup by adjacent tissue was overcome.

Case History 3: Metastatic Ovarian Carcinoma to the Pelvis with Rectal Compression

JP is a 36-year-old white female patient who presented with intestinal obstruction at an ileoproctostomy anastomosis with a history of prior subtotal colectomy. Rather than do an ileostomy in this patient, which was refused by her, and with full recognition of the experimental nature of the procedure, the pelvic tumor was vaporized with a Nd:YAG free beam laser at 90 W. This was done under a saline pool in the pelvis to prevent damage to adjacent tissue from lateral heat absorption. Complete mobilization of her rectum was achieved inasmuch as the tumor proved to be compressive but not invasive. Her postoperative course was benign with complete relief of preoperative crampy abdominal pain and restoration of full alimentation (Fig. 7.4).

This case has special significance because it represents the emergence of alternative surgical methods strictly because of the laser. Conventional methods would not allow such surgery because of the blood loss involved with scalpel-cautery methods. Further, it showed that quite apart from lasers, one should not assume full knowledge of the pathological process until it is proven. In this case, tumor compression did not mean invasion, and thus, the success of the operation.

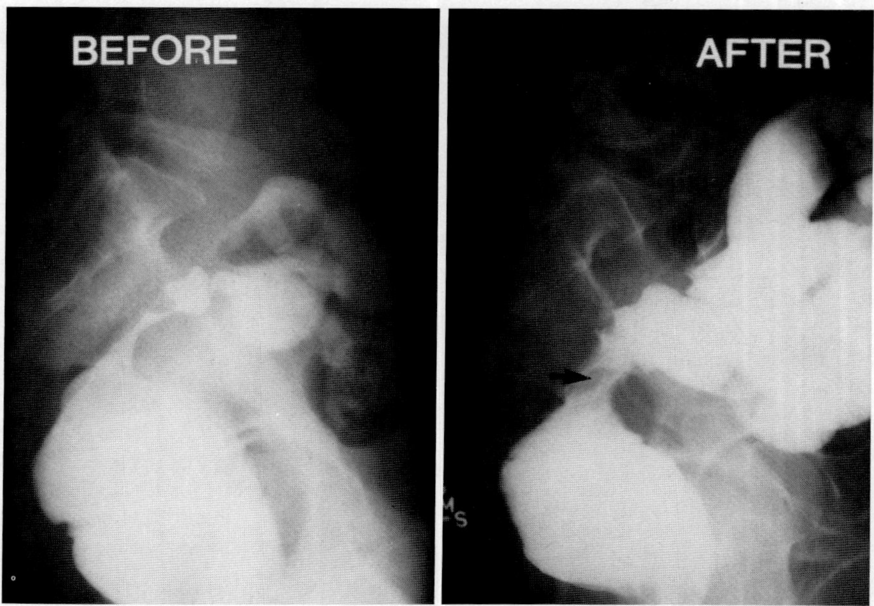

Figure 7.4. Case history 3. Pre- and postoperative barium enema exams indicating widened lumen after use of the free beam Nd:YAG laser (*arrow*). (Reproduced with permission of Alan R. Liss, Inc. Publ., New York.) Reproduced with permission from Schultz LS, Hickok DF, Graber JN, Stephens WE, Eds. Laser Medicine and Sugery News. New York: Alan R. Liss, Inc., 1987.

LASER SCALPEL

As detailed elsewhere in this text, Joffe and Daikuzono introduced the laser scalpel to American surgery (8). Developed by Daikuzono in Tokyo based upon the recommendations of Joffe and Sankar, the scalpel represented the solution to the two remaining problems in laser surgery; that of loss of the sense of touch, and heat absorption by adjacent tissue as a price for improved hemostasis with the Nd:YAG laser.

One of the most difficult things that the neophyte laserist must contend with is learning to operate on tissue without touching it. In essence, the surgeon loses the sense of touch when the beam travels through the air. The laser scalpel restored this quality to surgery and thereby eliminated a major obstacle to the acceptance of lasers by general surgeons, who have always been "hands on" specialists. Like the steel scalpel, subtle pressure differences caused direct tissue effects, something to which the general surgeon could easily relate. Heat absorption was eliminated by use of the contact scalpel because energy was concentrated at the tip rather than over a wider area. The scalpel served to contain the heat generated by the laser beam within the device itself.

With these obstacles overcome, the device was easily accepted and led to increased popularity of the Nd:YAG laser in general surgery. Not only did it once again allow the surgeon to feel the tissue, but it also improved further the evident laser virtues of precision and hemostasis without deep thermal penetration. An additional advantage of the laser blade is that it requires significantly less energy than when a free beam is used. Thus, a lesser power laser can be used at significantly less cost to the purchaser.

As the significance of these factors became appreciated, surgical efforts with the Nd:YAG laser broadened as the implications of this new technology were explored.

Incisions

Although the laser scalpel now concentrated the power of the laser to a minute area (the tip of the device with a diameter of 0.2–1.2 mm) without extensive lateral dispersion of the heat, initial experiences with skin incisions soon presented limitations.

Unlike the CO_2 laser, where incision was an instantaneous event, the scalpel ''cut'' in a time-dependent fashion. Thus, if the skin was thin as with breast, axilla, and groin, procedure would be swift. However, if the skin was thick, edematous, or scarred, then the ''contact'' was prolonged before the tissue separated. Because thermal injury is a function of both power and time, it was found that wounds in ''tough'' skin developed thermal injury along the margins, which caused early delay in healing, although the ultimate result was the same; i.e., a proper scar of suitable tensile strength. The early edema and erythema seen, however, dissuaded the authors from its continued use on any but the thinnest of skin, with incisions made at 15–17 W, continuous mode.

At this time, the usual custom is to cut the skin with a scalpel and then to use a laser scalpel thereafter for other abdominal wall layers. The wound is dry. Power settings of 20 W are used for these deeper layers to speed the surgery along. Clinical wound healing is normal.

Intraabdominal Use

Once within the abdominal cavity, the true virtue of the scalpel becomes evident. Setting the power at 15–20 W (always start low and gradually increase the wattage), adhesions are lysed with confidence and ease. Bleeding is rarely a problem. To prevent excessive heat buildup on the blade, the laser is turned on only when the scalpel is in contact with tissue and shut off when not actually being used. Further, it is always put on a moist towel when not in use and never on exposed skin or drapes since the residual heat in the blade may cause a burn. Naturally, care is taken not to touch the hands of operating personnel inadvertently with the blade for the same reason. Should the blade need to be cleaned of carbon buildup, a moistened sponge is used, which is also utilized if the blade needs to be changed.

Usually, a clear, nonetched blade of 0.6–0.8 mm in diameter is initially used to make the abdominal incision, whereas the etched blade of 0.8–1.2 mm is used for the intraabdominal work. The etching produces some enhancement in hemostasis. During the switchover in blades, the machine should be placed on standby to prevent any accidental activation of the free laser beam and, of course, safety lenses should be used throughout the course of the operation.

Once the target tissue is defined and moist laps are placed over adjacent tissue, the laser blade is used as a dissective tool. With the power set at approximately 20-25 W, the surgeon allows the blade to ''linger'' on vascular tissue before incising, and moves rapidly across tissue of a less vascular character. For example, adhesions or fat are rapidly incised while hepatic tissue is cut at a slower pace.

One technical point that deserves mention is the dissection of tumor off of tubular structures such as ureters, nerves, and major blood vessels. Learned from earlier work with the axillary vein dissection during mastectomy, it became apparent that vascular injury can occur if the laser scalpel is allowed to cut directly over a blood vessel. Thus, it is advised that such work be done at an angle, moving the blade along the ''edge'' of such structures. (The following two case histories will demonstrate these two techniques.)

Case History 4: Metastatic Adenocarcinoma of the Appendix in the Right Lower Quadrant

CL is a 64-year-old white male patient who was operated on in September of 1986. He presented with symptoms of right flank pain and right ureteral obstruction, which had been managed with a ureteral stent. He had previously undergone right hemicolectomy. At surgery, he was found to have a recurrent tumor mass in the right lower quadrant and had an incontinuity resection of this tumor in the right flank and right retroperitoneum using the Nd:YAG with laser scalpel at 20 W of power. The 1-mm ''frosted'' scalpel was used for the dissection, which included dissection of the tumor tissue off the ureter. He was readmitted approximately 1 week after discharge for a partial small bowel obstruction that was treated nonoperatively, and was discharged 3 days after readmission.

The true value of the laser scalpel is especially evident here because of its superiority in excising tumor that is embedded in muscle. The dryness of the surgical field was extrordinary in contrast to blood loss usually incurred with conventional methods, and the ability of the scalpel to create surgical ''planes'' where none existed has proven especially advantageous in these cases.

Of significant note as well in this case was the presence of postoperative obstruction. When major resections involving removal of serosa that cannot be resurfaced are done, we have seen a significant occurrence of a specific complication; that of small bowel obstruction occurring 3–4

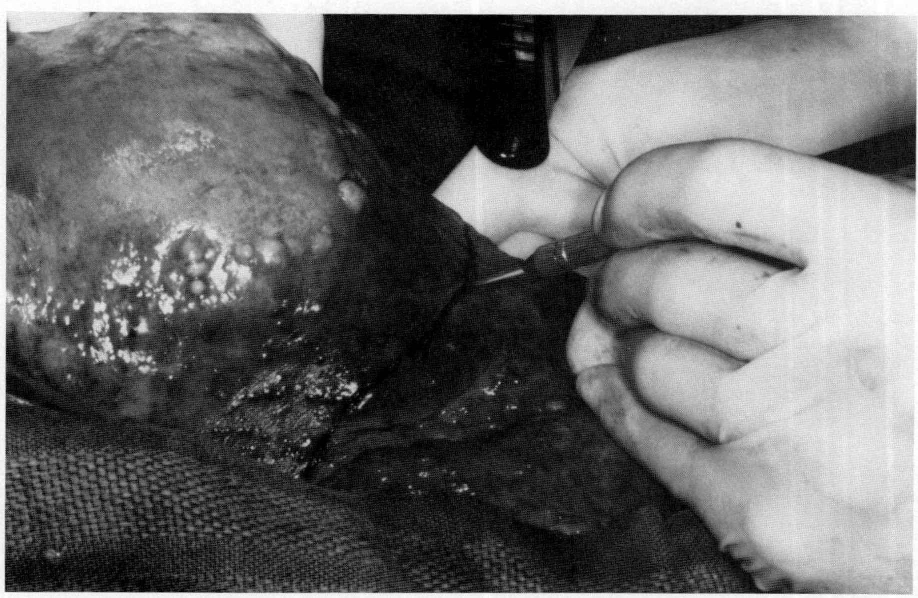

Figure 7.5. Case history 5. The Nd:YAG laser scalpel is being used to perform the hepatic resection. Hilar dissection has already been completed. No compressive clamps were required.

weeks postoperatively. It is believed that the reason for this, based on early attempts at operative release, is the adherence of bowel to denuded surfaces concomitant with a severe inflammatory reaction. Inadvertent enterotomies may complicate aggressive intervention, with resultant enteric fistulas. For this reason, the authors have concluded that the appearance of small bowel obstruction in the follow-up period is best treated nonoperatively, including nothing by mouth (NPO) status, nasogastric decompression, and intravenous steroids if the first two factors do not lead to resolution within 3 days.

If complications of cancer were the reason for the initial resection, nutritional therapy should be supportive for the first few days and not used aggressively if at all possible. The reason for this is that usually there is no protective anticancer therapy available, so that tumor growth will be favored by overly enthusiastic nutritional support such as with a total parenteral nutrition program.

Case History 5: Extended Right Hepatic Lobectomy

SM is a 79-year-old white male patient who presented with right upper quadrant pain. The workup indicated a hepatoma involving the right lobe with vena caval compression. Preoperative coagulation studies and serum bilirubin were normal. At exploration, three sites of bleeding from the tumor were noted with moderate hemoperitoneum. A palliative extended right hepatic lobectomy was performed with a formal hilar dissection. Tumor in the right branch of the portal vein was seen. Parenchymal resection was done with a 1.2-mm "frosted" laser scalpel and a Nd:YAG laser (Fig. 7.5) at 24 W. Hepatic ooze was minimal. Structures wider than 2–3 mm in diameter were clamped and ligated. The cut surface was dry at the conclusion of the procedure.

The comparison of laser versus ultrasonic scalpel (CUSA) resection in a case such as this deserves some discussion. Although both tools achieve the desired effect, i.e., a clean-cut surface, it is indeed safe to say that the laser heat seals parenchyma whereas the CUSA does not. Thus, the need for ligating intrahepatic structures is less with the laser and the field is drier than with the CUSA. Should prior hilar vessel ligation not be desired, however, and a nonanatomic resection be necessary (case 2), then the recommendation would be to use a CUSA scalpel.

At present, as the authors' clinical experience with laser technology has grown (Table 7.1), and

Table 7.1. Operative Summary[a]

Patient	Age (years)	Sex	Date of Surgery	Laser Used	Scalpel Used Yes	Scalpel Used No	Postoperative Discharge Day
NC	88	M	Sept 1985	CO_2			16
HK	86	F	Oct 1985	CO_2Nd:YAG		X	12
MK	61	M	Oct 1985	Nd:YAG		X	15
JT	36	F	Nov 1985	Nd:YAG		X	10
BM	54	F	Jan 1986	Nd:YAG	X		11
RB	63	F	June 1986	Nd:YAG	X		14
AL	59	F	July 1986	Nd:YAG	X		12
CL	64	M	Sept 1986	Nd:YAG	X		10
LH	63	M	Sept 1986	Nd:YAG	X		8
JR	43	M	Feb 1987	Nd:YAG	X		9

[a]Reproduced with permission from Schultz LS, Hickok DF, Graber JN, Stephens WE, Eds. Laser Medicine and Surgery News. New York: Alan R. Liss, Inc., 1987.

their confidence in its advantages expands, they have concluded that the Nd:YAG with contact scalpel is their preferred method for intraabdominal resections of both benign and malignant tumors.

ETHICAL CONSIDERATIONS

As the laser has enabled "inoperable" cases to be operated successfully, a heightened concern has arisen regarding the wisdom of performing such surgeries. As can be seen by the follow-up results in Table 7.2, not all patients receive significant benefit; in fact, many cancer patients receive palliative benefit only and, in some cases, it is evident that a quicker demise results from major surgical intervention. In fact, only 50% of them survive more than 1 year. Whether this represents significant palliation is a matter of personal judgment. Such judgment must be based upon a realization that

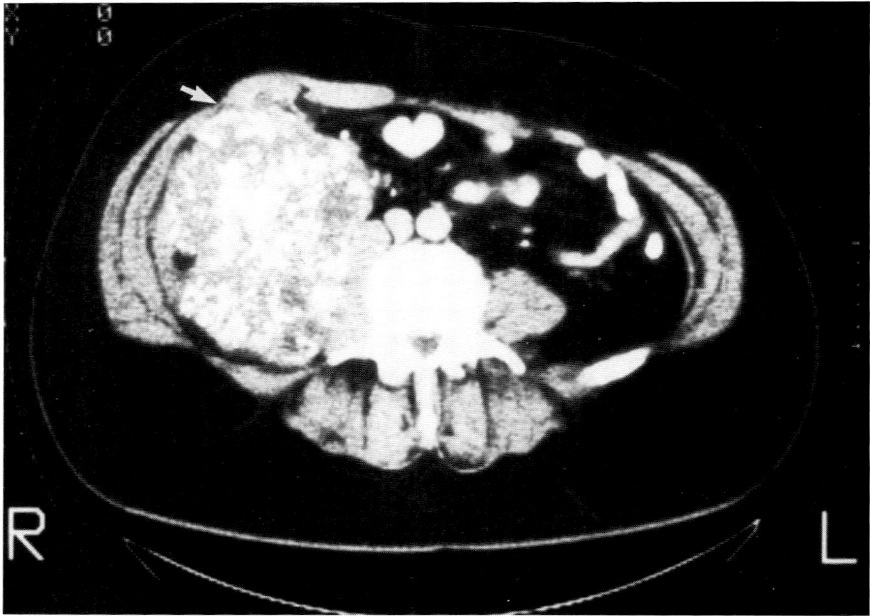

Figure 7.6. Case history 6. CAT scan of chondrosarcoma attached to the right ilium (*arrow*). (Reproduced with permission of Alan R. Liss, Inc. Pub., New York.) Reproduced with permission from Schultz LS, Hickok DF, Graber JN, Stephens WE, Eds. Laser Medicine and laser scalpel.

Table 7.2. Clinical History Summary[a]

Patient	Presenting Complaint	Postoperative Complications	Preoperative Chemotherapy Yes	Preoperative Chemotherapy No	Postoperative Therapy Chemo-therapy	Postoperative Therapy Radio-therapy	Follow-up
NC	Right lower extremity	None		X		X	Right iliac vessel obstruction relieved; died from disease 4 months postoperatively
HK	Upper intestinal obstruction	None		X	X		Died from disease 11 months postoperatively
MK	Upper abdominal tenderness	Right upper quadrant abscess drained with percutaneous catheter	X		X		Doing well
JT	Small bowel obstruction	None	X		X	X	Sept 1986, recurrent small bowel obstruction relieved with ileostomy; doing well
BM	Partial lower bowel obstruction and pain	None	X		X	X	Oct 1986, left nephrectomy for ureteral obstruction secondary to tumor; doing well
RB	Peritone-ovaginal fistula Partial small bowel obstruction	None	X		X		Transient small bowel obstruction
AL	Small bowel obstruction	None	X				Aug 1986, reoperated for small bowel obstruction; postoperative enterocutaneous fistula; died from disease 3 months postoperatively
CL	Right lower quadrant pain	None	X		X		Transient small bowel obstruction, doing well
LH	Small bowel	None	X		X	X	Spine metastases being treated with radiotherapy
JR	Right hemi-abdominal mass	None		X			Doing well

[a]Reproduced with permission from Schultz LS, Hickok DF, Graber JN, Stephens WE, Eds. Laser Medicine and Surgery News. New York: Alan R. Liss, Inc., 1987.

all such patients are seen very late in their disease, after their anticancer therapies have failed; thus, laser surgery represents a last resort for them. This is made very clear to patients, but they already realize the desperation of their clinical status. In fact, patients are very appreciative of the efforts made on their behalf because all have significant complications of their disease such as ureteral and/or gastro-intestinal obstruction, and they are aware that they are facing death in the presence of these disabling symptoms.

Experience with these patients has led to the conclusion that relief of these symptoms with a chance for a nonhospitalized existence with few, if any complications after their surgery is justification for doing the procedures.

One must also consider that lessons learned from these efforts have and will continue to lead to benefits for patients with less crucial needs.

Case History 6: Chondrosarcoma Arising from the Right Ilium

JR is a 43-year-old white male patient who presented with a large right hemiabdominal mass. Workup indicated a chondrosarcoma arising from the right ilium (Fig. 7.6). The mass was removed using the Nd:YAG with 1.0- and 1.2-mm frosted laser scalpels at 20 W of power (Fig. 7.7). He had no complications in his postoperative course and was discharged from the hospital on his 9th post-operative day.

This patient benefited from the information learned from prior experience and had a successful extirpation of a complicated tumor using laser methods with only minimal blood loss and an uncomplicated postoperative course.

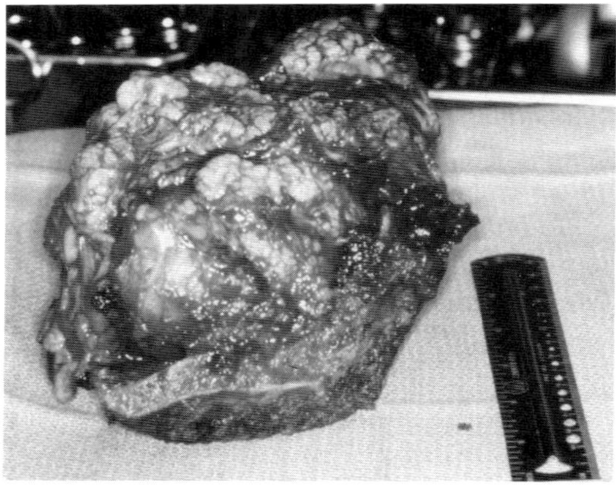

Figure 7.7. Case history 6. Specimen after complete excision with Nd:YAG laser and laser scalpel.

THE FUTURE

As general surgeons apply themselves to innovative uses of laser technology, there is little doubt that they will make significant advances in reduction of patient pain and morbidity through less interventional surgical techniques. The cases described above represent an attempt at enhancement of palliative care in much the same manner as photodynamic therapy and laser endoscopy have done. Ultimately, the aim is to use such methods to aid the less sick so that improved cure rates in malignancy can be achieved.

REFERENCES

1. Daniell JF, Brown DH. Carbon dioxide laparoscopy: Initial experience in experimental animals and humans. Obstet Gynecol 1982; 159:761-769.
2. Keye WR Jr, Dixon J. Photocoagulation of endometriosis by the argon laser through the laparoscope. Obstet Gynecol 1983; 62:383-386.
3. Ascher PW, Cerullo LJ. Neurosurgical applications of lasers. In Dixon JA, ed. Surgical Applications of Lasers. Chicago, Year Book Medical Publishers, 1983, p 163-173.
4. Jako GJ. Laser surgery of the vocal cords. Laryngoscope 82:2204-2209, 1972.
5. Schultz L, Hickok D, Graber J, Stephens W. Nd:YAG with contact probe in excision of major abdominal tumors (abstr.) American Society for Lasers in Medical Surgery Abstract 1987; 7:86.
6. Schultz LS, Hickok DF, Graber JN, Stephens WE. The use of lasers in general surgery. A preliminary assessment. Minn Med 1987; 70: 439-442.
7. Nims TA, McCaughan JS Jr. Clinical experience with CO_2 laser vaporization of neoplasm. Lasers Surg Med 1983; 3:265-268.
8. Daikuzono N, Joffe SN. Artificial sapphire probe for contact photocoagulation and tissue vaporization with the Nd:YAG laser. Med Instrum 1985; 19:173-178.
9. Joffe SN, Brackett KA, Sanker MY. Resection of the liver with the Nd:YAG laser. Surg Gynecol Obstet 1986; 153:437-442.
10. Iwasaki M, Sasako M, Konishi T, Maruyama Y, Wada T. Nd:YAG laser for general surgery. Lasers Surg Med 1985; 5:429-438.

CHAPTER

8

Carbon Dioxide Lasers in Surgery

B. L. Aronoff

The carbon dioxide (CO_2) laser was discovered by Kumar Patel and extensive research was done by Dr. McCord. It was believed that this was the "silver bullet" for cancer therapy. There were several adaptations of the CO_2 laser. Polyani and Jako made one of the first, a large instrument with a delivery system that was better adapted to a microscope. American Optical Company produced the machine. Isaac Kaplan, with the help of Oozie Sharon, changed the instrument and produced a delivery system marketed by Laser Industries in Israel. The beam was reflected through mirrors and eventually through a focusing lens contained in the handpiece. At first, this instrument had no directional beam, so a helium-neon (He-Ne) laser was added to the original 791 Sharplan laser. It was later incorporated into the instrument. Wattage on the early model was about 35. Newer models deliver up to 100 W. The CO_2 laser may be used as a continuous beam or may be pulsed at various intervals of a second. It may also be used in the superpulsed mode. The early instrument had to use extraneous water. New models have the system enclosed so they are semiportable. The power requirements vary with the manufacturer.

There are several advantages to the CO_2 laser and these are more important if one is dealing with cancer. The laser may be used as a surgical knife. It may be used freehand or through a microscope for greater precision. The usual freehand incision is 0.3 mm in width. There is a zone of change on either side of approximately this same width. The beam is absorbed by water so one must keep the area dry in order to make an incision. This beam will seal blood vessels up to 1 mm in diameter, maybe a little larger if the vessel is clamped. This is of particular importance if one is operating in a vascular area, depending on the part of the body. The bleeding is a bothersome complication if operating in an irradiated area. This fact may make surgery very difficult or impossible with conventional means. The laser will seal these vessels and there will be no delayed bleeding. Thrombocytopenia may interfere with surgery, whether due to idiopathic thrombocytopenic purpura or acquired due to chemotherapy. The sealing of vessels with ability to accomplish surgery is very gratifying. There have been operations on hemophiliacs and the Factor VIII requirement is much less.

Infection sometimes is severe enough to require days or weeks to control before conventional surgery is possible. Infected tumors, such as neglected cancer of the breast, may be removed. Grafts or flaps placed to cover the defect immediately have excellent "takes."

The use of the laser through the microscope is particularly useful in several organs, particularly the larynx. Here, one can destroy polyps, leukoplakia of carcinoma in situ, and some small cancers, particularly the exophytic lesions. Debulking may be accomplished in large or obstructing tumors so that conventional surgery may be accomplished as an elective. The increased mortality rates of emergency surgery are well known. In addition, debulking with the microscope and laser may be used in most parts of the body on inoperable cases or in cases where conventional therapy would fail (Fig. 8.1 A and B). This makes the life of the medical and radiation oncologist much easier or it indicates that the patient is a candidate for photodynamic therapy.

There are reports constantly that we are on the brink of discovery of a flexible fiber to carry the CO_2 beam. At the moment, the ideal fiber is not available. There are hollow waveguides of fairly smaller diameter. These are flexible to a minimal

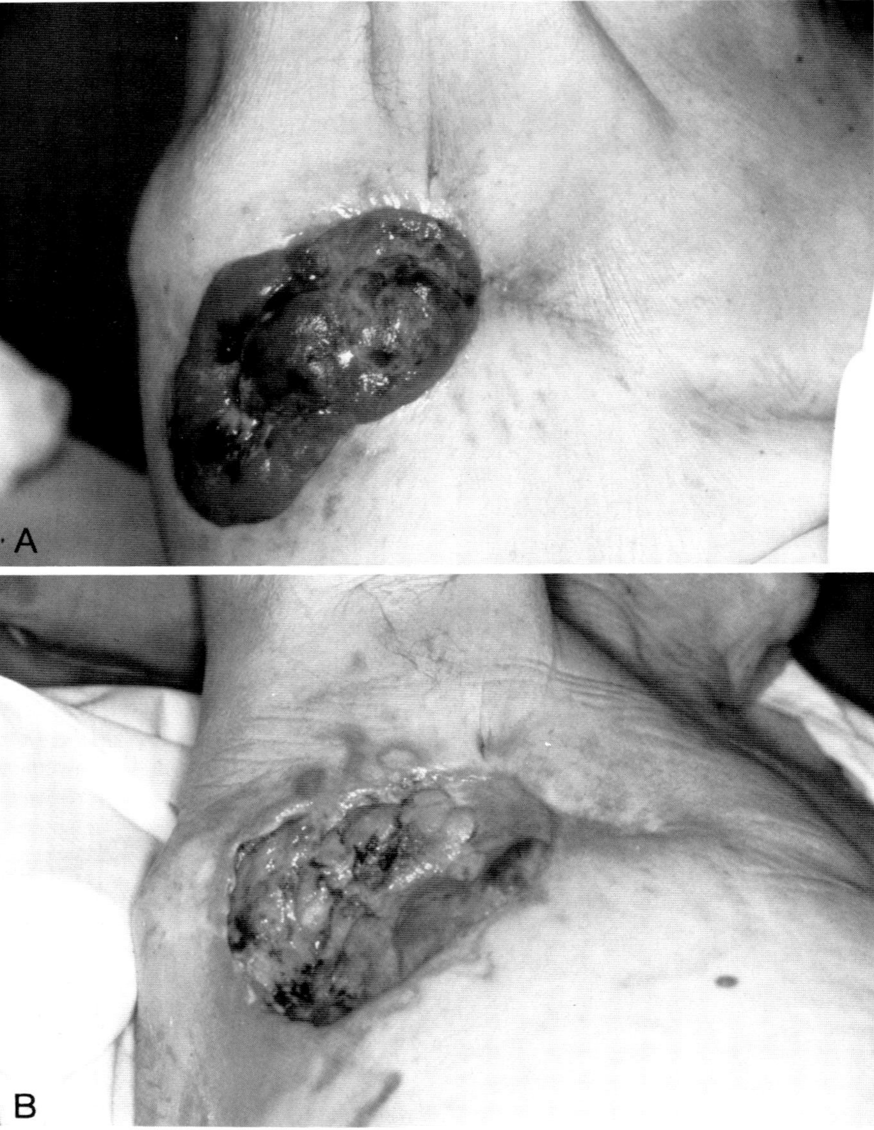

Figure 8.1. **A,** Recurrent carcinoma of the breast on the chest wall. **B,** This tumor was reduced in size with the CO_2 laser. The patient was subjected to photodynamic therapy.

extent and most endoscopes will not permit their passage. They may be used for many procedures and the power loss will usually be acceptable.

The sealing of lymphatics in cancer surgery (Fig. 8.2) is of paramount importance. The small invisible vessels are sealed spontaneously by the laser. This is very important in dealing with tumors and preventing seeding of the wound. There is no way to prevent milking of the tumor into lymphatics, even with minimal handling. The laser closes the end of the vessels immediately. There are recent publications that compare excising tumors with the knife to excision with the laser, and finally, to excising with the laser and then vaporizing the base. There is a marked decrease in the recurrence with the latter method.

CANCER SPREAD

1. Lymphatics
2. Direct via fascial planes
3. Spontaneous seeding
   Iatrogenic seeding
4. Blood
5. Transcelomic

Figure 8.2. The spread of cancer.

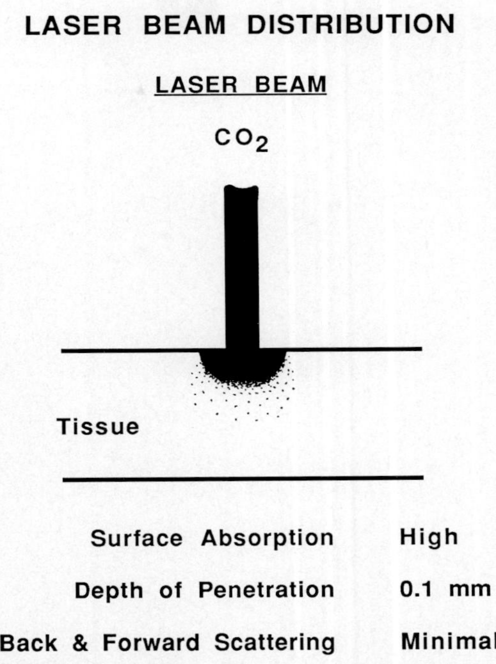

Figure 8.3. The action of the laser on tissue. Absorbed at the surface, there is minimal penetration and no scattering.

This should make the CO_2 laser an ideal instrument for performing cancer surgery.

When one discusses using the laser or the cold steel knife, many aspects must be considered. The first problem is the cost. A CO_2 laser will range from \$20,000–\$100,000 or more. This is certainly more expensive than a knife blade. If the hospital has lasers, there are still problems. Is it the correct laser? Does the surgeon want CO_2, argon, Nd:YAG, or a dye laser? Does this particular available laser have enough power? Is the laser available at the preferred time? Is the laser working? Most institutions have a biomedical department that can do emergency repairs. Occasionally, a back-up laser is available.

Another problem is the surgeon who has used the scalpel for so many years that it seems foolish to change. The most frequent question is, "why not use the cautery?" If the surgeon has no experience with the particular laser, he or she should not use it. One must take a didactic course and have hands-on experience. A preceptorship is then necessary. Finally the laser should be used under the observation of a qualified teacher. The surgeon must understand the effect of the laser on tissue, that there could be delayed healing. This may be too much of a chore for the scalpel user.

The attributes of the CO_2 laser will be pointed out in this chapter. Cases where the laser is preferrable to make the surgery safer and easier are reported. Another group of examples describe where the laser is indispensible. Situations where the laser is not necessary and, finally where it should not be used are listed.

Consider the action of the CO_2 laser on tissue. The infrared beam has a high absorption at the surface. One drop of water or blood will absorb the beam and will be vaporized. This means that the field must be kept relatively dry. The penetration of the beam is about 0.1 mm (Fig. 8.3) and there is very little fore- or backscatter. This is with the beam in focus and the incision will be between 0.1 and 0.3 mm in width. In using the CO_2 laser, heat is an important factor in tissue injury. A high wattage beam may be used for a short period of time or the superpulsed beam, which creates a series of high energy impulses of very short duration, may be used. The heat is dissipated rapidly, but the laser effect is secured. Now if the handpiece is backed away for 2–3 cm, then the beam becomes much wider and the power density much less. This will tend to vaporize the tissue. Again, the intensity will depend on the diameter of the beam and the wattage. One must understand the physics and, particularly, the tissue reaction.

SAFETY

Before embarking on the use of any laser, but particularly the CO_2, one must understand the usual precautions, but must realize that any tissue that is impacted with the laser will be injured. Also, the beam may be reflected by a shiny, smooth material. For example, in doing a simple

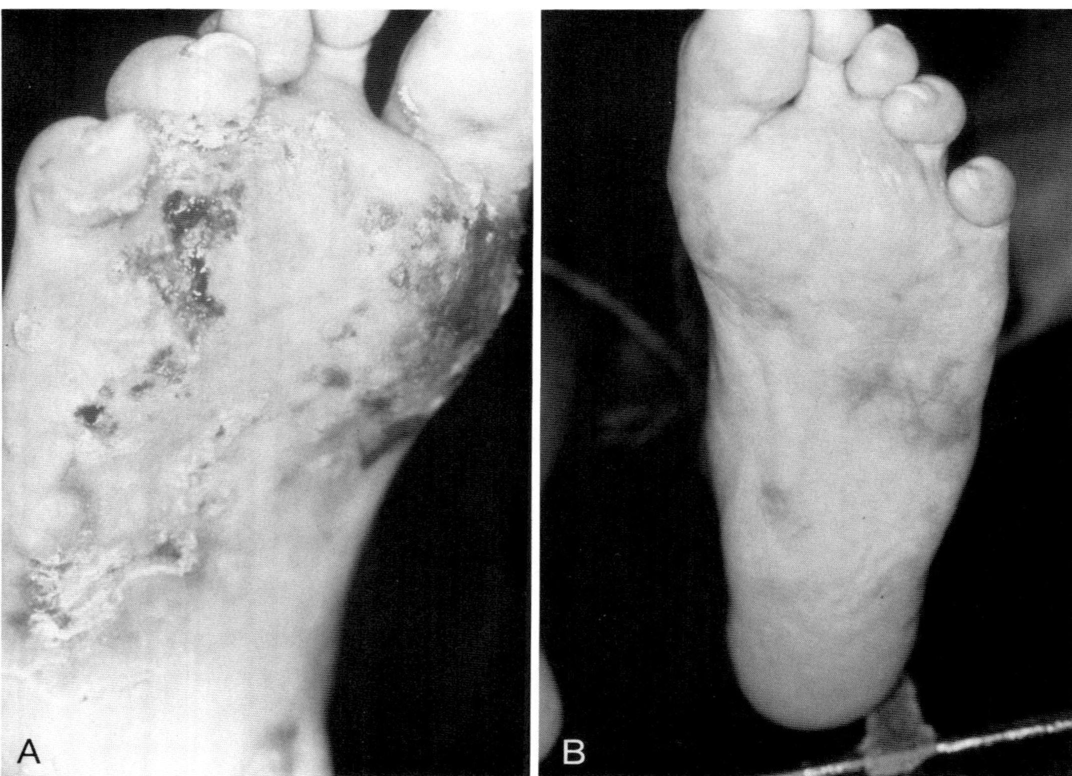

Figure 8.4. **A,** A patient with extensive disabling verruca is treated with CO_2 laser. **B,** Healing took a couple of months and was complete. The patient was able to walk thereafter.

V-excision of the lip, if the beam is directed toward the oral cavity, one must protect the tongue, teeth, and mucosa. If the upper lip is being incised, care of the skin that may be exposed, such as the nose, chin, or neck, likewise needs a dripping wet sponge. In the larynx and pharynx, the anesthesiologist must know the possibility of explosion with very damaging injuries. Several patients have needed extensive surgery for repair of these injuries. At the other end of the alimentary tract, methane gas may explode and injure the anus or vulva. A wet sponge placed in the anal canal may prevent injury. Despite all of these complications, the CO_2 laser is a very useful addition to the armamentarium and has many useful advantages.

SKIN

There are many lesions of the skin that may be removed with the scalpel or the CO_2 laser. With the popularization of the laser by the media, an increasing number of patients demand the use of the laser. This will definitely increase the cost of the procedure. Let us examine certain benign and malignant lesions of the skin. Starting with small angiomas that occur on skin of the trunk and extremity, certainly the CO_2 or argon laser does an excellent job and is preferable to the knife or cautery. If many of these lesions are present, the patient is taken to outpatient surgery, given a general anesthetic, and the lesions are treated. Upon recovery from general anesthesia, the patient is discharged. The common wart may be treated with cryosurgery, cautery, or excision. Many times, the lesion recurs and is sometimes stimulated. These cases are amenable to laser therapy but the patient is always informed of the fact that this may not be successful. Very large lesions that may partially recur have been treated and, usually with persis-

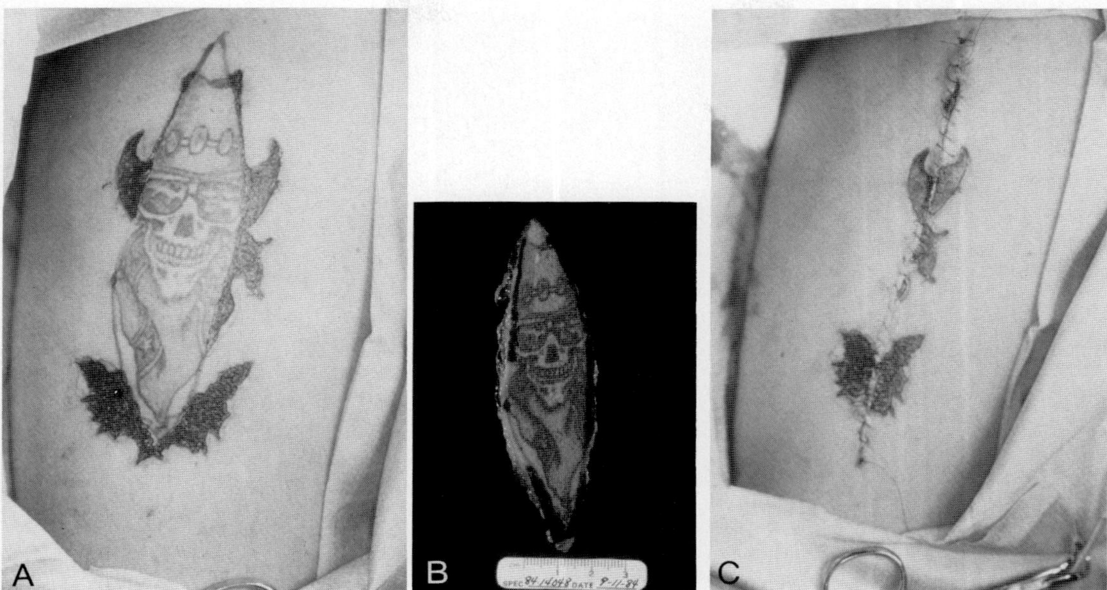

Figure 8.5. **A,** A tattoo on the deltoid area. **B,** Partially excised with the CO_2 laser, the remaining areas are treated with it. **C,** Plastic repair of the defect.

tance, the treatment has been successful (Fig. 8.4*A* and *B*).

Keratoses are usually treated with excision so as to obtain a specimen and cauterized in the office. Extensive lesions may be treated with the CO_2 laser but all lesions are biopsied. Most port wine stains and strawberry nevi are treated with the argon laser. A 577 Candella laser has now been obtained for this purpose. There are some individuals who use the CO_2 laser.

Tattoos that resulted from a "night on the town" may be treated with the CO_2 or the argon laser. In comparing results, the CO_2 laser is found to be faster and certainly removes the dye. Patient response to pain is mixed. It will be several years before a definite statement comparing the cosmetic results will be available (Figs. 8.5*A-C* and 8.6*A* and *B*). Large vascular anomalies may be benefited by the CO_2 laser, particularly tumors with predominantly capillary components (Fig. 8.7*A-C*). If they are large vascular tumors with cavernous components, the laser may open large channels that will be difficult to control. Pressure will have to be maintained while other modalities are used to stop hemorrhage. These include excision, ligation of feeding vessels, embolization, or the use of vasoconstrictors by arterial infusion. These tumors may demand all the modalities one has learned during residency and clinical experience. These fall into the group of "malignant benign" lesions and certainly cause plenty of problems. They occur in all parts of the body, including head and neck and extremities, but may also involve any organ, including the liver.

There are a group of these malformations that have so much blood flowing that there is cardiac dysfunction due to the shunt. These are pulmonary and cardiac cripples. Some of these tumors are mixed lymphangiohemangiomas (Fig. 8.8*A* and *B*). These, in the author's experience, are amenable to excision with the CO_2 laser. They seem to have large feeding vessels that may be clamped and ligated but not the medusa of large vessels around the edges.

Lymphangiomata are then encountered possibly involving large areas of the tongue. They may be vaporized with the CO_2 laser with good sealing and destruction of the tumor, which tends to be permanent. On the extremities, particularly in the upper thighs, it has frequently been necessary to exise or incise the offending area and find the large lymphatics and destroy them at the base.

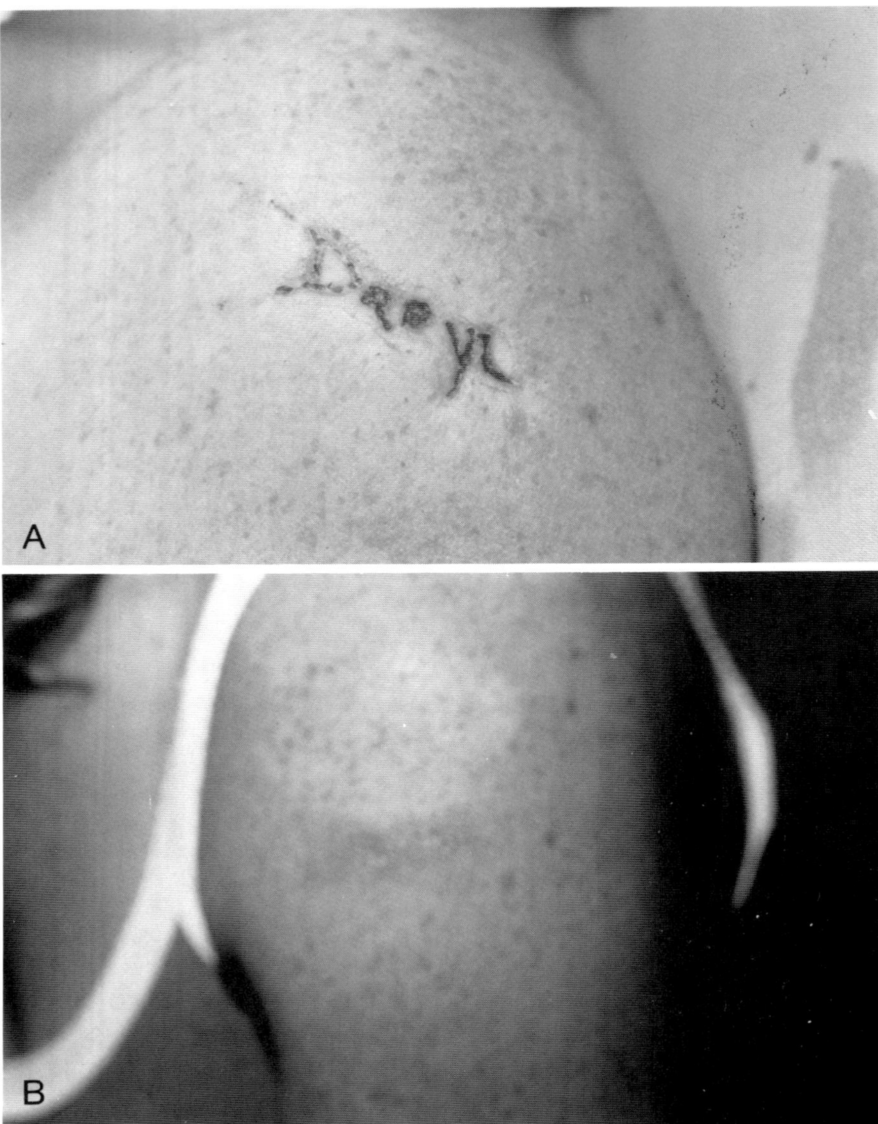

Figure 8.6. **A,** A small tattoo, **B,** easily ablated with the argon laser.

In dealing with malignant lesions, a frozen section is necessary to ascertain margins. The CO_2 laser may be used but is not necessary in many cases. Frequently, the lesions are excised using the laser instead of a knife. Then, frozen sections are available. These lesions are not vaporized (Fig. 8.9*A-C*). Originally, it was believed that melanoma would be a prime target. Communication with Isaac Kaplan of Israel confirmed that a prospective study he had recently finished showed no advantage for the laser.

The main indication for the laser is in those recurrent cases that have failed irradiation. Here, the sealing of blood vessels is quite beneficial.

A malignant variation of skin lesions that is so common in people with AIDS is Kaposi sarcoma.

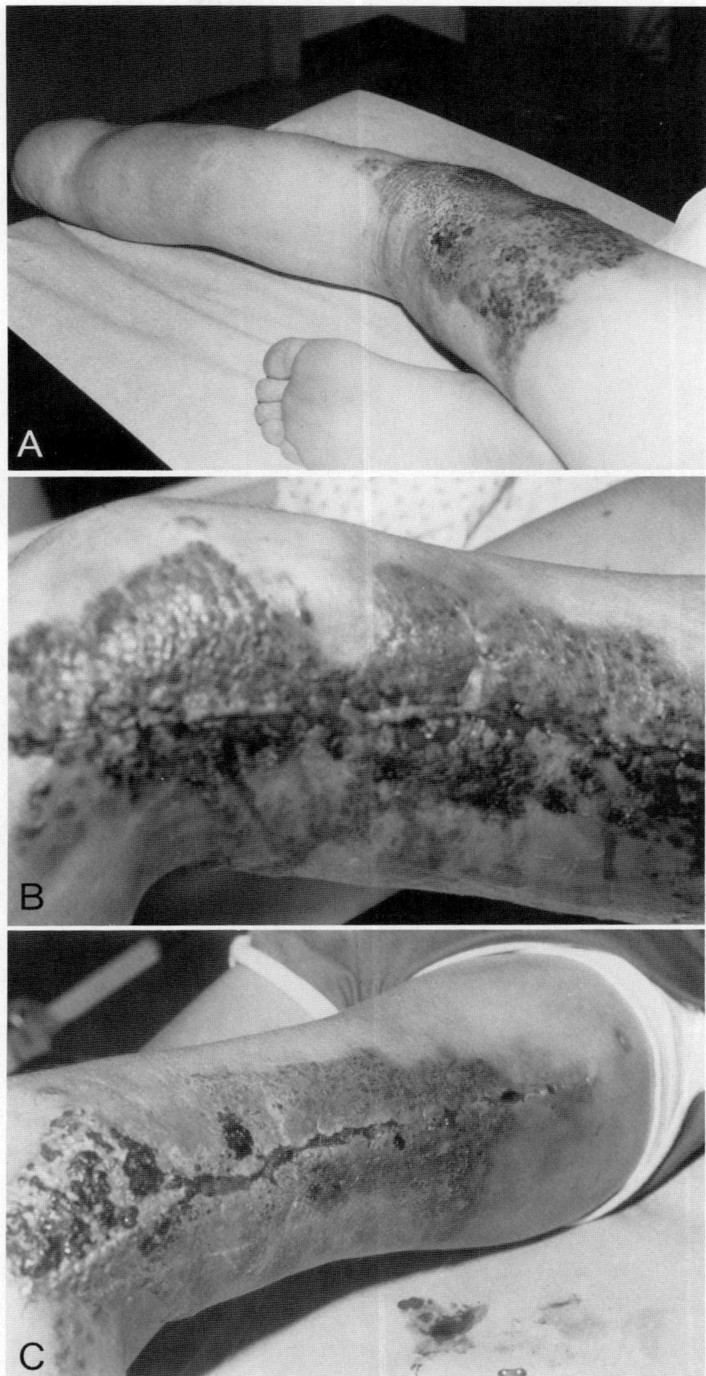

Figure 8.7. **A,** A large vascular anomaly was treated previously. **B,** Partial excision of skin with destruction of vessels in the subcutaneous area and closure are illustrated. **C,** Later, the argon laser was used to remove superficial vessels.

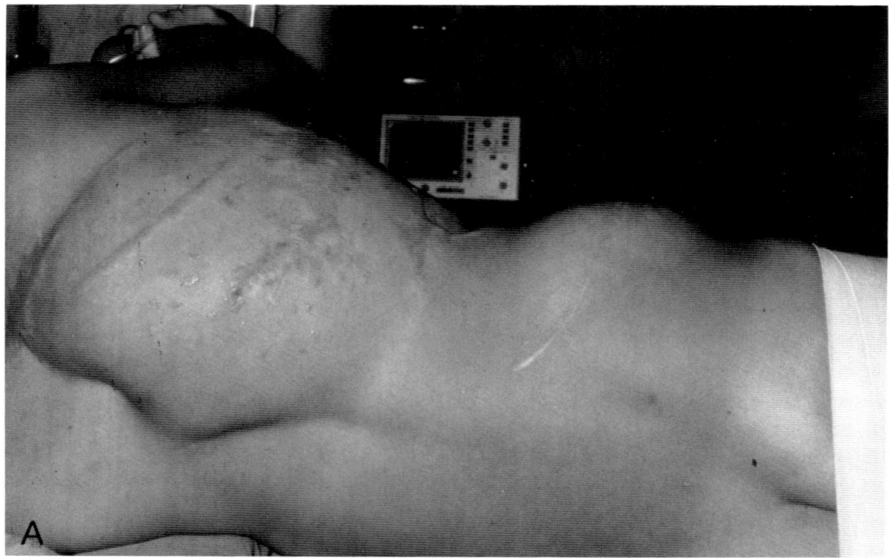

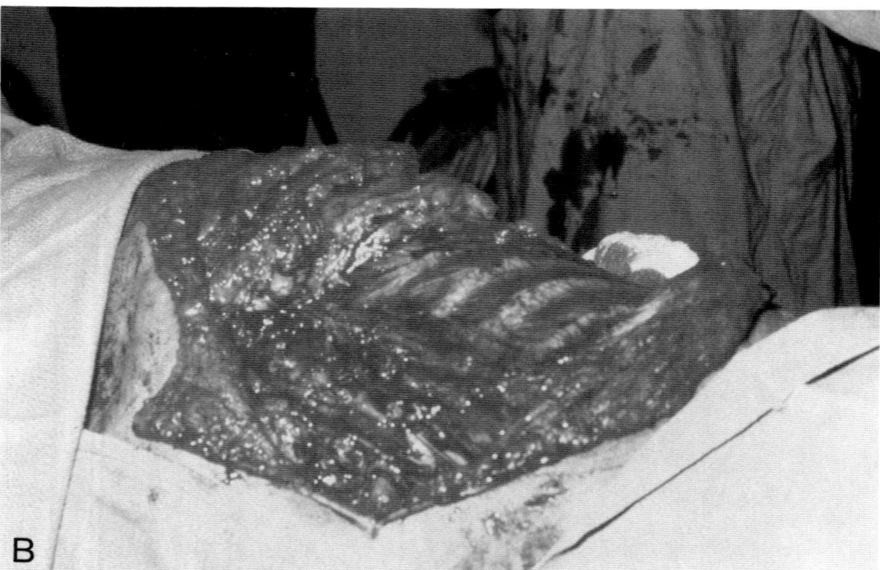

Figure 8.8. **A,** Hemangiolymphangioma of chest wall, **B,** resected with CO_2 laser.

Vaporization of these lesions has been attempted. First, there is a large subcutaneous component and usually, when destroyed, the defect must be sutured. Very limited experience has given very mixed results. It seems that these tumors are connected by subcutaneous communication.

An unusual tumor of the skin is the platelet-entrapping hemangioma (Fig. 8.10*A-D*) (Kasabach-Merritt syndrome). This, as in other platelet deficiencies, is very successfully treated with the CO_2 laser. A limited experience has produced an excellent result with large tumor cure.

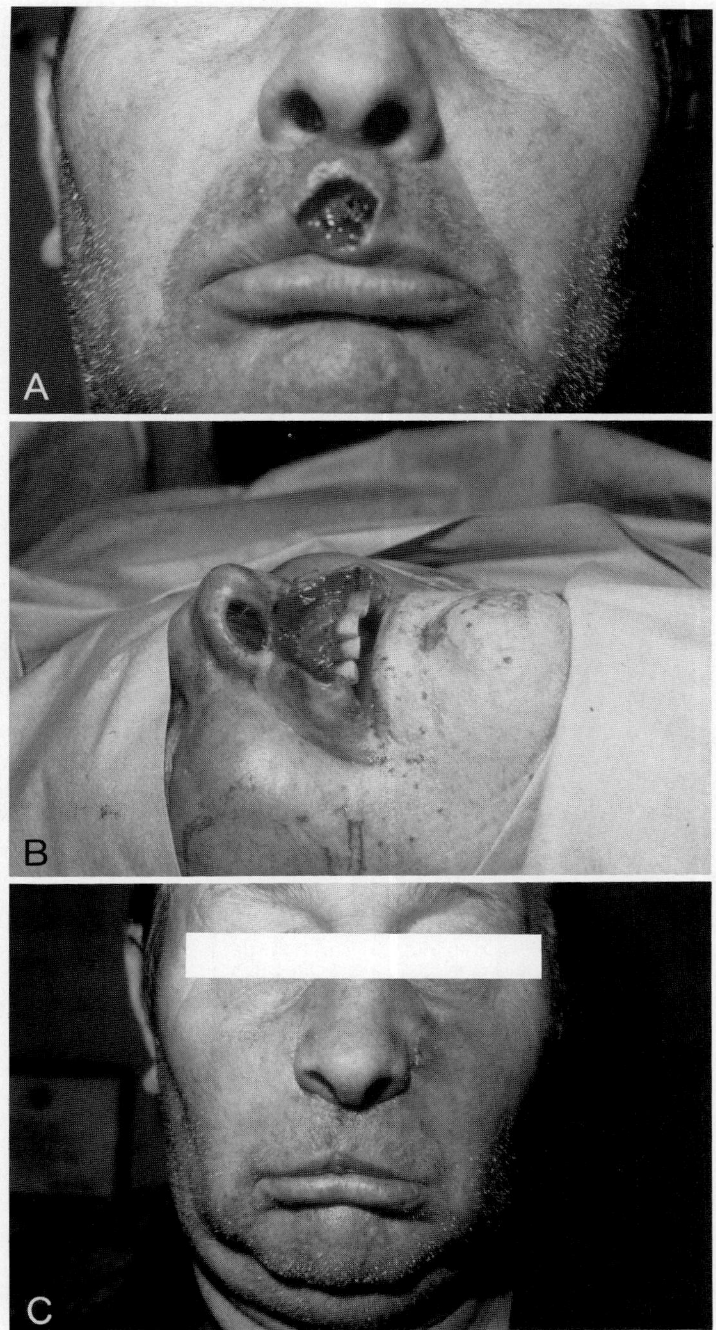

Figure 8.9. **A,** Recurrent carcinoma of the lip after irradiation. **B,** Excision; ala nasae flap developed with CO_2 laser. **C,** The patient after 2 weeks.

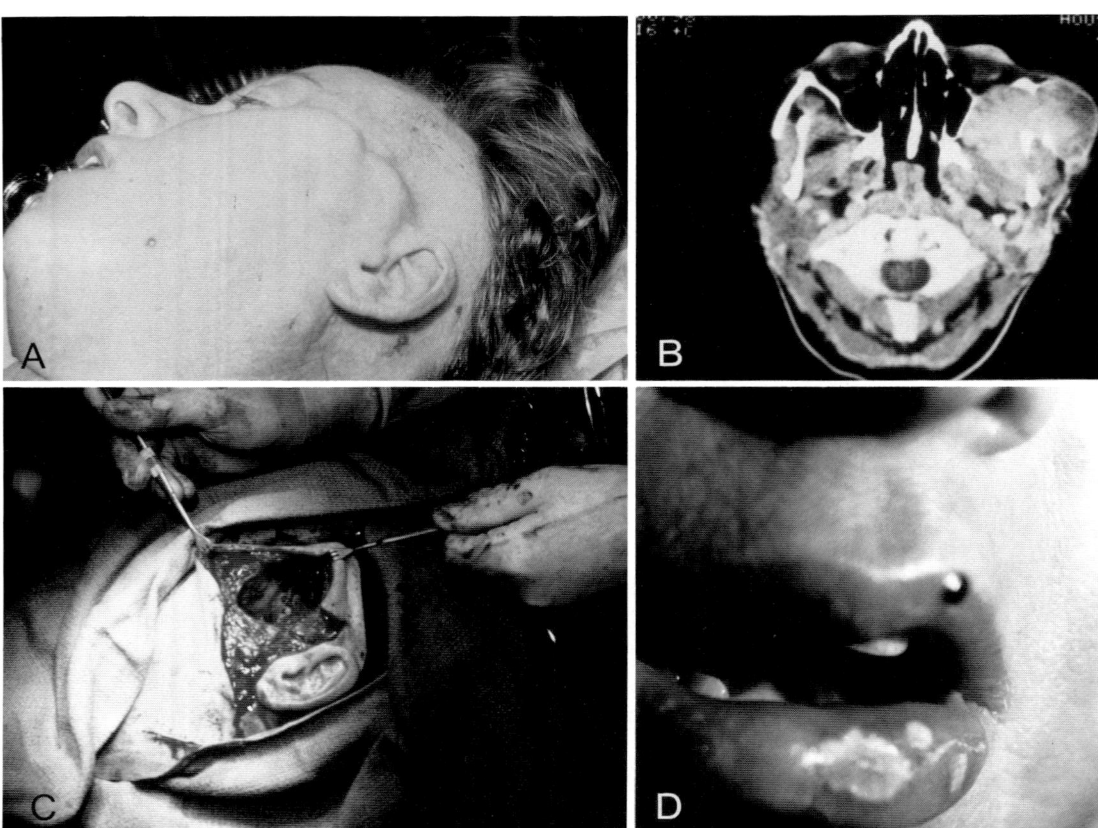

Figure 8.10. **A,** The patient with Kasabach-Merritt (platelet-entrapping hemangioma) syndrome. **B,** CT scan shows extent of tumor. **C,** Easily excised with the CO_2 laser, the blood loss is minimal. **D,** Lesion of the lip is treated with the argon laser.

As mentioned, when one operates on irradiated skin, the bleeding is minimal. The same is true in any of the platelet deficiencies for whatever cause.

HEAD AND NECK

Cutaneous lesions have already been discussed. Excision of tumor with superficial spread to the mastoid bone has worked well. Here the tumor (Fig. 8.11*A* and *B*), with or without neck dissection, is removed along with the outer table of the bone and mastoid air cells. The wattage is increased to 50 W or more and then the base is vaporized. This has been used as an alternative to temporal bone resection (Fig 8.12*A-C*). Adjacent flaps frequently are turned immediately. In the oral cavity, vaporizing leukoplakia and carcinoma in situ is preferred. The area includes all suspicious areas with a good margin. No graft is necessary and the results are excellent. Excision of lesions invading the palate may be accomplished with the laser. Partial glossectomy and pharyngectomy is performed, using the laser as a scalpel. The use of the laser in the larynx with the microscope for polyps, leukoplakia, and invasive cancer has been mentioned. Certainly, it may be used to debulk obstructing tumors. Thyroidectomy is not usually a procedure for the laser. Recurrent laryngeal nerves and parathyroids may be dissected out. If the specimen shows carcinoma, and particularly, if the margin is narrow, the thyroid bed, is vaporized but the recurrent nerves and parathyroids are always preserved and protected.

The turning of flaps for neck dissection in an unirradiated case rarely saves time or blood. It is so easy to dissect in a relatively avascular plane that the laser is not used. Frankly, it is rare to use the laser in any part of a neck dissection. A comparative

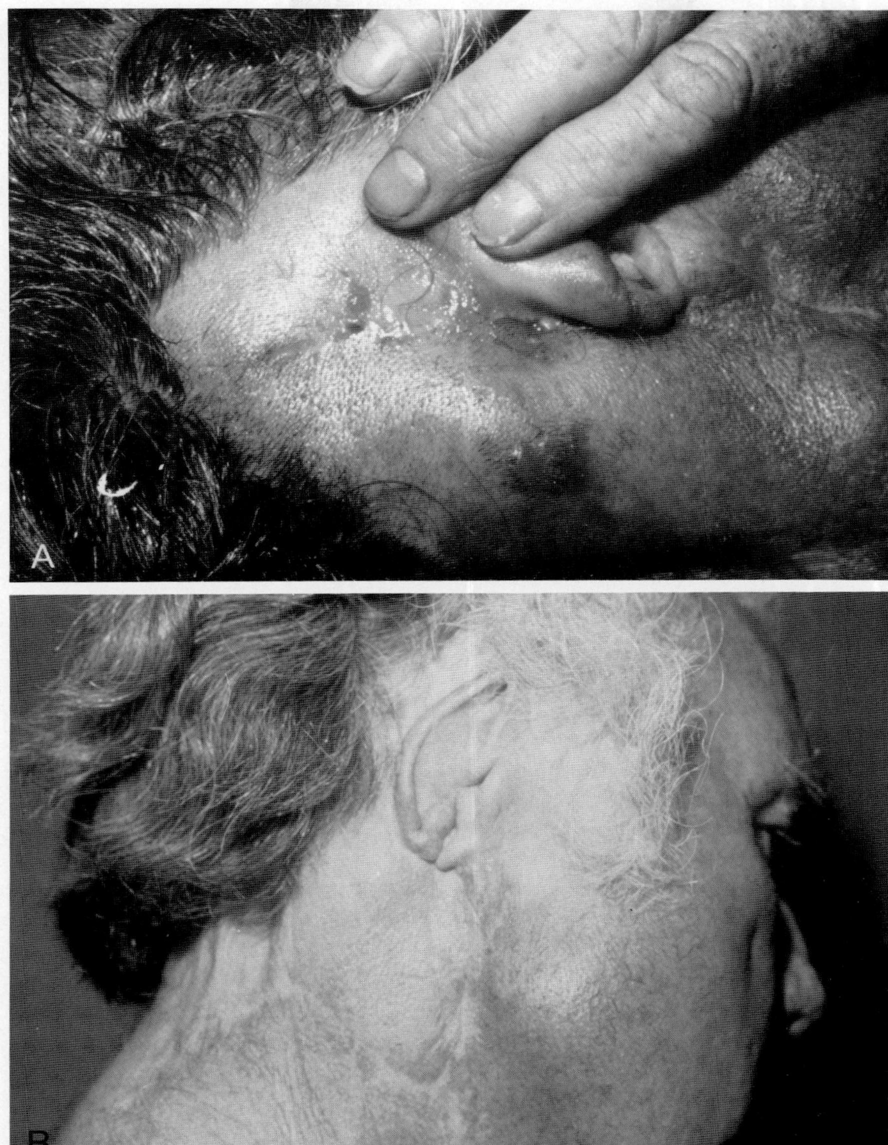

Figure 8.11. **A,** Basel cell invades the mastoid. It is resected and the outer table is excised. **B,** The adjacent flap is turned.

study found that no time was saved. The blood loss was minimal with either modality. The flap failure and suture line dehiscence was rare and fluid under the flaps was no different with either modality.

BREAST

Local excision of breast tumors for diagnosis or treatment is a relatively simple operation. The benign tumor or cancer is excised or biopsied. Estrogen receptors are done on the malignant lesions. The patients are then subjected to proper care. Most breast cancers are treated with modified radical mastectomy. The modality of turning flaps is varied and very little, if any difference is seen. The breast is removed along with the pectoralis fascia and this is done with the laser.

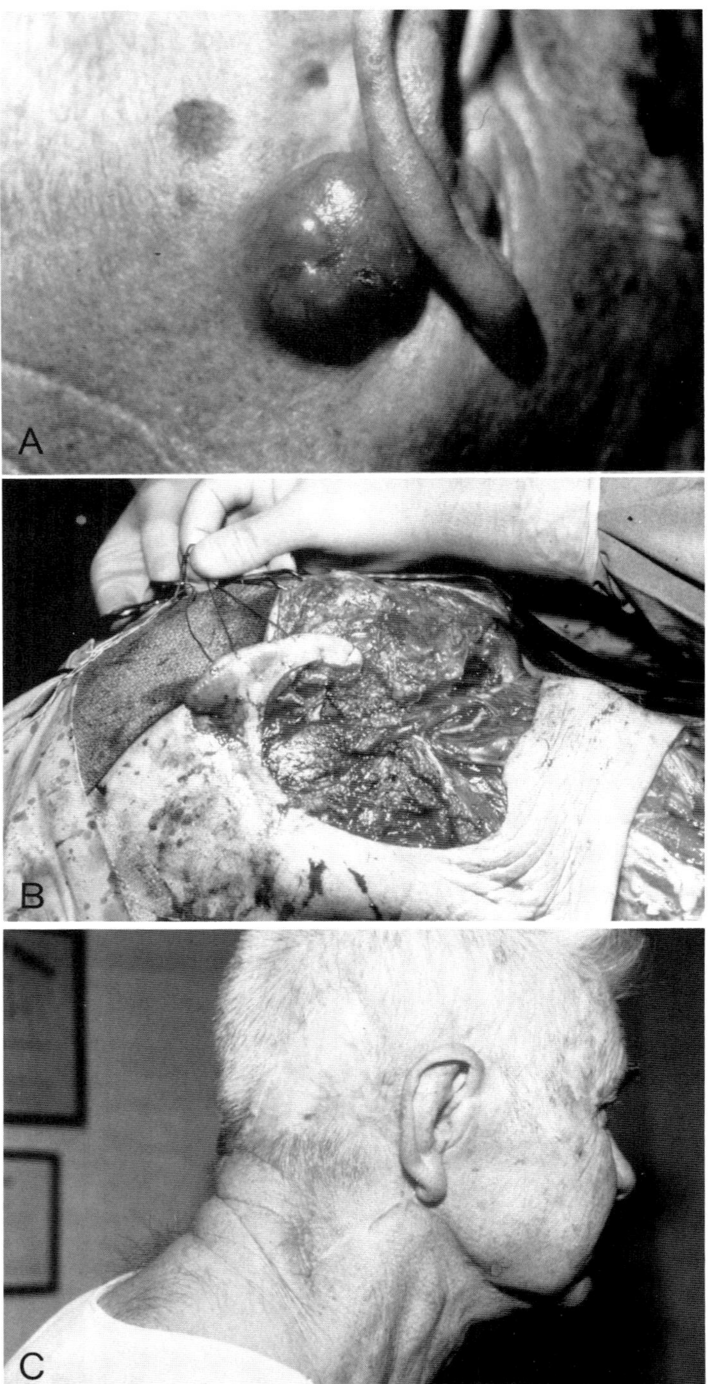

Figure 8.12. **A,** Sweat gland cancer of the mastoid area. **B,** Radical neck, parotidectomy, and excision of tumor with adjacent flap. **C,** Results of the procedure.

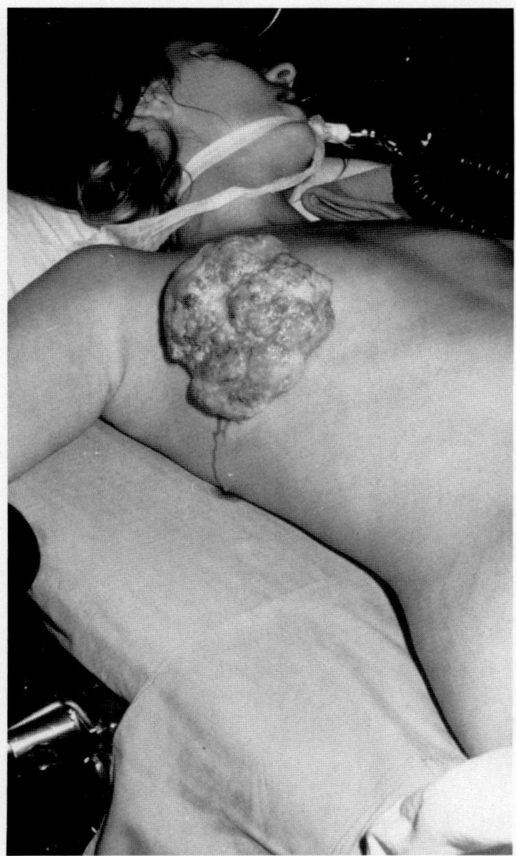

Figure 8.13. Ulcerated carcinoma of breast, treated with excision and a split graft. Two years later, axillary dissection is performed metastatic to lung 6 years after the first surgery.

The first part of the axillary dissection may be done with the CO_2 laser but, more commonly, with the scalpel. The lateral pectoral nerve is carefully preserved. The tendon of the pectoral minor muscle may be divided and the laser used to dissect most of that muscle away. The author certainly does not use the laser on the medial end of the axillary dissection, which is at the chest wall; a conventional scalpel excision is performed. However, with the advent of a CO_2 fiber, it will be used in this dissection.

The patient with ulcerated infected cancer that is a candidate for toilet mastectomy certainly is a prime candidate for laser (Fig. 8.13). A skin graft is immediately applied with excellent results. If the patient has a chest wall recurrence that has failed chemotherapy and/or irradiation, the bulk of tumor may be reduced with the CO_2 laser and then photodynamic therapy (dihematoporphyrin ether with dye laser destruction of the tumor) may be used.

Many reduction mastectomies have been performed with the CO_2 laser in many institutions.

HERNIA

There seems to be little merit to the use of lasers in hernia surgery. Rarely has the laser been used and then only when the patient demands it.

HEMORRHOIDS AND FISSURES

The laser is excellent in dealing with hemorrhoids, fissures, and fistulas. The author's method is to use the CO_2 laser and, usually, local anesthesia (occasionally, general). A stitch is placed at the apex of the hemorrhoid. The vessel mass is then dissected out, leaving most of the mucosa. It is then approximated with a fine absorbable suture. External hemorrhoids are vaporized until destroyed. Rarely, there is a small bleeder that is sutured. It is certainly much less painful than conventional hemorrhoidectomy and most patients leave the outpatient surgery in a matter of hours. Fistulas and polyps are frequent and can be removed with the laser.

Experience with perineal and perianal condylomata and warts has been gratifying. The larger lesions are excised down to the skin and the base is vaporized (Fig. 8.14*A-C*). Smaller lesions are simply vaporized. Many more of these lesions are seen in patients with AIDS. Certainly, with any of the viral type diseases, precautions are used to protect exposed skin, and the nose and mouth. Gowns and gloves with hood head-cover, goggles, and masks are mandatory for the surgeon and other personnel.

ABDOMEN

General surgeons have been very slow to accept the CO_2 laser. In the peritoneal cavity, there are a few areas in which the laser is very helpful. CO_2 lasers have been used on the liver for 13 years. The first laser would only generate 35 W. Segments of liver could be excised but it was necessary to control bleeding. The policy was to outline the area with through-and-through sutures and, after excision, to close the defect. In the laboratory, simultaneous delivery of CO_2 and argon or CO_2 and Nd:YAG laser therapy was possible. Better hemostasis was achieved with the argon

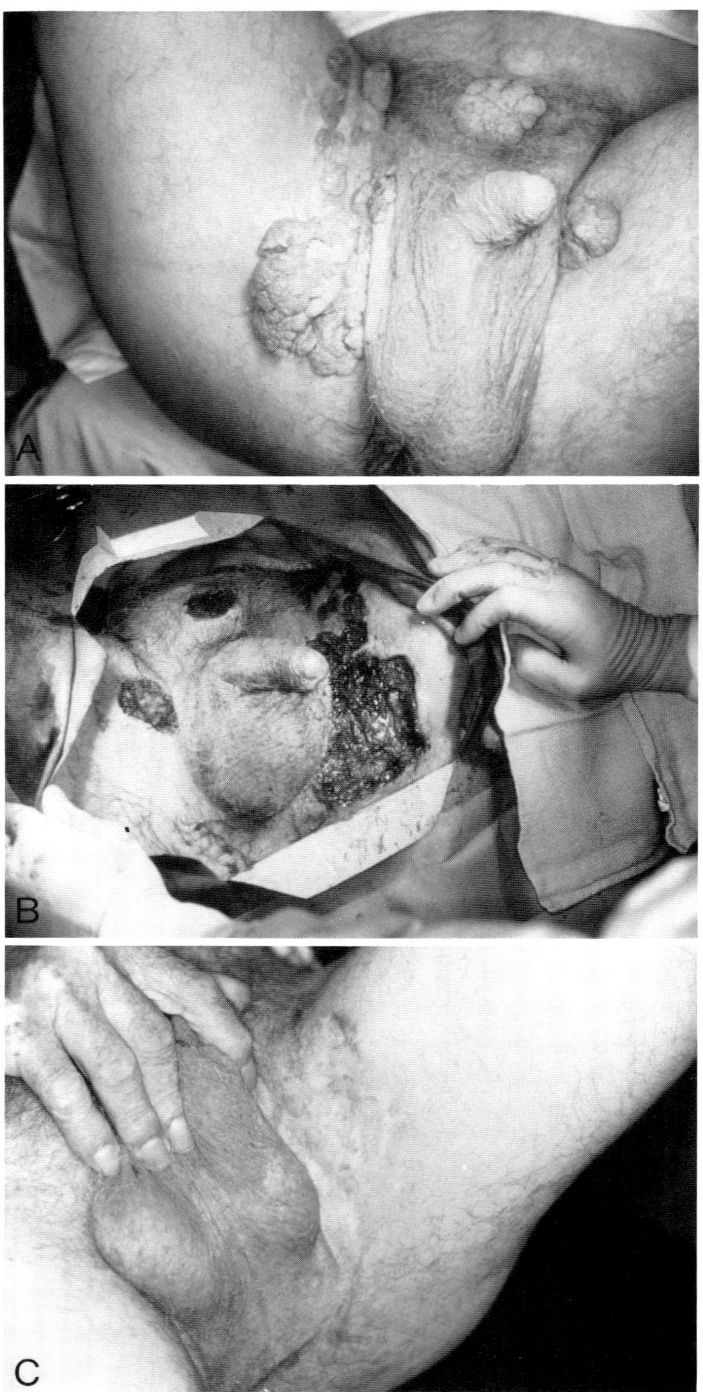

Figure 8.14. **A,** Condylomata. B, Condylomata are excised and the base is vaporized. **C,** Healing with some scar.

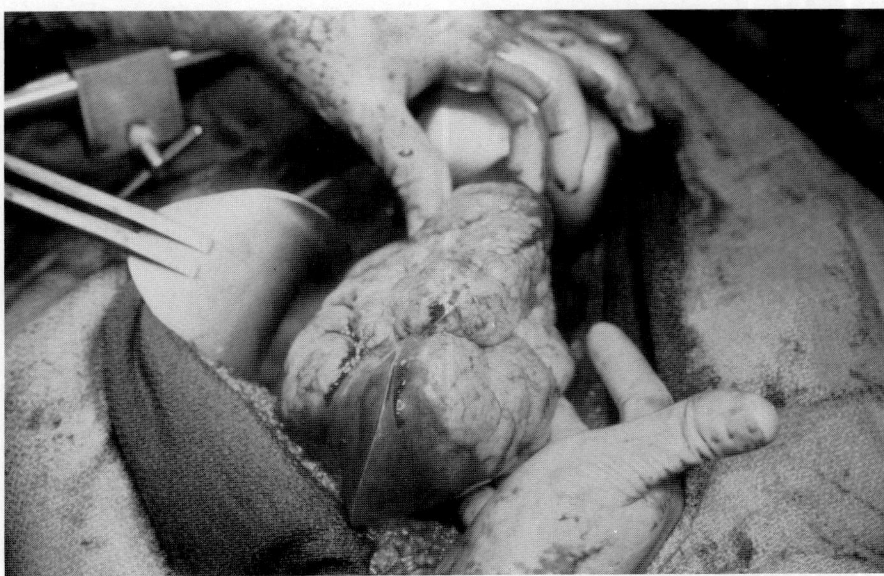

Figure 8.15. Metastatic adenoid cystic adenocarcinoma of tongue to liver, excised with the CO_2 laser.

and CO_2 combination. Bleeding from deeper vessels was more pronounced with the CO_2 and Nd:YAG. This was a very limited experience.

With increasing CO_2 wattage, better hemostasis is found (Figs. 8.15 and 8.16). If a lobectomy on trisegmentectomy is performed, the appropriate vessles are ligated and a T.Y. Lins clamp is slipped over the liver. The surgery is performed and the few large vessels controlled as the clamp is removed. The raw surface is covered with omentum. The drains are placed, but blood and bile drainage is limited and the drains may be removed early. The use of the Nd:YAG laser, particularly with the sapphire tip, will be discussed in Chapters 5, 7, and 9.

The CO_2 laser in distal pancreatectomy works well. The area is isolated and staples are placed across the pancreas. Cuts are then made with the CO_2 laser. Again, drainage is minimal. Frequently cuts with the laser are across the stomach (Fig. 8.17), or the small or large intestine. The sealing of blood vessels is gratifying. The mesentery or retroperitoneum are not dissected with this instrument. Abdominal perineal resections may be assisted by the CO_2 laser. We particularly use it in the perineal portion of the procedure.

Many people popularize the use of the CO_2 laser in cholecystectomy. The author has never believed it to be necessary and if one tried to use it around the common duct, complications may develop. With the excellent standard procedures for gallbladder removal, there is no inclination to use the laser. The one exception would be in cancer of the gallbladder with or without liver invasion; this organ could be removed with the adjacent liver and frozen section secured with confirmation or adequacy of excision.

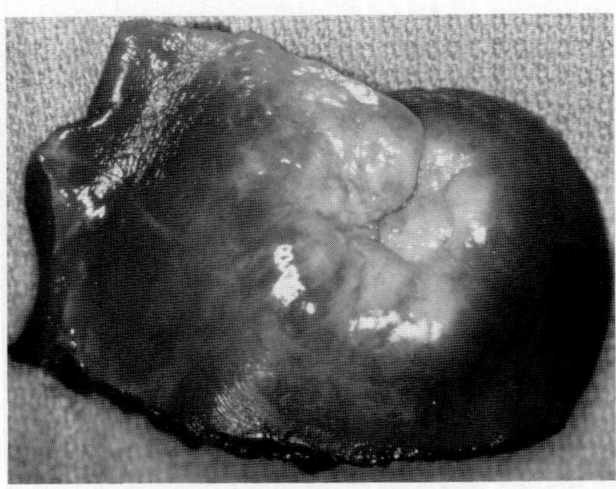

Figure 8.16. Metastatic carcinoma of breast to liver 20 years after primary surgery. Lobectomy with CO_2 laser.

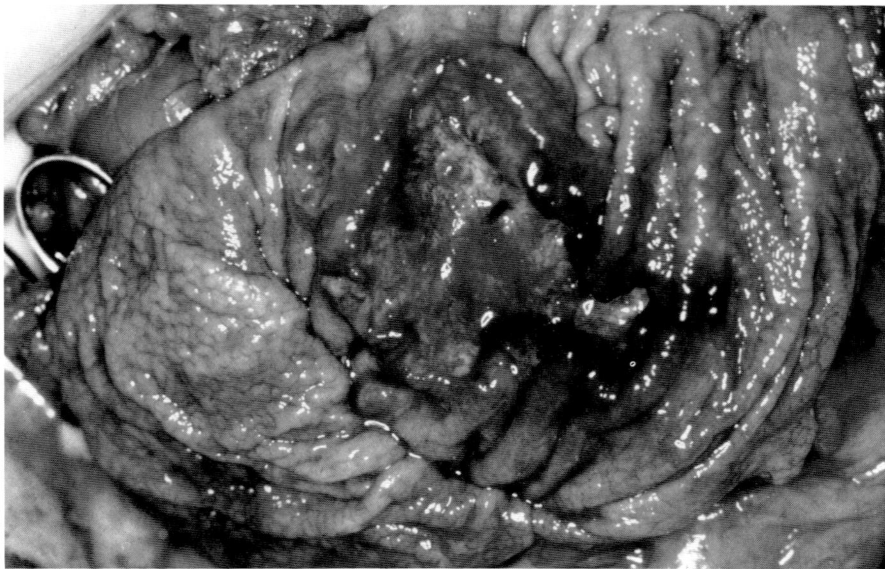

Figure 8.17. Carcinoma of the stomach invading the pancreas. Total gastrectomy, distal pancreatectomy, and splenectomy. Repair with jejunal roux-en-Y loop. The patient was alive 4 years postsurgery.

Appendectomy does not indicate laser surgical intervention.

Lastly, there are retroperitoneal tumors (Fig. 8.18*A-C*). The laser is used wherever it seems safe and great care is taken to avoid injury to kidney, ureter, small intestine, and blood vessels. Recurrent or irradiated tumors are more easily removed with the assistance of the CO_2 laser.

SARCOMAS

The sarcoma is an excellent model for the use of the laser. CO_2 lasers will cut through tissue well with minimal blood loss. The laser seals lymphatics and tissue planes and seems to prevent iatrogenic seeding. Further, the bed from which the tumor was removed can be vaporized. Frozen sections are easily available to confirm the adequacy of excision. Primary closure or skin grafts or flaps may be performed with an expectation of success. Not enough cases have been performed to evaluate the benefit in reduced recurrence. A nationwide survey would be quite beneficial.

MISCELLANEOUS

Amputations have not been discussed. All soft tissue work is done with the CO_2 laser but conventional means are used on large bones. Fingers and toes can easily be partially or totally removed with the laser. Many other procedures are accomplished with this modality.

CONCLUSION

The CO_2 laser, at the present, is the workhorse for general surgery. Excellent work with the YAG 1.312 and the Nd:YAG laser with the sapphire tip has been reported. Other lasers should soon be useful and are now being tried. The use of the argon fiber, either percutaneously or through the endoscope, to remove retained common duct stones is being used on a limited basis. The Trimedyne (hot-tipped) laser to create a passage in Klatskin tumors or other obstructive lesions in the bile duct is being explored. One is able to leave a stint to keep the duct patent. Many lesions are removable by endoscopy with the Nd:YAG laser to secure palliation or cure. There is still a need to expand photodynamic therapy by new dyes or chromophores so that the laser will penetrate through normal tissue and destroy cancer that is metastatic to the lung, liver, and other sites. Much research into all of these areas is progressing and should produce procedures to help in the attack on many cancers. The future is bright.

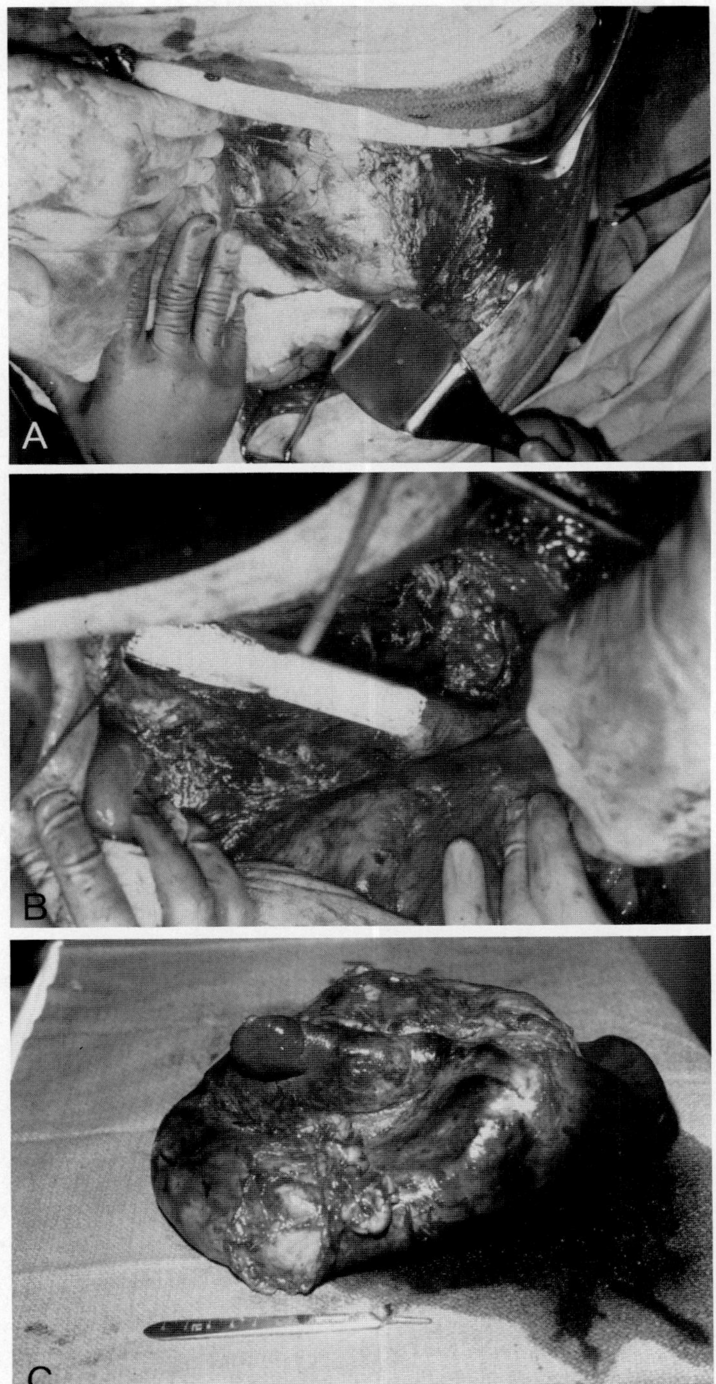

Figure 8.18. **A,** Previous surgery and irradiation for malignant histiocytoma. The tumor with the right kidney and vena cava excised. **B,** Vena cava graft by vascular surgeon. **C,** Specimen.

CHAPTER

9

Liver Resection

Stephen N. Joffe

Despite well-standardized techniques for liver resection, operative mortality rates ranging from 5–40% are reported (1, 2). Postoperative complications include liver failure, bleeding, infection, and sepsis. These complications are frequently related to intraoperative bleeding, extent of necrotic liver tissue, and bile leakage. Operative techniques in performing a liver resection are important factors in preventing these complications. Lasers as a surgical tool may offer an improvement in decreasing morbidity and mortality.

The CO_2 laser was first used in liver surgery in 1975 (3) and, subsequently, an experimental study used a CO_2 and a Nd:YAG laser in performing a partial liver resection (4). This combined laser system was effective in both cutting and coagulating the liver parenchyma. A subsequent clinical report presented 15 patients who underwent a liver resection (5). The CO_2 laser was used in 10 patients, in one the Nd:YAG laser alone and in four cases, both lasers were used. The CO_2 laser provided good cutting effects but hemostasis was inadequate. Whereas the noncontact Nd:YAG laser provided good coagulation, the necrotic zone of the liver surface was 5–6 mm. When the latter was combined with the CO_2 laser, the damage was decreased to 1.8 mm. A prototype combined a noncontact Nd:YAG handpiece using high powers of 100 W and the CO_2 at equally high powers of 80–90 W.

A study comparing an ultrasonic dissector, the noncontact Nd:YAG laser with a conventional finger fracture blunt dissection technique, showed the Cavitron ultrasonic aspirator (CUSA) was superior to the finger fracture technique by causing less postoperative tissue damage and reduced bleeding (6). The noncontact Nd:YAG laser had poor cutting properties and, although it produced hemostasis, the depth of tissue damage was considerable.

Contact Nd:YAG Laser Scalpels and Probes (Surgical Laser Technologies, Inc., Philadelphia, PA using synthetic sapphires have been developed (Fig. 9.1) (7). This device has proven to be effective and safe in both endoscopic and open general surgery (8) and requires a stable medium- to low-powered Nd:YAG laser system (Fig. 9.2) that delivers a sufficient power density when the probe is in direct contact with the tissue (Fig. 9.3).

An experimental study comparing the contact and noncontact air delivery Nd:YAG laser has shown the contact method to be much more effective (9). The SLT Contact Laser System required only low-power ranges (5–24 W) (Fig. 9.4) and approximately 75% less total energy (Fig. 9.5) for a rapid hepatic lobe resection. Noncontact resection at low power (10–20 W) caused uncontrollable bleeding leading to death in the experimental animals (Fig. 9.6). At power density ranges greater than 30 W, successful resection of a lobe of the liver could be done, but as the power increased, there was greater tissue damage. Light microscopy showed thermal tissue necrosis of 0.5 mm with the contact method with evidence of healing, fibrosis, and minimal necrotic material at 15 days. In the noncontact group, thermal damage was 2–3 mm in depth with accumulated necrotic material encapsulated by fibrous tissue at 15 days (Fig. 9.7) Both the amounts of smoke produced during the operative procedure (Fig. 9.8) and adhesion formation at 15 days postoperatively (Fig. 9.9) were less.

One problem with the contact Nd:YAG laser in major liver surgery is the potential difficulty in identifying the largest central hepatic veins before partial perforation without obtaining adequate he-

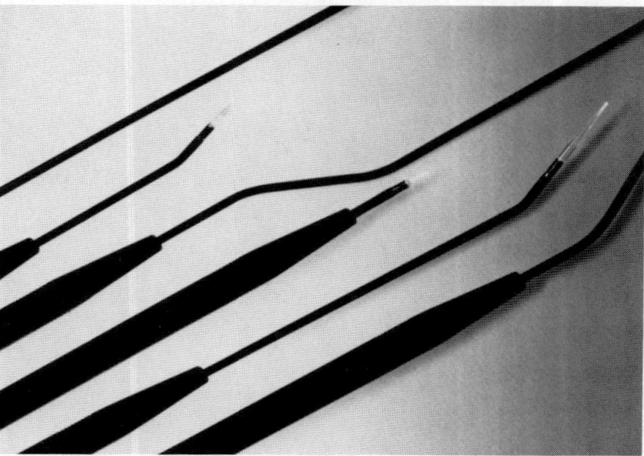

Figure 9.1. SLT Contact Laser Scalpels and Probes consisting of sterile disposable surgical handlepieces and reusable probes. (Surgical Laser Technologies, Inc., Malvern, PA, USA)

mostasis. The SLT Contact Laser System is able to coagulate 80–85% of the blood vessels during a liver resection. The remaining large vessels must be suture ligated. This finding was followed by the development of a new and modified technique for performing contact laser liver resection (10). In this technique a disposable plastic ''strapper'' is used as a proximal tourniquet to control the larger hepatic vessels (Fig. 9.10). The proximal resection surface is compressed by the strapper and the liver parenchyma distal to the tourniquet is resected with the SLT Contact Laser System (Fig. 9.11). This gives a completely hemostatic resection without any bleeding and a liver resection can be completed within 30 min. Thereafter, all large vessels could be visualized and ligated before and during the gradual release of the strapper. Histological studies showed that this method did not cause more damage to the resected liver surface than the earlier reported contact laser method (Fig. 9.12).

ANATOMY

Traditionally the liver has been demarcated by the falciform ligament into right and left lobes. This concept delayed surgical advances until it was recognized that the true line of division between the arterial, portal, and ductal systems lay

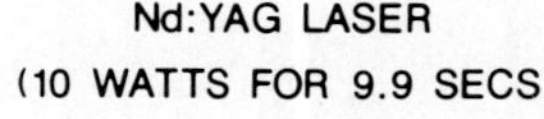

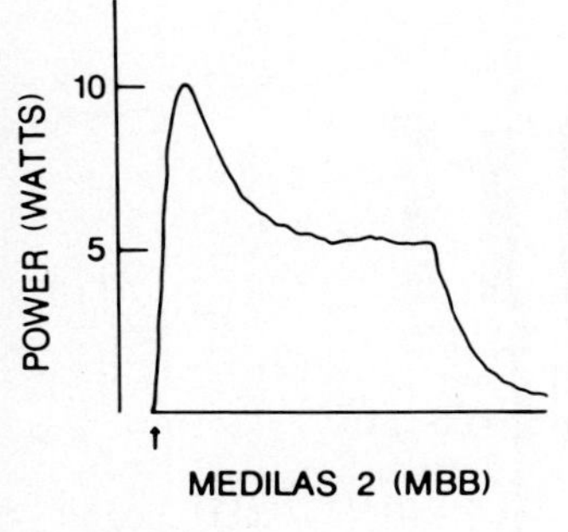

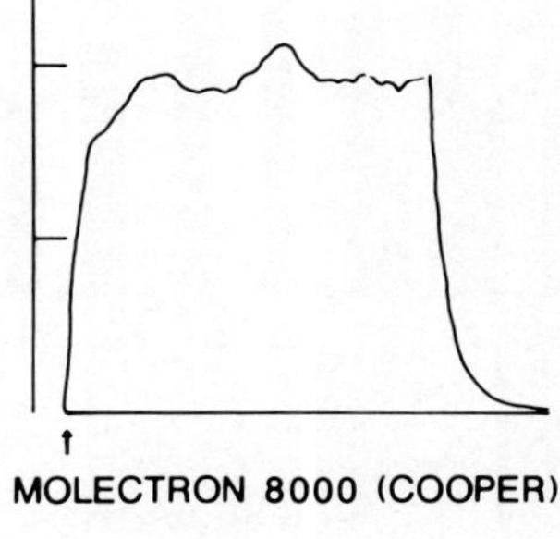

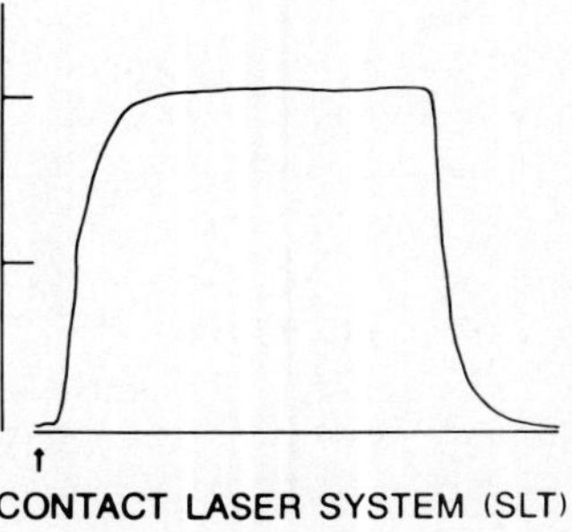

Figure 9.2. A comparison of the stability of three commercially available Nd:YAG lasers at 10 W for 9.9 sec.

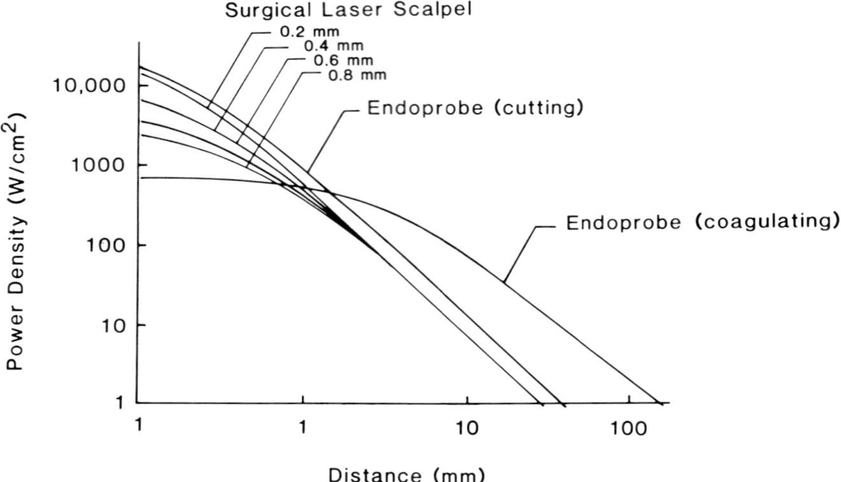

Figure 9.3. Power density delivered to tissue by laser surgical scalpels with distal tip diameters of 0.2–0.8 mm. The maximum power is delivered when the probe is in direct contact with tissue but rapidly decreases as the probe is moved away from the tissue.

well to the right of this ligament. Across this line little, if any, anastomosis took place. Five ligaments attach the liver to the anterior abdominal wall and the diaphragm. Four are peritoneal folds: the falciform, coronary, and two triangular ligaments; the fifth is a fibrous cord, the round ligament (Fig. 9.13).

The liver is divided into eight segments by three main fissures and by the distribution of its vascular and ductal anatomy. The main fissure

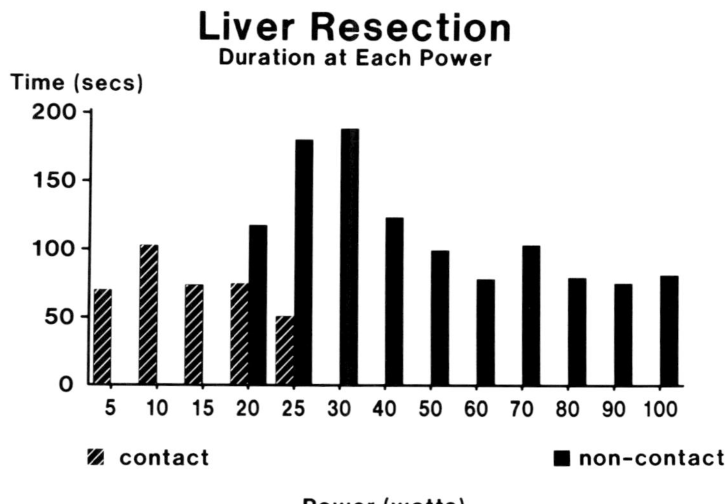

Figure 9.4. Operating time to perform a liver resection using either contact or noncontact methods of laser energy delivery at different power levels.

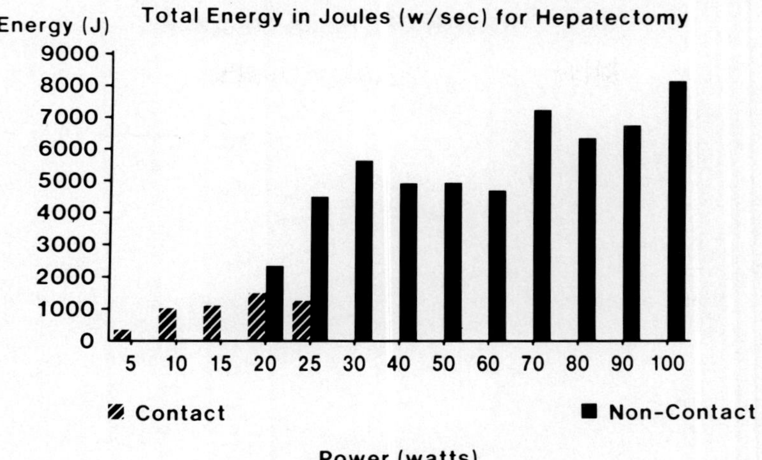

Figure 9.5. Total energy required to perform a hepatectomy using either contact or noncontact methods of laser energy delivery.

passes from the upper end of the inferior vena cava superiorly to the gallbladder fossa inferiorly. The left (umbilical) fissure corresponds to the attachment of the falciform ligament and the right fissure passes in a coronal plane from the right lateral surface to the vena cava. The vascular pedicles play a part in delineating the segments. The portal triad (hepatic artery, portal vein, and bile duct) branch primarily at the porta and then continue to branch intrahepatically. They are contained in a perivascular fibrous capsule (Glisson) in their intrahepatic course. The hepatic veins have very little perivascular investments and lie in more intimate contact with the liver tissue anterior to the triad throughout much of their course.

INDICATIONS (TABLE 9.1)

Hepatic resection is indicated for hepatic carcinoma, cysts, and adenomas, gallbladder or bowel carcinomas in continuity, hemangiomas, or traumatic rupture of the liver parenchyma. Metastases within the liver are solitary lesions or, if multiple, are technically easy to resect provided the primary colon carcinoma has been removed. Possible hemorrhage associated with the giant hemangi-

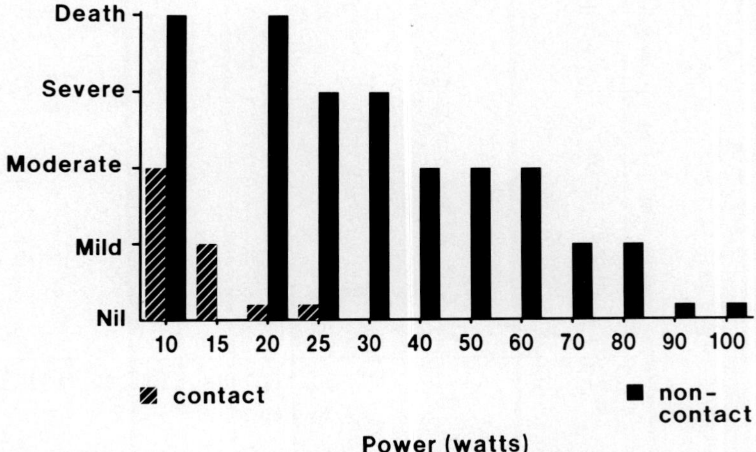

Figure 9.6. Blood loss in performing a liver resection in experimental animals (rats).

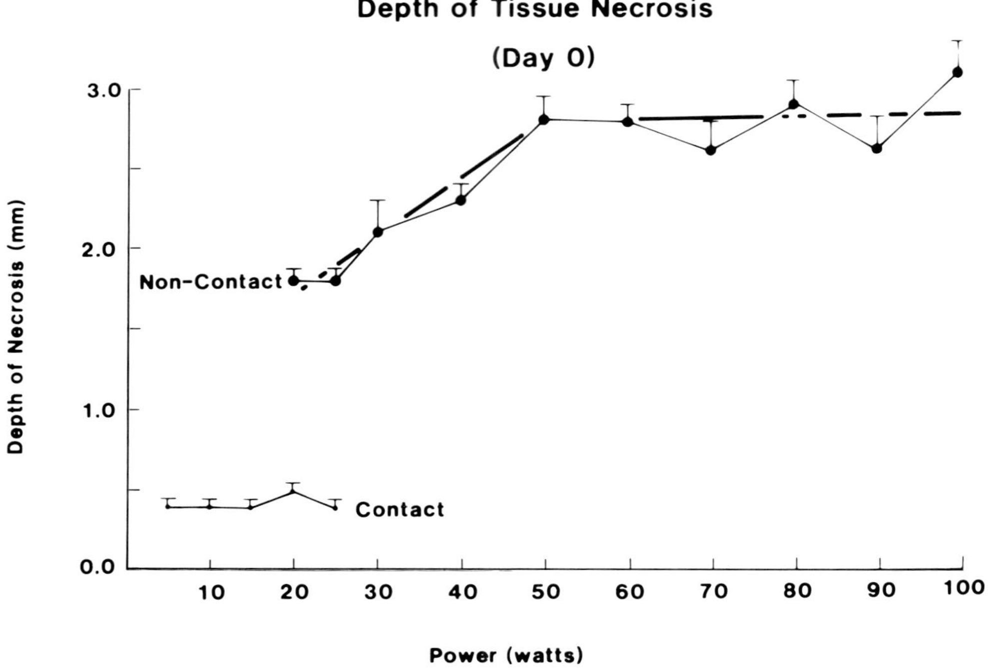

Figure 9.7. Depth of thermal tissue necrosis (mm) during resection of the liver (zero hours) with the contact and noncontact methods using the Nd:YAG laser at various power levels. The tissue damage is measured lateral to the resection edge.

omas and the probability of malignant degeneration in adenomas are the main reasons for their excision. Resection for massive traumatic rupture confined to an anatomic lobe is usually preferred if multiple mattress sutures are inadequate in controlling blood loss.

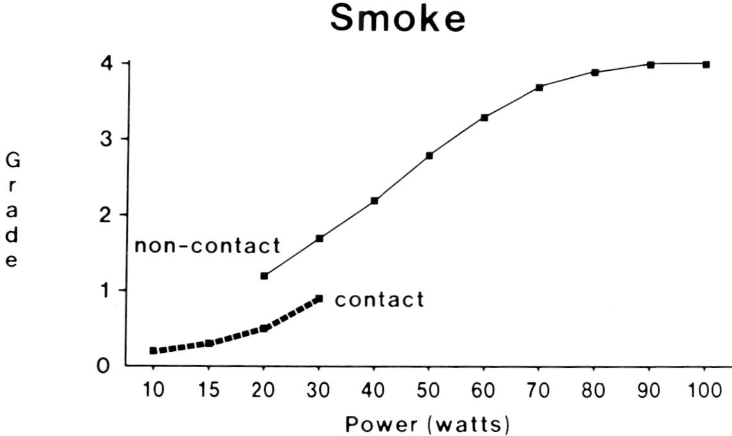

Figure 9.8. Smoke produced (''laser plume'') during liver resection. Graded semiquantitatively from grade 0, no smoke, to 4, which was malodorous requiring a smoke evacuator.

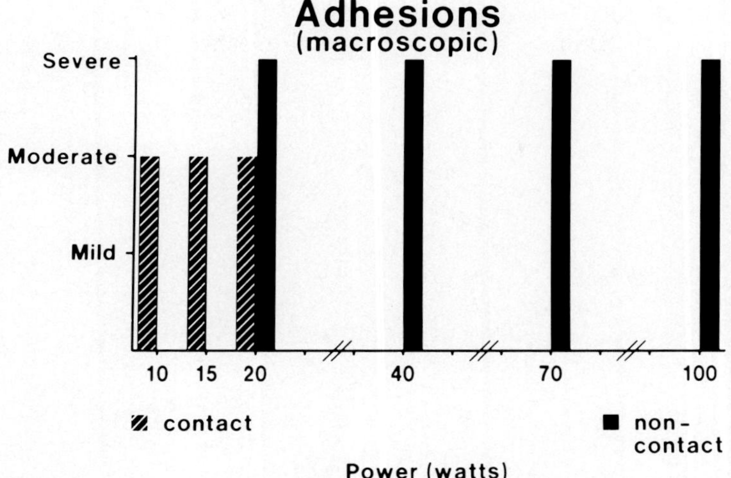

Figure 9.9. Adhesions to resected liver surface found at 15 days postoperatively. Graded semiquantitatively from mild, flimsy attachments, to severe which required sharp dissection with bleeding to separate adhesions from the liver surface.

PREOPERATIVE PREPARATION

In patients with liver trauma, the primary preoperative considerations are maintenance of an adequate blood volume and assessment and treatment of associated injuries. The majority of patients undergoing elective hepatic resection have normal liver function. Evaluation includes ultrasound, computed tomography (CT) scanning, nuclear magnetic resonance imaging (MRI) scan, and hepatic angiography. Full bowel preparation, vitamin K, propolylactic antibiotics, and correction of clotting factors should be undertaken. A percutaneously ultrasound-guided fine needle aspiration for both histological and cytological examination will often give a preoperative diagnosis (11). Laparoscopy may help in the assessment.

ANESTHESIA

Careful preoperative preparation, control of blood volume and blood pressure, venous and arterial pressure monitoring, Swan-Ganz catheters for pulmonary wedge pressures, monitoring of urinary output, and avoidance of hypoxia are im-

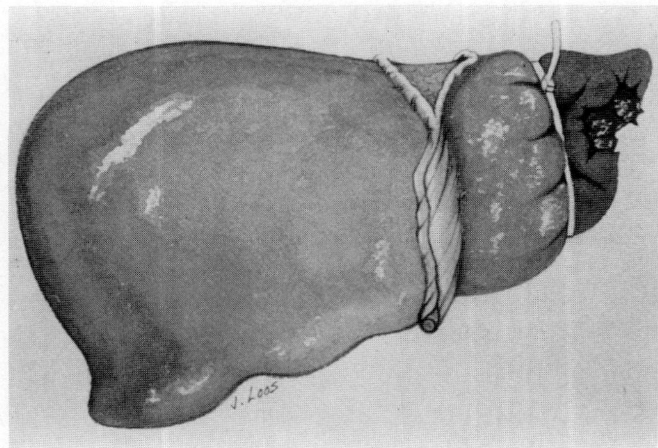

Figure 9.10. Liver strapper for use as proximal tourniquet.

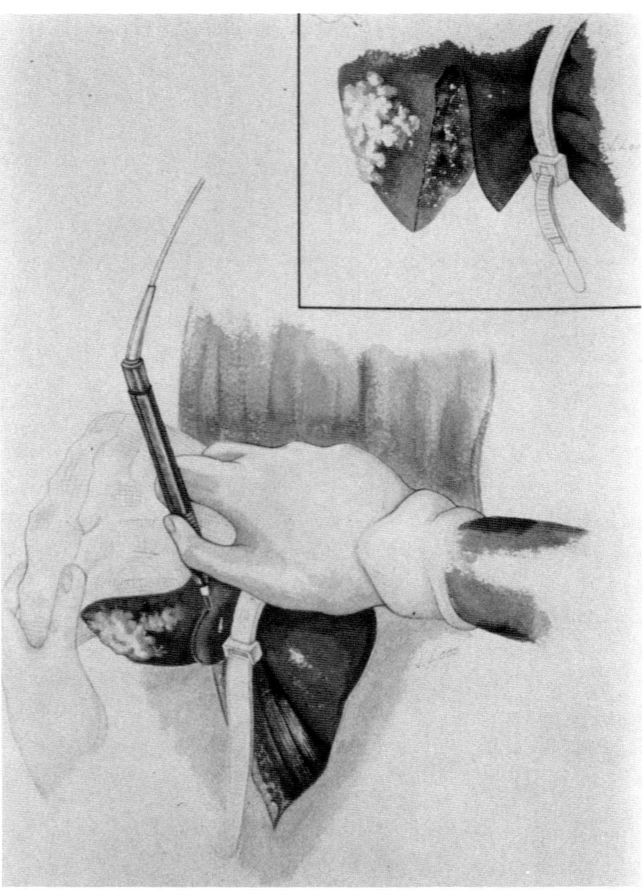

Figure 9.11. Hepatic resection with contact laser scalpel with proximal liver strapper.

portant. Potentially hepatotoxic drugs should not be used in patients undergoing massive liver resection. Adequate amounts of fresh whole blood and fresh frozen plasma must be available.

INCISION AND TECHNIQUE

Several incisions can be used but a bilateral subcostal (rooftop) or transverse supraumbilical incision is preferred. This can be extended into the chest through the seventh or eighth ribs on the right side. The diaphragm is incised and the phrenic nerve preserved to prevent diaphragmmatic paralysis. A midline abdominal incision extended up as a median sternotomy also provides good exposure.

The SLT Contact Laser Scalpel with a 0.2- to 0.4-mm diameter SLT Frosted Probe is used for the incision of subcutaneous tissue, muscle, fascia, and peritoneum. Skin is either incised with a steel scalpel or the laser scalpel. Power settings are 12–20 W with the laser set in the continuous wave (CW) and controlled by the foot switch. Coaxial air or CO_2 is used to cool the interphase between the quartz fiber and the synthetic sapphire probe. Water is never used.

The *principles* of using the SLT Contact Laser System are as follows:

1. Laser power is *on* as the probe of the scalpel comes into contact with tissue and the laser is *off* as the probe comes off the tissue. If probe sticks to tissue it means that the power via the foot pedal was disengaged before the probe came off the tissue. One must not pull the

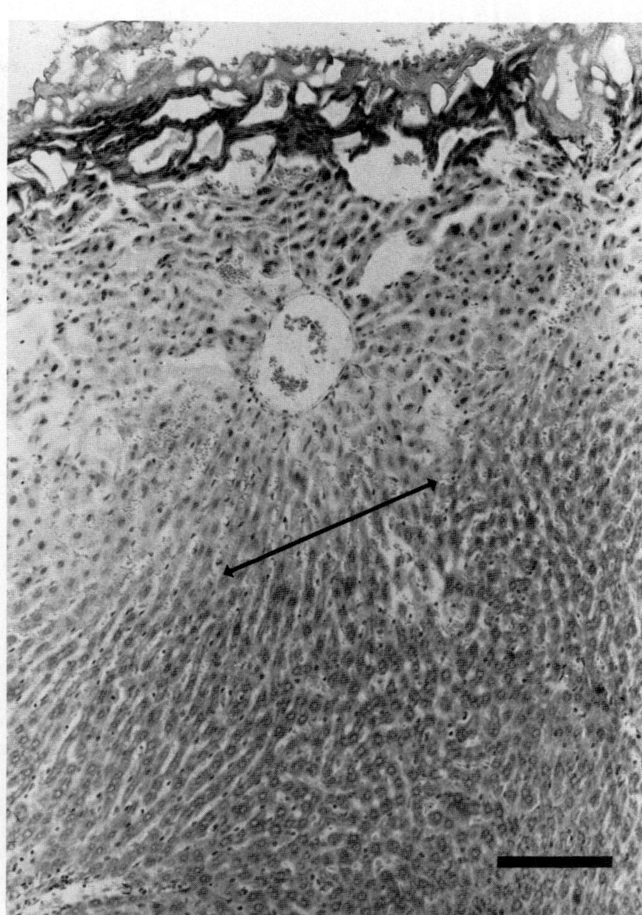

Figure 9.12. Contact laser-resected liver sample (Eosin stain) taken at time of operation using 20 W of laser power. The surface is composed of dense structureless protein coagulum containing minimal carbon deposits. Beneath the surface layer are highly condensed hepatocytes with pyknotic nuclei. Fluid-filled vesicles are present in these two layers. A band of eosinophilic killed cells extends approximately 0.5 mm (*arrow* is transition zone). The bar represents 85 μm.

probe off the tissue. Re-engage the laser and the heat will allow the probe to come off the tissue easily. Furthermore, laser power must not be on while the probe is not in direct contact with tissue. This may cause irreversible damage to the crystalline structure of the probe. If the probe begins to glow a white color at its distal tip the laser must be immediately disengaged. If not, within several seconds the tip will melt into a globular shape and the laser effect will be significantly diminished. If this occurs, the probe should be discarded and replaced with a new proble. The globular shape can be both seen as well as felt digitally.

2. Tissue adherent to the probe can be easily wiped off with a dry gauze swab. However, this is not usually necessary because adherent tissue does not cause much impairment to the laser function. The adherent tissue will become carbonized and burn off. Immediately after use the probe is hot and should be allowed to cool for 20-30 sec before being wiped with a wet sponge dipped in sterile water, saline, or hydrogen peroxide. Alcohol should not be used nor should the probe be cleaned with an abrasive material during the procedure.
3. The laser scalpel is not a mechanical cutting instrument. A ''light touch'' technique with gentle pressure is required to obtain cutting and coagulating effects. The laser energy must be allowed to do the incising. The more mechanical pressure used the less effective is the instrument. The probe, therefore, moved slowly and gently over the

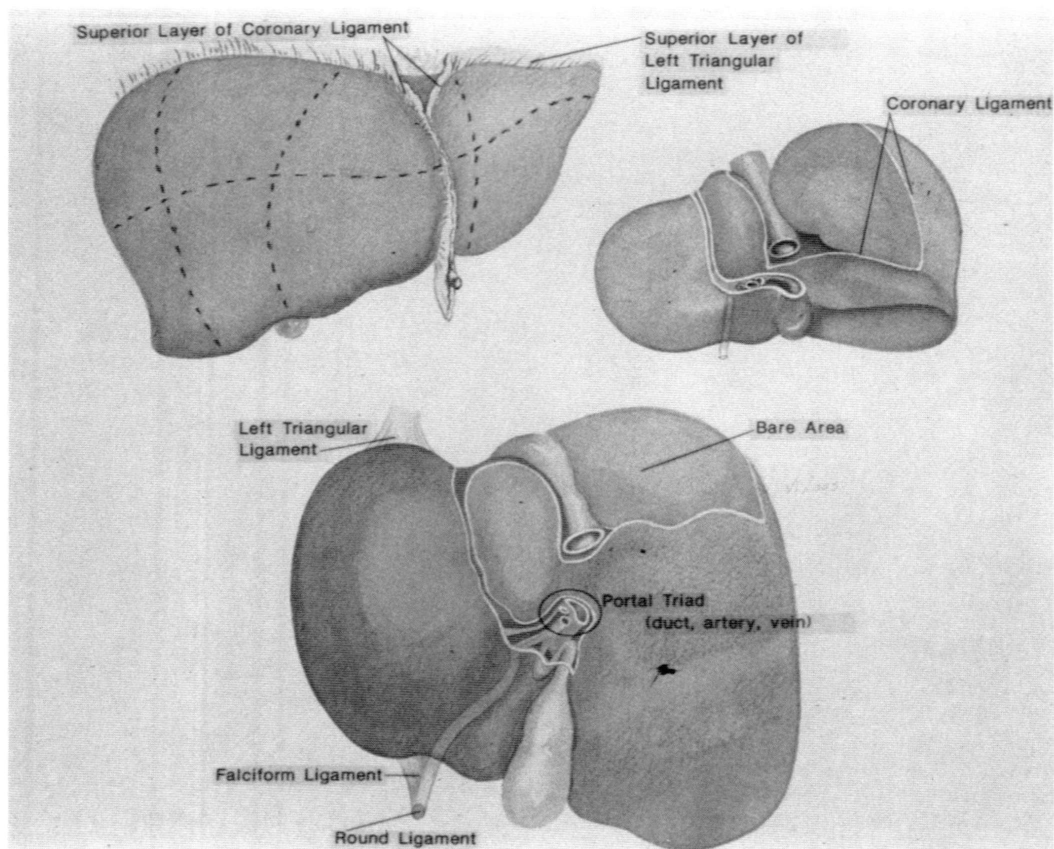

Figure 9.13. Normal anatomy of liver showing ligaments, portal triad, and anatomical liver lobes.

tissue in a continuous motion without "scratching."

4. Traction and countertraction must be maintained at right angles to the incision at all times either by manual pressure or using retracting instruments.
5. The laser power is controlled by the laser foot pedal in the continuous wave (cw) mode. This requires the surgeon to use an "eye-hand-foot" coordination.
6. The laser power is set initially at 15 W and the power is increased or decreased at 2-W increments until the desired tissue effect is obtained. The frosted laser probe with a tip diameter of 1.0–1.2 mm is used for liver resections.
7. Major blood vessels are ligated or clipped. The technique for coagulating vessels 1–3 mm in size is to run the probe initially parallel to and on either side of the vessel to allow shrinkage and coagulation before transsection. If bleeding occurs, this can be stopped using the lateral side of the frosted probe by "painting" or the vessel is caught in a hemostat and the side of the probe is applied directly to the transsected vessel surface.
8. Initially, the cutting process will appear slower than a steel knife but the major advantage is a *hemostatic* incision that does not need electrocautery or sutures. Increasing the speed of cutting can be obtained by increasing the power.

The technique of contact laser surgery is rapidly learned and experience is obtained by using the equipment frequently.

Table 9.1. Indications for Liver Surgery Using SLT Contact YAG Laser System

Tumors
  Benign
    Solid
      Hepatic cell adenoma
    Cystic
      Hemangioma
  Malignant
    Primary
      Hepatocellular carcinoma
      Cholangiocarcinoma
    Secondary
      Colon
      Carcinoid
Cysts
  Nonparasitic
  Parasitic
    Hydatid
Abscess
Trauma
  Blunt
  Penetrating

PROCEDURES

Resection of the liver with the SLT Contact Laser System can either be anatomical or nonanatomical (Table 9.2).

Anatomical Liver Resection

Right Hepatic Lobectomy

The line of liver resection extends from the gallbladder bed to the inferior vena cava. Dissection is begun in the hilar region. The gallbladder is removed after division of the cystic artery and duct. The branches of the hepatic artery, portal vein, and bile ducts are carefully identified. The right hepatic duct and artery are ligated. If in doubt, a temporary occlusion is performed. If both the arterial and venous supply to the right lobe are occluded, a line of color demarcation corresponding to the anatomical division between the right and left lobes extending from the midpoint of the gallbladder fossa to the inferior vena cava is seen.

The right branch of the portal vein is doubly ligated and divided. The liver is rotated down and to the left to expose the inferior vena cava and the right hepatic veins. The right hepatic vein is ligated and divided carefully as it is extremely short and easily torn. The line of liver resection is now marked out using the laser scalpel leaving a margin of avascular liver for later identification of the middle hepatic vein.

Dissection with the activated laser scalpel is begun just to the right of the center of the gallbladder fossa. The dissection is continued at a slight angle toward the left, following the trunk of the middle hepatic vein in the interlobar fissure.

Contact laser dissection is continued more into the liver substance, controlling the tributaries of the heptatic veins as they pass into the right lobe. This dissection is then carried down to the vena cava. This technique leaves a small amount of devitalized liver tissue along the margin with preservation of the middle hepatic vein in the interlobar fissure. After the vena cava is reached, the right lobe is freed of its remaining attachments and removed. The new surface of the liver, if oozing, is "painted" over with the side of the laser scalpel. Large bleeding vessels are suture ligated and decompression of the biliary tree with a T-tube is not necessary. Catheter-type sump drains are placed in the wound and the incision is closed in layers.

Left Hepatic Lobectomy

The preoperative preparation, anesthesia, position, incision, and exposure are the same as for the right hepatic lobectomy. The middle hepatic vein is the guideline for resection within the hepatic parenchyma and should be preserved. Mobilization of the ductal structures proceeds in the same order as for the right lobectomy. It is convenient to remove the gallbladder early on. The left triangular ligament is divided to mobilize the superior surface of the left lobe. By medial and downward traction on the liver, the hepatic veins are exposed. The left hepatic vein is carefully dissected into the liver substance. This locates the entrance of the middle hepatic vein. The left hepatic vein is carefully ligated and divided. Contact laser dissection is used to divide the liver substance, beginning just to the left of the gallbladder fossa and proceeding to the vena cava, leaving behind a border of the left lobe. The left lobe is freed of its remaining attachments and removed.

Left Lateral Segmental Resection

The same incision as done previously is used. The left branches of the portal triad *must not be ligated* or divided as it results in devitalization of the medial segment of the left lobe. The line of

Table 9.2. Operative Procedures in Liver with SLT Contact YAG Laser System

Disorder	Morbidity and Mortality	Treatment
Hepatic adenoma	Secondary intraabdominal hemorrhage	Resection
Hemobilia	20% mortality	Resection of hepatic segment with fistula
Hemangioma	Usually incidental; if large, will rupture	Resection if large
Hepatocellular carcinoma (hepatoma)	High mortality	Resection
Metastatic nodules	Depends on primary malignancy and time interval	Enucleation if single and no other sites of metastases; resection if multiple and technically possible
Unknown lesions	Depends on pathology	Excision, incision, biopsy, or wedge resection
Hydatid cyst	Cyst rupture and infection	Excision
Amebic abscess	Spread	Drainage
Pyogenic abscess	Fatal if untreated	Drainage
Trauma	Depends on extent and associated injuries	Nothing to major resection

laser dissection should be approximately 1 cm to the left of the falciform ligament to avoid damaging the structures of the medial segment of the left lobe and the left branch of the portal vein. In this resection, the laser scalpel obviates the need for blunt dissection or multiple sutures through the liver. Individual large vessels are ligated. The falciform ligament can provide a peritoneal surface for covering the raw area of the liver. If oozing persists, the cut surface of the liver can be gently "painted" over using the side of the frosted laser scalpel.

Mesohepatectomy

A median hepatectomy is a method for resection of hilar cholangiocarcinomas, obtaining access to bile ducts for anastomosis or in the treatment of carcinoma of the gallbladder. The contact laser scalpel facilitates this anatomical procedure.

Nonanatomical Liver Resections

Benign Solid Tumor

Surgical resection of hepatic adenomas is recommended due to the high incidence of hemorrhage, rupture, or both. If ruptured, emergency surgical resection of the tumor-bearing liver with the laser scalpel is necessary to control bleeding. Wedge resection or hepatic lobectomy, resulting in complete removal of the tumor, can be accomplished with a minimum of risk (Fig. 9.14).

Nonparasitic Cysts

Small cysts discovered incidentally at surgical exploration or on CT scans require no treatment. Large cysts causing symptoms can be treated by surgical excision. If the cyst contains clear fluid and is difficult to excise because of the proximity to vascular or ductal structures, the cyst may be unroofed with the laser scalpel. Cystadenomas, cystadenocarcinomas, and cysts associated with other neoplasms are excised with the laser scalpel.

Hemangioma

A cavernous hemangioma is the most common benign tumor of the liver and small symptomatic lesions require no treatment. The SLT coagulating or SLT vaporization contact laser probe can be used. Symptomatic lesions require resection and the procedure depends on site and size. Pedunculated lesions are easily resected with the laser scalpel whereas large sessile tumors may re-

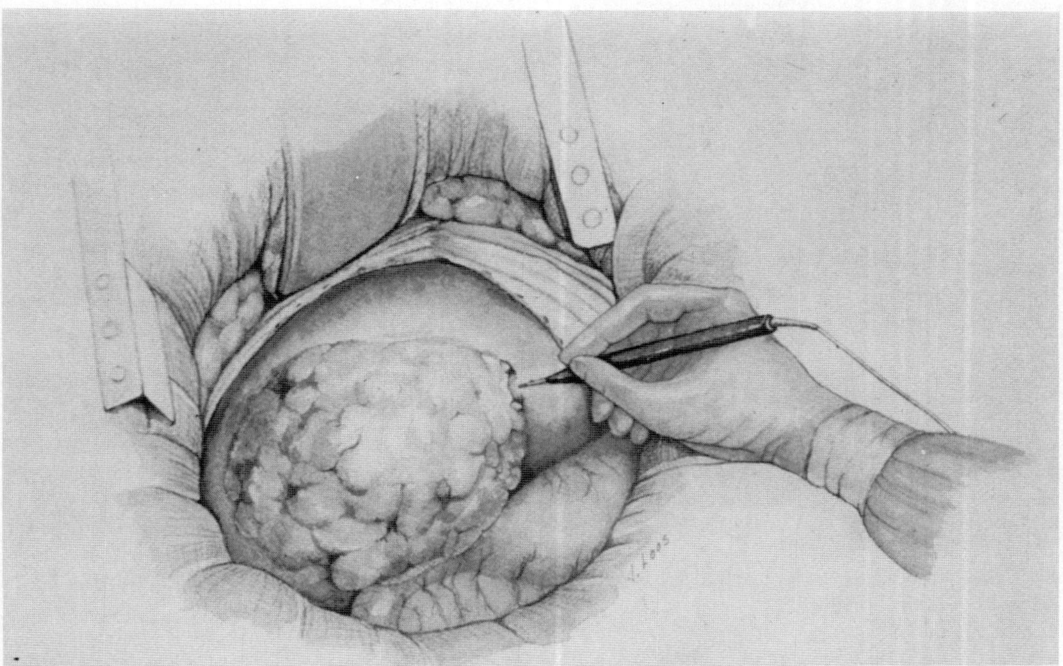

Figure 9.14. Schematic representation of a nonanatomical right hepatic resection of a solid tumor using the contact laser scalpel.

quire an anatomical resection. Multiple small superficial lesions are easily excised by multiple wedge resections with the frosted laser scalpel.

Hepatocellular Carcinoma

Tumors less than 3 cm in diameter should be resected nonanatomically with a good margin of normal liver. Results of local wedge resection versus lobectomy are similar. For larger symptomatic tumors, the goal is to excise the tumor if possible. A standard laser hepatic lobectomy or extended hepatic resection is performed. However, in the case of extrahepatic spread or where resection is not advisable, patients are treated with chemotherapy or radiation therapy or both. The prognosis in this group is not good.

Metastatic Tumors

The most common metastatic tumor is from the colon. The 5-year survival rate in patients with resectable hepatic metastases is reported as high as 22% after concomitant hepatic resection (either during the initial surgery or as a staged procedure). The degree of liver involvement has been correlated with the survival rate: (*a*) patients with less than 25% of the liver replaced by tumor; (*b*) patients with 25–75% of the liver replaced by tumor; and (*c*) patients with greater than 75% of the liver replaced by tumor. The median survival in groups *a*, *b*, and *c* is 6.2 months, 5.5 months, and 3.4 months, respectively. Improved survival after surgical resection of hepatic metastases at 3 years is 73%, 60%, and 29% in groups *a*, *b*, and *c*, respectively. Carcinoembryonic antigen (CEA) determination should be periodically performed in the follow-up care of these patients. Any sudden rise may indicate a new metastatic lesion.

Surgical treatment improves survival when the hepatic lesion is the only metastatic lesion. Complete curative resection of the primary lesion and resection of the metastases, therefore, are recommended. When hepatic metastases involve both lobes of the liver or when extrahepatic spread exists, surgical resection is not always indicated. Tumor debulking and excision of multiple liver metastases has been carried out using the laser scalpel with minimum blood loss (Fig. 9.15).

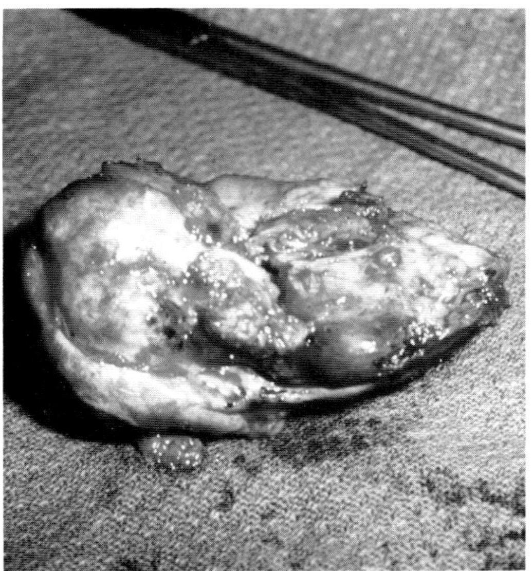

Figure 9.15. Nonanatomically resected hepatocellular carcinoma with surrounding normal liver tissue.

These patients may also receive chemotherapy. Direct intrahepatic artery infusion is occasionally used to treat the liver metastases. The ultimate prognosis is guarded, and the mean survival time is about 8–10 months but may be prolonged with resection of the metastases. Multiple liver metastases can be enucleated with a surrounding rim of normal liver tissue (Fig. 9.16) and superficial metastases can be vaporized using the "rounded" contact probe.

Trauma To The Liver

The overall mortality rate in blunt hepatic injury is about 9%. Mortality rates have improved over the last several decades, directly related to better prehospital transportation, resuscitation, operative management, and postoperative care.

A rapid intraabdominal exploration is performed and the liver is carefully inspected for lacerations and active bleeding. Posterior inspection requires mobilizing the liver after the triangular and falciform ligaments are divided. In small, superficial lacerations hemostasis is obtained by simple tamponade and by using the painting technique with the side of the frosted laser scalpel. Larger and deeper lacerations may require suture ligatures and laser photocoagulation to achieve hemostasis. Drainage is necessary postoperatively.

In central deep hepatic injuries with active bleeding, laser hepatotomy may be necessary to expose the depth of the wound and to identify the bleeding vessels. Suture ligation of larger vessels is performed and smaller vessels are laser coagulated. If ischemic, nonviable fragments of injured hepatic parenchyma are detected, resectional debridement is performed with the laser scalpel. A formal lobectomy or segmentectomy is rarely

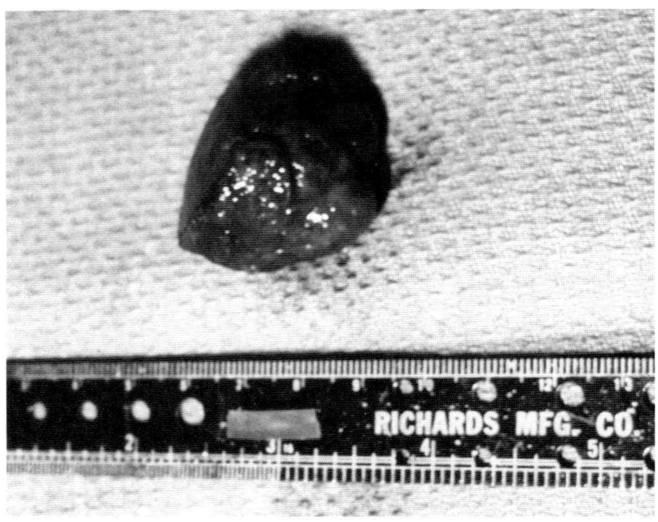

Figure 9.16. Local excision of a liver metastasis using the contact laser scalpel. Multiple metastases can be enucleated from both right and left lobes.

necessary (<10%), except when extensive parenchymal damage is encountered.

POSTOPERATIVE CARE

Careful attention should be given to postoperative blood volume maintenance. Arterial, central venous, and Swan-Ganz pressure catheters are useful. To avoid hepatic anoxia, ventilation should be adjusted using arterial blood gases as a guideline. Serial hematocrit and coagulation profiles should be obtained. Copious drainage may be encountered from the operative site and, therefore, the drain sites must be inspected ensure that they are draining freely. Delayed hemorrhage is considerably reduced using the SLT contact YAG laser system.

Each patient having undergone a massive liver resection should be treated postoperatively as if hepatic insufficiency existed. Albumin (50–75 daily) should be given and vitamin K administered parentally daily. Hyperalimentation is necessary to ensure adequate calories and intake of amino acids, vitamins, and minerals. Antibiotics that have high concentrations in bile are given. Serial blood sugars should be obtained to determine the early onset of postresection hypoglycemia. Serial determinations of SGOT, SGPT, LDH, alkaline phosphatase, and total bilirubin should be obtained to detect early signs of hepatic decompensation, in which event vigorous treatment must be instituted.

After major hepatic resection, significant enlargement of both splenic and hepatic remnants may occur secondary to a reduction in hepatic outflow. Although splenomegaly may be demonstrated radiographically for 6–8 weeks, clinically apparent hypersplenism does not develop. Rapid liver regeneration occurs which is easily followed using serial ultrasound and CT scans.

In conclusion, liver resections can be technically difficult and associated with problems in control of bleeding. All new techniques need to be critically evaluated. The use of the strapper with the SLT Contact YAG Laser System appears to be the most promising. Larger clinical studies are needed to evaluate its application in human liver surgery.

REFERENCES

1. Sisto ME, Vogt DP, Herman RE. Hepatic resection in 128 patients: A 24 year experience. Surgery 1987; 102:846-851.
2. Bradpiece HA, Benjamin IS, Halevy A, Blumgart LH. Major hepatic resection for colo-rectal liver metastases Br J Surg 1987; 74:324-326.
3. Fidler JP, Hoeter RW, Polyani TG, et al. Laser surgery in exsanguinating liver injury. Ann Surg 1975; 181:74-80.
4. Meyer H-J, Haverkampf K. Experimental study of partial liver resection with a combined CO_2 and Nd:YAG laser. Lasers Surg Med 1982; 2:149-154.
5. Sultan RA, Fallouh H, Lefebvre-Vilardebo M, Ladouch-Badre A. Separate and combined use of Nd:YAG and carbon dioxide lasers in liver resections: A preliminary report. Lasers Med Sci 1986; 1:101-105.
6. Tranberg KG, Rigotti P, Brackett KA, Bjornson HP, Fischer JE, Joffe SN. Liver resection. A comparison using the Nd:YAG laser, ultrasonic aspirator, or blunt dissection. Am J Surg 1985; 151:368-372.
7. Daikuzono N, Joffe SN. An artificial sapphire probe for contact photocoagulation and tissue vaporization. Med Instrument 1985; 19:173-178.
8. Joffe SN. Contact neodymium:YAG laser surgery in gastroenterology: A preliminary report. Lasers Surg Med 1986; 6:155-157.
9. Joffe SN, Brackett KA, Sankar MY, Daikuzono, N. Resection of the liver with the Nd:YAG laser. Surg Gynecol Obstet 1986; 163:437-442.
10. Schroder T, Sankar MY, Brackett KM, Booth A, Joffe SN. Major liver resection in the pig using contact Nd:YAG laser—a new technique. Third International Nd:YAG Laser Symposium, Tokyo, November 1-3, 1986.
11. Craggs-Hall MA, Lees WR. Fine needle biopsy: Cytology, histology or both? Gut 1987; 88:233-236.

CHAPTER

10

Lasers in Pancreatic Surgery

Tom Schröder, O. Juhani Rämö

The extended knowledge of pancreatic diseases has increased the indications for pancreatic surgery. The trend in recent years for the treatment of pancreatic carcinoma and, occasionally, for pancreatitis has been toward total pancreatectomy. Total pancreatectomy with duodenal preservation has also been recommended for the treatment of chronic pancreatitis, but the technique used in this procedure should be refined (1). In addition, the pancreas is now also being harvested for transplantation. Pancreatic operations, however, are often associated with technical difficulties due to the anatomy and blood supply of the pancreas. Clinical operations are time-consuming and blood loss can be considerable (2, 3). Thus, any operative technique that can reduce operating time, blood loss, and associated morbidity and mortality would be advantageous.

The ability of the laser to cut tissue without attendant hemorrhage makes it a promising tool for resection of highly vascularized solid organs, such as the pancreas (4). Many different types of lasers are currently available, but they have different effects on the tissue of the pancreas and all of them are not suitable for pancreatic surgery.

EXPERIMENTAL PANCREATIC SURGERY

Total pancreatectomies are performed in experimental studies of pancreatic transplantation and also to evaluate new techniques that may later be used in clinical situations (5). Most of these studies have been performed in dogs because they are easy to house and they can be used for long-term studies. The pig is considerably cheaper as an experimental animal and easy to handle, but only few groups have reported studies using pigs in total pancreatectomies (5–7).

In the dog, the uncinate process lies free in the mesentery (Fig. 10.1). The most difficult region to dissect in the dog is surrounding the pancreaticoduodenal vessels, i.e., the duodenal part. This anatomical relationship between the blood vessels and the pancreas is not seen in the pig or human (Fig. 10.2). There is a recent report, however, that the operation in the dog could be performed by resecting the pancreaticoduodenal vessels with the pancreas if only the duodenal branch is identified and spared (8). Total pancreatectomy can be done easily in the pig and the anatomy is much like that of humans (Fig. 10.3). The pancreas lies close to the caval and the portal veins, and the uncinate process is under the portal vein where it joins the body of the pancreas.

The laser has been suggested to offer a new therapeutic modality in the performance of tedious and often difficult pancreatic surgery (4). The Nd:YAG laser diminishes operating time and the number of ligatures required in total pancreatectomy in dogs (9). Furthermore, the new contact Nd:YAG method has been demonstrated to be as precise and safe as conventional techniques in the dog (10) and it has been used successfully in total pancreatectomy in the dog and pig (11).

The CO_2 laser has been used as a laser scalpel since it was first introduced into surgery. It has also been used in experimental studies on pancreatic surgery (12), but its hemostatic effect has been found to be unsatisfactory (13). The development of the contact Nd:YAG laser added a new dimension to surgery. The contact method provides a precise incision and dissection by the use of a sapphire tip and the good coagulation properties of the Nd:YAG laser (14). Recently, the contact Nd:YAG laser technique was compared with the noncontact Nd:YAG method and with the conventional electrocautery technique. Proximal pancreatectomy was performed in dogs and only a small portion of the pancreatic tail was left in situ.

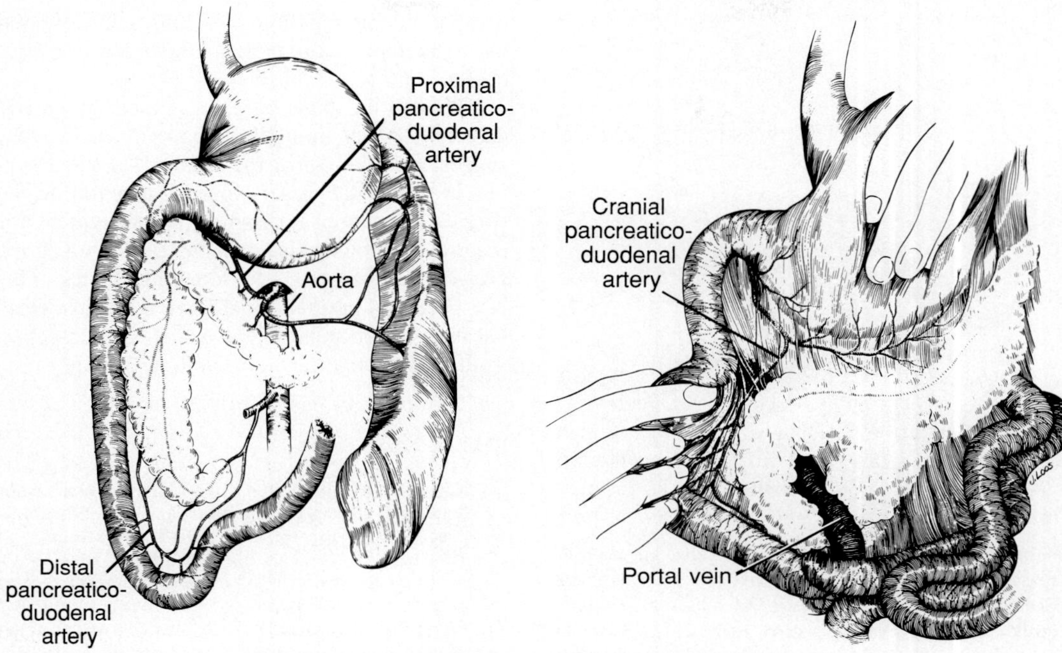

Figure 10.1. The pancreas of the dog is composed of two lobes. The right lobe receives its blood supply from the distal mesoduodenal arcade and the mesoduodenal vessels. The proximal part of the right lobe encloses the main pancreatic duct and the proximal pancreaticoduodenal vessels. (From Schröder T, Rämö OJ, Joffe SN: Laser pancreatectomy—a comparison between the dog and pig. Res Exp Med 1988; 227–233.)

Figure 10.2. The pancreas of the pig is closely related to the portal vein. The cranial pancreaticoduodenal artery supplies the head and body of the pancreas, whereas the tail of the pancreas receives its arterial supply from branches of the splenic artery. (From Schröder T, Rämö OJ, Joffe SN: Laser pancreatectomy—a comparison between the dog and pig. Res Exp Med 1988; 227–233.)

The electrocautery technique (''bovie'') was used, which is a modification of the conventional ligature technique. The small vessels were coagulated, and vessels that were too big to coagulate were ligated. Both the bovie and the contact Nd:YAG laser were technically superior to the noncontact Nd:YAG. The latter was slower and caused more bleeding and smoke than the other methods.

Histologically, the thermal injury to the pancreas by the contact Nd:YAG was milder in comparison with the noncontact Nd:YAG method (10). No severe acute time damage was seen in the pancreatic stump that was left at the operation. On the contrary, after cutting with the two other devices, extensive coagulative energy had to be applied to the resected surface to stop bleeding, which resulted in a thick, necrotic pancreatic stump. This was probably the reason for hemorrhagic pancreatitis resulting in death in two animals in the noncontact and bovie groups (10).

A recent study in rats demonstrated that electrocautery and various lasers have almost similar tissue effects on the pancreas (13). The thermal damage, however, was most extensive after the use of the noncontact Nd:YAG laser, whereas the contact method of this laser caused thermal injury at a significantly deeper level than did electrocautery or CO_2 laser. Based on the results of this experimental study, it seems that the noncontact Nd:YAG laser may not be suitable for pancreatic surgery.

CLINICAL PANCREATIC SURGERY

The data concerning the use of lasers in clinical surgery of the pancreas are limited. Until now, only one report can be found in the literature in which 2 patients with pancreatic disease had been treated with the Nd:YAG laser (4). One was a young man with an insulinoma at the junction of

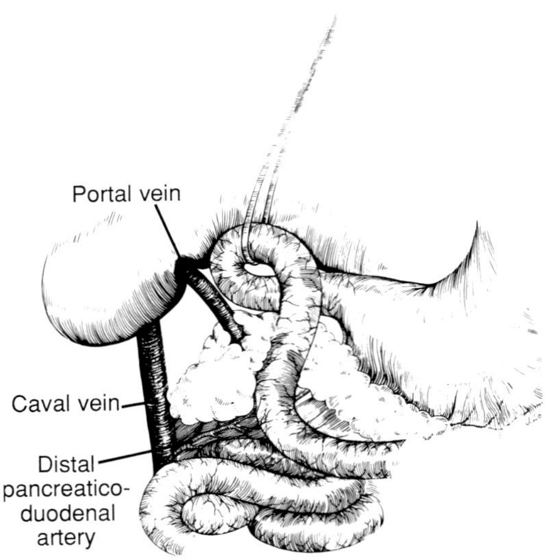

Figure 10.3. The uncinate process of the porcine pancreas continues under the portal vein to join the body of the pancreas. The uncinate process receives its arterial supply from the distal pancreaticoduodenal artery. (From Schröder T, Rämö OJ, Joffe SN: Laser pancreatectomy—a comparison between the dog and pig. Res Exp Med 1988; 227–233.)

the body and neck of the pancreas, and the other one was a young woman having protracted pancreatobiliary problems caused by chronic pancreatitis. Both of them underwent pancreatic resection (50% and 80%, respectively) with preservation of the head of the pancreas and the duodenal loop. After lifting the pancreas from its inferior border, the dissection of the superior border was performed easily using the noncontact Nd:YAG laser. The power was between 60 and 70 W for 1–2 sec in duration.

The postoperative period was uneventful in both patients. The acute histology of the resected human pancreas demonstrated the similar tissue effects as reported in experimental studies with the exception of the depth of penetration of the acidophilic cells in zone 3, which reached a depth of 3.5 mm (4).

It seems that the Nd:YAG laser using the contact probe may relatively easily resect the head of the pancreas with preservation of the duodenum. However, no clinical data on this procedure are yet available. Other innovative procedures include drainage of pancreatic pseudocysts by performing an endoscopic laser cystogastrostomy and endoscopic papillotomies, but more research has to be done before these methods can be evaluated.

Although the experiences in clinical pancreatic surgery are very limited, the experimental results suggest that the use of the contact Nd:YAG system in pancreatic surgery offers a new tool to the surgical armature. It provides an instrument for precise dissection and coagulation with good preservation of normal surrounding tissues. This is especially important in surgery of the pancreas because the procedure involves delicate dissection from vitally important surrounding vessels.

REFERENCES

1. Rossi RL, Breasch JW, O'Bryan EM, Watkins E Jr. Segmental pancreatic autotransplantation for chronic pancreatitis. Gastroenterology 1983; 84:621-626.
2. Traverso LW, Tomkins RK, Urrea PT, Longmire WP Jr. Surgical treatment of chronic pancreatitis. Ann Surg 1979; 190:312-319.
3. White TT, Slavotinek AH. Results of surgical treatment of chronic pancreatitis. Ann Surg 1979; 189:217-224.
4. Joffe SN, Sankar MY. Lasers in hepato-biliary and pancreatic surgery. In: Shapsay SM, Ed. Endoscopic Laser Surgery Handbook. New York: Marcel Dekker, 1986.
5. Kretschmer GJ, Sutherland DE, Matas AJ, Payne WD, Najarian JS. Autotransplantation of pancreatic fragments to the portal vein and spleen of totally pancreatectomized dogs: A comparative evaluation. Ann Surg 1978; 187:79-86.
6. Hoorn van WA, Vinik AI, Hoorn-Hickman R, Terblanche J. The effect of feeding and starvation upon immunoreactive glucagon in the pancreatectomized pig. Endocrinology 1978; 102:653-656.
7. Kiviluoto T. Transplantation of pancreatic microfragments in totally pancreatectomized pigs. Eur Surg Res 1985; 17:119-127.
8. Eloy R, Bouchet F, Clendinnen G, Daniel J, Grenier JF. New technique of total pancreatectomy without duodenectomy in the dog. Am J Surg 1980; 140:409-412.
9. Berlatzky Y, Muggia-Sullam M, Munda R, Joffe SN. Use of Nd:YAG laser in pancreatic resections with duodenal preservation in the dog. Lasers Surg Med 1985; 5:507-514.
10. Schröder T, Brackett K, Joffe SN. Proximal pancreatectomy: A comparison of electrocautery with the contact and non-contact Nd:YAG laser techniques in the dog. Am J Surg 1987; 154:493-498.
11. Schröder T, Rämö OJ, Joffe SN. Laser pancreatectomy—a comparison between the dog and pig. Res Exp Med 1988; 227-233.
12. Orda R, Bara J, Orda S, Wiznitzer T. Partial distal pancreatectomy with a hand-held CO_2 laser. Arch Surg 1980; 115:869-873.

13. Schröder T, Brackett K, Joffe SN. An experimental study of the effects of electrocautery and various lasers on gastrointestinal tissue. Surgery 1987; 101:691-697.

14. Daikuzono N, Joffe SN. An artificial sapphire probe for contact photocoagulation and tissue vaporization. Med Instrum 1985; 19:173-178.

CHAPTER

11

Abdominal and Anorectal Surgery

Raymond A. Sultan, Jean-Luc Boulnois

The first experimental and clinical reports on the use of lasers in open surgery appeared in 1968–1972. The pace of these events may seem both rapid and sluggish: rapid because this field is not even 20 years old, and sluggish because the development of a new medical technology is always slow and cautious. In fact, early knowledge of laser surgical indications began with the first Meeting of the International Society for Laser Surgery in 1975. Since then, training and information for surgeons has spread through professional journals and conferences restricted only to a small community. However, initiation to optical physics as well as laser surgery is not yet fully organized. In the meantime, medical laser technology itself has demonstrated an outstanding evolution with the outcome of new wavelengths, new modalities, new handpieces, photodynamic therapy, etc. Finally, material costs may also explain the "wait and see" attitude of many potential practitioners. Nevertheless, 1990 will certainly see a marked improvement in surgical laser activity due to currently rising interest.

This chapter concerns surgical laser applications in abdominal open surgery and in most usual anorectal indications. Oncological surgery is predominant but not exclusive. Experimental and clinical aspects are presented and emphasis on the use of lasers is enhanced when appropriate. Consequently, the chapter is divided in two main parts: *technical aspects* of the various laser surgical procedures; and *clinical indications* in the abdominal and anorectal fields.

LASER PLATFORM

Operative Theaters

Management of laser treatments may be performed in various modalities. Some are common to physicians and surgeons, others are completely different: some require operative theaters, general anesthesia, and sometimes emergency safety environments; others are undertaken on an outpatient basis with or without analgesia.

A Laser Platform is a particularly constructive environment. Since 1979 such a Platform has been developed in Rueil-Malmaison (Fig. 11.1) (1). The aim was three-fold: to mix medical and surgical teams, to promote laser applications, and to reduce the cost of investments through a multidisciplinary approach.

The three operative theaters of the *aseptic area* are for abdominal, thoracic, oncological ears, nose, and throat, and orthopaedic surgery. There are two high-power CO_2 lasers (70 and 90 W, respectively) and one Nd:YAG laser (80 W). The theaters are instrumented with an operative microscope, an intraoperative ultrasonograph, and video cameras for surgery, laparoscopies, and arthroscopies. The two operative theaters of the *septic area* are for proctology, dermatology, gynecology, bronchopulmonary and gastroenterological operative endoscopies under general or neuroleptic analgesias. At their disposal, these theaters have a CO_2 laser and a Nd:YAG unit, an operative microscope, and now expect a videoendoscopy. Outpatient endoscopies as well as endoscopic retrograde cholangiopancreatography (ERCP) or esophageal prosthetic intubations are performed close to the Radiology Department.

For 8 years now, this kind of Platform has proved its effectiveness. But a Laser Research Center in the vicinity would certainly enhance those modalities. In fact, all over the world, more and more Laser Centers are being developed. One of the most attractive is the new Beckman Laser Institute & Medical Clinic, in Irvine, CA, which associates treatment units, a central surgical com-

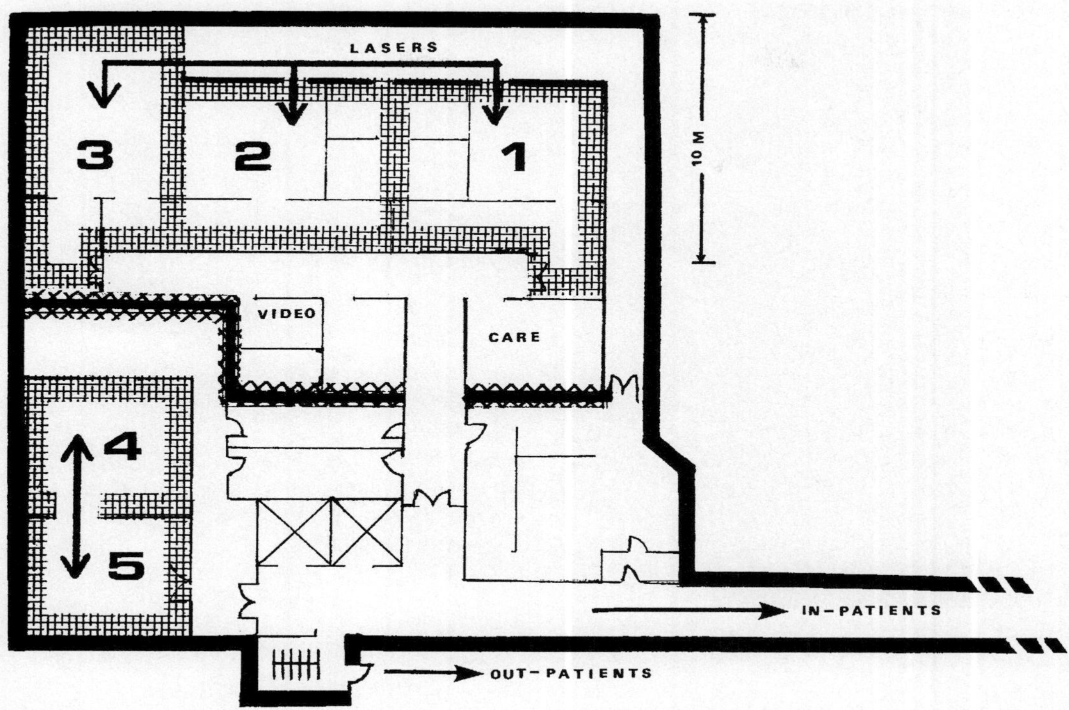

Figure 11.1. Operative theaters in the Laser Platform in Rueil-Malmaison: Aseptic areas (*1, 2, 3*); septic areas (*4, 5*); *arrows* indicate access to the lasers.

plex, and all research facilities in a special unit, together with a conference center and a research library. All types of lasers are gathered for multidisciplinary use and patients are treated on an outpatient basis. Of course, in open laser surgical oncology, connection with a hospital must exist for any Laser Center.

Lasers and Handpieces

In order to be protected against infection, lasers should stay in their respective areas (see Fig. 11.1). Surgical high-power CO_2 lasers must have a long and light optical arm, must be handy, and easily moved from one operative theater to another in the same area. Precise locations are predetermined for each type of operation, even when both CO_2 and Nd:YAG lasers are used in combined delivery (Fig. 11.2). Cooling systems must exist in each theater for each system, particularly the Nd:YAG laser unit.

Several handpieces with a wide range of focal lengths, for example, 50, 125, 150, and 200 mm for the CO_2 laser, and 50 or 100 mm for the Nd:YAG laser are commonly employed in the noncontact technique. They must be presented ready to use under sterile paper bags attached to a flexible tube for the protection of the CO_2 laser optical arm sterility. Similarly, optical fiber handpieces together with their various tips are presented ready when using the contact surgical technique.

Endoscopic Team

The presence in the same Platform of an endoscopic team essentially using the Nd:YAG laser is very useful. It is easy for surgeons to follow complementary therapy for common patients in bronchology and gastroenterology. Intraoperative endoscopies may also be requested when needed. On the other hand, complications of endoscopic treatments, if any, at once find surgical advice and cooperation.

LASER-TISSUE INTERACTIONS

The major effect of argon and/or Nd:YAG lasers on normal fundic walls, widely described in

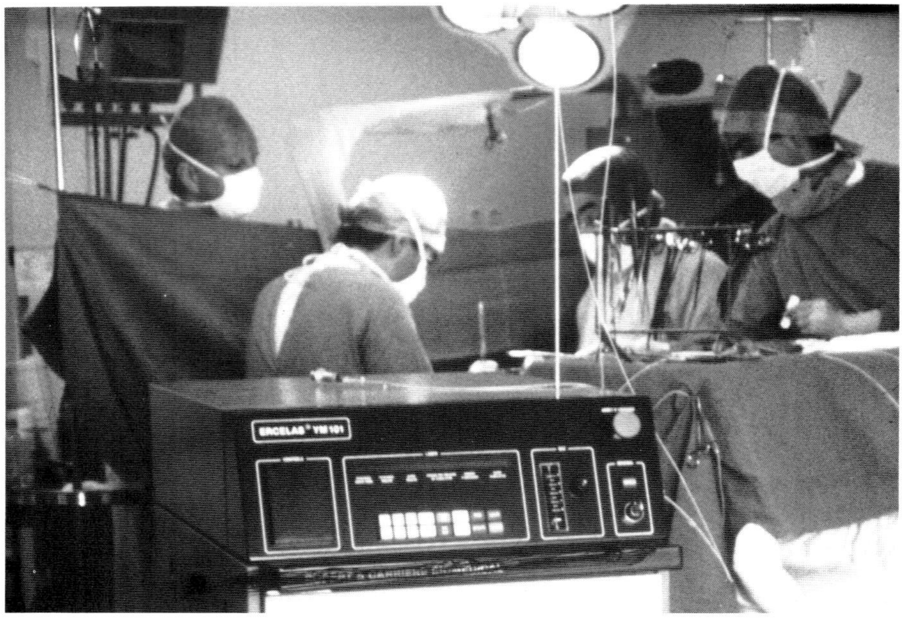

Figure 11.2. Operative theater with Nd:YAG and CO_2 lasers working in abdominal open surgery.

dogs and rabbits (2, 3), is to promote laser photocoagulation of bleedings in the upper gastrointestinal tract without damage and/or perforation. In open surgery, hazards usually do not follow these paths, and a permanent visual evaluation by the surgeon is necessary, bearing in mind the underlying structures in the areas that are exposed to radiation. The tissue susceptibility of these structures depends on the respective differences of penetration of the CO_2 and the Nd:YAG laser radiations.

Noncontact Technique

Human tissues have a high water content, and the 10.6-μm CO_2 laser radiation is well known to be very strongly absorbed by this molecule. Therefore, a focused beam will permit very precise incisions while a defocused beam will perform a bloodless tissue vaporization without danger for proximal or subjacent structures. Of course, width and depth of laser-tissue interaction will vary with laser power density and duration of exposure at a given location. On the contrary, the Nd:YAG radiation at 1.06 μm exhibits a low absorption coefficient in most tissues and, hence, a high degree of penetration; the surgeon may use long exposure times and low-power densities to obtain tissue retraction, coagulation necrosis, and a hemostatic effect. Finally, high-power densities and variable exposure times achieve tissue vaporization. The combined action of both radiations resulting in hemostasis followed by vaporization is sometimes useful in highly vascularized tumors.

When focusing a CO_2 laser with a short focal length (50-mm handpiece) on the *skin*, a cut similar to a scalpel incision is obtained because the width of the laser spot is about 0.1 mm at focus. But the nature of the skin is not comparable on the face, anterior and posterior part of the neck, abdomen, thorax, and back. Therefore, the power density to achieve a perfect incision is different in each case. In the abdominothoracic field, histological findings concerning series of CO_2 laser cuts at various powers (i.e., 20, 40, and 60 W) and various beam-tissue angles (i.e., 30°, 60°, and 90°), showed no significant difference as a function of angle. Comparable features with scalpel cuts were also obtained with high powers (60-70 W) and long focal lengths (125 and 150-mm handpieces, respectively).

Fat tissues need the greatest power densities to achieve effective vaporization. It is certainly the tissue that produces the greatest amount of smoke;

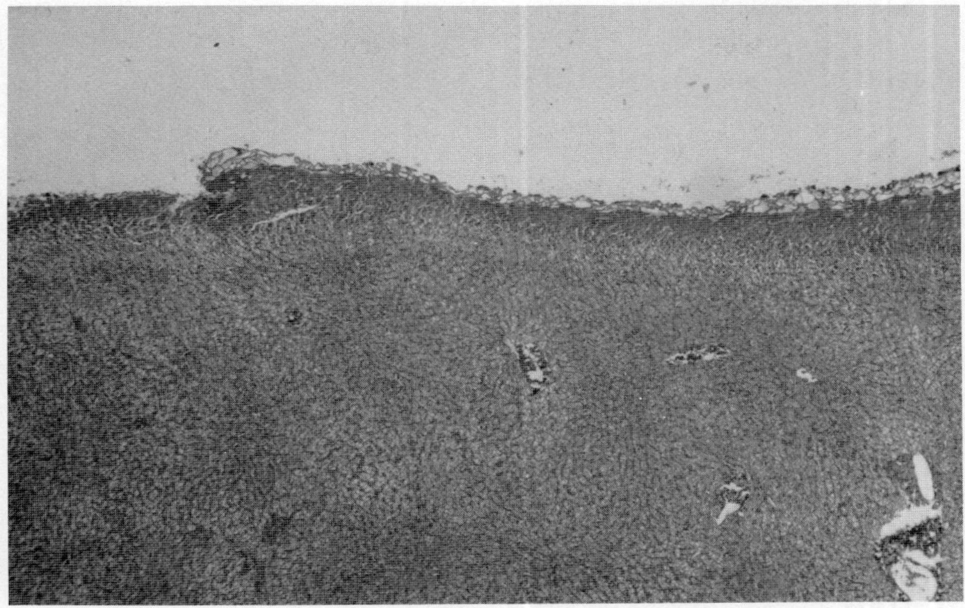

Figure 11.3. CO_2 laser cutting in liver.

surgical efficacy can be achieved with high power and an efficient smoke suction system. Thus, thick subcutaneous layer can be easily cut with the CO_2 laser in a bloodless fashion.

The same laser performs perfect *muscle transections* without any contraction or fibrillation as is the usual awkward case with electric cautery. This is very useful during various wall incision procedures through muscle layers, such as subcostal and/or transversal laparotomies, thoracotomies, and lombotomies. On the other hand, surgeons will unfortunately not be warned when approaching a motor nerve as is the case with the electric cautery.

Visceral transections, such as in the stomach and colon, have a small necrotic zone not exceeding 400 μm deep with CO_2 laser radiation, thus permitting safe manual procedures. In the liver, thermal damage shows a narrow carbonization overhanging a superficial necrotic layer with tiny cavities evenly scattered. Between this layer and normal tissue lies a thin edematous layer with identified structures whereas the whole thermal damage does not exceed 2 mm. It is worth noticing that such findings are obtained on resected human liver specimens under compression or blood inflow interruption, which increases the damage depth (Fig. 11.3). The Nd:YAG laser in liver transections produces four layers well described by Godlewski and co-workers (4). Such liver damage is shown on Figure 11.4. Here the whole lesion reaches 5.0–5.5 mm deep. At last, combined action of focused CO_2 laser radiation onto a defocused Nd:YAG laser spot (5), reduces significantly the residual necrotic zone to 1.6-1.8 mm as shown on Figure 11.5. The increase in Nd:YAG laser-induced necrotic zone under hepatic pedicle clamping has also been described: it enhances the safety of liver cutting in oncology (6, 7).

Contact Technique

Here the laser-tissue interaction only exists when a contact between an optical crystalline probe (currently sapphire) and the tissue is effective. The resulting high-power densities at the tip of the probe allow for perfect cutting with a Nd:YAG laser in a much smaller power range (5–25 W).

In a recent study (8), 57 samples of various tissue as detailed in Table 11.1 have been analyzed. For the sake of comparison, a 0.2-mm sapphire tip was used in all instances. In all except two cases, the range of induced necrotic zones

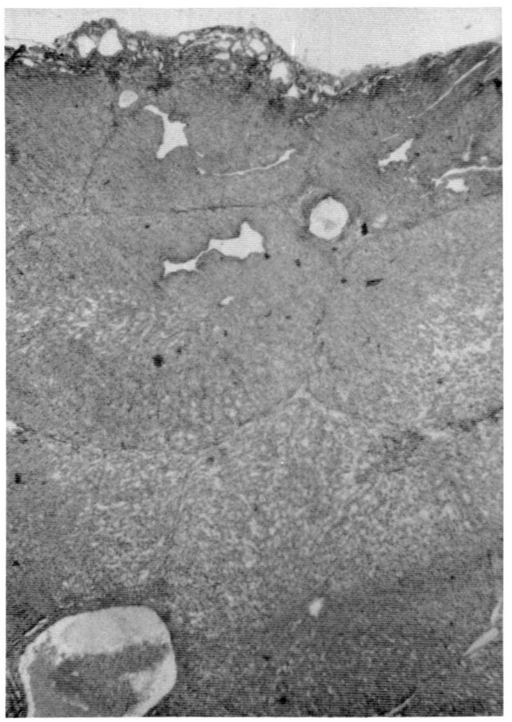

Figure 11.4. Nd:YAG laser cutting in liver.

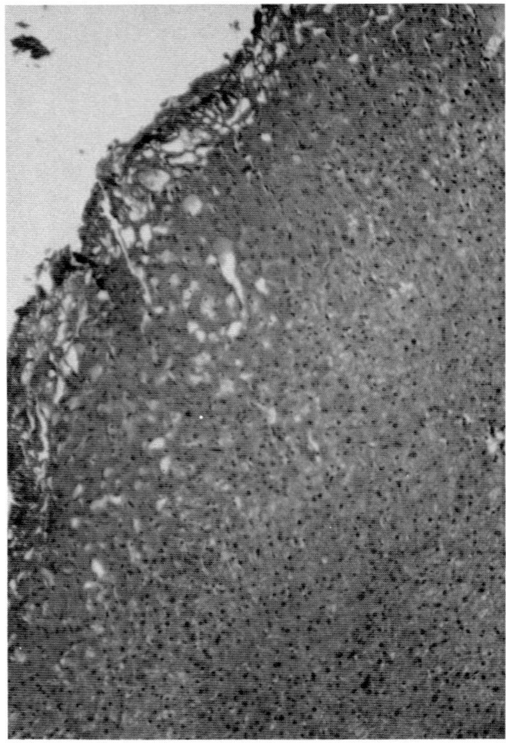

Figure 11.5. Combined laser delivery cutting in human liver.

remained between 0.11 mm at 10 W (32 kW/cm^2) and 1 mm at 20 W (64 kW/cm^2). The two extremes were 0.09 and 1.4 mm at 5 and 40 W, respectively. In most samples the necrotic zone was close to that obtained with CO_2 lasers in the same tissue. A statistical analysis of the corresponding data is given in Figure 11.6; it exhibits a quasilinear relationship of ''depth of necrosis'' vs. ''power density.''

TECHNICAL ASPECTS

In this section, attention is drawn to particular technical aspects in the use of lasers in abdominal and anorectal surgery, which constitute basic elements in the training of surgeons practicing contact or noncontact laser techniques.

In the forthcoming, the nominal value of power mentioned corresponds to the power setting on the instrument; it is not the actual power delivered to the tissues because of inherent propagation losses within the optical system (typically 10–20%). Also, for most practical noncontact handpieces, the beam focus, materialized by a prong, is always located between the handpiece tip and the target tissue.

Laparotomies

Typically, abdominal incisions at 20 W with a CO_2 laser and a 125-mm handpiece (approximately 10-20kW/cm^2) are performed rather slowly, not very satisfactorily, and the healing time is delayed to about 15 days. However, under these conditions, no wall healing failure has been reported. Higher power densities (30–60 kW/cm^2) allow for the recovery of usual wall opening times as well as usual healing times (i.e., about 9 days) (9).

Skin incision is always undertaken at focus and cutting velocities can reach nearly 2 cm/sec, simultaneously yielding a good hemostasis. Subcutaneous tissues, aponeuroses, and muscles are incised with a defocused beam from a handpiece maintained more or less 5 cm away from the target tissue. During the process of laser cutting,

Table 11.1. Results of Histological Findings Using a 0.2-mm Sapphire Tip Contact Nd:YAG Laser Probe

Samples	N = 57	W	Depth of necrosis (mm)
Cutaneous	12	15–25	0.23–0.50
Subcutaneous	1	20	0.46
Aponeuroses	2	15	0.12–0.23
Muscles	2	15	0.23
Tendons	2	20	0.115–0.46
Hygroma	2	20	0.23–0.46
Synovial ganglions	7	10–15–40	0.12, 0.23, 1.4
Neurolemmas (in neurolysis)	4	5–10–15–20	0.092, 0.115, 0.23, 0.345
Anterior carpal ligament	2	20	0.23–0.345
Skin necrosis, burns	3	15	0.23
Cutaneous metastases	2	15	0.23–0.34
Ureterolysis	2	15	0.23
Mesenteric / Mesocolic / Peritoneal } dissections	10	15–20	0.35–0.50
Liver biopsies	3	15, 20	0.23, 0.50–1.0
Colon section	1	10	0.23
Miniconization	2	20	0.11–0.23

muscles do not start as with electric cautery, and phrenotomy may be accurately accomplished without bleeding. Tissue vaporization is easily appreciated visually and a small change of the position of the handpiece with respect to the tissues, farther or nearer, at once delivers less or more energy density according to the surgeon's will. This provides safety and control of the beam penetration. Lateral pulls are recommended with all tissues during laser cutting to enhance the process. Upper tractions of the wound to facilitate air penetration in the peritoneal cavity will provide complete safety when opening the peritoneum. Use of wet packs inside the abdominal cavity is common to protect the viscera.

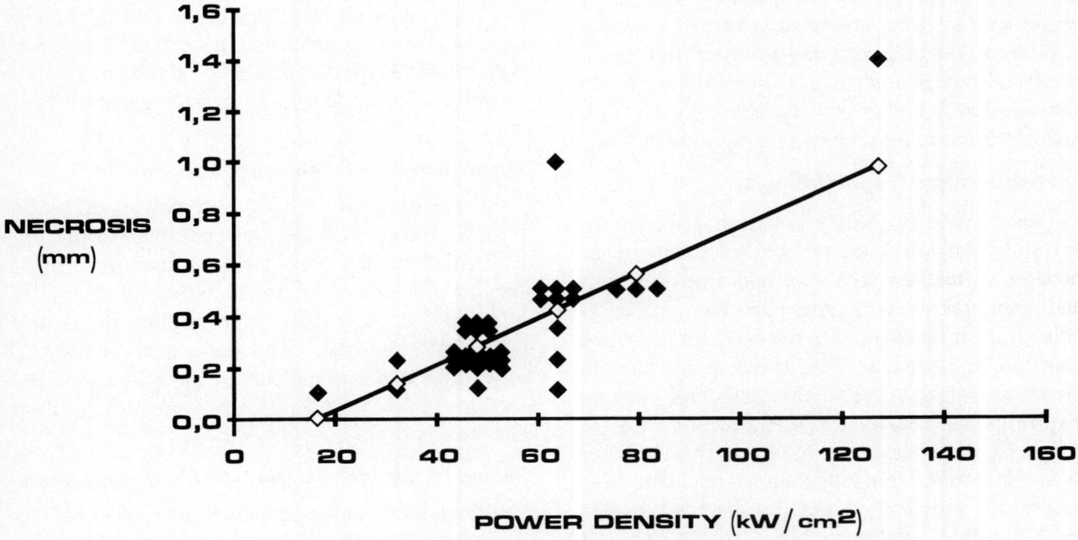

Figure 11.6. Correlation depth of necrosis versus power density with a sapphire tip.

Using this procedure, only a few vessels will need specific hemostasis; this is usually done with a Nd:YAG laser defocused beam at 5 cm from the target, at a power about 80 W, or with electric cautery.

The major drawback is the production of smoke, especially with fat patients.

Intraabdominal Dissections

This is the field in which the particular behavior or feeling of each surgeon will be put to test. Performing dissections with lasers in a noncontact approach ("no-touch") is not obvious at once and requires adaptibility. Clearly, the arrival of contact probes and their associated methodologies restores a tactile feedback.

The *CO_2 laser* with 125- or 150-mm handpieces is used at various powers, generally ranging from 20–40 W in soft and proximal peritoneal areas, and 50–60 W when excising the rectum ampulla, but always with a defocused beam.

In noncontact techniques, the *Nd:YAG laser* is used at higher powers (80 W) with small focal lengths (50-mm handpiece), mainly to achieve or complete hemostasis, also with a defocused beam. The contact 0.2-mm sapphire tip at 20 W has been preferred for the last 3 years, especially in high-risk areas (10, 11). The laser must absolutely start when the tip is in contact with the tissue, and sufficient coaxial gas flow must be supplied (2 liters/min) to ensure proper cooling of the tip; if contact is not established, illumination of the tip may occur and the diameter of the probe is then modified, generating a substantial loss in power density. Larger tips, (1.0 or 1.2 mm) may also be used at higher powers, about 30–40 W, in low risk areas to allow for more rapid dissections.

Intraabdominal Vaporizations

Vaporization of tumors is an attractive feature specific to the CO_2 and Nd:YAG lasers in the noncontact method. The spot size, power setting, and temporal mode (continuous wave [CW] or pulsed) must be adapted to the size, location, and nature of the tumors. With these indications the lasers are always used with defocused beams. Typical parameters are a power range of 30–80 W with a CO_2 laser and long focal length handpieces (125–150 mm), generating spot sizes from 2–6 mm (750 and 250 W/cm^2, respectively). The Nd:YAG laser power range is 60-80 W, with shorter focal length handpieces of 50–100 mm and 2- to 4-mm spot sizes (1500 and 500 W/cm^2, respectively).

Peritoneal Vaporizations

During surgery, the operator will assess the effective power densities really needed according to the tissue response while vaporizing. As already mentioned, defocused beams provide safety when beginning the irradiation. It is always possible to come closer to focus if more power density is needed. Only when larger powers are required on larger spots should the power setting be increased (12). Vaporization is easy in small tumors; however, large tumors may require laser resections at beam focus, the dissected area being finally irradiated with a large spot for complementary sterilization. The CO_2 laser is most frequently used because of its active and effective results. Its small penetration gives the surgeon an accurate depth of tissue destruction and also allows for the assessment of underlying structures. In unresectable tumors or nodes or in residual diseases after incomplete vaporizations due to anatomic constraints, irradiation with the Nd:YAG laser may be performed after exact evaluation of the depth of the remaining disease to be destroyed. Penetration of the Nd:YAG laser radiation being deeper, necrosis can be reached up to an extra depth of 5–6 more mm in the following days. Metallic clips are inserted to define the area where such residual diseases can be left to facilitate exact targeting in postoperative radiotherapy. In some high-risk areas with subjacent large vessels or bowel, preference is given to a precise contact microdissection with the 0.2-mm sapphire tip at about 10 W, namely, a power density in the vicinity of 25 kW/cm^2.

Vaporizations in Pathological Tissues

In pathological tissues, low-power densities (around 200 W/cm^2) are preferred in order to sterilize all dissected areas. This procedure is performed after the clearance of lymph nodes in all territories, e.g., celiac, iliac, and/or along the aorta and vena cava. The same methodology is also suitable during the cure of intraabdominal infectious areas, abscesses, or parasitic diseases (13–15).

Spread Prophylaxis in Dukes C Rectal Carcinoma

Techniques and parameters are identical to those described above. In the anterior resection of the rectum, the defocused beam must irradiate the

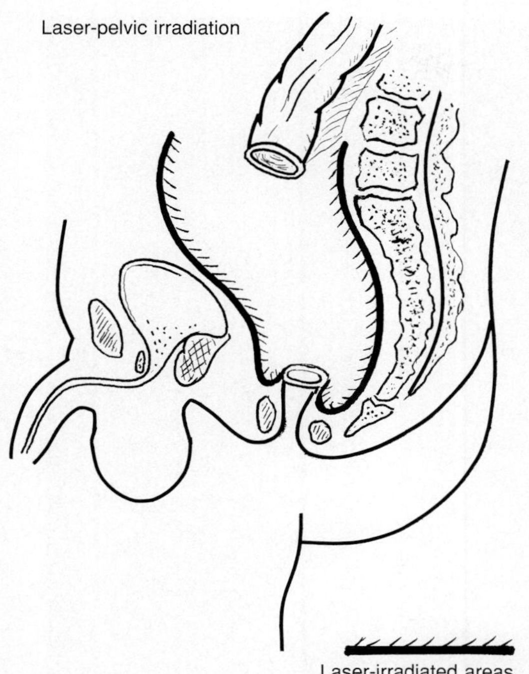

Figure 11.7. Area of pelvic irradiation in anterior resection of the rectum.

whole pelvic cavity, including the anterior face of the sacrum and the dissected areas up to the ligated inferior mesentric artery (Fig. 11.7). The latter resected pedicle must be studied by the pathologist before irradiation. In the Miles operation, the irradiation protocol will be the same, but should also be performed in the perineal wound before closure.

Liver Surgery

Liver Cutting in Humans

Lasers have made new contributions to liver surgery. However, it should be stressed that the essential rules of liver surgery remain of prime importance and might never be avoided even with the new methodology.

The largest body of experience with lasers has been in *noncontact surgery*. Several procedures have been successively employed.

The CO_2 laser, at about 70-90 W, has long focal lengths (125-mm handpiece). It is very important to recall that even a high-power CO_2 laser is unable to cut a human liver because bleeding occurs, blocks the beam, and shields the tissue. Liver cutting with a focused CO_2 beam is only possible under hepatic pedicle clamping or under parenchymal compression with a soft surgical clamp. Naturally, velocity increases with power. Although this could be considered satisfactory, once the clamping or the compression is released, all the liver edge hemostasis remains to be undertaken, sometimes in poor conditions when there are large resections. It might be acceptable for small partial or wedge resections but not for lobectomies or hepatectomies where hemostasis could become tedious and sometimes dangerous. An improvement is to cut under clamping, slowly, at 30 or 40 W. This would obtain a hardened liver allowing for easier ligation of vessels during and after cutting (5, 16). On the other hand, if the main vessels have to be regularly ligated, a defocused beam at similar powers, 3 cm away from the target, is able to stop effectively any minor oozing, and gives a very clean edge.

Nd:YAG lasers have also been used, but require short focal lengths (typically 50 mm). At about 55 W, liver cutting is slow and not satisfactory, yielding a charring of the tissue that slows the cutting process. At 80 W, cutting is acceptable and, at 110 W, it is greatly improved. The main purpose in using this wavelength is to obtain large necrotic zones (5 mm) in which the photocoagulation gives a correct hemostasis. Repeated action with lateral pulling is usual and leads to a parenchymal cut. In the future, it is expected that more powerful Nd:YAG lasers will be useful in this particular field (17).

In the third approach, the *combined use of CO_2 and Nd:YAG* lasers was experimentally proposed in 1982 (18). This application was achieved in the human either with two separate handpieces and two surgeons with the CO_2 laser beam following the path of the Nd:YAG laser beam (Fig. 11.8). It was also successfully implemented with a combined delivery device of a focused CO_2 beam inside a defocused Nd:YAG laser spot (Fig. 11.9). In this procedure, cutting with the CO_2 beam inside the Nd:YAG laser-induced necrotic zone is more effective. Generally, clamping of the pedicle is not undertaken but the main vessels remain to be ligated. Nevertheless, in major resections, preparation of the clamping and access to the hepatic veins near the vena cava are performed before resection in order to keep emergency vascular exclusion possible.

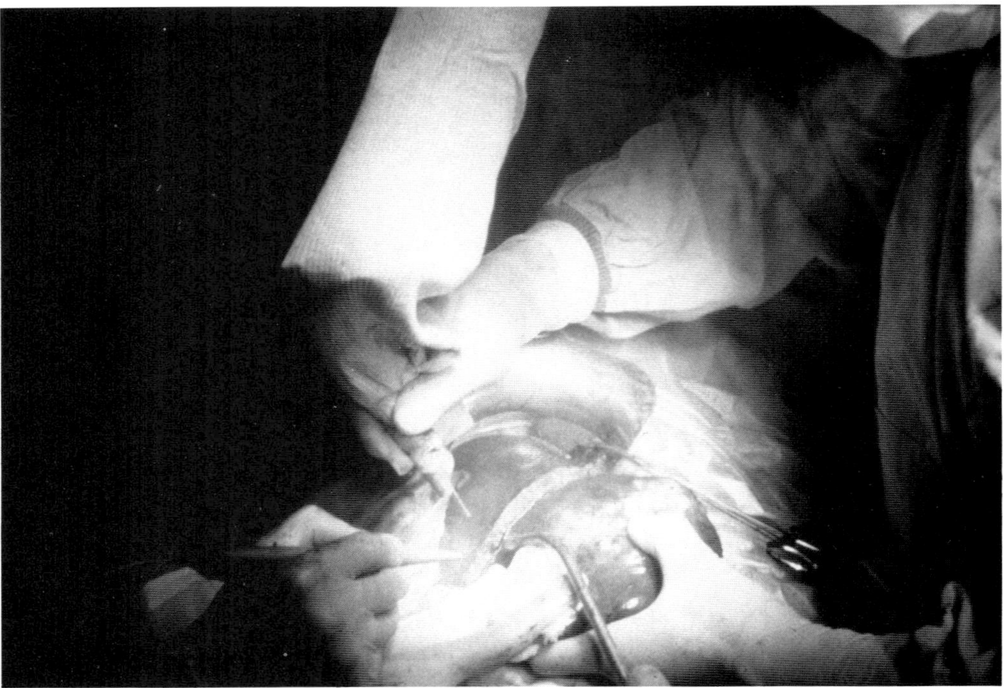

Figure 11.8. Combined laser delivery with two surgeons, two separate handpieces, and one target.

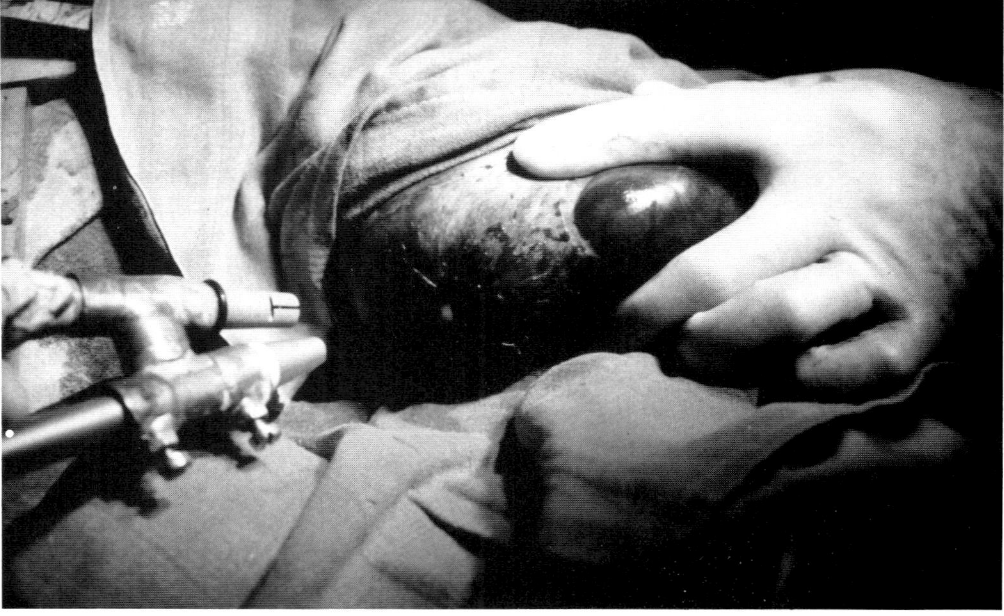

Figure 11.9. Combined delivery device holding the two handpieces (Nd:YAG and CO_2 lasers).

Bile leakages: When identified during the cutting process, segmental bile ducts have to be ligated. When a complementary cholecystectomy is recommended, a test with methylene blue using the cystic duct is advisable at the end of the cut. Remaining open bile ducts must then be spotted and ligated. Despite these precautions, bile leaks may occur 2-4 days postoperatively. If the main bile duct has been operatively controlled to be free, leaks will spontaneously stop before day 15. Hence, postoperative drainage is fully required because these leaks become a complication only if drainage was not efficient or if the main bile duct is not free.

One of the main features of the *ultrasonic surgical aspirator (USA)* is the safety obtained when approaching hepatic veins. It is not at all comparable to the laser action that may cut, vaporize, or photocoagulate every structure. On the contrary, USA dissociates and absorbs hepatic parenchyma except for skeletonized vessels and biliary structures. A comparison between USA, noncontact Nd:YAG laser, and blunt dissection in experimental liver resections confirms the efficacy of USA in the vessels and in bile duct control. The Nd:YAG laser reduces the resection time but enlarges the tissue necrosis and may increase the percentage of bacterial infection (19). A combined action of USA as a first tool, followed by Nd:YAG laser photocoagulation of the skeletonized vessels is possible and interesting, but the process is time-consuming.

In conclusion, preference is given to the combined laser delivery at high power densities. After identification by intraoperative ultrasonography, the main vessel structures have to be dissected with USA before ligation.

In *contact surgery*, the first surgical contact probe is the Doty and Auth silica blade (20), used in particular with the Nd:YAG laser at 70 W (21). This probe seems not to have had further developments. On the contrary, a comparative experimental study in rat livers between contact sapphire tips, contact bare quartz fiber, noncontact Nd:YAG laser, and electrocautery states the hemostatic and cutting qualities of the sapphire tips (22). Another comparative study on rats between noncontact and contact Nd:YAG laser techniques establishes that liver resections are performed with much lower power densities, less bleeding, less smoke, and less tissue necrosis (23). With the sapphire 0.2- to 0.8-mm tips, Nd:YAG laser radiation has been used at a mean power of 15 W (range 10–20 W) in humans (24).

As indicated in Table 11.1, the induced depth of necrosis with the 0.2-mm tips does not exceed 1 mm at 20 W without interruption of the blood flow in the liver. Such a low penetration may lead to an unsuccessful hemostasis because the process is very close to the one obtained by the CO_2 laser radiation. Finally, a sapphire tip frosted on 4 mm has been developed in order to increase the necrotic zone up to that of a noncontact result in order to enhance hemostasis: no data have yet been reported.

Liver Tumor Vaporizations (LTV)

The main principles have been discussed but some aspects should be presented in more details.

1. Various *responses* are obtained depending on specific histological structures (25). This determines the wavelength and power setting to be employed. CO_2 is sometimes used alone, more often simultaneously with the Nd:YAG laser (see page 19).
2. *Vaporizations* of tumors are undertaken from the center toward the periphery. Generally, there is no bleeding while vaporizing solid tumor tissues, but it occurs when reaching the liver parenchyma. In liver metastases, malignant islets are often present in the peripheral border of the tumor, beyond its limits, 1 cm inside the parenchyma (Fig. 11.10). Upon reaching this moment in LTV, the hepatic pedicle is clamped because it is easier to evaluate the thickness of peritumoral hepatic tissue to be destroyed (Fig. 11.11). As discussed in liver transection (see page 4), temporary occlusion of the pedicle increases the Nd:YAG laser-induced necrotic zone providing more oncological safety.
3. Small *biliary ducts* may be severed during the peripheral phase in LTV; in this case, ligations are required.
4. *Hepatic and portal veins* are identified with intraoperative ultrasonography. The distance to the vessels appears on the screen. Here again, if the deepest part of the tumor is adjacent or displaces the main vessels, USA can be used more safely than the laser.
5. Once *LTV is achieved*, collagen packs, impregnated with fluorouracil (5-FU), can be inserted in the residual crater(s) within the liver.

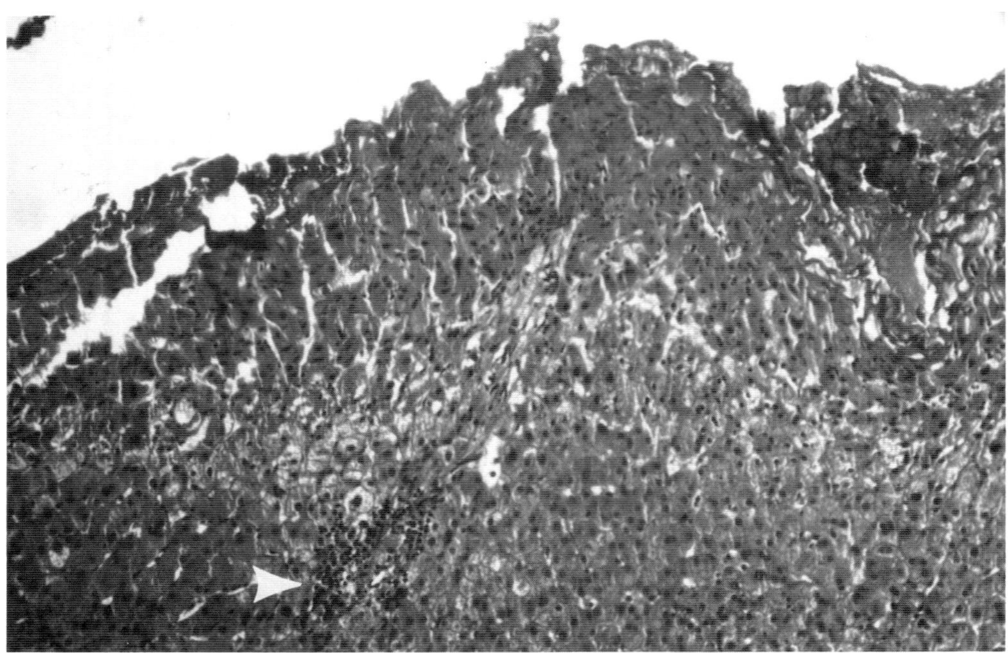

Figure 11.10. Malignant islets visible beyond the tumoral destruction border (bottom left)

Anorectal Surgery

Proctology

In this field, CO_2 laser radiation (typically 20-40 W and 125- to 150-mm handpiece) has been used since the very beginning of its medical applications and is still the most widespread technique (26–29). Nd:YAG laser has been used concurrently with cryotherapy (30, 31), but the adjunct of the CO_2 laser for external anal pathology enhances postoperative comfort (32). Nevertheless, the outcome of Nd:YAG laser sapphire surgical contact probes may change the outlook. At present, no comparative studies exist to appreciate an eventual significant difference. But due to the weak penetration of the Nd:YAG laser radiation in the contact technique, such studies should appear very soon in the literature.

Operative Positions. The routine operative position is the gynecological position, with a small table between patient and surgeon sitting with elbows resting on the table for comfort and precision. The laser optical arm is located between the patient legs (Fig. 11.12). Pilonidal sinuses are operated upon in the ventral position.

Surgical Techniques. All conventional techniques have been adapted to the laser technology. Consequently, an excellent specimen is also available for examination by the pathologist. Specific laser vaporizations where specimens do not exist are only proposed in anal warts. The oncological vaporizations to be described in the Endorectal Surgery and Anal Conservative Surgery sections below are different because they are performed after tumor identification. Skin is opened in the focus of a CO_2 laser, but the whole operation is performed in the defocused mode, 3–5 cm from the tissues. Hence, it is easy to follow the tissue dissociation and vaporization during the noncontact dissection, for example, Parks ligament in hemorrhoidectomies, leiomyotomy in anal fissures and sometimes in hemorrhoidectomies, tract(s) in anal fistulas, abscess cavities, or pilonidal sinuses.

Endorectal Surgery

Intraoperative direct access to the lower rectum implies a good exposure, otherwise surgery cannot be performed. Exposure depends on several factors.

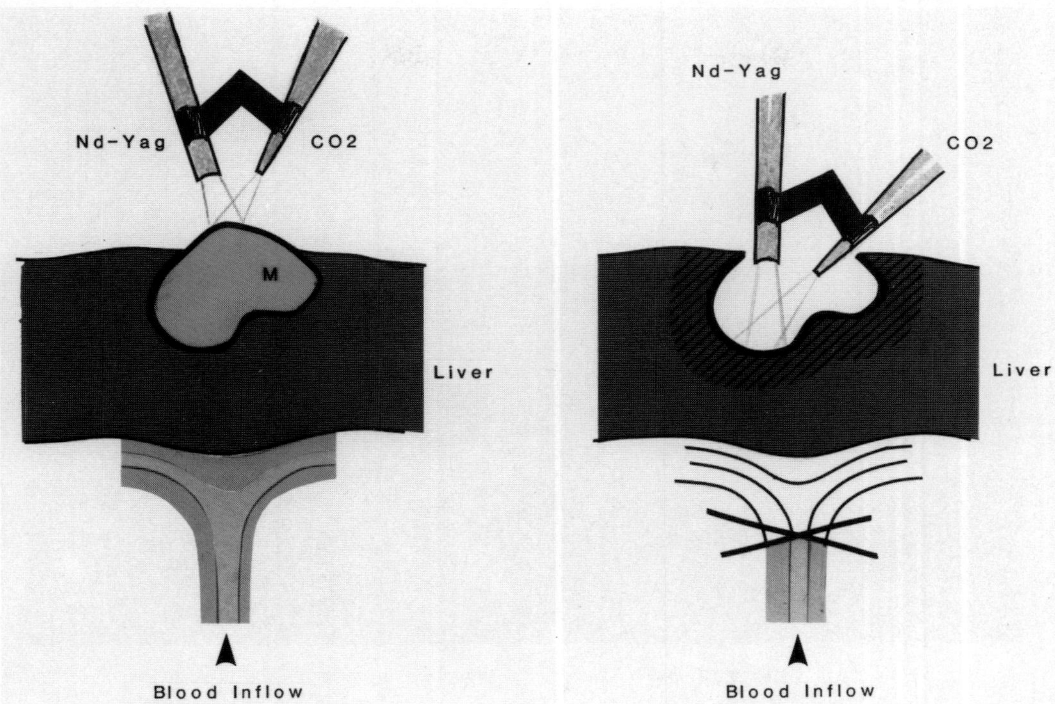

Figure 11.11. Laser tumor vaporization technique: Tumor is vaporized using a combined delivery until apparently healthy parenchyma is reached; bleeding occurs at this moment. Hepatic pedicle is clamped: irradiation is pursued and vaporizes more than 1 cm of liver all around the tumor site; under clamping, Nd:YAG laser-induced necrotic zone is increased.

1. *Anesthesia* might be sphinteric, spinal, or general, according to the anesthetist's proposals and acceptance by the patient.
2. *Division of the sphincter* has been proposed as a means of excellent exposure with full continence after accurate restoration (33). Such indications may be suggested in situations where there is difficult access to curable lesions, but certainly not in palliative carcinoma treatments.
3. A large *operative anuscope* or rectoscope, able to remove smoke, has been used for electrocoagulation (34) or with a microscope for a laser procedure (35). Introduction of this 35-mm diameter anuscope follows a gentle sphincteric dilation progressively made with the fingers of both hands. The large Storz anuscope presently available with smoke removal is suitable, its funnel allows full vision while introducing the laser handpiece. At times, the Parks retractor is useful for better exposure, depending on the site and size of the tumor. Since all tumors do not have the same response to CO_2 laser radiation depending to the tissue reaction, powers ranging from 40 to 60 W are used. Recommended handpieces should be bent although straight instruments are more common. A long focal length is required, typically with a 200-mm lens (Fig. 11.13). Radiation from a 1.06-m Nd:YAG laser may be used to photocoagulate if bleeding occurs or to vaporize the tumor subsequently. A 1.32-m Nd:YAG laser radiation seems to be promising in the treatment of adenomas. Finally, contact sapphire probes may help when part of the tumor has to be dissected before or after vaporization, or during large control biopsies.
4. *Endorectal ultrasonography* (ERUS) can be successfully performed with an ultrasonic echographic probe (36). Its applications are

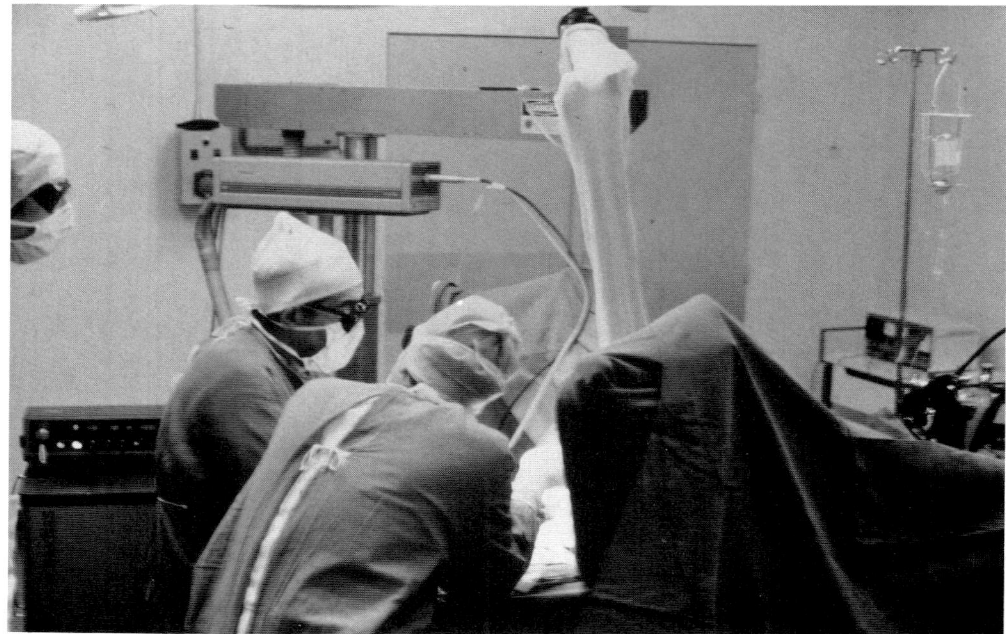

Figure 11.12. Operative position in anal surgery.

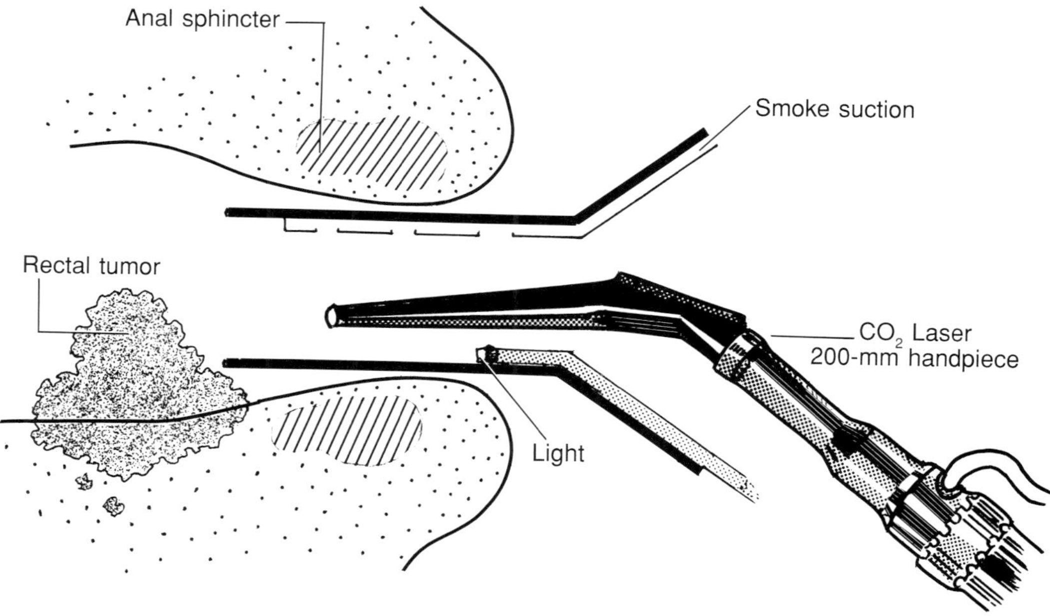

Figure 11.13. Operative anuscope and CO_2 laser with a 200-mm bent handpiece.

found in several instances: *(a)* preoperative period for assessment of length, extent, and depth of the tumor and perirectal tissues or nodes, which permits an assessment of a Dukes stage; *(b)* intraoperative time, the only actual means to control and assess laser destruction during and at the end of the treatment; *(c)* postoperative follow-up in order to discover an asymptomatic recurrence in the perirectal tissues, even if endoscopic control and biopsies look negative. In any cases, comparative video sonograms are very useful.

At the end of the laser session, after the latest biopsies, the residual crater(s) is cleaned with a rectal irrigation. Sterilization of stools is recommended. Antibioprophylaxis is ongoing during the operation and 2 days after; the patient is discharged with an oral medication for a week. Mean healing time for craters takes about a month, depending on the size.

Anal Conservative Surgery

Clinical digital examination of the carcinoma is essential and gives very important information. Endoanal procedures, e.g., anuscopy, direct or transrectoscopic ERUS, are undertaken if the tumor is small, not too painful, and without stenosis. Otherwise endoanal procedures as well as digital examinations must be performed, under anesthesia, pre- or intraoperatively. Because poorly differentiated squamous cell carcinomas may have a rapid intrapelvic extent, according to the histology, the stage, or the volume, a scanner is recommended. Detection of nodes is very important. ERUS is becoming more accurate in the diagnosis of nodes but its spatial field is actually limited to 14 cm from the anal verge because the probe is rigid. Current expectations are the nuclear magnetic resonance (NMR) and computerized immunoscintigraphy.

Tumors Smaller than 2 cm. The CO_2 laser is first used at 20–40 W with the 125- to 150-mm handpiece to excise the tumor (see Proctology, page 11). At the end of the resection, a defocused irradiation at 20 W is performed to achieve wound sterilization. The pathologist gives the information concerning the tumoral extent on the boundaries of the specimen. Healing will occur within 4–5 weeks. Then, external radiotherapy is undertaken with Co-60 and/or preferably 25 Mev photons. Curative dosimetry is recommended.

Tumors 2-4 cm. Radiotherapy is primarily performed in these tumors. Dosimetry is 30-35 Gy, and it is preferable to wait 5–6 weeks to obtain the full effect of radiation before using the lasers. Under local, spinal, or general anesthesia, according to anesthetist's proposals and acceptance by the patient, a complete finger examination is necessary to explore the anal canal, the sphincter, and the perirectal tissues in order to detect eventual residual nodules. Intraoperative ERUS is very useful here. The anal canal is a difficult area to explore with usual ultrasonic probes but the recent 7 MHz probe manufactured by Brüel & Kjaer allows direct tissue contact in the anal canal and provides better imaging. Dissection to approach residual tumoral diseases are performed with CO_2 laser radiation or sapphire contact Nd:YAG laser probes to reach the site(s). Photocoagulation and vaporization are then undertaken combining successively the high power radiations of both the Nd:YAG and CO_2 lasers. Hence, Nd:YAG-induced necrosis is vaporized, leaving a clean, non-necrotic wound. Final irradiation at 20-30 W with the CO_2 laser will heat the wound without charring or popcorn effect. Healing occurs within 4–6 weeks. In both cases, a follow-up every 3 months during the first 2 years is necessary (R.A. Sultan, unpublished observations).

Tumors Larger than 4 cm. No conservative surgery is recommended at this stage.

ABDOMINAL INDICATIONS

Thoracolaparotomies

All open abdominal surgery starts by opening the wall. In order to perform a complete laser oncological surgery, it appeared suitable to use the laser at the onset of the operations and thereby develop a no touch technique with simultaneous wound sterilization. Laser laparotomies as well as thoracotomies or thoracophrenolaparotomies are mostly performed on patients with digestive carcinomas requiring surgical assessment and intraoperative laser treatment. Surgical technique and parameters have been discussed in the previous section, Technical Aspects.

Achievement and reconstruction of such openings are actually well established. This quite bloodless surgery gives intraoperative comfort to the surgeon and postoperative comfort to the patient, with minimal edema or hematoma, minimal pain and/or inflammation. The procedure can be performed under anticoagulant treatment. At the end of operation the wound remains clean and dry.

Comparative series with and wothout lasers have been performed to assess healing, infectious complications, and immediate as well as long-term parietal solidity (9). In these series, no statistically significant difference was found but in the laser group no infectious complications or parietal deficiencies occured. For example, a gallbladder carcinoma with partial liver resection of segments IV and V with a CO_2 laser now reaches a 5-year follow-up (5). Results with scar cosmetics are variable but none has subcutaneous fibrosis.

Intraabdominal Laser Dissections (ILD)

Here CO_2 laser-defocused beams allow for the dissection of peritoneal areas, such as cologastric omentum, freeing left and right mesocolon, opening inflammatory pelvic peritoneum, and excising the rectum ampulla in anterior resection of the rectum or in a Miles operation. In the latter, perineal wounds were also performed with lasers as described for the first time in 1978 (37). Naturally, lateral pedicles near the pelvic wall need ligations.

Surgical resection of the pyloric antrum, ulcerectomies, gastrotomies, and pyloroplasties may be performed using a noncontact CO_2 beam. Manual sutures can be safely used without any postoperative leaks.

An alternative to hyperselective vagotomy was experimentally tested on dogs, combining a posterior truncal vagotomy with an anterior lesser curvature argon laser myotomy; results were promising and long-term trials are indicated (38). Similar techniques, using either CO_2 laser radiation or sapphire contact tips are perfectly able to give favorable surgical results with a precise dissection, particularly in obese patients.

Today, *preference is given to sapphire tips* for intraabdominal dissections. The actual indications for use are adhesiolyses, small bowel- and viscera-freeing in second look operations, dissection of hepatic cysts, hydatic liver cysts, inflammatory or neoplastic implants in advanced ovarian carcinomas, complete ureterolysis through a peritoneal spread from a digestive carcinoma, and preparation of anastomosis verges before intestinal sutures.

Intraabdominal Laser Vaporizations (ILV)

Indications in abdominal surgery were defined by Nims and McCaughan in 1983 (12). These authors used the CO_2 laser exclusively as a vaporizing instrument for a useful adjunct therapy. Targets are advanced ovarian carcinomas and liver tumors.

Advanced Ovarian Carcinomas

In advanced ovarian carcinomas the aim is to try to remove all visible disease in the peritoneal cavity. It is an admitted truth that survival of these patients is a function of the residual tumor size. Therefore, surgeons have to be as complete as possible without generating a major complication such as a colostomy. Implants in this particular disease are scattered throughout the peritoneal cavity. Sometimes resection of the whole peritoneal serosa, i.e., subdiaphragmatic, lateral, pelvic, is recommended but it seems more attractive to associate resections with vaporizations of implants (39). Of course, the technique must be adapted to specific locations. Spots and power must be increased with the distance to the targets, for example, subdiaphragmatic spread needs more power, typically 80 W and 6-mm spots. On the other hand, with respect to the underlying structures, such as abdominopelvic vessels, ureter, and bowel, specific procedures are proposed, e.g., use of 0.1-sec pulse at 30 W CO_2 laser radiation (12) and use of 0.2-mm contact Nd:YAG sapphire tip at 10 W in high-risk areas (40). As defined in the Technical Aspects section, the noncontact Nd:YAG laser can also be employed for *unresectable malignancies* and/or *nodes*.

Peritoneal spread of digestive carcinomas is another useful indication. Diffusion of the disease in inflammatory colonic or rectosigmoid carcinomas in the lower part of the peritoneal cavity is generally destroyed using one laser or the other in succession. Intraoperative biopsies give the exact assessment of the destruction and the orientation or limits of the irradiation.

Clearance of Lymph Nodes

Clearance of lymph nodes in gastric, colonic, or rectal carcinomas performed with conventional techniques or with the help of sapphire contact probes have to be completed by defocused irradiation with the CO_2 laser only at low-energy densities (see Vaporizations in Pathological Tissues). This will heat all of the dissected areas and consequently seal the microlymphatics to avoid the spread of cancer cells. If unresectable residual disease exists, then the Nd:YAG irradiation appears to be the best procedure to generate postoperative necrosis. Chemotherapy and/or radiotherapy are generally combined according to the histological types of carcinomas.

The same procedure has been applied for the management of contamined or infected wounds in other areas (13, 14) and is suitable in *intraabdominal infectious and parasitic pathology*.

Subdiaphragmatic, sub- or intrahepatic abscesses during surgical treatment, once the cavity(ies) is(are) void, are wholly irradiated with a defocused CO_2 beam at nearly 40 W. Caution must be exercised and perioperative antibiotherapy is advisable. In liver hydatic disease, once the contents have been evacuated as usual, the protruding portion of the cyst(s) is(are) resected using a sapphire tip before vaporizing the whole internal surface. Similar successful procedures in two cases of alveolar enchinococcosis have been reported (15).

Pelvic Irradiation in Carcinomas

Experimental comparative work using a CO_2 laser in a defocused mode ($\approx$4-mm spot size) versus a scalpel, clearly demonstrated effective results in the reduction of local recurrences (41). Also, in advanced ovarian carcinomas, the photoirradiation of the pelvis has been undertaken after removal of the pelvic peritoneum (39).

Dukes C carcinoma of the rectum is now assessed preoperatively by means of scanner, NMR, and ERUS. When the perirectal tissues are involved, local recurrences are expected within 10–36% (42). Identification of recurrent disease occurs when following up several criteria: CEA and CA 19-9 levels, ERUS after an anterior resection of the rectum, and/or scanner after Miles operation, and/or, when possible, by NMR or computerized immunoscintigraphy. Endoscopy is frequently negative because the recurrences arise in the perirectal environment and its negativity might be a factor of time loss.

The aim of intraoperative laser irradiation (see Spread Prophylaxis in Dukes C Rectal Carcinoma, page 7) is to obtain the *sterilization of all dissected areas* and prevent spread of cancer cells. The main purpose is the reduction of local recurrences. The method is simple and not time-consuming (typically about 10 min). It is easier to perform than intraoperative radiotherapy (43). The procedure applies even if a preoperative radiotherapy has been undertaken and does not hinder postoperative radiotherapy if asked by the surgeon, because the two forms of energy deposition are not cumulative. First results are encouraging but prospective studies on a larger scale are ongoing.

Liver Surgery

Laser Liver Resections (LLR)

First experiments on animals were promising regarding the capability of CO_2 lasers in liver parenchymal cutting (44–47). The quality of cutting was enhanced by compressing of parenchyma or by clamping the blood inflow. Then it was demonstrated that satisfactory liver cutting with a Nd:YAG laser was achievable with a better hemostasis than with the CO_2 laser (4, 48, 49). Experiments with an effective output of 120 W at the end of the handpiece were reported to produce positive results (50). A very attractive procedure was proposed in 1982; CO_2 and Nd:YAG lasers were experimentally combined in a single spot and this delivery system associated the advantages of each wavelength (18).

The first successful cases in humans were reported with a Nd:YAG laser in 1981 (51) and in 1985 (21). It was confirmed that the use of the CO_2 laser alone was not satisfactory (51, 52). Then, in 1986, preliminary results were reported using noncontact surgery and also combined delivery (5), and later, the contact sapphire probes (24).

In humans, interest in *noncontact LLR*, lies in various aspects.

1. The *possibility of a precise cut* with an efficient hemostatic control is of interest (see Liver Cutting in Humans, page 8). The procedure gives comfort to the surgeon and saves blood, which is salutary for patients and beneficial for the cost of pathology.
2. *Wedge resections and/or hepatectomies* performed with combined lasers are now well established; their achievement is time-saving and may require pedicle clamping according to local reasons.
3. *Temperature* in the path of the Nd:YAG laser beam is higher than 200°C (53), and decreases rapidly to 70°C at a radius of 4 mm delimiting the thermal damage zone. Godlewski and co-

workers demonstrated in pigs that the clamping leads to temperature increases and also to a thicker necrotic zone, i.e., 7–8 mm (54). It is acceptable to presume that these effects are favorable from an oncological point of view, particularly when cutting is close to the visible limit of the tumor(s). In addition, it has been proved that this does not generate severe complications related to the lasers, but may be contraindicated if current liver deficiency exists. According to Godlewski et al., a neovascularization appears in the repaired area in the first 2 postoperative months, which may enhance local chemotherapeutic efficacy by means of a drug delivery implantable device in the gastroduodenal artery.

4. *Liver cutting with combined laser delivery* has been observed to lead to a reduction of the necrotic zone (see Noncontact Technique, page 3). Theoretically, liver regeneration may be enhanced but it is really difficult to appreciate this process in humans because postoperative investigations are limited to ultrasonography and scanner. In the case of major resections, liver regeneration may be followed by regular assessments of gamma GT and alkaline phosphatase levels that slowly (sometimes after months) reach normal levels.

In *contact LLR in humans*, reported by Iwasaki and co-workers (21), the laser silica blade at 70 W was used under inflow occlusion. Capability of cutting cirrhotic liver has been reported with a velocity comparable to the electric cautery. No significant hemorrhage when reopening the blood inflow shows a difference with the CO_2 technique. Iwasaki et al. report a necrotic zone smaller than 2 mm, very close to the CO_2-induced zone and slightly superior to reported findings with a 0.2-mm sapphire probe (Table 11.1). Joffe has reported LLR with similar probes, also with satisfactory results (24). No data with the "frosted tips" have yet been reported in liver. This new contact probe was initiated to obtain a useful greater hemostatic zone for hypervascularized tissues. In fact, considering the quasilinear relationship shown in Figure 11.6 (see Contact Technique, page 5), a greater power density should induce a larger necrotic zone. Actually, the sapphire probes must be used at powers less than 25 W, because higher powers usually lead to probe impairments.

No hemorrhagic complications relating to the use of lasers have been reported by the different investigators. Bile leaks may occur despite meticulous detection during the liver edge management and are not hazardous if drainage is efficient and the main bile duct is controlled free operatively (5).

A particular aspect of liver surgery may occur in heavy liver injuries. In first hand surgery, the aim should be to maintain the greatest amount of hepatic parenchyma and, after vascular control, the lasers are used as in regular LLR. In the possible case of second hand patients, liver necrosis may exist. The interest in lasers here lies as well in wound sterilization as in necrotic area vaporizations, until normal bleeding occurs again.

Liver Tumor Vaporizations (LTV)

The first experimental technique of combined therapy with Nd:YAG and CO_2 lasers was applied successfully on malignant animal liver tumors in 1981 (55). At the same time, tumoral vaporizations in human livers were reported and considered as formal indications of intraoperative laser treatment (1). More accurate data were later given in 1983 concerning the power and technique suitable in liver metastatic disease (size range: 1–8 cm) from colon and gallbladder carcinomas (12). In 1986, the place of surgical tumoral vaporizations in oncology, their management and limits, their risks, possibilities of improvement, and follow-up have been fully described, and histological structures of liver tumors have been shown to modify their responses to laser radiation (25).

Liver metastases from squamous cell carcinomas (i.e., esophagus, bronchus, anus), do not require high-power densities to be easily and rapidly destroyed with CO_2 alone at 40 W or about 0.25 kW/cm^2. It is similar for daughter nodules in primary hepatocarcinoma and liver nodules in Hodgkin disease. Nevertheless, as expected, higher power reduces operating time. On the other hand, high-power densities are necessary to achieve vaporization of metastases from colonic, pancreatic, and especially gastric carcinomas: CO_2 at 80 W, and better if combined with Nd:YAG at 80–110 W (or more if available).

Vaporizations are easy when tumors are visible and/or peripheral in the liver, in a size-range of some 2–3 cm. But other tumors, for example, posterior in segment VIII, or in the subhilar portion of segment IV, or in a size-range of 4–6 cm, are sometimes tedious to destroy completely if high-power lasers are not available. Moreover, these tumor vaporizations may be dangerous with respect to underlying structures (25). Intraoperative sonography, which identifies hepatic and portal veins, and also smaller nodules not seen at the preoperative examinations has been a major help. USA is recommended in cases of contiguity between veins and tumors, both techniques being complementary. No hemorrhagic complications nor biliary leakages are mentioned by authors. Of course, biliary surgery rules prescribe that the freedom of the common bile duct be controlled. Implantation of a drug delivery system aimed at remnant liver protection, generally in the gastroduodenal artery, completes the protocol. Local insertion of collagen packs impregnated with 5-FU in residual liver craters has also been proposed.

Pancreatic and Splenic Surgery

Pancreas

In 1979, Giler and co-workers compared partial pancreatic resections in dogs with scalpel, electric cautery, and CO_2 lasers at 20 W, and indicated that laser beams sealed pancreatic ducts and appeared as a ''relatively safe procedure'' in partial pancreatectomies and biopsies (56). Di Donna in 1981 described a total pancreatectomy technique in dogs, using CO_2 laser radiation (57). Berlatzky and co-workers in 1985 achieved total pancreatectomies in dogs with a Nd:YAG laser and a fiber delivery system versus conventional operative procedures. They found a significant reduction in operative time, the blood loss and duodenal viability being similar (58). They noticed the surgical drawback of beam divergence at the fiber tip (10°), also mentioned in reports on liver surgery (4), and suggested the use of a ''constant and variable focusing mechanism.'' These conclusions lead to the ulterior use of the sapphire tip as the constant focusing mechanism whereas the lens handpiece affords a variable focusing. Brackett and co-workers in 1986, using a similar Nd:YAG device with progressive increments of power densities, have demonstrated that high power produces damages beyond the exposed area leading to the early death of animals (59). Results suggest the use of lower power levels, which is the performing range of the contact probe.

In 1986, Joffe used a Nd:YAG contact laser scalpel to perform six pancreatectomies in humans for chronic pancreatitis (i.e., three total, two distal, and one insulinoma excision) with excellent results and no complications (24). More data are expected to determine the promising place of contact Nd:YAG lasers in difficult pancreatic surgery.

Spleen

In splenic surgery, no specific laser surgical experience in humans has been reported yet.

Since the first paper in 1952, ''Susceptibility to infection after splenectomy performed in infancy'' (60), and numerous works on the high incidence of postsplenectomy infection (61–63), interest in saving total or part of the spleen has been widely discussed. Anatomy of the spleen, blood supply, distribution, territories, and spleen segmentation have been very well defined (64–66). Techniques of splenic conservation have resulted from these investigations (67, 68). In 1979, Giler and co-workers undertook partial splenectomy in mongrel dogs with the CO_2 laser at 30 W without clamping the splenic pedicle, but using manual compression and, sometimes, ligation of large blood vessels (69). Another technique, described by Dixon and co-workers in 1980, associates suction, aspiration, and Nd:YAG laser radiation. Segmental splenectomies have been performed in mongrel dogs, using a 600-μm fiber, 8° divergence, and at a power of 55 W. The laser was considered useful to control peripheral vessel bleeding but not for intermediate or central vessels (70). The possible enhancement of the process by using the Auth contact silica blade was mentioned in the report by Dixon et al. (70). Spleen inferior pole resections in pigs after ligation of the gastroepiploic artery and the inferior branches of the splenic artery were performed in 1986 using a Nd:YAG laser, a 600-μm fiber with a 8° divergence, and placement of the tip 10 mm from the tissues. Cutting results were quick, easy, and yielded no complications with a 2- to 4-mm thermal damage (71).

A comparative study was presented by Schröder and co-workers in 1986 (72). The CO_2 laser at 25 W, 0.5-mm spot size versus the Nd:YAG laser with a contact-frosted 1.2-mm sapphire tip at 10 W. The spleen was divided in the widest diameter with no previous ligations. Significant results in favor of the Nd:YAG laser radiation pertain to ligatures posttransection ($P<0.01$), operating time, and blood loss ($P<0.05$) (72).

In humans, operative circumstances are obviously different regarding the volume and form of the spleen; the nature of the disease, namely, cyst, tumor, or surgical laceration during abdominal surgery; or traumatic injury (Barrett's type I to IV). The surgeon's decisions depend on those circumstances, but individual experience together with the availability of different laser equipment will also play a critical role.

ANORECTAL INDICATIONS

Proctology

Obviously, the most common disease is hemorrhoids, but presently only 5% of the medically treated piles undergo surgery. Most have injections, rubberband ligations, cryotherapy, infrared photocoagulation, and surgery is proposed on failures of these treatments.

In this field, progress is undeniable. Most surgeons operate only on Stage III prolapsed hemorrhoids under general, peridural, or spinal anesthesia. Reduction of pain, minimal postoperative edema, less medication, shortened hospitalization stays, minimal short- and long-term complications, earlier return to professional activity, and satisfactory long-term follow-up are the unvaried items one can find in all reports on laser anal surgery (26–30).

Comparative studies between CO_2 lasers and conventional surgery (27) or between CO_2 laser surgery and cryotherapy (73) give the preference to the laser. Recent data show that more and more patients are undertaken on an outpatient basis (74). Tendancy to operate on Stage II or even Stage I hemorrhoids by laser excision under local anesthesia on a similar basis is clearly visible. Such acts are painless, without complications or stenoses, and are at least as efficient as other medical methods and will reduce the treatment duration for the patients.

In strangulated prolapses or circumferential thromboses, the first step for most authors remains medical treatment, namely, hospitalization for local cure, radiotherapy against edema and pain for some, and delayed operation according to the risk of stenosis. Laser technique brings other advantages: early surgery; saving pain, time, and cost; and producing no long-term complications.

Remnant anal benign pathology may be divided into three categories:

1. *Noninfectious:* Anal fissures, inferior transphincteric fistulas, and skin tags, hypertrophic papillas are treated on an outpatient basis under local anesthesia.
2. *Infectious:* For superior transphincteric fistulas, anal verge abscesses that need intraoperative dye-identification of the causal tract, and pilonidal sinuses, general anesthesia with short hospitalization is more advisable.
3. *Anal warts:* Anal warts are usually vaporized in outpatients under local sphincteric anesthesia allowing for a complete anal canal exposure. Recurrences, if any, come from unrecognized sites. Massive and giant circular varieties are vaporized in one session under general anesthesia. Results are excellent but in any case, within a month, a control under microscope is recommended.

Rectal Tumors

In benign or malignant rectal tumors, endoscopic Nd:YAG laser therapy is widely performed in elderly and/or nonsurgical patients.

In *adenoma*, success rates vary with tumor size (i.e., 94% with tumors smaller than 2 cm to 24% with tumors larger than 4 cm) and recurrence rate at 2 years is 38% (75). New 1.32-μm Nd:YAG laser radiation, highly absorbed in high-water content tissues, is considered satisfactory in broad-based adenomas (76), but more data are expected.

In *rectal carcinoma*, the same procedure has also been widely applied, mostly in palliative treatment against rectal syncrome: bleeding between one and five sessions and/or bowel obstruction, two to five sessions. In practice, vaporizing tumors necessitates two to three sessions at 48-hour intervals and follow-up every three months during the 1st year, combining laser and dilators every 6 months or at request, with a routine liver control by ultrasonography.

Direct access to the lower part of the rectum has also been used widely by surgeons with conventional means and techniques, for example, excisions with or without electric cautery, tracted flaps, "parachute," cryotherapy, etc. But is there a *place for a surgical laser technique*? In visible tumors that are 3–9 cm from the anal verge, the answer is yes.

In *adenoma* and *adenocarcinoma*, Guyot and co-workers (77), using a CO_2 laser at 20–30 W with a 5- to 8-cm defocused beam through an anuscope, achieved the treatment of residual disease after endoscopic Nd:YAG therapy. Irradiation was painless and without significant bleeding. Destruction was complete in adenoma, incomplete in adenocarcinoma. Pfeffermann and co-workers (78) also performed CO_2 resection en bloc in villous adenomas and vaporizations in adenocarcinomas. In the latter indication, Pfeffermann et al. also reported incomplete destruction and applied the method in patients with contraindications for open surgery and in palliative treatments. However, no power parameters are given.

Endorectal ultrasonography has demonstrated an accurate assessment of rectal layers and perirectal tissues (36, 79–81). Exact depth and volume of tumors are now available preoperatively and give useful information in the treatment of local rectal tumors. Indications must be reserved to controlled benign tumors and palliative treatments in unoperable adenocarcinomas. The method is exposed in the Technical Aspects section (see Endorectal Surgery, page 12). Use of direct access allows for easy visualization of the tumor and achievement of vaporization with a bent 200-mm handpiece at 40–60 W. Differences in power densities come from accessibility to the tumor and the need to complete vaporization. Lateral and posterior tumors are not hazardous. On the contrary, anterior tumors require great care. No complications have been reported yet with the surgical use of the CO_2 laser radiation, but rectovaginal fistulas occurred with the endoscopic protocol (82). Intraoperative ERUS gives excellent assessment and allows complete destruction in many instances. The operative time-range is 30–90 min, but the aim is the total destruction in one session, which is not possible with the endoscopic treatment. The surgical approach represents a definite improvement for the patient, not to mention the cost.

On the other hand, Nd:YAG laser radiation, as expected, generates a tumor's surface carbonization, which modifies light absorption and stops radiation efficacy. If this laser is used surgically in a noncontact method with a short 50-mm handpiece, carbonization will also occur but the successive use of the CO_2 laser radiation will enable vaporization of the necrosis and allow the pursuit of tumoral destruction. Nd:YAG contact laser surgery may also be considered to complement this surgical technique.

Intraoperative biopsies and immediate pathological answers are available to complete ERUS informations and control the destruction, which is also not possible in the endoscopic way because of the size of the biopsies. Pain is nonexistent except if the Nd:YAG laser has been used markedly. The mean hospitalization stay is 1-2 days. When total destruction has been achieved, a 3-month follow-up is proposed, including liver ultrasonography.

In these endorectal protocols, lymph node involvement is not discussed. Of course, preoperative ERUS and scanner will assess the disease spread, but the surgical laser technique is mostly targeted at patients with surgical contraindications. According to the stage of tumors, a complementary radiotherapy treatment can be proposed to achieve a more complete palliative treatment.

Anal Carcinomas

In this section, squamous cell carcinoma and adenocarcinoma of the juxtaanal area involving or able to involve the anal sphincter will be considered.

Adenocarcinoma of the lower part of the rectum with successive spread to the anal canal will be treated by Miles operation if operable (see Intraabdominal Laser Dissections, page 15) or by palliative laser technique (see Rectal Tumors, page 23). Similarly, squamous cell carcinoma or Bowen's disease arising from the skin of the external perianal area, whose extent may slowly involve lower anal canal superficial layers only, will have a local excision considered here as an excellent treatment (83). Of course, it is a good indication for laser surgery, for example, CO_2 laser or sapphire contact Nd:YAG laser probes (see Intraabdominal Dissections, page 6).

As very well described by Papillon (84), anal canal squamous cell carcinomas generally present an early involvement of the sphincter and extensive spread leads to a malignant sphincteric stenosis. In reported data, inguinal and pelvic nodes are involved at 10-40% and 10-46%, respectively. Also, the adenocarcinomas arising in the juxtaanal area will infiltrate the sphincter early because of their predominant ulcerative configuration (85).

Before treatment, a clinical assessment must be undertaken as indicated previously (see Anal Conservative Surgery, page 13). Selected cases, for example, only those that are histologically well differentiated and or with no evidence of pelvic node involvement, will enter in present indications. The question arises again: where is there a place for a *laser conservative surgery*? In order to answer this question, four points must be examined.

1. From an oncological point of view, the *Miles operation* appears to be the most suitable solution. But, in case of the elderly patient, definitive colostomy is often not advisable and very badly accepted. In comparative data, the mean 5-year survival rate is 49.2% with a mean operative mortality rate of 6.7% and, when pelvic nodes are involved, the 5-year survival rate drops to 27.6% (86).
2. In such tumors, when the sphincter must be widely removed, conventional conservative surgery is generally excluded. Only small carcinomas are still proposed to *local excision* and most surgeons undertake postoperative radiotherapy to reduce the outcome of local recurrences.
3. Actually, it is admitted that *radiotherapy must keep the main place* in the *conservative treatment of anal carcinoma*. The different methods and results of radiotherapy, which are fully reported in Papillon's monography (87), will not be discussed in this chapter. But even in the best and most valuable series, the rate of local failures and/or severe radionecrosis that leads to a definitive colostomy must be taken in account. Rousseau and co-workers (88), and Eschwege and co-workers (89) report 20% and 34%, respectively. Using Co-60 and iridium 192, Papillon, whose series are considered as the most successful ones, relates excellent results at 5 years, however, with an 18% rate of such complications.
4. *Lasers*, instead of iridium, *might usefully suppress radionecrosis* and allow for a controlled destruction of the residual disease, even intrasphincteric disease. The limits of this therapeutic policy appears in the following preliminary study. In an early sample of 13 patients with anal carcinomas involving the sphincter (i.e., six squamous cell carcinomas and seven adenocarcinomas), lasers were used before radiotherapy for surgical resections of small tumors. For larger tumors, radiotherapy anticipated the laser treatment. Results are summarized in Tables 11.2 and 11.3. Local failures concern patients with tumor size larger than 4 cm who refused Miles operation. In these cases the protocol was applied on recurrence of disease, 1-2 years after radiotherapy, curietherapy, or 1 year after an endoscopic laser treatment. The patients having no previous therapy have been successful with no sphincteric impairment; 6 patients are alive with the survival indicated in Tables 11.1 and 11.2, 2 died by disease spread, and one died by cerebral hemorrhage at 91 years of age.

It is worth mentioning that in patients with recurrences after radiotherapeutic treatment, lasers must only be considered as a palliative treatment and will not avoid radical surgery whenever possible, advisable, and accepted. On the other hand, in small carcinomas, lasers allows precise dissection but must always be followed by complete external radiotherapy. Preoperative radiotherapy is indicated in tumors that are 2-4 cm in size followed 6 weeks later by laser surgery to remove and/or to vaporize residual tumors or nodules under intraoperative sonographic control.

Concerning lymphatic involvement, 2 patients had early inguinal metastases and 3 had massive pelvic metastases in the follow-up, and belong to the failures. The method is contraindicated in local recurrences in which pelvic spread must be accurately assessed, and also in tumors larger than 4 cm. The quality of the method is limited in early inguinal involvement, but the prognosis is bad with any other method. On the contrary, conservative laser technique looks promising in selected patients as defined by results, but of course, more prospective data are necessary.

CONCLUSIONS AND FUTURE PROSPECTS

In this chapter, the actual indications of surgical laser intraoperative procedures in abdominal and anorectal fields have been summarized. Most of these indications hold established protocols and recognized results. These indications have brought another approach to surgery, particularly in surgical oncology, in highly vascularized tissues, in hemophilia, or in patients under anticoagulant treatment.

Liver tumoral vaporizations have been proved feasible, useful as an adjunct therapy, and techniques to avoid hazards have been described. However, as far as the quality of life in the sur-

Table 11.2. Squamous Cell Carcinomas[a]

	Sex	Age (years)	Previous treatments	Tumor size	Protocol	Follow-up	Anal sphincter	Survival rate (months) Died	Alive	Cause of death
Failures	F	48	Recurrence 1 year after RT and curie therapy	3 cm	CO_2 + Nd:YAG	Persistent pelvic spread, APR accepted	Failure	20 post APR		Massive pelvic involvement
	M	68	Recurrence 2 years after RT and curie therapy	4 cm	CO_2 + Nd:YAG	Persistent pelvic spread	Failure	24 post APR		Massive pelvic involvement
	F	80	No, but inguinal mestastases	3 cm	CO_2 pelvic and inguinal RT	Inguinal recurrence, Local excisions	Normal	25		Pleuropulmonary metastases
Successes	F	62	No	3 cm	CO_2 RT postoperatively	Twice a year	Normal		61	
	F	57	No	3 cm	CO_2 + Nd:YAG RT postoperatively	Every 4 months	Normal		28	
	F	91	No	4 cm	RT preoperatively CO_2 + Nd:YAG	Every 4 months	Normal		39	

[a]Abbreviations used in table: RT, radiotherapy; APR, abdominoperineal resection.

Table 11.3. Anal Canal Adenocarcinomas[a]

	Sex	Age	Previous treatments	Tumor size	Protocol	Spread and follow-up	Anal sphincter	Survival rate (months) Died	Alive	Cause of death
Failures	M	60	RT 1 year before 1-year laser endoscopic therapy	4 cm	CO_2 + Nd:YAG	Liver metastases, APR + liver tumor vaporizations	Failure	26 post APR		Pulmonary tuberculosis
	M	64	No	4 cm	RT preoperatively CO_2 + Nd:YAG		Normal	19		Cerebral metastases
	M	61	Recurrence after RT; APR refused	4 cm	CO_2 + Nd:YAG	Tumor not controlled, APR accepted	Failure	24		Massive pelvic recurrence
Successes	F	82	No	3 cm	RT preoperatively CO_2	Twice a year	Normal		58	
	H	69	No	4 cm	RT preoperatively CO_2 + Nd:YAG RT postoperatively	Twice a year	Normal		54	
	F	62	No	4 cm	RT preoperatively CO_2 + Nd:YAG	Twice a year	Normal		49	
	F	87	No	3 cm	RT preoperatively CO_2 + Nd:YAG		Normal	36		Cerebral hemorrhage at 91 years of age

[a]Abbreviations: RT, radiotherapy; CO_2, CO_2 laser therapy; YAG, Nd:YAG laser therapy; APR, abdominoperineal resection.

vival of such patients has been demonstrated, effective, prospective studies are still needed. Assessment of their enhanced role in the destruction of these localizations remains to be improved.

Similarly, intraoperative irradiation of the pelvic cavity and of the lymph node clearance areas in Dukes C carcinoma of the rectum seems attractive and promising; both the lower rate of local recurrences and the prophylaxis of cancer cell spread during surgery have to be confirmed by further studies. Such a protocol does not prevent a previous, a simultaneous, or a successive radiotherapy. It is obvious that laser irradiation of the wounds and of all dissected areas at the end of a surgical oncological procedure appears suitable and attractive in all fields after tumoral excision. Confirmation of the results presented in this chapter will certainly enlarge laser intraoperative applications.

In the search for higher power densities, one should expect more powerful lasers to be useful in noncontact liver surgery. Tumor destructions will be less time-consuming, the necrotic zone being not very different from today's achievements. Chinese scientists have started to open these new vistas, describing applications with a 200-W Nd:YAG laser (17), but no other report has been published yet. Of course, such lasers should be under the control of experienced teams, but the results of the effects they may induce are of utmost interest.

CO_2 and Nd:YAG lasers coexist already in a unique apparatus with the possibility of emitting beams through the same optical arm; but it is not possible to have the two beams simultaneously. This will happen soon and will greatly facilitate the combined delivery.

Photodynamic therapy has not been raised in this chapter because it is not an open surgical procedure. But, in a Laser Platform, the presence of dye (pulsed or CW), pulsed-Nd:YAG, excimer, and metal vapor lasers should open opportunities of finding and applying new techniques that will generate progress.

REFERENCES

1. Sultan RA, Etienne J, Raimbert P, Fallouh H, et al. Multidisciplinary centre for laser surgery. Report in connection with 515 cases. In: Atsumi K, Nimsakul N, Eds. Laser Tokyo '81. Tokyo, Inter Group Corp, 1981; pp 20-23.
2. Etienne J, Dorme N, Ladouch-Badre A, Raimbert P, Berthier JP, Sultan RA. Comparative study of the effects of Argon and Neodymium-YAG laser beams on the normal fundic wall in the beagle dog. Digest Dis Sci 1982; 27:425-433.
3. Joffe SN, MacLeod IA, Rao SS. Influence of Nd:YAG laser power density and coaxial CO_2 on the gastric wall. Lasers Surg Med 1984; 4:247-259.
4. Godlewski G, Ginoves P, Chincholles JM, et al. Hepatic resection with an Nd:YAG laser in pigs. Lasers Surg Med 1983; 3:217-224.
5. Sultan RA, Fallouh H, Lefebvre-Vilardebo M, Ladouch-Badre A. Separate and combined use of Nd:YAG and carbon dioxide lasers in liver resections: A preliminary report. Lasers Med Sci 1986; 1:101-105.
6. Godlewski G, Rouy S, Gay G, Bureau JP, Eledjam JJ. Influence du clampage pédiculaire dans les resections hrépatiques partielles au laser Nd:YAG. J Chir (Paris) 1984; 121:667-672.
7. Godlewski G, Rouy S, Eledjam JJ. Thermal and morphological effects of hepatic bloodflow variations during liver resections with the Nd:YAG laser. Lasers Med Sci 1986; 1:41-46.
8. Sultan RA, Philandrianos G, Fallouh H, Boulnois JL. Multidisciplinary surgical experience of sapphire contact probes. Lasers Med Sci 1986; 1(A):295.
9. Sultan RA, Fallouh H, Marinov V. Chirurgie digestive: Quels lasers pour quelle chirurgie? Ann Gastrol Hepatol 1987; 23:389-392.
10. Joffe SN, Daikuzono N. Contact laser surgery in gastroenterology. An update on the endoscopic and open surgical applications. Lasers Surg Med 1986; 6(A):200.
11. Steger A, Hira N, Moore KC. Lasers in gastrointestinal tract surgery. Lasers Surg Med 1986; 6(A):279.
12. Nims TA, McCaughan JS. Clinical experience with CO_2 laser vaporization of neoplasm. Lasers Surg Med 1983; 3:265-268.
13. Hinshaw JR, Herrera HR, Lanzafame RJ, Pennino RP. The use of carbon dioxide laser permits primary closure of contamined and purulent lesions and wounds. Lasers Surg Med 1987; 6:581-583.
14. Chegin VM, Skobelkin OK, Brekhov EI. Laser surgery for soft tissue purulent diseases. Lasers Surg Med 1984; 4:279-282.
15. Partensky C, Champetier P, Bretagnolle M, Valette PJ, Paliard P. Traitement de l'échinococcose alvé olaire he patique. Utilisation du laser CO_2 en complément de l'hépatectomie palliative. Med Chir Dig 1987; 16:131-133.
16. Sultan RA, Lefebvre-Vilardebo M. Could the CO_2 laser be involved in the hepatic tumoral localizations treatment? 1rst Congress of the European Laser Association. Cannes: Tech Digest, 1982; p 55.
17. Yegin Y, Zhaoyou T, Xinda Z. High power Nd:YAG laser in the treatment of liver cancer. Experimental and clinical study. Lasers Surg Med 1986; 6(A):276.
18. Meyer HJ, Haverkampf K. Experimental study of partial liver resection with a combined CO_2 and Nd:YAG laser. Lasers Surg Med 1982; 2:149-154.
19. Tranberg KG, Rigotti P, Brackett KA, Bjornson HS, Fischer JE, Joffe SN. Liver resection. A comparison

using the Nd:YAG laser, an ultrasonic surgical aspirator, or blunt dissection. Am J Surg 1986; 151:368-373.

20. Doty JL, Auth DC. The laser photocoagulating dielectric waveguide scalpel. IEEE Trans Bio Eng 1981; 28:1-9.
21. Iwasaki M, Sasako M, Konishi T, Maruyama Y, Wada T. Nd:YAG laser for general surgery. Lasers Surg Med 1985; 5:429-438.
22. ReMine SG, Aretz TH, Shapshay SM, Setzer MD, Setzer SE. Sapphire tip contact Nd:YAG laser vs other cutting techniques for hepatic resections. Lasers Surg Med 1986; 6(A): 200.
23. Joffe SN, Brackett KA, Sankar MY, Daikuzono N. Resection of the liver with the Nd:YAG laser. Surg Gynecol Obstet 1986; 163:437-442.
24. Joffe SN. Contact Neodymium-YAG laser surgery in gastroenterology: A preliminary report. Lasers Surg Med 1986; 6:155-157.
25. Sultan RA, Fallouh H, Lefebvre-Vilardebo M. Lasers et volatilisations tumorales chirurgicales. In: Champault G, Malafosse M, Eds. Actualités Chirurgicales; Vol 1. Paris: Masson, 1986, Vol 1, p 153.
26. Riedlinger J. The surgical treatment of hemorrhoids by means of the carbon dioxide laser. In Atsumi K, Nimsakul N, Eds. Laser Tokyo '81, Tokyo, Inter Group Corp, 1981, pp 30-31.
27. Sultan RA, Fallouh H, Raimbert P. Proctology with the CO_2 laser. In connection with 75 cases. In Atsumi K, Nimsakul N, Eds. Laser Tokyo '81, Tokyo, Inter Group Corp, 1981, pp 39-42.
28. Morselli M, Buttazzi A, Manenti A, Stacca R, Farinelli FF. Outpatient treatment of hemorrhoids by CO_2 laser. Lasers Surg Med 1985; 5(A):144-145.
29. Zadeh AT. Three hundred fifty hemorrhoidectomies using carbon dioxide laser Lasers Surg Med 1985; 5(A): 145.
30. Eddy HJ. Treatment of hemorrhoids with the Nd:YAG laser. A preliminary report. Lasers Surg Med 1983; 3(A): 155.
31. Eddy HJ. Treatment of hemorrhoids with the Nd:YAG laser—100 cases. Lasers Surg Med 1984; 3(A):337.
32. Eddy HJ, Yu JC, Eddy EC. Dual laser hemorrhoidectomy. Lasers Surg Med 1986; 6(A):201.
33. Mason AY. Transphincteric surgery of the rectum. Prog Surg 1974; 13:66-97.
34. Crile G, Turnbull RB. The role of electrocoagulation in the treatment of carcinoma of the rectum. Surg Gynecol Obstet 1972; 135:391-396.
35. Verschueren R, Oldhoff J. Laser surgery on polyps and tumors of the rectosigmoid colon. A preliminary report. In Kaplan I, Ed. Laser Surgery. Jerusalem, Jerusalem Academic Press, 1976, p 70.
36. Hildebrandt U, Feifel G. Preoperative staging of rectal cancer by intrarectal ultrasound. Dis Colon Rectum 1985; 28:42-46.
37. Shafir R, Zweig A, Slutzki S, Bornstein LA. Use of the carbon dioxide laser in an abdominoperineal resection for epidermoid anal carcinoma: A case report. Br J Surg 1978; 65:565-566.
38. Hunter JG, Dixon JA. Lesser curvature laser myotomy: A potential treatment in peptic ulcer. Lasers Surg Med 1984; 4(A):362.
39. McCaughan JS. Multilaser approach to management of malignancies. Lasers Surg Med 1983; 3(A):123.
40. Sultan RA, Philandrianos G, Fallouh H, Boulnois JL. Dix-huit mois d'expérience des pointes saphir en chirurgie de contact au laser Nd:YAG. La Presse Med 1987; 16:636.
41. Lanzafame RJ, Rogers DW, Naim JO, DeFranco CA, Ochej H, Hinshaw JR. Reduction of local tumor recurrence by excision with the CO_2 laser. Lasers Surg Med 1986; 6:439-441.
42. Rao AR, Kagan AR, Chan PM, Gilbert HA, Nussbaum H, Hintz BL. Patterns of recurrence following curative resection alone for adenocarcinoma of the rectum and sigmoid colon. Cancer 1981; 48:1492-1495.
43. Dubois JB, Joyeux H, Solassol C, Pujol H. La radiothérapie peropératoire dans le traitement des cancers. La Presse Med 1986; 15:1397-1399.
44. Mullins F, Jennings B, McClusky L. Liver resection with the continuous wave carbon dioxide laser: Some experimental observations. Am Surg 1968; 34:717-722.
45. Hall RR. Haemostatic incision of the liver: Carbon dioxide laser compared with surgical diathermy. Br J Surg 1971; 58:538–540, p 33.
47. Fidler JP, Hoefer RW, Polanyi TG, et al. Laser surgery in exsanguinating liver injury. Ann Surg 1975; 181:74-80.
48. Königsmann G, Köster K. Lasers in surgery. Battelle Frankf Inf 1978; 27:26-30.
49. Tranberg KG, Rigotti P, Joffe SN. Liver resection. A study comparing the Nd:YAG laser, CUSA, and conventional 'finger fracture'. Lasers Surg Med 1984; 3(A):362.
50. Meyer HJ, Haverkampf K, Frank F, Ostertag H, Neuhaus R, Newhaus P. Surgery of the liver with a new high power Nd:YAG laser. Lasers Surg Med 1985; 5(A):148.
51. Maruyama Y, Iwasaki M, Sasako M, Wada T. Nd:YAG laser for general surgery. In: Atsumi K, Nimsakul N, Eds. Laser Tokyo '81, Tokyo: Inter Group Corp, 1981, pp 26-29.
52. Gagna G, Massaioli N, Fausone G, et al. The CO_2 laser in general surgery. Lasers Surg Med 1985; 5(A):147.
53. Bödecker V, Buchholz J, Drake KH, Grotelüschen B: Influence of thermal effects on the width of necrotic zones during cutting and coagulating with laser beams. In: Kaplan I, Ed. Laser Surgery. Jerusalem: Jerusalem Academic Press, 1976, p 101.
54. Godlewski G, Rouy S, Eledjman JJ. Thermal and morphological effects of hepatic blood flow variations during liver resections with the Nd:YAG laser. Lasers Med Sci 1986; 1:41-46.
55. Nagasawa A, Kato K, Nishikawa K, Atsumi K, Arai K. Combined YAG laser with CO_2 laser therapy applied to malignant tumors. In: Atsumi K, Nimsakul N, Eds. Laser Tokyo '81, Tokyo: Inter Group Corp, 1981, pp 38-41.
56. Giler S, Gassner S, Ben Uri R, Kaplan I. The CO_2 laser surgery of the pancreas: An experimental study. In: Kaplan I, Ascher PW, Eds. Laser Surgery III, Part 1, Tel-Aviv: OT-PAZ, 1979, p 211.

57. Di Donna G. Total pancreatectomy with CO_2 laser. In: Atsumi K, Nimsakul N, Eds. Laser Tokyo '81, Tokyo: Inter Group Corp, 1981, pp 43-45.
58. Berlatzky Y, Muggia-Sullam M, Munda R, Joffe SN. Use of the Nd:YAG laser in pancreatic resections. Lasers Surg Med 1985; 5:507-514.
59. Brackett KA, Sankar MY, Joffe SN. Effects of Nd:YAG laser photoradiation on intra-abdominal tissues: A histological study of tissue damage versus power density applied. Lasers Surg Med 1986; 6:123-130.
60. King H, Schumacker HB. Splenic studies. Susceptibility to infection after splenectomy performed in infancy. Ann Surg 1952; 136:239-242.
61. Diamuno LK. Splenectomy in childhood and the hazards of overwhelming infection. Pediatrics 1969; 43:886-889.
62. Eraklis A, Filler RN. Splenectomy in childhood: A review of 1413 cases. J Pediatr Surg 1972; 7:383-388.
63. Gopal V, Bisno AL. Fulminant pneumococcal infection in normal asplenic hosts. Arch Intern Med 1977; 137:1526-1530.
64. Michels NA. The variational anatomy of the spleen and splenic artery. Ann Anat 1942; 1:21-73.
65. Nguyen H. Territoires artériels de la rate. Etude expérimentale. Possibilités de résection partielle réglée de la rate. La Presse Med 1956; 64:63-64.
66. Pina JA. Territorios Arterios Asplenicos. Lisbon; University Press, 1979.
67. De Boer J, Summer Smith G, Dawnie H. Partial splenectomy. Technique and some hematologic consequences in the dog. J Pediatr Surg 1972; 7:378-381.
68. Morgenstern L, Shapiro SJ. Techniques of splenic conservation. Arch Surg 1979; 114:449-454.
69. Giler S, BenBassat M, Gassner S, Kaplan I. The CO_2 laser surgery of the spleen: an experimental study. In: Kaplan I, Ascher PW, Eds. Laser Surgery III Part 1. Tel-Aviv: OT-PAZ, 1979, p 217.
70. Dixon JA, Miller F, McCloskey D, Siddoway J. Anatomy and techniques in segmental splenectomy. Surg Gynecol Obstet 1980; 150:516-520.
71. Godlewski G, Rouy S, Eledjam JJ, Cousineau J, Pradel P, Bureau JP. Partial splenectomy with the Nd:YAG laser in pigs. Lasers Med Sci 1986; 1:147-151.
72. Schröder T, Foster J, Brackett K, Joffe SN. Splenic resection with the CO_2 laser and the contact Nd:YAG scalpel. Lasers Med Sci 1986; 1(A):293-294.
73. Rausis C, Amato M. Haemorrhoidal proctitis: from cyrogenic treatment to surgery with CO_2 laser. Lasers Med Sci 1986; 1(A):296.
74. Zadeh AT. Outpatient haemorrhoidectomy using the CO_2 laser in 750 cases. Lasers Med Sci 1986; 1(A):296.
75. Lambert R, Sabben G. Laser et tumeurs du tube digestif. In: Girardeau-Montaut JP, Lambert R, Eds. Les Lasers et Leurs Applications Médicales. Lyon: Ed Medicales Internat, 1987, p 315.
76. Sander R, Pösl H, Strobel M, Ünsold E, Frank F, Spuhler A. The Nd:YAG laser in gastroenterology: Initial results of experimental and clinical studies with a wavelength of 1.32 μm. Lasers Med Sci 1986; 1(A):282-283.
77. Guyot P, Lambert R, Sabben G, Chavaillon A, Boustière C, Bonvoisin S. CO_2 vs Nd:YAG laser in the treatment of rectal neoplastic lesions. Lasers Med Sci 1986; 1(A):294.
78. Pfeffermann R, Merhav H, Rothstein H, Simon D. The use of laser in rectal surgery. Lasers Surg Med 1986; 6:467-469.
79. Beynon J, Foy DMA, Roe AM, Temple LN, McC Mortensen NJ. Endoluminal ultrasound in the assessment of local invasion in rectal cancer. Br J Surg 1986; 73:474-477.
80. Mosnier H, Guivarc'h M, Barbagelata M. L'échographie endorectale: Appréciation de l'extension loco-régionale des cancers du rectum. Gastr Clin Biol 1987; 11:307-311.
81. Sultan RA, Faure JC. Intéret des échographies endorectales. Med Chir Dig 1986; 15:259-264.
82. Naveau S, Poitrine A, Zourabichvili O, Poynard T, Chaput JC. Endoscopic Nd:YAG laser therapy for palliative treatment of rectal adenocarcinoma: Immediate results, follow-up and parameters affecting tumor destruction. Lasers Med Sci 1986; 1(A):284.
83. Papillon J. Rectal and Anal Cancers. Berlin: Springer-Verlag, 1982, p 181.
84. Papillon J. Rectal and Anal Cancers. Berlin: Springer-Verlag, 1982, p 116.
85. Papillon J. Rectal and Anal Cancers. Berlin: Springer-Verlag, 1982, p 95.
86. Papillon J. Rectal and Anal Cancers. Berlin: Springer-Verlag, 1982, p 129.
87. Papillon J. Rectal and Anal Cancers. Berlin: Springer-Verlag, 1982, p 130.
88. Rousseau J. Mathieu G, Fenton J: Résultats et complications de la radiothérapie des épithéliomas du canal anal. Etude de 128 cas traités de 1956 à 1970. Gastr Clin Biol 1979; 3:207-208.
89. Eschwege F, Breteau N, Chavy A, Lasser P, Wibault P, Kac J. Complications de la radiothérapie transcutanée des épithéliomas du canal anal. Gastr Clin Biol 1979; 3:183-186.

CHAPTER

12

Anorectal Disorders

Norman Sohn

It is natural that advances in laser science and technology would be applied to the treatment of anorectal disorders. Indeed, lasers have a profound effect on the therapy of anorectal disorders. Contact Nd:YAG lasers, in particular, facilitate anorectal surgery by effecting a dramatic reduction in postoperative pain. This extends the possibility of anorectal operative therapy, employing standard operative techniques, to groups of patients for whom it would not have been considered previously. Conditions that are amenable to contact Nd:YAG laser surgery include hemorrhoids, fissures, fistulas, pilonidal sinuses, condylomata acuminata, and various benign and malignant neoplastic conditions. These entities and their therapy using contact Nd:YAG lasers will be discussed. The laser is a tool that can substitute for the scalpel and electrocautery. It enables the surgeon to work more efficiently and results in less postoperative pain. The basic principles of therapy of these disorders has not changed. In order to maximize the benefits available from laser anorectal surgery, the principles underlying treatment of these conditions will also be covered. This chapter will not delve into the management of rectal or colonic carcinoma.

HEMORRHOIDS

Hemorrhoids are pads of tissue that line the anorectum (1). This concept is most consistent with many observations on the nature and behavior of hemorrhoids. The former theory, regarding hemorrhoids as mere varicosities, is incompatible with current knowledge. Hemorrhoids serve to produce complete closure of the anal canal by acting as compressible sponges lining the lower rectum. They are always present when a rectum is present. Therapy is directed toward symptomatic treatment of hemorrhoids. Asymptomatic hemorrhoids require no treatment.

The author prefers to classify hemorrhoids into five major types depending primarily on the symptoms they produce and secondly on their location; hemorrhoids can be internally or externally positioned (2). The traditional hemorrhoid classification into grades I, II, III, and IV applies only to the capability of internal hemorrhoids to protrude or to external hemorrhoids. This classification fails to account for hemorrhoids whose major symptom is bleeding. It also groups thrombosed hemorrhoids and the "acute attack" with other hemorrhoid types with which these have little in common.

The five groups of hemorrhoids are bleeding, internal, external, thrombosed, and the acute attack of piles.

In treating patients with bleeding hemorrhoids, it is most important to exclude the possibility of other etiologies for the bleeding. Bleeding hemorrhoids are usually internal hemorrhoids. These can be simply treated by injection sclerotherapy, rubber band ligation, or infrared photocoagulation. Laser photocoagulation and newer modalities of electrotherapy are now used in the management of bleeding hemorrhoids. However, any new modality will have to rival the safety, efficacy, and economy of the simpler methods mentioned.

Internal hemorrhoids can cause symptoms of protrusion, bleeding, or a sensation of incomplete evacuation of the rectum. The classical classification of hemorrhoids as grades I, II, III, and IV pertain to protruding hemorrhoids in which grade I hemorrhoids do not protrude, grade II protrude but reduce spontaneously, grade III require manual reduction, and grade IV are irreducible. Internal hemorrhoids respond to rubber band ligation. Protruding internal hemorrhoids rarely respond to infrared photocoagulation or injection sclerotherapy. Those that fail to respond to rubber band ligation require operative hemorrhoidectomy. This will be described later in this chapter. In some cases, part or all of the circumference of the lower rectum everts during defecation. This configuration of hemorrhoids does not respond to conservative modalities and is best treated operatively.

External hemorrhoids may be asymptomatic, may produce symptoms of a cosmetic nature, or cause difficulty in maintaining personal hygiene. When there is a significant internal component, rubber band ligation can be curative. Those that fail to respond to rubber band ligation or those in which there is an insignificant internal component are optimally treated by operative hemorrhoidectomy.

In assessing patients with hemorrhoids, it is advisable to examine them immediately after defecation. This is accomplished by administering a phosphate enema and performing a rectal examination shortly after it is expelled. This is an essential part of the examination and significant pathology, often revealed by this maneuver, can otherwise be overlooked.

Thrombosed hemorrhoids are hemorrhoids in which a thrombus has formed. In treating this condition it must be remembered that this is a spontaneously resolving condition. The pain that is present resolves over a period of a few days and the thrombus is reabsorbed over a period of 2–8 weeks. Only when it is causing excessive pain should the thrombosed hemorrhoid be excised. The Nd:YAG laser is helpful in these excisions.

Pruritus ani often has nothing to do with hemorrhoids. It can usually be corrected without performing a hemorrhoidectomy and, conversely, an operative hemorrhoidectomy often has no effect on pruritus ani. When specific pathology has been excluded, pruritus ani usually responds to a regimen of local anal hygiene and topical flurandrenolide cream.

The acute attack of piles is a startling event in which the hemorrhoids are edematous and contain multiple thrombi. This, again, is a self-curing condition. The pain is maximum at the outset and then usually resolves spontaneously. In the exceptional case where the condition fails to improve, operative hemorrhoidectomy could be considered.

Most anorectal operations can be performed with local anesthesia. The author prefers the prone jackknife position for anorectal surgery. Multiple subcutaneous injections of ½% bupivacaine with 1:200,000 epinephrine containing 150 units of hyaluronidase for each 15 ml of solution are made. A wheal is raised continuously around the anus. A 25 to 30-gauge needle is utilized. Then in the left and right midlateral positions, and anterior and posterior midline positions, a 22-gauge, 1½-inch long needle is passed up to the hub and 2.5 ml of the anesthetic solution are deposited. Because these injections are painful, the patients are sedated with meperidine and midazolam.

An operative hemorrhoidectomy utilizing a contact-type Nd:YAG laser is performed by first introducing local anesthesia. A Hirschmann anoscope is placed in the anal canal. Four lubricated gauze pads (4 × 8 inch) are passed through the anoscope. The latter is then removed. The gauze pads are then gradually withdrawn. This causes the internal hemorrhoids to prolapse. This can disclose hitherto unrevealed pathology. In general, there are three major hemorrhoids: in the right anterolateral position, the right posterolateral position, and the left lateral position. The anal canal is then examined with Parks and Hill-Ferguson retractors to search for any other pathology (Figs. 12.1 and 12.2).

The hemorrhoid to be dissected is exposed with a Parks retractor. This dilates and shortens the anal canal facilitating dissection of the hemorrhoid, which is grasped with an Allis clamp. A second Allis clamp is placed at the peripheral margin of the hemorrhoid. A 00 Vicryl suture ligature is placed just proximal to the hemorrhoid pedicle and tied (Fig. 12.3*A*). This suture marks the proximal extent of the dissection and reduces bleeding.

The borders of the excision are outlined with a vaporization probe using 17-19 W of power (Fig. 12.3*B*). This is done slowly and deliberately, particularly proximally, just distal to the previously placed suture ligature, in order to obliterate the underlying vasculature. A 1.2-mm scalpel probe, at 17-19 W is next used to dissect the hemorrhoid off the underlying internal sphincter and to divide any residual hemorrhoidal attachments laterally or proximally (Fig. 12.3*C*). Any residual bleeding sites can be suture-ligated or coagulated with a coagulation probe at 8-9 W.

After all of the hemorrhoids have been excised, the Parks retractor is replaced by a Hill-Ferguson

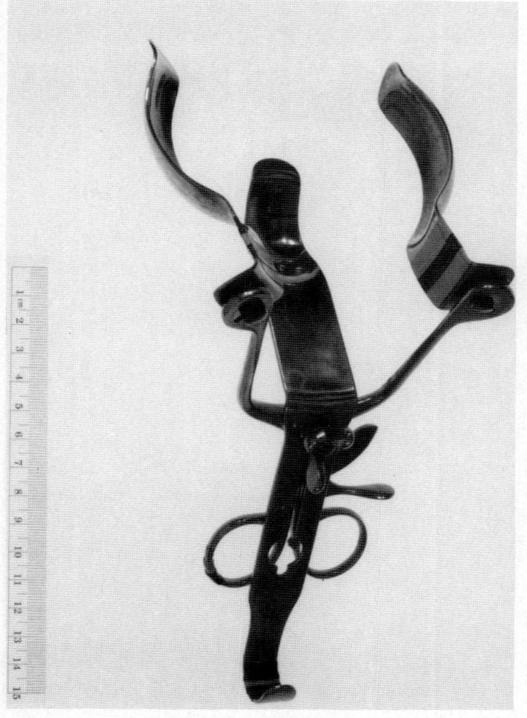

Figure 12.1. Parks retractor.

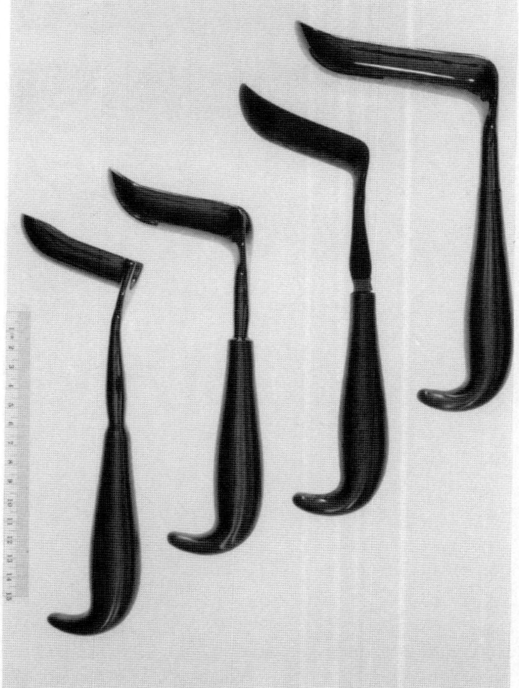

Figure 12.2. Hill-Ferguson retractors.

retractor. The latter serves to lengthen the anal canal and to coapt the mucosal edges, which facilitates mucosal and skin closure. A running 00 Vicryl suture is used to repair the defect in the mucosa and skin (Fig. 12.3*D*). Any other residual or minor hemorrhoids are excised and repaired transversely.

Patients are cautioned about the following potential postoperative complications: (*a*) bleeding; (*b*) fever; (*c*) inability to urinate; and (*d*) bowel movements and fecal impaction.

Patients are watched carefully for approximately 1 hour after the procedure to ascertain that there is no active bleeding. They are also cautioned against the use of aspirin or aspirin-containing products because these may promote postoperative bleeding. Acetaminophen or compounds containing acetaminophen are encouraged instead.

Postoperative fever is not to be expected. There was one case when a patient had a fever of 38.3°C on the first postoperative evening. The patient was give amoxicillin, 500 mg every 8 hours. The fever promptly resolved. Its specific etiology was never elucidated.

Postoperative pain is managed with acetaminophen or codeine. More severe pain is controlled with oxycodone-acetaminophen.

Difficulty urinating is more likely to occur in males, particularly those over 60 years of age. However, it is possible for this to occur in younger patients as well as in women. In the author's series, two patients, both men, required a single catheterization, in the postoperative period. To encourage urination, patients limit the oral intake of fluids until they are urinating, take adequate analgesics, and take sitz baths. In addition, bethanecol chloride in an oral dose of 25 mg four times a day is prescribed unless there are contraindications.

Patients undergoing hemorrhoidectomy, particularly extensive hemorrhoidectomy, tend to be constipated in the postoperative period. In order to encourage defecation, the patients are placed on dioctyl sodium sulfosuccinate in a dose of 600 mg day and psyllium seed supple-

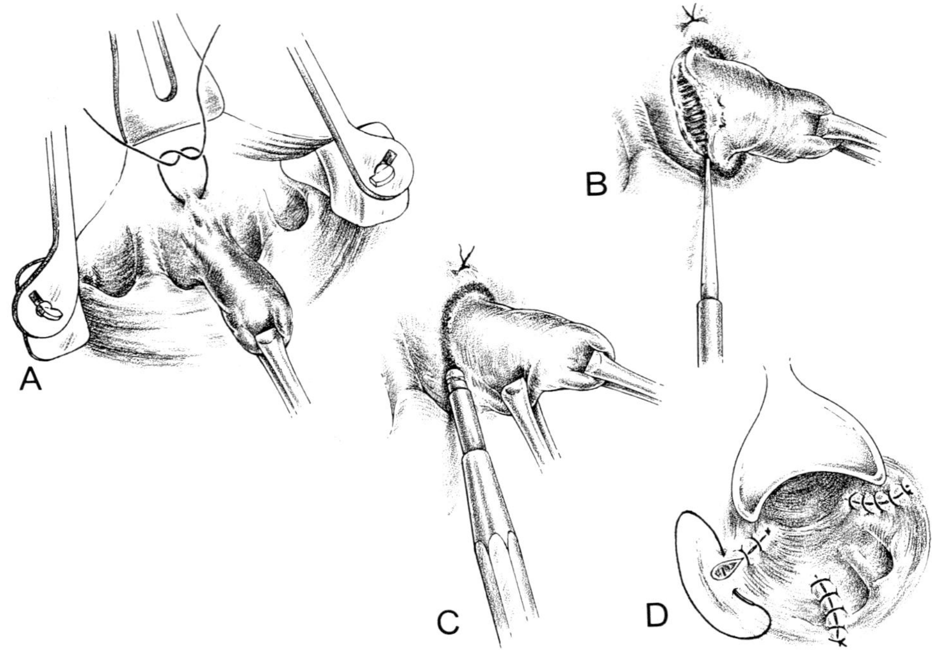

Figure 12.3. Hemorrhoidectomy. **A.** A hemorrhoid is grasped in an Allis clamp. A 00 Vicryl suture is being tied just proximal to the hemorrhoid pedicle. **B.** Excision borders are outlined with a vaporization probe. **C.** The hemorrhoid is dissected off the underlying internal sphincter with scalpel probe. **D.** The Hill-Ferguson retractor is in place. Three hemorrhoidectomy wounds are sutured.

ments. In addition, they are given bisacodyl tablets in a dose of 10–15 mg on the first postoperative day. This is repeated on the second postoperative day if there has not been a bowel movement. If there is still no bowel function by the end of the third day, the patients are given 300 ml of magnesium citrate. In the author's series, two patients developed postoperative fecal impactions that required disimpaction. This was accomplished utilizing local anesthesia and an impaction evictor.

After the immediate postoperative period, the patients are seen at approximately 2- to 4-week intervals until the operative wounds have healed fully. Working people are advised that they will be out of work for up to 10 days after a hemorrhoidectomy.

FISSURE IN ANO

An anal fissure is an ulcer in the posterior or anterior midline locations. Rarely will they be located other than in the midline. Under these circumstances a specific etiology must be sought, such as Crohn's disease, syphilis, or tuberculosis. There is frequently an enlarged anal papilla or an enlarged sentinel pile and hypertrophy of the internal sphincter.

Patients with anal fissures have internal anal sphincter dysfunction (3, 4). The sphincter pressure tends to be normal or elevated at rest but with an exaggerated response after distension of the sphincter. The pain pattern of a fissure is that of pain which occurs with defecation or a variable period of time later, persists for several minutes to several hours, and then usually subsides until the next defecation. This pattern reflects the underlying pressure in the rectum and is assumed to be due to spasms of the anal sphincter.

Adequate operative treatment of an anal fissure involves a step that interferes with function of the internal sphincter. In the past, dilatation of the anal sphincter was commonly performed. This was believed to exert its effect by causing a temporary paralysis of the sphincter, breaking up the cycle of sphincter spasm that is known to interfere with healing of the fissure.

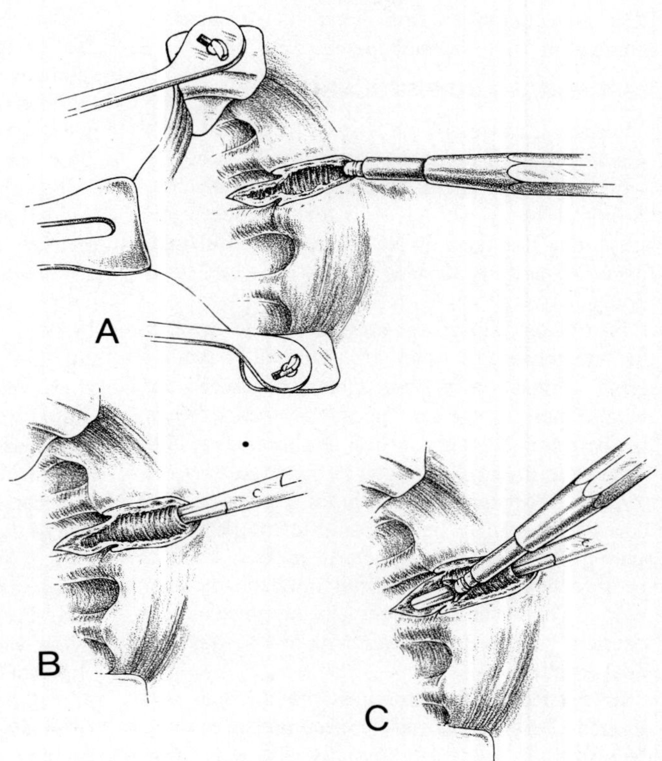

Figure 12.4. Internal anal sphincterotomy. **A**, The Parks retractor is in place. Incision is made in mucosa and skin from dentate line to intersphincteric groove. If hemorrhoidectomy was performed, mucosa is retracted to display midlateral position of internal sphincter. **B**, The internal sphincter is dissected off external sphincter with hemostat. **C**, The internal sphincter is incised with a vaporization probe from the dentate line to its lower border.

More recently, an internal anal sphincterotomy has been favored (5). This again interferes with the cycle of spasm and permits the fissure to heal. This is performed in the lateral position where it is alleged to have a lesser effect on anal continence than a posterior midline sphincterotomy. The latter can be associated with a ''keyhole'' deformity with minor impairments of continence.

The etiology of a fissure is not certain. It may be related to direct trauma from a bowel movement or to stretching of the anal sphincter in order to accommodate a large or hard stool. Most fissures will heal on a conservative regimen consisting of bulk laxatives, stool softeners, and bland suppositories. Only when they cause severe symptoms, fail to heal, or persistently recur is operation indicated.

In operating on anal fissures, the local anesthetic technique is as described previously. A concomitant hemorrhoidectomy can be performed if indicated. Exposure of the midlateral position, either right or left, is obtained with a Parks retractor. This puts the thickened internal sphincter under stretch. If a hemorrhoidectomy has been performed, before repair of the hemorrhoidectomy wound, the sphincterotomy site is selected by retracting the mucosa in order to expose the midlateral position of the internal sphincter (Fig. 12.4*A*). The internal sphincter is dissected off the external sphincter bluntly with a hemostat (Fig. 12.4*B*). It is then incised utilizing the vaporization probe, at 17–19 W, from the dentate line out to its lower border (Fig. 12.4*C*). Hemostasis is completed with coagulation probe.

If no concomitant hemorrhoidectomy is being performed, an incision is made from the dentate line out to the lower border of the internal sphincter with the vaporization probe (Fig. 12.4*A*). The internal sphincter is dissected off the external sphincter with a hemostat (Fig. 12.4*B*). It is incised with the vaporization probe as described previously (Fig. 12.4*C*). An anal dilatation is performed by administering local anesthesia and then maintaining the Parks retractor in an open position for 5 min. The postoperative course and care is the same as that described for hemorrhoids.

Less postoperative pain than in a hemorrhoidectomy is to be anticipated.

ABSCESSES AND FISTULAS

Perirectal abscesses and fistulas represent ends of a spectrum of perirectal infection. The abscess is the acute undrained infection. The fistula is a chronic draining wound. A fistula frequently results after drainage of an abscess. Intermediate forms of partially drained abscesses occur commonly.

Fistulas and abscesses are believed to arise in the intersphincteric space (6). Normally, the internal sphincter represents a barrier between the rectal lumen and the deep perirectal tissues. When this barrier is breached, fistulous abscesses result. Where the internal sphincter is penetrated by the crypts of Morgagni a breach in this barrier occurs. This is believed to be the route to the perirectal space. Once an intersphincteric abscess occurs, the infection can spread throughout the perianal region. The abscess may remain intermuscular in location, causing severe pain with no obvious perianal swelling.

A perirectal abscess must be incised and drained. This can be easily accomplished when the abscess is palpable externally. The skin overlying the area to be incised and drained can be infiltrated with local anesthetic and an incision can be made using the laser scalpel probe. A cruciate incision is made and the edges are excised to produce an adequate drainage. The perirectal abscess is drained as close as possible to the anal orifice to reduce the length of any subsequent fistula. An intermuscular abscess is drained by performing a partial internal anal sphincterectomy as described below.

Inasmuch as fistulas arise in the intersphincteric space and then may penetrate through the external sphincter, their treatment can involve incision of the sphincter and possible loss of continence. Small amounts of external sphincter can be divided without compromising continence. However, the traditional approach in anal fistula surgery advising incision of the sphincter mechanism up to but not including the anorectal ring, has been associated with a significant percentage of patients losing some continence (7).

A short fistula coursing through a minimal amount of external sphincter can be treated by simple fistulotomy. A complex fistula or one in which fistulotomy would involve severing a significant portion of the external sphincter mechanism is best treated by a partial internal anal sphincterectomy. This serves to unroof and drain the intersphincteric component of the fistula that is its origin. This permits the fistulous tract to close and to heal completely.

In performing either a fistulotomy or a partial internal anal sphincterectomy, the laser can be effectively utilized. In the proposed excision or incision site, any large vascular structures are first obliterated utilizing the vaporization probe at 17–19 W. The remainder of the incision is performed utilizing the 1.2-mm scalpel probe at 18–19 W, after which any residual bleeding can be controlled with a coagulation probe.

In performing anal fistula surgery, it is important to identify the internal origin of the fistula. This can be identified by probing the external orifice of the fistula or by probing the internal orifice if it exists. This is done with a crypt hook. In many cases, there is no internal orifice of a fistula. The origin of the fistula is then represented by an intersphincteric infection.

When the course of the fistula has been determined, a decision can be made regarding a simple fistulotomy or partial internal anal sphincterectomy. If fistulotomy involves division of only a small amount of the external sphincter, it is performed. Local anesthesia is administered as described previously. In addition, subcutaneous injections are made around the external orifices and along the proposed incisions. A probe is passed from the external orifice of the fistula up to its origin, either in the intersphincteric space or within the rectal lumen. The fistula is unroofed using a 1.2-mm scalpel probe at 17–19 W (Fig. 12.5*A*). Wound edges are excised using the same laser technique to produce a saucerized wound (Fig. 12.5*B*).

When fistulotomy involves division of a larger portion of the external sphincter, a partial internal anal sphincterectomy is performed. The origin of the fistula is determined by probing its external orifice or the crypts (Fig. 12.6*A*). A 1-cm wide segment of mucosa and skin, centered on the presumed crypt of origin and extending from the intersphincteric groove up to 3 mm proximal to the dentate line is excised using a 1.2-mm scalpel probe at 17–19 W (Fig. 12.6*B*). The internal sphincter within those same limits is dissected off the external sphincter with a hemostat and excised (Fig. 12.6*B*). The fistula's origin can be identified

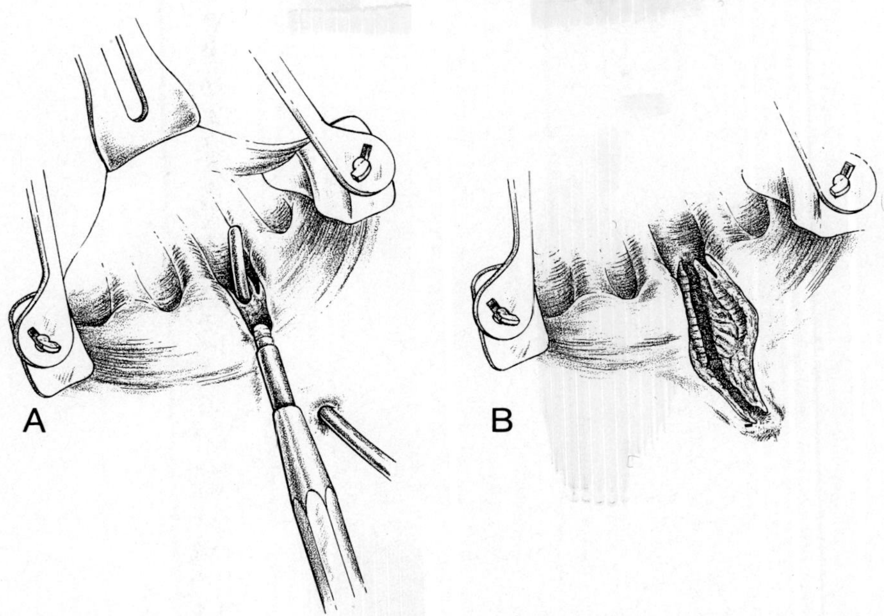

Figure 12.5. Fistulotomy. **A**, The Parks retractor is in place. A probe is passed from the external orifice through the internal orifice. The overlying tissues are divided with a vaporization probe. **B**, The wound edges are excised to produce a saucerized wound.

in the intersphincteric space. Hemostasis is completed with a coagulation probe at 7–9 Watts or by suture ligation. Large fistulous tracts or abscesses may require additional drainage in the form of ¼-inch Penrose drains placed between the sphincterectomy site and the fistulotomy site (Fig 12.6*C*).

The partial internal anal sphincterectomy is particularly applicable to the patient with Crohn's disease (8). A small, predominantly intrarectal incision is utilized. This protects the patient from the effects of poor healing. Limiting sphincter incisions to its internal component also minimizes any adverse effects on continence.

CONDYLOMATA ACUMINATA

Condylomata acuminata or venereal warts occur perianally or intraanally. Warts are caused by a virus and commonly spread venereally. They also occur in the absence of sexual transmission. Warts can be treated with topical medications including podophyllum or bichloroacetic acid. Those that fail to respond to topical medication can be treated with laser photocoagulation, cryosurgery, or electrocautery. Topical 5-FU cream can also applied at intervals, once every 1–3 days, in patients with recurrent condylomata acuminata.

The cryosurgical treatment of anal condylomata has not been popular and has not been very successful. Electrocautery destruction of warts is associated with severe postoperative pain. Laser photocoagulation appears to be the most effective way to treat these. Most of the experience thus far has been with the CO_2 laser. However, the Nd:YAG laser with contact probes is associated with less pain than electrocautery, permitting greater use of ambulatory therapy. Preliminary experience suggests that this form of laser therapy is more effective than electrocautery in reducing recurrences. There are no studies comparing Nd:YAG and CO_2 lasers in this setting.

In the laser treatment of warts, the principles of local anesthesia and sedation are as described previously. The warts are totally destroyed utilizing a vaporization probe at 19 W.

PERIANAL NEOPLASMS

Perianal neoplasms lend themselves to treatment with the Nd:YAG laser. Bowen's disease or

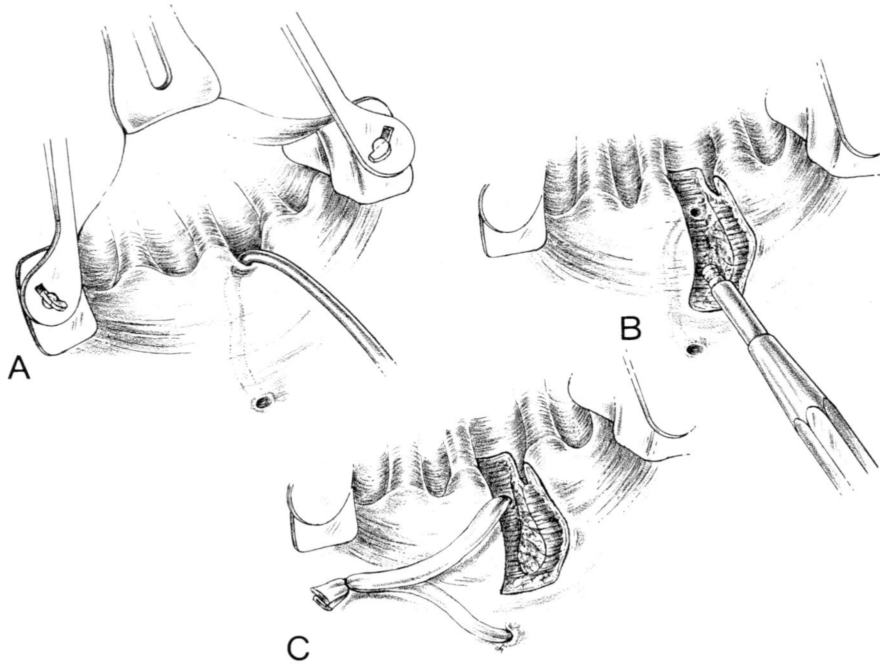

Figure 12.6. Partial internal anal sphincterectomy. **A**, The Parks retractor is in place. A crypt hook is seen in a crypt communicating with an anal fistula. **B**, The overlying mucosa and internal sphincter are excised exposing the intersphincteric space with the internal orifice of the fistula. **C**, A ¼-inch Penrose drain placed between the sphincterectomy site and the peripheral margin of fistula/abscess.

Bowenoid papulosis can be excised. The diminution in postoperative pain makes it possible to perform these procedures on an ambulatory basis. Other perianal neoplasms that would normally be treated by excision can be excised with the Nd:YAG laser. Intrarectal neoplasms have not been included in this discussion.

PILONIDAL SINUS

Pilonidal sinuses usually occur in the sacrococcygeal region. Most are due to hair that gains access to the subcutaneous tissue causing an acute or chronic infection. Midline "pits," which represent the entrance point for the hairs, can be found (Fig. 12.7*A*). The author has found that excision of the pilonidal sinus can be effectively performed utilizing the Nd:YAG laser.

A probe is placed in a pit and passed as far as possible. Alternatively, the probe can be placed in any sinus tract or an incision can be made with an 0.6-mm scalpel probe at 17–19 W to permit entry of the probe. The tissues overlying the cavity thereby defined are incised with the laser (Fig. 12.7*B*). All tracts are similarly opened up. Then the wound edges are excised, incorporating all of the midline pits, to produce a saucerized wound (Fig. 12.7*C*). Hemostasis is completed with the coagulation probe at 7–9 W. This permits limited but total excision of the pilonidal sinus.

The wounds are left open and allowed to heal by second intention. Patients are seen at intervals of 2–4 weeks until the wounds have fully healed. At these visits, hair is shaved for 1 inch around the wound. Complete wound healing takes 4–10 weeks. The laser permits this surgery to be performed with less postoperative pain. Preliminary data suggest that wound healing is more rapid as a result of laser use.

AUTHOR'S SERIES

The author and his associates have performed 125 anorectal and pilonidal sinus operations employing contact Nd:YAG lasers since November, 1986. There were 80 male patients and 45 female

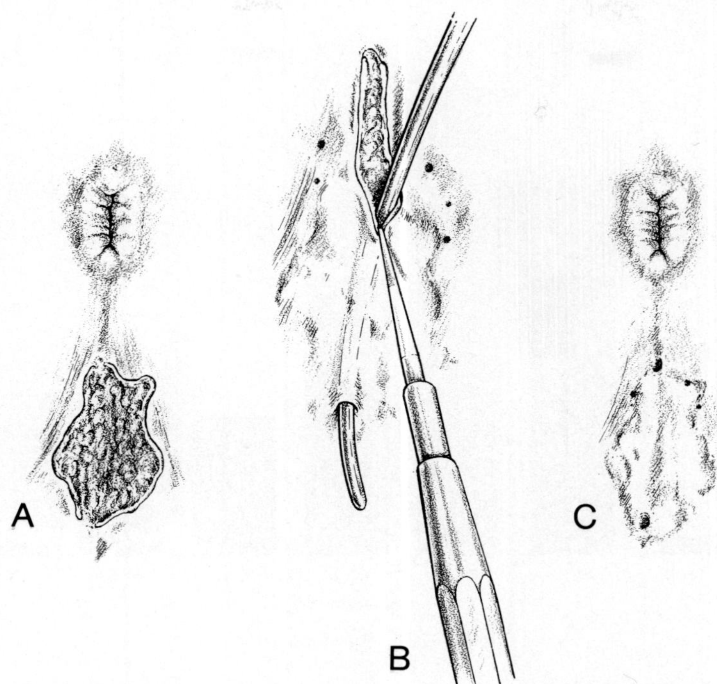

Figure 12.7. Pilonidal sinus. **A**, "Pits" are clustered on or just off midline. **B**, The probe is passed through the pit or sinus and the overlying tissue is incised with a scalpel probe. **C**, Wound edges are excised to produce a flat, saucerized wound.

patients. The ages ranged from 18–77 years and were distributed as in Figure 12.8. The diagnoses included hemorrhoids, anal condylomata acuminata, fissure, fistula, pilonidal sinus, anal Bowen's disease, perianal nevus, and anal skin tags. This distribution is shown in Table 12.1. The number of diagnoses exceeded the number of patients because some patients had more than a single diagnosis.

The operations performed are listed in Table 12.2. Where more than one procedure was performed, the procedure was classified as that which was likely to cause the most postoperative pain.

The most dramatic effect of the use of the laser was in the reduction of postoperative pain. Pain was classified as grade 1 when it was controlled with acetaminophen or nothing; grade 2 patients required codeine for pain relief; grade 3 patients required oxycodone-acetaminophen; and grade 4 patients had severe pain despite the oxycodone-acetaminophen (Table 12.3). Of the hemorrhoidectomy patients, 35% were classified as having grade 1 pain, 27% were grade 2, 23% were grade 3, and 10% were grade 4 (Fig. 12.9*A*). One patient in the latter group required hospitalization for 1 day to control pain. He had undergone an extensive hemorrhoidectomy.

The reason for the diminution in postoperative pain remains to be explained. It has been suggested that the Nd:YAG laser surgery is associ-

Table 12.1. Diagnoses

Diagnosis	No. of Patients
Hemorrhoids	58
Condylomata acuminata	24
Fissure	20
Fistula	19
Fissure and fistula	7
Fissure and hemorrhoids	4
Anal Bowen's disease	2
Perianal nevus	1
Fissure, fistula, and warts	1
Fissure, hemorrhoids, and warts	1
Fissure, fistula, and hemorrhoids	1
Fistula and warts	1
Skin tag	1
Pilonidal sinus	13

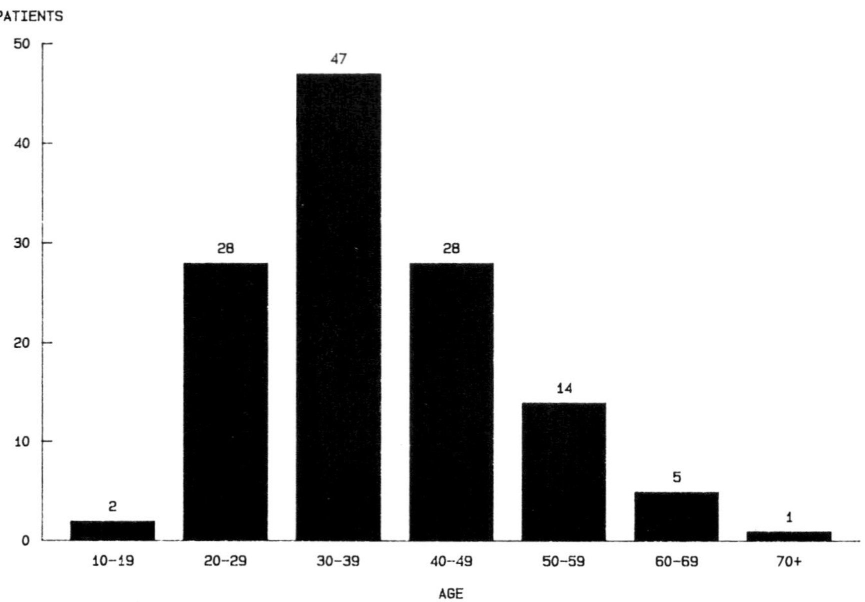

Figure 12.8. Age distribution.

ated with diminished tissue trauma, less postoperative wound edema, and sealing of severed nerve endings. Any of these factors, or perhaps other factors, may be responsible for the marked reduction in pain after anorectal surgery.

Two hemorrhoidectomy patients required a single urinary catheterization. This was carried out on an outpatient basis. Two hemorrhoidectomy patients required disimpaction.

Table 12.2. Procedures

Procedure	No. of Patients
Hemorrhoidectomy	52
Laser destruction of condylomata acuminata	21
Fistulotomy	19
Sphincterotomy with excision hemorrhoid or sentinel pile	10
Internal anal sphincterotomy	4
Anal dilatation with excision sentinel pile	1
Partial internal anal sphincterectomy	1
Excision perianal Bowen's disease	2
Excision perianal nevus	1
Excision postoperative skin tag	1
Pilonidal Cystotomy	13
Total	125

Of the patients who underwent laser destruction of condylomata acuminata, postoperative pain in 24% was classified as grade 1, 43% were grade 2, 29% were grade 3, and 19% were grade 4 (Fig. 12.9*B*). When sphincterotomy was combined with excision of a hemorrhoid or sentinel pile, pain was classified in 60% as grade 1, 30% were grade 2, and 10% were grade 3 (Fig. 12.9*C*). Fistulotomy patients were grade 1 in 32%, grade 2 in 63%, and grade 3 in 5%. The sphincterotomy, pilonidal cystotomy, and perianal excision patients all had minimal pain.

Postoperative care included the use of bulk laxatives, stool softeners, and mineral oil; saline cathartics; or stimulant laxatives as required in order to produce bowel movements daily or every other day. This is continued for 2 weeks. Before the institution of this aggressive program of laxative use, fecal impaction requiring disimpaction

Table 12.3. Postoperative pain classification

Grade 1	Controlled with acetaminophen or nothing
Grade 2	Codeine required
Grade 3	Oxycodone-acetaminophen required
Grade 4	Severe pain despite oxycodone-acetaminophen

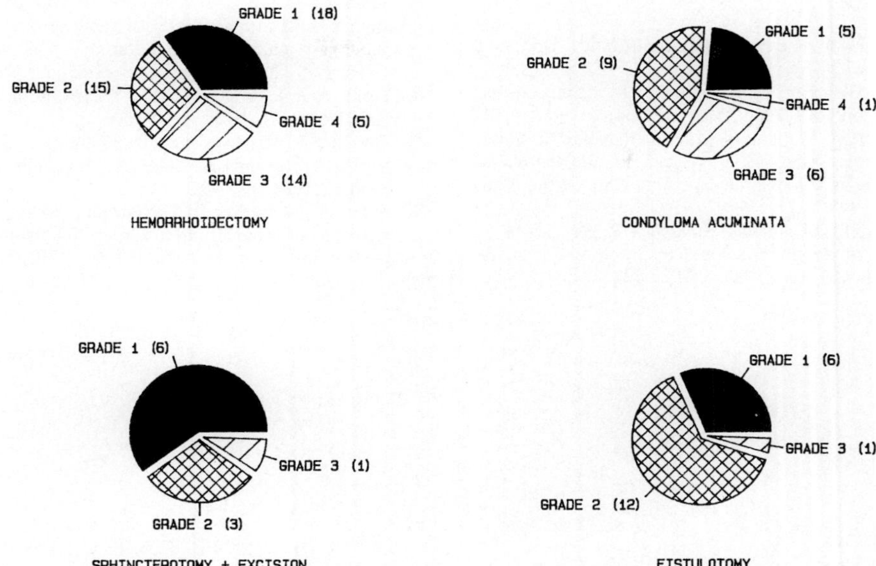

Figure 12.9. Grades of postoperative pain after laser anorectal surgery.

occurred in two patients who underwent extensive hemorrhoidectomies.

Of the 52 hemorrhoidectomy patients, several (particularly in the early part of the series) were operated upon for single or simple hemorrhoids. As further experience was accumulated, very extensive hemorrhoidectomies were performed.

Patients were selected for laser destruction of condylomata acuminata who had failed on other therapy or who had extensive lesions. Eighteen patients who underwent contact Nd:YAG laser therapy of condylomata acuminata were followed for periods of 3–9 months. Thirteen were male homosexuals, three were heterosexual males, and two were women. Seven patients, including five male homosexuals, did not develop any recurrences during the follow-up period. Nine developed few recurrences that were easily managed by repeat laser destruction or topical medications. Two of the 18 developed extensive recurrences.

In this population of patients who either had failed prior therapy or who had very extensive lesions, total wart eradication with a single treatment is better than would be expected from electrodestruction. In addition, it is more difficult to cure warts in male homosexuals than in heterosexuals or in women. The total eradication of warts after a single treatment in the five male homosexuals is of particular significance.

Data on wound healing, both in anorectal wounds and in pilonidal wounds, is too preliminary to report at this time.

Contact Nd:YAG lasers thus have become a very valuable tool to assist the physician in the care of patients with anorectal disorders. It can be substituted for the scalpel or the electrocautery using standard operative techniques. Others are reporting uses of the laser in the management of hemorrhoids basing the treatment on concepts that are unproven, such as destroying "feeding arteries" of hemorrhoids. Others are simply using laser energy to produce necrosis of internal hemorrhoids. This appears to achieve what is generally accomplished with rubber band ligation. The preference of the laser over the rubber band ligator will depend on studies comparing the efficacy, safety, and cost of each modality.

The contact Nd:YAG laser is a wonderful tool for performing anorectal operations. The reduction in postoperative pain is extraordinary. Future developments in laser technology and new applications for them are to be anticipated.

REFERENCES

1. Thomson WH. The nature of haemorrhoids. Br J Surg 1975; 62:542-552.
2. Sohn N, Weinstein MA, Robbins RD. Anorectal disorders. Curr Prob Surg 1983; 20:1-66.
3. Hiltunen KM, Matikainen M. Anal manometric evaluation in anal fissure. Effect of anal dilation and lateral subcutaneous sphincterotomy. Acta Chir Scand 1986; 152:65-68.
4. Abcarian H, Lakshmanan S, Read DR, Roccaforte P. The role of the internal sphincter in chronic anal fissures. Dis Col Rect 1982; 25:525-528.
5. Abcarian H. Surgical correction of chronic anal fissure: Results of lateral internal sphincterotomy vs. fissurectomy-midline sphincterotomy. Dis Col Rect 1980; 23:31-36.
6. Parks AG. Pathogenesis and treatment of fistula in ano. Br Med J 1961; 1:463-469.
7. Goligher J. Fistula-in-ano. In: Goligher J: Surgery of the Anus, Rectum and Colon, ed 4. London, Bailliere Tindall, 1984, p. 178.
8. Sohn N, Korelitz BI, Weinstein MA. Anorectal Crohn's disease: Definitive surgery for fistulas and recurrent abscesses. Am J Surg 1980; 139:394-397.

CHAPTER
13

Contact Nd:YAG Laser Hemorrhoidectomy

M. Y. Sankar

Hemorrhoids have afflicted mankind since ancient times, noted in the Egyptian papyrus (1) and surgically treated in ancient Rome and Greece (2). The disease may be asymptomatic at times, being only recognized on routine rectal and proctoscopic examinations. The incidence of hemorrhoids increases with age and is said to affect at least 50% of people over the age of 50 years. Hemorrhoids occur at all age groups but appear more common in men.

The word "hemorrhoid" is derived from the Greek adjective "haimorrhoides," meaning bleeding (*haima*—blood, *rhoos*—flowing), which places the emphasis on the prominent symptom of bleeding. The term "pile" is derived from the Latin word meaning "a ball;" some cases having a swelling around the anus during some stage of the disease. The terms hemorrhoids and piles are frequently used synonymously.

CLASSIFICATION

Hemorrhoids are divided into *internal* and *external* types. The internal type arises in the upper two-thirds of the anal canal, which is lined by columnar epithelium. External hemorrhoids arise in the lower third of the anal canal, which is covered by squamous epithelium of the skin. This type of classification may fit the description in the early stages, but later, when the hemorroids have enlarged sufficiently, the internal hemorrhoids may present externally at the anus.

According to Graham-Steward (3), internal hemorrhoids can be further divided into two categories: (*a*) vascular hemorrhoids, which consist mainly of distended vessels and are seen in the younger age group; and (*b*) mucosal hemorrhoids that are composed of thickened mucosa and encountered in older patients.

In the early stages, the internal hemorrhoids protrude slightly into the anal canal as congested veins. These are called first degree hemorrhoids. With the passage of time, they become larger and descend toward the anal orifice. The piles then may be found externally, especially on straining at defecation, and spontaneously regress into the anus at the end of the effort. These are second degree hemorrhoids. Later, the internal hemorrhoids protrude not only during defecation but may stay prolapsed until they are digitally reduced and are called third degree hemorrhoids. Finally, longstanding piles, especially in the elderly, become very large, covered by skin, and remain prolapsed permanently outside the anal canal. These irreducible masses are known as fourth degree or complicated third degree hemorrhoids and are seen as interoexternal hemorrhoids.

Shafik (4) suggests that there is no true anal canal but rather a continuity of the rectum to the perianal skin. The failure of remodeling and persistence of anorectal band results in the narrowing of the lower rectal neck, which initiates the hemorrhoid disease. The increase in rectal neck pressure and straining during defecation eventually leads to prolapse of rectal mucosa and venous congestion.

CLINICAL FEATURES

The prominent symptoms of internal hemorrhoids are *bleeding* and *prolapse*. Apart from these two main symptoms, the patient may suffer from a discharge leading to soiling of underclothing, anal irritation, and symptoms of secondary anemia. Severe pain is only present in complicated cases with irreducible prolapse, thrombosis, or with an associated perianal fissure. A history of slight pain was elicited by Bennett et al. (5) in 86% of 138 patients suffering from hemorrhoids and was the presenting complaint in 18% of these cases.

On clinical examination, proctoscopy is the essential step in confirming the presence of internal hemorrhoids. Barium enema followed by sigmoidoscopy and/or colonoscopy are mandatory in patients over 40 years of age with rectal bleeding.

TREATMENT

The treatment of internal hemorrhoids includes the following major categories.

1. *Conservative:* This is useful for first degree hemorrhoids, especially when discovered during a routine examination. The treatment consists of regulation of bowel habits, administration of mild laxatives, and advice regarding inclusion of high-fiber diets. The local use of suppositories and ointments providing symptomatic relief are probably not valuable.
2. *Injection treatment:* In selected cases, injection therapy is of great value. The two important effects include:
   a. Formation of fibrous tissue that surrounds, constricts, and obliterates blood vessels in the submucosa; and
   b. The fibrosis increases the fixation of the hemorrhoid and the mucosa to the underlying tissues, thus preventing prolapse.

   Beneficial results are obtained with first and second degree hemorrhoids that have bled. Third and fourth degree hemorroids cannot be cured by injection treatment. The procedure is done in the office and can be repeated as necessary. The fibrous reaction after repeated injections makes further injections more difficult. During the injection therapy of the scleroscent agents (e.g., phenol in almond oil, sodium tetradecyl), the patient may experience some discomfort. Late necrosis of the injection site may lead to ulcer formation and other rare complications, including submucous abscess formation, hematuria, prostatic abscess, and portal vein embolism.
3. *Operative Treatment:* The multiple operations available for the treatment of hemorrhoids include:
   a. Ligation and excision (6-8);
   b. Submucosal hemorrhoidectomy (9);
   c. Excision of individual hemorrhoid with primary suture (10, 11);
   d. Excision of the entire pile-bearing area with suture (12);
   e. Clamp and cautery technique (13);
   f. Rubber band ligation (14, 15);
   g. Maximum dilatation of the anus (16);
   h. Cryosurgery (17, 18);
   i. Infrared coagulation (19);
   j. Laser hemorrhoidectomy.

The increasing number of techniques mentioned above for dealing with hemorrhoids attests to the lack of universal satisfaction with those currently available. Furthermore, hemorrhoidectomy is considered to be a painful operation (9). Parks even suggested that patients will conceal rectal bleeding because of the dread of an operation (9).

Under these circumstances, the management is not only selected according to the individual patient's specific problem, but other factors, like associated morbidity (e.g., pain, bleeding), long-term complications (e.g., anal incontinence or stricture, recurrence), hospital stay, and cost-effectiveness, are also important.

LASERS IN SURGERY

The first reports on the use of lasers in medicine were in the early 1960s (20) with the CO_2 laser being used in general surgery. In 1973, the first flexible laser waveguide was developed, which made the use of lasers possible during fiberoptic endoscopy (21). Lasers produce an intense beam of light of uniform wavelength and color that can be precisely focused to deliver high levels of energy to small areas. The most important interaction between laser radiation and tissue is the absorption of light with conversion of the light energy into heat. In performing a laser hemorrhoidectomy, both the CO_2 laser and the Nd:YAG laser have been tried with various degrees of success. The CO_2 laser, operating at a wavelength of 10,600 nm and with an energy output of 100 W, is effective in cutting but not so adept in performing coagulation. On the other hand, the Nd:YAG laser, operating at a wavelength of 1064 nm and with energy output up to 150 W can vaporize tissues at higher powers and coagulate bleeding points at relatively low powers, including blood vessles up to 2–3 mm in diameter. Current Nd:YAG laser light transmission systems use a flexible quartz fiber that delivers laser energy at a distance of 0.5–1.5 cm from the tissue. This noncontact system has distinct disadvantages regarding beam irradiation, backscatter, and damage to the quartz tip should it come into contact with tissue or blood. Furthermore,

Nd:YAG laser, due to its depth of penetration into tissue, in its noncontact mode, is used primarily for coagulation but has poor cutting capabilities and may cause excessive tissue damage resulting in perforation.

A synthetic sapphire crystal has been developed that is easily attached to the end of the quartz fiber using a universal metal connector allowing contact irradiation. The geometric shape of these contact synthetic sapphire provides the desired effect of coagulation of bleeding points and/or vaporization, as well as precise incision of tissues (22). Furthermore, the contact probes prevent backscattering of Nd:YAG laser light, reduce the depth of tissue damage, and allow for much lower powers of laser energy to be used. A longer probe attached to a handpiece, the laser scalpel, allows for open surgery to be performed with ease. The power density at the tip of the contact probe is related to the distal probe diameter and the results obtained are comparable to the average power density values of different spot sizes and power levels found with the CO_2 laser beam. The contact cutting probes thus combine the coagulating properties of the Nd:YAG laser with incising capabilities previously only seen with the CO_2 laser.

Laser Hemorrhoidectomy

In the USA, at present, over 150,000 conventional surgical hemorrhoidectomies are perfomed per annum with an average inpatient hospitalization stay of 5 days. The laser offers an alternative method of treating hemorrhoids as an outpatient procedure under local, regional, or short general anesthesia.

CO_2 Laser

Eddy et al. (23) has performed 150 procedures using the CO_2 laser and claims that the incidence of postoperative pain was much less and, therefore, narcotics were seldom needed. Complications such as urinary retention and constipation were not even seen in the elderly and poor risk patients. Mokhniuk et al. (24), from the Proctological Division of the Kiev Medical Institute in Russia, has treated 352 patients suffering from hemorrhoids between 1976 and 1980. Of these, 281 were women. In 80% of the total 352 patients, a modified Milligan-Morgan procedure was performed. In another 9% of the patients, the hemorrhoids were vaporized using the CO_2 laser employing a power of 60 W in a continuous mode with a focused beam diameter of 0.2 mm. Epidural anesthesia was used and a clamp or hemostat was applied to the base of each hemorrhoid before removing the hemorrhoid. After removal of the hemostat, no bleeding was observed. In the immediate postoperative period, edema was minimal and appeared much less than that observed after the conventional ligation and excision operation for hemorrhoids (Table 13.1). Pain was almost absent and no discharge was noted from the operated site. The laser may have sterilized the wound surface, preventing infection during the postoperative period. In cases of hemorrhoids with thrombosis, Mokhniuk, et al. (24) recommend cryosurgery but without supporting evidence. Rausis (25) has also used the CO_2 laser and found less pain in the postoperative period. Of Rausis' 21 proctological procedures using the CO_2 laser, 12 were for third degree hemorrhoids. The laser hemorrhoidectomy followed the same principles of the Milligan-Morgan procedure and there was a decrease in the postoperative complaints, bowel movements were normal, and postoperative bleeding was negligible. Healing was complete after 2 or 3 weeks. No incontinence of flatus or feces was observed nor was there any anal stenosis. The follow-up of 1.5 months is too short for evaluating recurrences.

Denis and Lemarchand (26) have carried out 150 hemorrhoidectomies using the CO_2 laser, 150 cases by conventional operative methods, and 47 using electrocautery within a period of 1 year. Results showed very little difference at the statistical 5% level between the CO_2 laser and the conventional type of hemorrhoidectomy when factors such as postoperative pain and wound healing are taken into consideration. Electrocautery, on the other hand, was worse regarding postoperative pain, leading to a higher analgesic intake. Furthermore, with electrocautery, wound healing was delayed, causing severe scarring and leading to anal stricture and stenosis (Table 13.2). The initial postoperative bowel movements were similar in producing discomfort in all three groups. They concluded that conventional surgery of hemorrhoids by high ligation and excision was just as effective as the laser.

In support of CO_2 laser hemorrhoidectomy, factors include more rapid healing, less scarring and fibrosis, therapeutic effectiveness regarding decreased recurrence with fewer complications

Table 13.1. Hemorrhoidectomy: Summary of Review of Various Procedures, Results, and Immediate Postoperative Problems[a]

		Modes of Therapy								
								Laser Hemorrhoidectomy		
									Nd:YAG Laser	
No.	Problems	Injection Therapy	Rubber Banding	MDA	Cryo-Surgery	Infrared Coagulation	Formal Conventional Hemorrhoidectomy	CO_2 Laser	Noncontact	Contact
1.	Pain	+ (2 days)	+/++ (2 days)	++/+++[b]	++/+++ (7 days)	+ (2 days)	++/+++ (7 days)	+/++ (5 days)	+/++ (5 days)	+ (2 days)
2.	Bleeding	+/++[c]	+/++[d]	±	+/++[d]	±	++/+++[d]	±	±	±
3.	Anal discharge	±	±	±	++/+++	+	+/++	±	±	±
4.	Urinary retention	–	–	±	–	–	+/++	–	±	–

[a]Symbols used in table: –, NIL or none; +, mild/minimal; ++, moderate; +++, severe.
[b]With subsequent daily passage of large anal dilator.
[c]Injection ulcer.
[d]Secondary/reactionary hemorrhage.

Table 13.2. Hemorrhoidectomy: Summary of Review of Various Procedures, Results, and Late Postoperative Problems[a]

		Modes of Therapy								
								Laser Hemorrhoidectomy		
									Nd:YAG Laser	
No.	Problems	Injection Therapy	Rubber Banding	MDA	Cryo-Surgery	Infrared Coagulation	Formal Conventional Hemorrhoidectomy	CO_2 Laser	Noncontact	Contact
1.	Wound healing	Good	Good	Good	Good (14-21 days)	Good	Good (21-28 days)	Good (14-21 days)	Good (14-21 days)	Good (7-14 days)
2.	Anal stricture	+ (Temporary)	–	–	–	–	+ +/+ + +	±	±	–
3.	Anal incontinence	–	–	+ +/+ + +	–	–	–			
4.	Recurrences	*/**	*/**	**	*/**	*	*/**	*	*	o
5.	Return to work	Straightaway (repetition of the procedure in most cases	Straightaway (repetition of the procedure in some cases)	7 days	7-14 days	3-7 days	5 days Hospitalization followed by recuperation at home (15-21 days)	within 5 days	within 7 days	3–4 days

[a]Symbols used in this table: –, NIL or none; +, mild/minimal; + +, moderate; + + +, severe; *, occasional; **, sometimes; *** frequent; o, no recurrences in 2.5-year follow-up.

and excellent patient acceptance (27). Zadeh (28) has carried out laser hemorrhoidectomy using the CO_2 laser in 350 patients in just over a year on an outpatient basis. Of 350 patients, 27% were second degree, 39% were third degree, and 34% were fourth degree hemorrhoids. Male patients accounted for 70% of the total and in the majority of cases, local infiltration of an anesthetic drug with intravenous sedation was used. The hemorrhoidectomy was performed in about 20 minutes at a power density between 38,200 and 47,000 W/cm^2 using a continuous wave mode. Postoperative pain was classified either as none (6%), minimal (29.8%), moderate (41.3%), or severe (22.9%), the average duration of postoperative pain was 5-6 days. They conclude that both routine as well as difficult cases can easily be treated using CO_2 laser as on an outpatient basis, which improved the cost-effectiveness and convenience of patient care.

Nd:YAG Laser

The Nd:YAG laser has been used for hemorrhoidectomy with success although the techniques described are different.

Noncontact Laser Technique. DeMarco (personal communication) applies the laser energy directly over the target tissue by the noncontact method. The patient is placed in the lithotomy position rather than the jack-knife position. General anesthesia was administered in 95% of the cases as this was particularly requested by these patients. The procedure could be done under local anesthetic infiltration with intravenous sedation. Low powers of 25 W for a short duration of 0.8 sec was used, as opposed to a higher power for a longer duration. An important step was to leave normal area of tissue in between the lasered sites. The total duration of the operation was about 1 hour. During the postoperative period, mild swelling, a little discharge, including bleeding, and a feeling of slight pressure was experienced by the patient. The complications that could occur include urinary retention, especially in the older age group, and bleeding of not more than a cupful including clots. In his series of 350 cases, the healing of the wound took about 3 weeks. Other possible complications include fistula formation, excessive scarring, and sphincter damage. The Nd:YAG noncontact laser technique then is a "hot knife," which is similar to the "cold knife" but with more advantages. These include less pain and the patient's return to work sooner. The procedure can be performed as an outpatient procedure.

Dwyer (29) in the University Center of Los Angeles, uses the Nd:YAG laser noncontact technique through a flexible fiberoptic colonoscope which is retroflexed in the rectum to visualize the internal hemorrhoids. The flexible laser guide is introduced through the operating channel and the hemorrhoidal veins are lasered from proximal to the distal areas.

Shude Zhao and Fengzao (personal communication), in the Laser Research Unit in Beijing, China, have treated 156 cases of hemorrhoids using the Nd:YAG laser noncontact technique under local anesthesia. Advantages in the method include safety, simplicity, and that it could be done as an outpatient procedure. The patients were able to return to work much earlier. In their experience, the postoperative complications have been less.

Contact Nd:YAG Laser. Since 1985, the author has performed laser hemorrhoidectomy using Nd:YAG laser by the contact technique. To date, 36 patients have been treated, of which 24 were men with the mean age of 49.5 years. The mean age of the 12 women was 46.6 years.

Technique of Contact Laser Hemorrhoidectomy. A low-residue diet is begun 2 days preoperatively and the patients report on the morning of the surgery to the surgicenter on an empty stomach. Anesthetic is either epidural, caudal, short general, or local with intravenous sedation, as indicated. In the lithotomy position, the anorectal region is examined. Flexible fiberoptic sigmoidoscopy and/or colonoscopy is performed to confirm or exclude associated colonic lesions. The nature and position of the internal hemorrhoids are noted on anoscopy.

Technique of Coaptation. Internal hemorrhoids of first and second degree are "coapted" by using the flat contact probe or coagulation probe (SLT, Inc., Malvern, PA), which is initially applied around the hemorrhoid and finally directly onto it (Figs. 13.1 and 13.2). The laser power used is between 5 and 10 W for a duration of 2–3 sec with coaxial water. Successful coapting is indicated by blanching of the tissue; the blood loss is nil. Care is taken not to use higher power levels that cause vaporization of the mucosa leading to a postoperative discharge per rec-

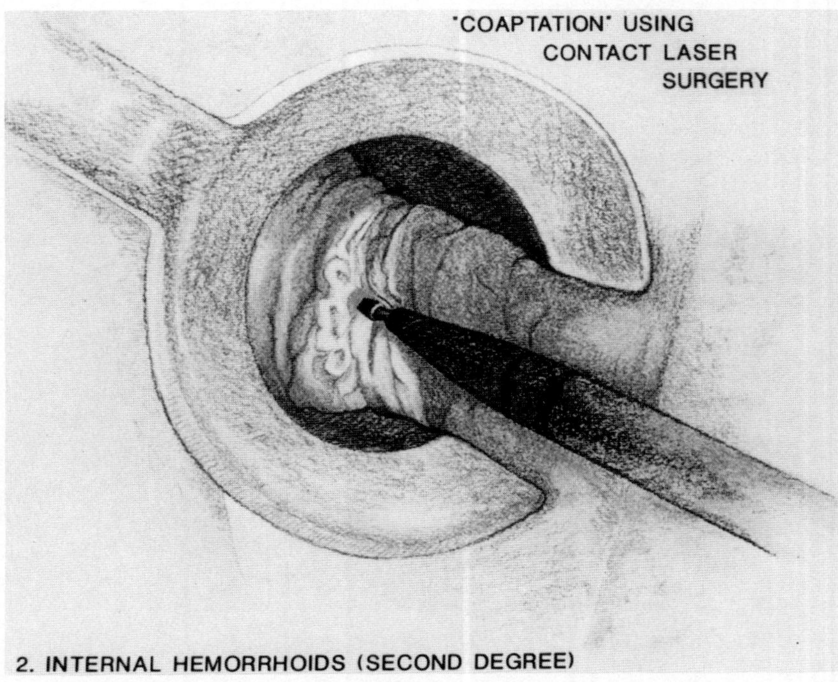

Figure 13.1. Diagram of 'coaptation' using contact laser surgery of first degree and small second degree internal hemorrhoids.

tum. Local infiltration of long-acting local anesthetic is carried out at the end of the procedure.

Sometimes a second degree hemorrhoid may be larger in size. It is suggested that internal hemorrhoids of more than 1.25 cm^2 surface area be treated by contact laser submucosal hemorrhoidectomy. When coapted, the larger sized hemorrhoids, even of second degree, tend to cause postoperative edema due to the large surface area of treatment. This may cause the tissue to prolapse, which may necessitate admission to the hospital for a short stay.

Technique of Contact Laser Submucosal Hemorrhoidectomy. Parks considered that the widely used operation of low ligation and excision (7) involved inclusion of the sensitive anal mucosa and, furthermore, pain was caused by large areas of denuded anal wall leading to spasm and painful bowel actions. He advocated a submucosal hemorrhoidectomy on the grounds that the hemorrhoidal tissue was ligated above the anorectal ring and the mucosal lining was preserved resulting in a less painful procedure. Following this principle we have been treating the internal hemorrhoids of third and fourth degree (and nowadays, the larger second degree internal hemorrhoids as well) by contact laser submucosal hemorrhoidectomy (Figs. 13.3 and 13.4).

A Fansler proctoscope is inserted and the hemorrhoid to be operated is brought under direct view. No maximal dilatation of the anus or infiltration of noradrenaline is carried out. The hemorrhoid is grasped and pulled toward the operator with gentle traction. A linear incision using the frosted laser scalpel (SLT, Inc., Malvern, PA) with a tip diameter of 0.2 or 0.4 mm, is made from the base of the pedicle outward (Fig. 13.5). The power used is in the range of 10-15 W in the continuous mode controlled by the foot pedal. The hemorrhoid is separated up to the pedicle and a high ligation is carried out using 0 chromic catgut or dexon suture (Fig. 13.6). The pedicle is then 'lased' distal to the ligature, leaving a comfortable sleeve, thus preventing any possible slipping of the ligature. After this, any bleeding points are lased, almost invariably resulting in a dry field (Fig. 13.7). The mucosal incision is approximated together without tension using 00

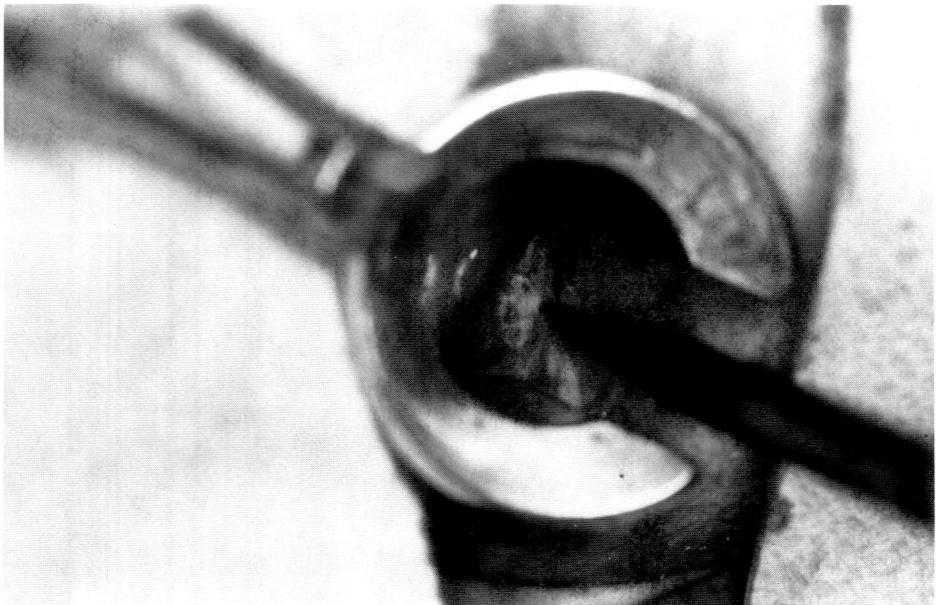

Figure 13.2. Operative procedure of 'coaptation.'

chromic catgut (Fig. 13.8). The procedure is repeated by laser excision of larger sized second, third, and fourth degree hemorrhoids or coapted if they are of smaller sized first or second degrees. At the end of the procedure, 0.5% marcaine or bupivacaine (10 ml) is injected around the sphincter region and the area is gently massaged. A dressing is applied and the patient is returned to the recovery area before discharge. The total blood loss during the submucosal hemorrhoidectomy by the Nd:YAG laser contact technique is less than 20 ml. The average duration of the procedure is less than 30 min. Patients are advised to take analgesics (acetaminophen) if and when they feel any discomfort. Broad spectrum antibiotics parenterally are given ½ hour before the surgical procedure and then continued for a period of 5–7 days. Patients are advised to go on a high fiber diet from day 1 and are seen at 1 week postoperatively as an outpatient.

Evaluation. *Pain.* The surgical treatment of hemorrhoids in the patient's mind carries with it a notorious reputation of severe postoperative pain. After contact laser hemorrhoidectomy and using the scoring system of Watts et al. (30), 97% of the patients were in the B category (less than average pain). The first night after the operation, they were able to sleep after taking 1-2 tablets of acetaminophen. All patients felt some discomfort during the first bowel movement, which ranged from a burning sensation to pain. This was of short duration and they were able to go about their daily chores without any further problem.

Retention of urine requiring catheterization has not occurred in this small series of cases. This may be partially related to the avoidance of local infiltration of noradrenaline before the procedure.

Hemorrhage. Postoperative bleeding, either reactionary or secondary, has not occurred.

Wound healing. The lesions produced in the anal canal itself cannot be visualized in the immediate postoperative period due to pain, discomfort, and apprehension of a conscious patient relating to the introduction of an anoscope. This method does not involve producing an actual wound over the skin area. Inspection at 15 days to 3 months reveals a healed wound without fibrosis.

Anal incontinence. No incontinence of flatus or feces with soiling of the underclothing has been observed. Maximal dilatation of the anus is avoided during the laser surgery for hemorrhoids to decrease this risk.

Formation of skin and mucosal tags. Any skin tag that is found during the laser operative proce-

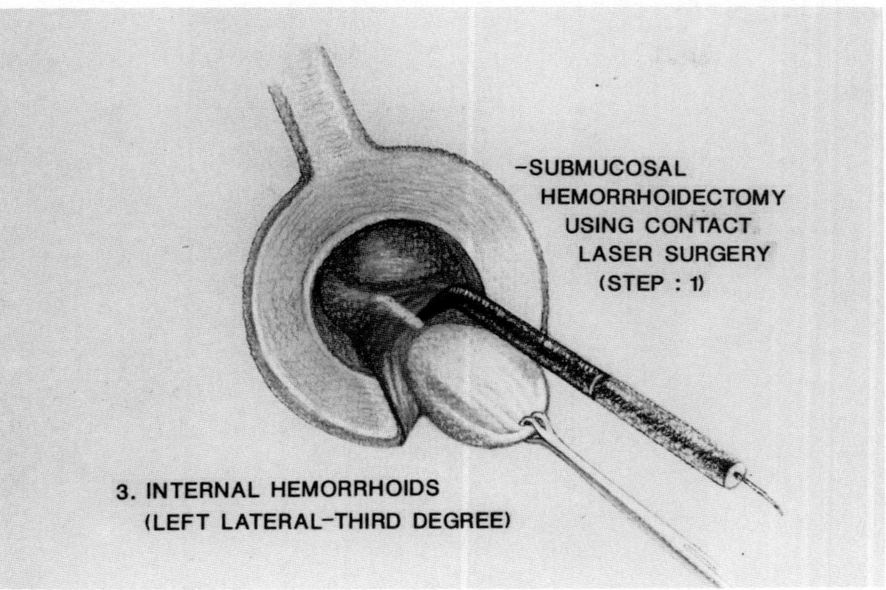

Figure 13.3. Diagram of submucosal hemorrhoidectomy using contact laser surgery (step 1) for third and fourth degree internal hemorrhoids.

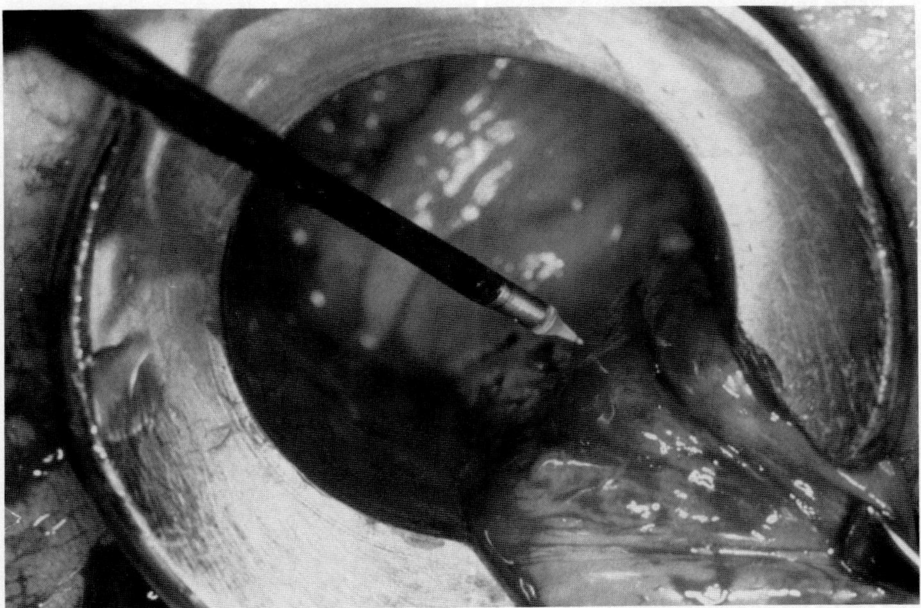

Figure 13.4. Operative procedure for submucosal hemorrhoidectomy using 0.4-mm tip diameter frosted contact laser scalpel (SLT, Inc., Malvern, PA).

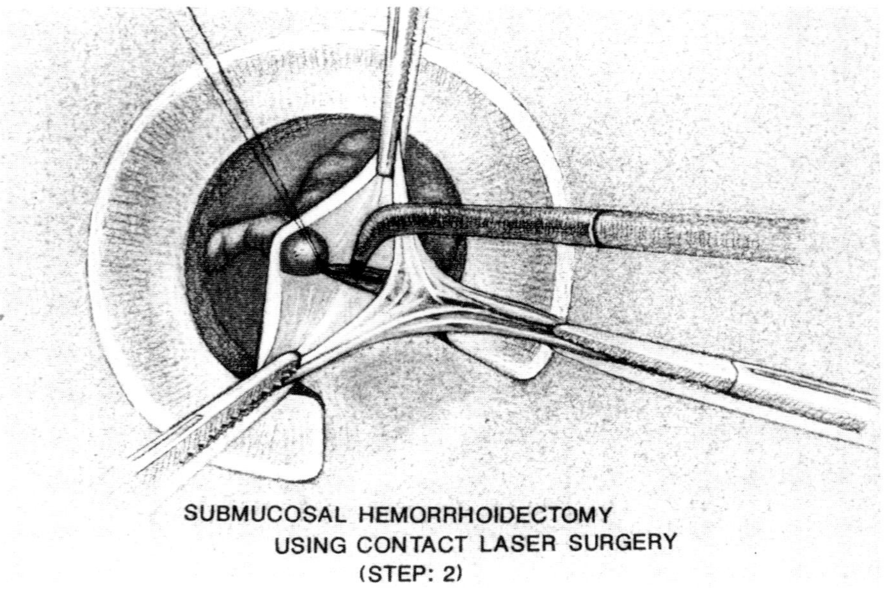

Figure 13.5. Diagram of submucosal hemorrhoidectomy using contact laser surgery (step 2).

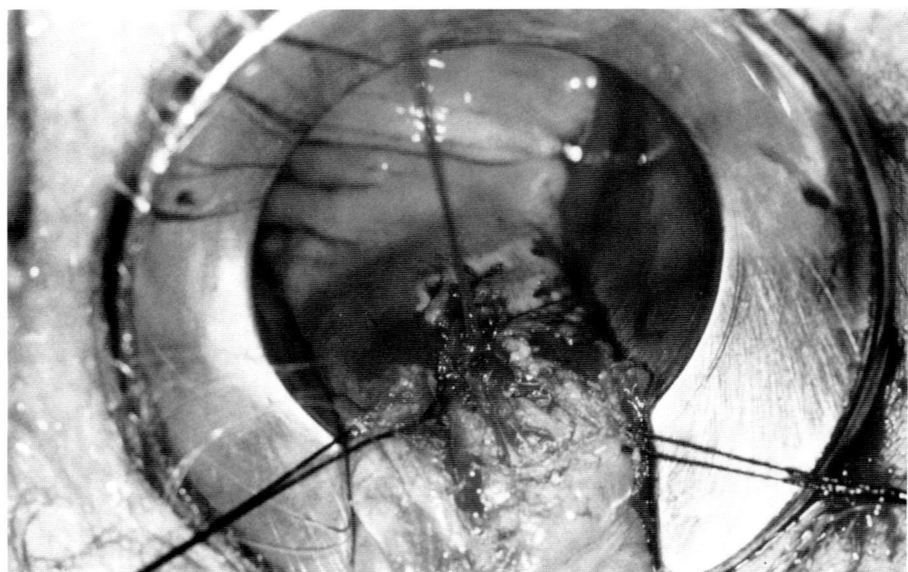

Figure 13.6. Operative procedure of submucosal hemorrhoidectomy—the bed of the hemorrhoidal tissue and the ligated pedicle.

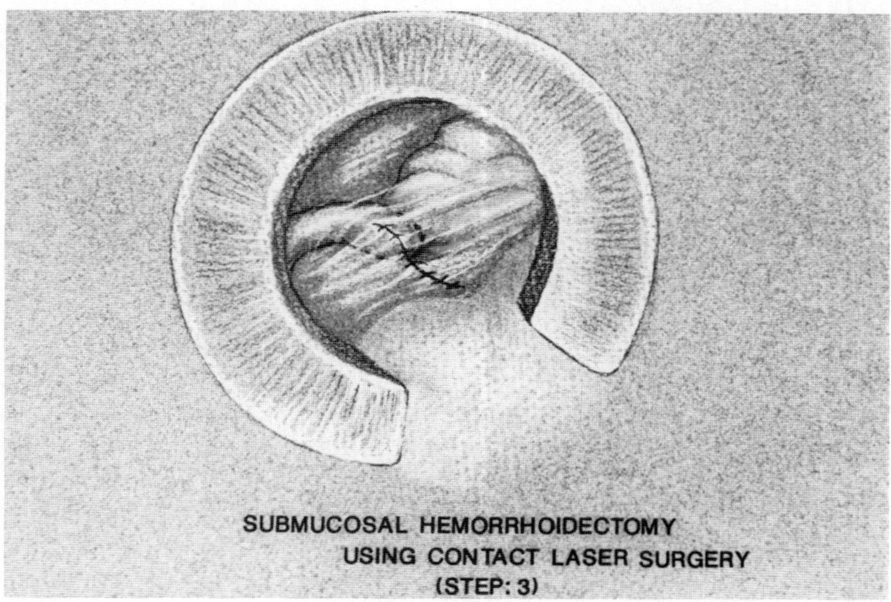

Figure 13.7. Diagram of submucosal hemorrhoidectomy using contact laser surgery (step 3).

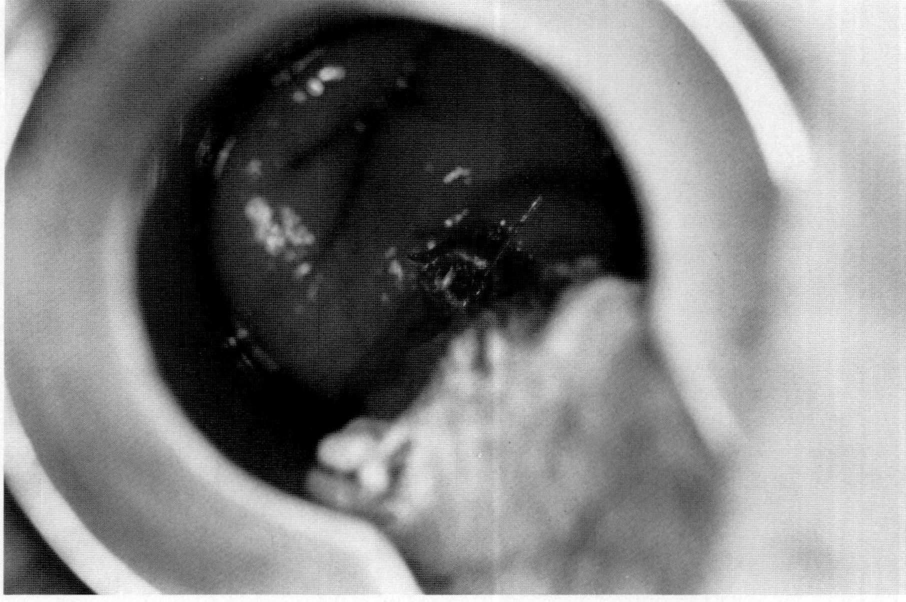

Figure 13.8. Operative procedure of submucosal hemorrhoidectomy—just before the closure of the mucosa overlying the ligated hemorrhoidal pedicle.

dure is excised using the contact laser scalpel. No new skin or mucosal tags have been observed after the laser procedure.

Recurrence of hemorrhoids. The first contact laser hemorrhoidectomy was performed in November 1985. A careful postoperative follow-up for 2.5 years of 36 patients showed no recurrences of internal hemorrhoids. One patient, however, returned with pain at 6 months due to the formation of posterior fissure in ano with severe constipation and external hemorrhoids. Neither were present at the first visit.

The main advantage of the submucosal hemorrhoidectomy as outlined by Parks (9) and modified by Goligher (31) is said to be the decrease in postoperative pain. The reason for this is that the ligature does not include any anal mucosa, which is particularly sensitive. Further, fibrosis or stricturing does not occur as neither the mucosa nor the skin is excised. The disadvantage of this operation is due to the difficulties in the dissection of the mucosa off the hemorrhoid because of bleeding, which may be troublesome and time-consuming. It appears that the use of Nd:YAG laser contact technique in performing submucosal hemorrhoidectomy eliminates this disadvantage. In a recent interesting paper by Roe et al. (32), the submucosal hemorrhoidectomy procedure was compared to the ligation-excision of the hemorrhoids from the viewpoints of anal sensation and sphincter manometry and postoperative pain and function. There were 18 submucosal hemorrhoidectomies compared to 22 ligation-excision procedures.

Anal sphincter manometry and anal mucosal electrosensitivity were measured preoperatively and 6 weeks after surgery. Postoperative pain was assessed by linear analogue scale. Anal sphincter pressures, which were high preoperatively, fell to normal after surgery. Neither operation was thought to affect functional sphincter length or the rectoanal-inhibiting reflex. Of the patients, 40% were recorded to have shown ultraslow waves on sphincter motility studies. These were associated with the highest pressures and in all but three cases disappeared after surgery. Roe et al. (32) found no differences in postoperative pain scores between the two techniques and this concurs with the findings of Watts et al. (30), but Singh and Lal (33) reported severe pain after submucosal hemorrhoidectomy only on the day of operation after which it was less painful than ligation-excision procedure in the next few days. In the author's small series, the postoperative pain is definitely much less after contact laser hemorrhoidectomy and it has become an ambulatory surgical procedure.

Roe et al. believed that submucosal hemorrhoidectomy preserved anal sensation better than ligation-excision technique although, according to them, this was not reflected in improved function. Minor leakage and anal soiling is reported in 50% of their patients from both groups, but all these symptoms resolved by 6 weeks after surgery.

Such studies of comparison of anal sensation and anal sphincter manometry have not yet been done after contact laser hemorrhoidectomy. Even though it may appear that contact laser hemorrhoidectomy could become the preferred treatment for hemorrhoids, further studies and information are required.

REFERENCES

1. Banov L. The Chester Beatty medical papyrus: The earliest known treatise completely devoted to anorectal diseases. Surgery 1965; 58:1037-1043.
2. Parks AG. De Haemorrhoids. Guy's Hosp Rep 1955; 104:135.
3. Graham-Steward CW. What causes hemorrhoids? A new theory of etiology. Dis Colon Rectum 1963; 6:333.
4. Shafik A. A new concept of the anatomy of the anal sphincter mechanism and the physiology of defecation, treatment of hemorrhoids: Report of a technique. Am J Surg 1984; 148:393-398.
5. Bennett RC, Friedman MHW, Goligher JC. The late results of hemorrhoidectomy by ligature and excision. Br Med J 1963; 2:216.
6. Lockhart-Mummery JP. Diseases of Rectum and Colon 2nd ed. London:Bailliere, 1934.
7. Milligan ETC, Morgan C, Naunton Jones LE, Officer R. Surgical anatomy of anal canal and operative treatment of hemorrhoids. Lancet 1937; 2:1119-1124.
8. Miles WE. Rectal Surgery. London: Cassell, 1939.
9. Parks AG. Surgical treatment of haemorrhoids. Br J Surg 1956; 43:337-351.
10. Mitchell AB. A simple method of operating on piles. BR Med J 1903; 1:482.
11. Ferguson JA, Heaton JR. Closed hemorrhoidectomy. Dis Colon Rectum 1959; 2:176.
12. Whitehead W. Surgical treatment of hemorrhoids. Br Med J 1882; 1:149.
13. Anderson HG. The after results of the operative treatment of hemorrhoids. Br J Med 1909; 2:1276.
14. Blaisdell PC. Prevention of massive hemorrhage secondary to hemorrhoidectomy. Surg Gynecal Obstet 1958; 106:485.
15. Barron J. Office ligation of internal hemorrhoids. Am J Surg 1963; 105:563.

16. Lord PH. A new regime for treatment of hemorrhoids. Proc R Soc Med 1968; 61:935.
17. Lewis MI. Diverse methods of managing hemorrhoids: Cryohemorrhoidectomy. Dis Colon Rectum 1973; 10:175.
18. Lloyd-Williams K, Haq IU, Glem B. Cryodestruction of hemorrhoids. Br Med J 1973; 1:666.
19. Leicester RJ, Nicholls RJ, Mann CV Infrared coagulation in the treatment of hemorrhoids. Gut 1981; 22:436.
20. Goldman L, Hornby P, Long E. Effect of the laser beam on the skin. Transmission of laser beams through fiberoptics. J Invest Dermatol 1964; 42:231-234.
21. Nath G, Gorish W, Kiefhaber P. First laser endoscopy with a fiberoptic transmission system. Endoscopy 1973; 5:203-218.
22. Daikuzono N, Joffe SN. Artificial sapphire probe for contact photocoagulation and tissue vaporization with Nd:YAG laser. Med Instrum 1985; 19:173-178.
23. Eddy HJ, Yu JC, Eddy EC. Dual laser hemorrhoidectomy (Abstract). Lasers Surg Med 1986; 6:201.
24. Mokhniuk YN, Baltaitis YV, Maltsev VN, Yurshenico VP, Korolenko VB, Korsunovsky AI, Bassel-Shabane. Comparative evaluation of methods of treatment of patients with hemorrhoids. Clin Surg 1983; 2(494):1-4.
25. Rausis C. Surgery of hemorrhoids by means of CO_2 laser (Chirurgie des hemorroides avec le laser CO_2). Schweiz, Rundschauc Med (Praxis) 1982; 71:177-180.
26. Denis J, Lemarchand N. The present day treatment of hemorrhoids (Etat Actuel due traitement des hemorrhoides). Revue de P'Infirmiere 1985; 3:49-51.
27. Riedlinger J. The surgical treatment of hemorrhoids by means of CO_2 laser. In: Atsumi K, Ed. Laser-Tokyo '81, Intergroup Corporation, Japan 1981; 23:30-31.
28. Zadeh AT. Three hundred and fifty hemorrhoidectomies using the CO_2 laser. Lasers Surg Med 1985; 5:145.
29. Dwyer R. The technique of gastrointestinal laser endoscopy. The Biomedical Laser, New York: Springer-Verlag, 1981, p. 255-269.
30. Watts JM, Bennett RC, Duthie HL, Goligher JC. Healing and pain after different forms of hemorrhoidectomy. Br J Surg 1964; 51:808-817.
31. Goligher J. Haemorrhoids or piles. In: Surgery of the Anus, Rectum and Colon 5th ed. London: Bailliere Tindall, 1984; pp. 123-125.
32. Roe, AM, Bartolo DCC, Vellacott KD, Locke-Edmunds J, Mcc. Mortensen NJ. Submucosal versus ligation excision hemorrhoidectomy: A comparison of anal sensation, anal sphincter manometry and postoperative pain and function. Br J Surg 1987; 74:948-951.
33. Singh J, and Lal P. Submucosal hemorrhoidectomy versus low ligation-excision. J Ind Med Assoc 1975; 64:111-114.

CHAPTER

14

Surgical Techniques in Perianal and Other Diseases[a]

Howard J. Eddy, Jr., Elizabeth C. Eddy

For many years attempts have been made to develop a method of treating rectal pathology that would provide a more comfortable postoperative course for the patient while maintaining a high degree of safety. As cost became a factor, rectal surgery became more of an outpatient procedure, and these two considerations—comfort and safety—assumed even greater importance.

Earlier methods (1), however, did not always eradicate the pathology completely or permanently, and even the most innocuous methods were not without possibly dangerous complications. Injections (2), which are a palliative procedure for internal hemorrhoids only, could cause serious allergic-type reactions. Rubber band ligations (3) could result in protracted pain or hemorrhage, either when the hemorrhoid sloughed off or if a rubber band came off prematurely. Although more effective than injections, this method also was only for internal hemorrhoids.

With cryosurgery (H.J. Eddy, unpublished information; 4), the mass of the large external hemorrhoid must be removed, preferably with electrocautery, before the base is treated with the liquid nitrogen. Otherwise, there can be a period of several weeks before the odorous discharge from the treated hemorrhoid ceases to be a major aesthetic problem. Because most surgeons who attempted to use rectal cryotherapy did not recognize the importance to the postoperative course of removing the bulk of the large external hemorrhoids before the application of the liquid nitrogen, the procedure was not well received in general. However, in the authors' experience of more than 3000 cases, patient acceptance was excellent due to the total eradication of all rectal pathology and a shortened, more comfortable postoperative course.

Infrared photocoagulation (5, 6) is also used for the palliation of moderate-sized internal hemorrhoids, but the results are less predictable and a greater possibility of bleeding exists.

Electrotherapy, in conjunction with cryotherapy, pointed the way toward the use of the laser as the ultimate method of eradicating rectal pathology. The Nd:YAG laser is a superior coagulating instrument, and it provides safe and effective "no-touch" control as well. The ability to regulate both the power output and the duration of exposure gives even more acccurate control. This has the advantage of avoiding extended depth of necrosis and damage to the adjacent tissue.

In 1983, the first total hemorrhoidectomies were performed using the Nd:YAG laser for the entire procedure (H.J. Eddy, unpublished information). With the addition of the CO_2 laser for the eradication of the external pathology, patient comfort was further improved and anatomical and physiological results were gratifyingly precise (Table 14.1).

Thus, the dual laser procedures described in this chapter were developed.

EQUIPMENT

The Nd:YAG laser machine is checked and tested according to the manufacturer's instructions by the operating room laser nurse. The power is set to deliver 22–24 W for pulses of either 0.4 sec or 0.6 sec. The CO_2 laser machine is also checked and tested, and its power is set to deliver 15 W at the setting marked "continuous"

[a] The authors acknowledge with sincere appreciation their partner, Jian Chu Yu, M.D.

Table 14.1. Distribution of Laser Rectal Surgery

Surgical Pathology	Laser Surgery Performed: Nd:YAG	Laser Surgery Performed: Dual: Nd:YAG and CO_2	Totals
Hemorrhoids	340	475	815
Hemorrhoids and fissures	147	282	429
Hemorrhoids and condylomata	18	26	44
Condylomata	18	24	42
Hemorrhoids and fistulae	15	26	41
Fissures	13	15	28
Fissures and fistulae	0	18	18
Fistulae	2	19	21
Pilonidal cysts and sinuses	5	9	14
Hemorrhoids, fissures, and fistulae	2	9	11
Hidradenitis suppurativa	1	2	3
Neoplasms, rectosigmoid	8	38	46
Totals	569	943	1512

and in the "superpulse" mode, if available. The superpulse mode delivers repeated short bursts of high power that produce greater energy and less heat. Although this mode causes less adjacent tissue trauma, it must be remembered that it produces less hemostasis.

A CSV II Bovie electrosurgical unit is set up as part of the surgical equipment. It is invaluable for hemostatis of the highly vascular rectal area both during surgery and for the prevention and treatment of postoperative bleeding. The Bovie has the advantage of arresting bleeding with the least adjacent tissue trauma. It has the necessary type of power in more than adequate amounts for hemostasis, which are features not generally possessed by the solid-state electrosurgical units. When hemostasis is attempted with the Nd:YAG laser, any previously blackened tissue greatly potentiates the energy being delivered by the laser beam. This is particularly true for larger vessels in the internal hemorrhoidal beds. It should be noted also that the CO_2 laser may be used for superficial external hemostasis with a defocused beam at a 15- to 20-W continuous setting. The superpulse mode should not be used for hemostasis.

A high-powered vacuum smoke evacuator and a conventional suction machine are prepared for use. The smoke evacuator removes smoke that consists of, among other things, vaporized tissue particles and bacteria.

PATIENT PREPARATION

The patient is given a complete rectal examination at the time of the first office visit. This includes taking the patient's history, abdominal palpation, a digital rectal examination, anoscopy, and rigid proctosigmoidoscopy.

Inasmuch as routine colonoscopy has resulted in finding neoplastic polyps and other pathology in 48% of the cases (H.J. Eddy, unpublished information), the patient is urged to have a colonoscopy before rectal surgery if the patient is over 40 years of age and has no family history of colon lesions or breast malignancy, or over 30 years of age if there is a family history of those lesions.

Complete laboratory studies, an electrocardiogram, and a chest x-ray are performed before the day of surgery. On the morning of the procedure, the patient takes two sodium biphosphate-sodium phosphate enemas at home; fasts for 8 hours; and omits regular medications unless there is a special condition, which must then be discussed with the surgeon.

Having read and signed the operative consent forms, the patient may be medicated preoperatively with 1–2 mg of lorazepam and 50–100 mg of hydroxyzine pamoate given orally, or parenteral medications may be administered as soon as the intravenous drip is in place.

The patient is placed in the prone position on the operating table, where a cardiac monitor, a pulse oximeter, and an electronic sphygmomanometer are connected. Both arms are placed on arm boards for comfort, and eye patches are placed securely over the eyes. The eye patches are imperative for protection from reflected laser energy.

The buttocks are taped apart and the area cleansed with a povidone-iodine scrub and a 10% povidone-iodine solution. The operative site is not shaved except for pilonidal surgery.

For sedation, 50–60 mg of meperidine and 1.0–3.0 mg of midazolam hydrochloride are injected into the venous catheter.

The local anesthetic consists of 5 ml of hyaluronidase injected into a 50 ml bottle of 0.25% bupivacaine hydrochloride (plain). Approximately 35 ml of this mixture is injected into the anal verge. The remainder of this mixture is usually injected at the end of the particular surgical procedure. The laser surgical procedures for each condition are described below.

SURGICAL TECHNIQUE

Hemorrhoids

The operative site is examined visually, and a digital rectal examination is performed, particularly checking the aperture size of the anorectal canal. For nearly 20 years, these authors have been using the digital anorectal dilatation procedure originated by Peter Lord (7), and have found moderate dilatation to be an invaluable adjunct, especially in younger male patients and others who tend to have a hypertonic sphincter. This anal dilatation is performed to accomodate two to three fingers. However, in women and in the elderly, it is usually unnecessary to dilate the anorectal area, because of hypotonicity and/or redundancy of the mucosa. The prime reason for the digital examination under anesthesia is to discover any previously undetected pathology.

An appropriate-sized, coated Hill-Ferguson retractor is inserted into the anus. Cotton balls or a pad of gauze are moistened and inserted into the rectum proximal to the pathology, and the internal hemorrhoids are treated in rotation as follows. The noncontact Nd:YAG laser is set at a power of 22–24 W for 0.4 to 0.6-sec pulses. It is used in this pulsed mode at a distance of 3–5 cm from the pathology, with a spot size of 2–3 mm, to establish a grid pattern of spots approximately 6–8 mm apart over the surface of each internal hemorrhoid. The purpose of this laser procedure is to create deep destruction and hemostasis. Previously, a brush technique, or closely spaced single applications of laser energy were used. This technique resulted in an unacceptable increase in levator and sphincter spasm postoperatively and, occasionally, anal stenosis. The distance of 6–8 mm between laser beam applications seems to be critical in reducing associated deep-tissue trauma, muscle spasm, and stenosis. The remainder of the destruction is accomplished with the CSV II Bovie at a coagulation setting of 50–60, which is also the setting needed for internal hemostasis. (External hemostasis is performed at a coagulation setting of 30–40.) Great care must be used with both the Nd:YAG laser and the Bovie to keep the destruction of the tissue proximal to the anorectal line. It is also important to preserve as much anoderm as possible.

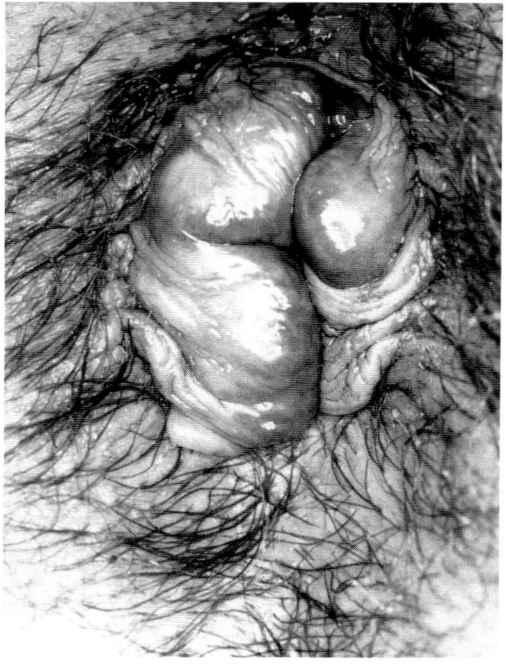

Figure 14.1. Massive preoperative hemorrhoids, internal and external, grade IV.

All pathology distal to the anorectal line is vaporized with the CO_2 laser at a "continuous" setting of 15 W using the superpulse mode if available, at a distance of 3–5 cm with a spot size of 2–3 mm. It is imperative to biopsy any questionable pathology before laser destruction.

In the case of massive external hemorrhoids, most of the mass of the hemorrhoid is excised by the CO_2 laser or the CSV II Bovie (Figs. 14.1–14.4). The remaining base of the tissue is carefully vaporized with the CO_2 laser in order to obtain a good anatomical and cosmetic result. During this procedure, a defocused beam with a spot size of 2–3 mm and a setting of 15–20 W in the continuous, nonsuperpulse mode, provides superficial hemostasis. For additional hemostasis, electrocautery is substituted. As stated previously, solid-state electrosurgical units do not generally provide the necessary type and amount of power for anorectal hemostasis.

Previous cryosurgical experience has proven the effectiveness of cryoanalgesia using liquid ni-

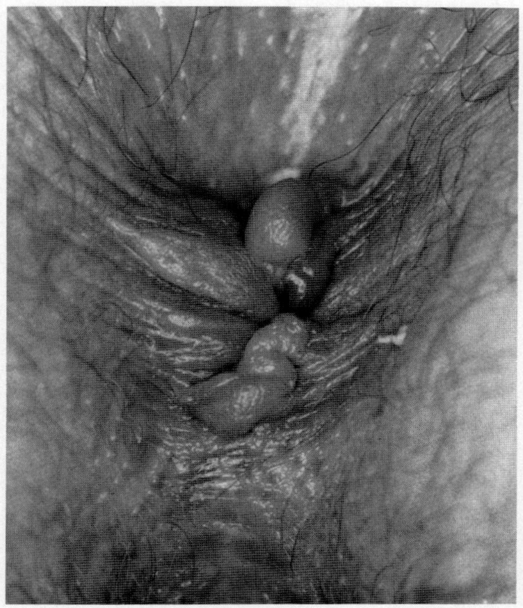

Figure 14.2. Preoperative hemorrhoids, grade III.

trogen for relieving postoperative pain (Figs. 14.5–14.7). The limited superficial application of liquid nitrogen to the external wounds appears to counteract the heat effect of the procedure, resulting in a much more comfortable postoperative course.

The operative site is then cleansed and coated with povidone-iodine solution, and 10–20 ml of 0.25% bupivacaine hydrochloride (plain) with hyaluronidase is infiltrated into the operative area.

Steroid ointment is applied internally and externally, and a medium or large cotton ball is placed against the anal opening. No taping or packing is used, and the patient is moved to the outpatient recovery room. Postoperative care is important to improve the patient's comfort. A family member, who will assist with the postoperative regimen, is shown the operative site and given a verbal description of the procedures to be followed. Written instructions and prescriptions are also given to this family member.

At this time, the patient is usually alert and is given a bland sandwich of peanut butter and jelly or cream cheese and jelly, and a soft drink or tea. No coffee product is allowed until healing has occurred, as it can be irritating to the anorectum.

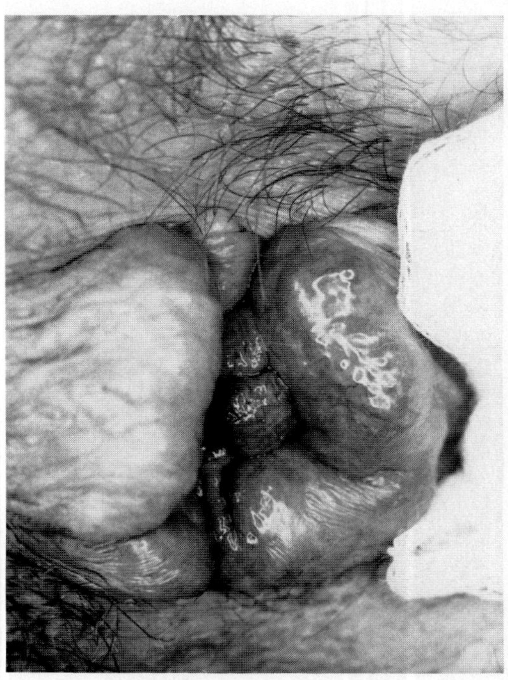

Figure 14.3. Massive preoperative hemorrhoids, internal and external, grade IV.

Patients are discharged into the care of a family member with printed instructions and prescriptions. They are scheduled to return in 1 or 2 days for an examination of the postoperative site, a review of perianal care, and to resolve any questions. They are seen at 4- to 7-day intervals until healing has occurred. This takes approximately 3–4 weeks.

Although it is advisable for the patient to recuperate before returning to work, the actual interval varies widely, depending on whether the patient is a housewife with children, an executive, a clerical worker, or self-employed. However, strenuous work or long distance commuting requires a longer period of recuperation. Also, the patient must have toilet facilities at work that allow for irrigation and application of medications.

The surgery itself causes relatively minor discomfort, and most patients have a bowel movement the morning after surgery. Topical anesthetic ointment is often the only analgesia required. In the majority of patients, discomfort is caused by wound secretions and injudicious diet, which cause irritating stools. Therfore, a

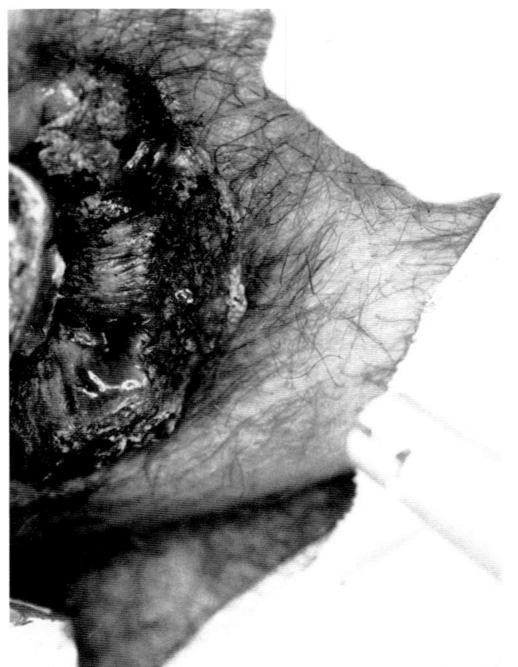

Figure 14.4. Total eradication of massive, grade IV internal and external hemorrhoids with the CO_2 laser.

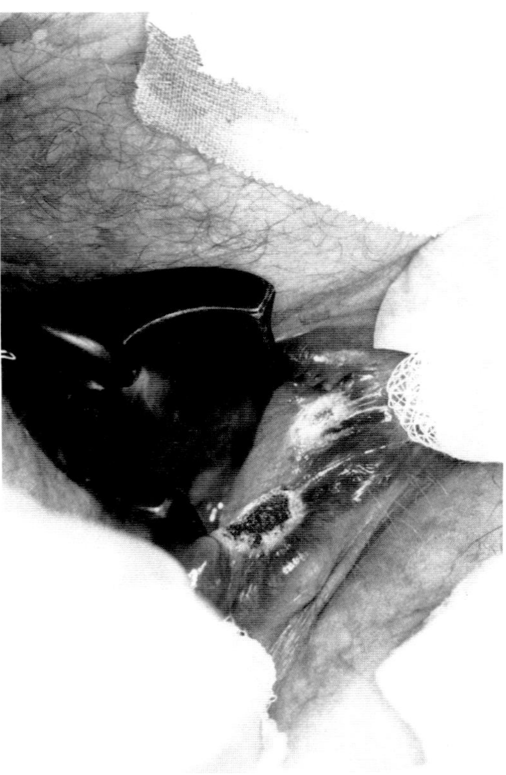

Figure 14.5. Initiation of liquid nitrogen cryoanalgesia at completion of CO_2 laser surgery.

careful and continuous round-the-clock regimen of cleanliness and perianal care is imperative. Warm, but not hot, normal saline sitz baths are taken for 10 min every 2 hours during the day and every 3 hours during the night. A portable sitz bath may be used. This is followed by external irrigation of the perianal area with normal saline solution in a bulb syringe or a Water-Pic. A steroid ointment is then inserted with a nozzle or injector into the anus, applied externally with the finger, and a dry cotton ball reapplied. The cotton ball may be changed between sitz baths if necessary, depending on the amount of secretions. The time intervals between treatments are increased as the secretions decrease. Soap is never used in the perianal area due to its irritating properties. A soapless rectal cleanser may be used if desired.

In order to establish a regular time for having a bowel movement each day and to prevent straining and bearing down, most patients are instructed to use a 120-ml oil enema, to be held for 15–20 min, and repeated once or twice if necessary. A 120-to 480-ml plain tap water enema or a glycerine suppository may be used if preferred, but soapsuds are never used. Usually, this procedure is suggested for the time of the patient's normal bowel movement, and it is preceded by the insertion of 5% lidocaine ointment approximatey 5 min before the enema. For the occasional patient who has spontaneous, urgent bowel movements, the lidocaine should be inserted at the first sign of an impending bowel movement.

Because part of the healing process requires the regular passage of normal-sized, well-formed stools, the patient must be instructed to eat regular, well-balanced meals, with adequate bulk and fluids. Alcohol, spices, fried or fatty foods, coffee, or citrus juices should be avoided during healing. Vitamins and a psyllium-seed powder are prescribed. Mineral oil preparations may also be ordered. Analgesia for discomfort includes propoxyphene napsylate with acetaminophen and, on rare occasions, oxycodone hydrochloride with acetaminophen.

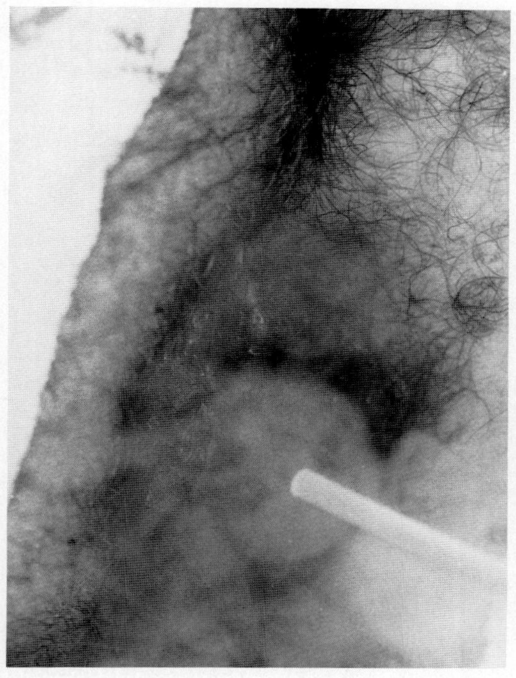

Figure 14.6. Smoky effect of liquid nitrogen cryoanalgesia after vaporization of massive external hemorrhoids with CO_2 laser.

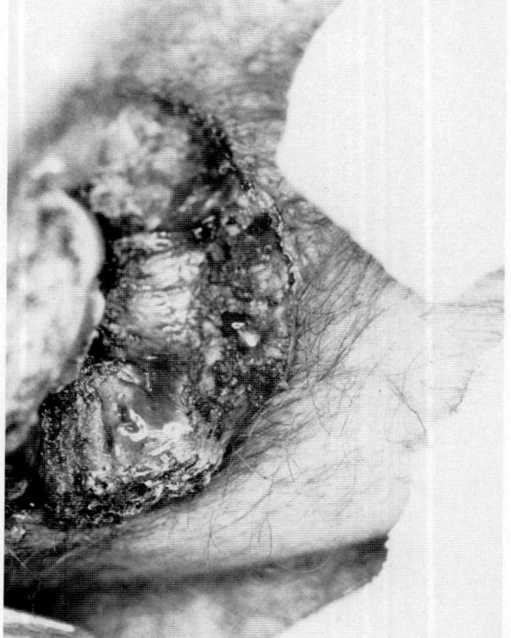

Figure 14.7. Liquid nitrogen cryoanalgesia nearly completed after vaporization of massive external hemorrhoids with CO_2 laser.

Fissures

Although the patient's main complaint may be the pain arising from the fissure, most of these patients will have associated hemorrhoids. If, at the time of surgery, these asymptomatic hemorrhoids are left untreated, they often become painful postoperatively. Therefore, with most fissurectomies, a hemorrhoidectomy is performed at the same time. The procedure is usually the same as that described above for the hemorrhoidectomy, but with the addition of the specific CO_2 laser therapy for the fissure (Fig. 14.8).

Instead of surgical excision of the fissure and its associated drainage area with the usual sphincterotomy, the CO_2 laser is used at a setting of 15 W continuous in the superpulse mode, at a distance of 3–5 cm with a spot size of 2–3 mm, for vaporization of the affected areas. This wound is more superficial than that occurring with surgical excision. As a result, it heals more quickly with less discomfort.

In cases of chronic, longstanding fissures, stenosis can develop with such a severity that the fifth digit is inserted anally with difficulty. This necessitates releasing incisions with the CO_2 laser through anal skin and scar tissue in three quadrants before the fissure in the fourth quadrant can be treated. These releasing incisions are performed with the CO_2 laser set at 15 W continuous in the superpulse mode at a distance of 3–5 cm, with a spot size of 2–3 mm. Any hypertrophied papillae or other pathologies are laser vaporized. Cryoanalgesia is performed with liquid nitrogen to all the external wounds distal to the anorectal line. A steroid ointment is inserted into the anus and the internal and external wounds, and cotton balls are applied to the site without tape or packing. Postoperative care is similar to that for hemorrhoidectomy.

Fistulae and Abscesses

For the classical fistula, a probe is passed from the external to the internal fistulous opening. With the probe in place, the tract is laid open with

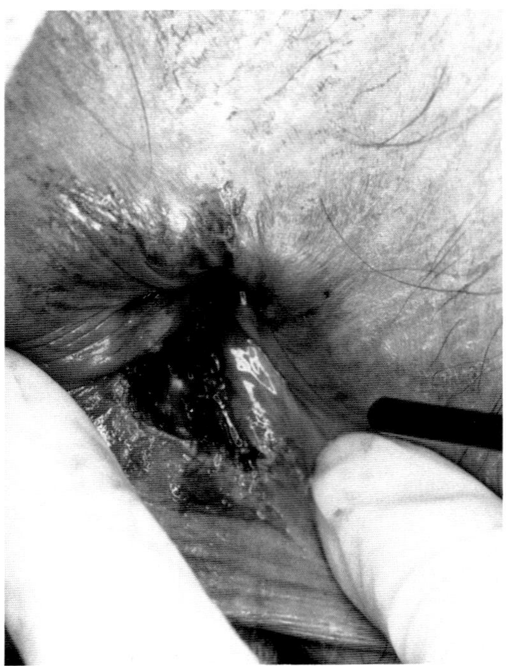

Figure 14.8. Treatment of anal fissure with CO_2 laser.

the CO_2 laser at a continuous setting of 15 W in the superpulse mode, at a distance of 3–5 cm and a spot size of 2–3 mm, increasing the power if necessary. A V-shaped area is then excised with the former tract as its base. This allows for adequate drainage and healing from the inside outward. Multiple tracts and extensions are handled in the same way. In the case of high anal fistulae, where the conventional approach is not possible without damage to the sphincteric muscle, with resulting fecal incontinence, the use of a nylon seton has been the method of choice. However, two cases have been reported by Slutzki et al. (8) where the probed tracts were cored out directly with the CO_2 laser beam.

Abscesses are opened with the CO_2 laser at a setting of 15 W continuous in the superpulse mode. A wide opening is established to promote continuous drainage and to prevent premature closing. It is frequently possible to locate an internal opening of the fistulous tract and to perform a laser fistulectomy, which saves the patient a second procedure. Any vessels that are not suitable for laser hemostasis are controlled with electrocautery. Cryoanalgesia with liquid nitrogen is applied to any wounds distal to the anorectal line. A steroid ointment is inserted into the anus and applied to the internal and external wounds. Cotton balls are used for dressings without pressure, taping, or packing. Postoperative care is similar to that for hemorrhoidectomy.

Pilonidal Cysts and Sinuses

After nearly 40 years of experience, these authors believe that the best results and least complications occur using the open technique, although healing may be prolonged.

Having shaved the operative site, the area is inspected, probed, and the main cyst and sinus tract(s) are laid open with the CO_2 laser at a 15-W continuous setting in the superpulse mode at a distance of 3–5 cm with a spot size of 2–3 mm. Higher settings can be used if necessary. Great care is taken to locate and lay open any additional pathology, especially any inferior, superior, or lateral extensions. All of these incisions are then debrided and beveled so that healing will occur from the inside out. Because large vessels may be encountered, electrocautery is frequently used for hemostasis. Cryoanalgesia using liquid nitrogen is applied to all wound edges. A steroid ointment and cotton balls are applied to the operative area without packing, pressure, or tape.

Postoperatively, normal saline sitz baths are taken at least four times a day with an optional one during the night. Irrigation is desirable. Steroid ointment and cotton balls are applied every 1–2 hours as needed, as drainage is usually profuse. The edges of the wound must be shaved every 3–5 days, and the depths of the wound must be wiped out three times a day with wet gauze (normal saline solution) starting at the seventh day and continuing until healing occurs. Cleanliness of the wound area is extremely important in order to prevent recurrence. Office visits should be weekly to prevent wound bridging. Shaving should be continued for several weeks after the area is apparently healed.

Condylomata

Although condylomata may be removed by surgical excision, electrocoagulation, or cryosurgery, CO_2 laser vaporization is, by far, the best method and gives the greatest patient comfort. These lesions present an extremely difficult problem for treatment, as they are not only perianal, intraanal, and intrarectal, but are also found on the genitalia of both male and female patients. Therefore, it is frequently necessary to refer the patient to a urologist or gynecologist for further treatment. The patient's sexual partner should also be examined and treated. These patients must be followed at increasing intervals for 6 months, and instructed to return immediately at the first sign of a recurrence.

Povidone-iodine scrub and solution are used to cleanse the operative area gently. Due to the possiblity of malignancy, multiple representative biopsies are taken before vaporization. The CO_2 laser is set at 15 W continuous in the superpulse mode at a distance of 3–5 cm with a spot size of 2–3 mm, and each condyloma is vaporized to its base. Cryoanalgesia with liquid nitrogen is then applied to all lesions distal to the anorectal line.

In an attempt to prevent the development of further condylomata, the operative site is lightly frozen, carefully avoiding cryodestruction. The long-term effect of this procedure is unknown.

A suitable steroid ointment and cotton balls or soft folded dressings are applied to the wounds without packing or pressure. Tape is not used unless a small amount is needed to hold the dressings in place. Postoperative care is similar to that for hemorrhoidectomy.

Hidradenitis Suppurativa

Usually, the patient with this unfortunate disease is referred to a specialist only after a variety of treatments have failed and the condition is far advanced. This suppurative process can extend over the surface of the buttocks bilaterally and can affect the axillae incidentally. Although the disease must be completely eradicated, if it is very extensive, it is usually best treated in stages.

The CO_2 laser is used at a 15-W continuous setting in the superpulse mode, at a distance of 3–5 cm with a spot size of 2–3 mm, for a combination of excision and vaporization of the pathology. Higher power may be needed. This is followed by liquid nitrogen cryoanalgesia. Previous experience with conventional surgical methods of treatment is important, as skin grafting may be required.

Neoplasms of the Rectum and Rectosigmoid

Most neoplasms are benign, but because of the increased number of small carcinomas being found, an excisional biopsy should be performed on all lesions 5 mm or larger, and smaller lesions should be biopsied if in doubt. Almost all of the small carcinomas have appeared macroscopically as benign lesions. It is advisable to perform the excisional biopsy with a hot forceps or electrosnare, making certain that the base of the lesion is dry. In this instance, there is no particular need for laser therapy, unless the lesion is sessile or when a larger villous lesion is being treated. For these lesions, the Nd:YAG laser is used.

It is important that the larger villous lesions be destroyed in stages. A number of complications are due to the surgery being performed at too high a laser power and attempting to destroy the entire lesion at one time.

Before each treatment, multiple biopsies of the polyp are taken. The Nd:YAG laser is set at 40–50 W with the time set at 4–5 sec. A brush technique is used, with a spot size of 2–3 mm, and treatment proceeds to the point of tissue blanching. If the villous lesion occupies one-third or more of the bowel lumen, each laser treatment should be limited to a quadrant. The operator must be conservative in the amount of power used and in the extent of the treatment at that particular session. Longitudinal lesions, on the other hand, maybe treated more aggressively at each session. Intervals between treatments vary, but 4–10 days is preferred.

For lesions distal to the peritoneal reflection, it is desirable to use a rigid proctosigmoidoscope. This allows for better suction of gasses, smoke, and removal of tissue debris. If a flexible fiberoptic instrument is used, extra suction may be provided by a tube taped to the colonoscope or flexible sigmoidoscope.

Frequent follow-up is essential, as recurrence is common and the risk of an undetected carcinoma is everpresent. Follow-up visits are every 10–14 days until healing occurs; then every 14–21 days for 2 months; every 3 weeks for 3 months; every month for 3 more months, increasing to every 2 months, and then to once every 3 months.

This method is particularly desirable for elderly and poor-risk patients, especially those with recurrent lesions. However, it may be that for surgeons who have had extensive experience formerly with electrocautery and more recently with laser, the procedure could be used for younger and healthier patients, thus saving them conventional surgery.

The indications for laser surgery for malignancy are basically similar to those above but with the addition of the problem of the advanced, encircling, or recurrent adenocarcinoma. In this event, the rectum can be kept patent in many cases by repeated destruction of the occluding tumor. However, tissue edema and inflammatory response may cause temporary obstruction after each treatment. This palliative procedure maintains the quality of life for the preterminal patient. The lack of associated morbidity with this therapy is a positive force toward good patient attitude during the final phase of the disease.

Squamous Cell Carcinoma of the Anus and Anal Canal

Squamous cell carcinoma of the anal area should be treated with conventional techniques. The CO_2 laser may be used for recurrence at a continuous 15-W setting in the superpulse mode, at a distance of 3–5 cm with a spot size of 2–3 mm.

One patient whose Paget's disease was treated 10 years ago has had the recurrences controlled by laser therapy at 6-month intervals.

COMPLICATIONS

The results of this dual laser technique are generally excellent, especially during the immediate postoperative period; in addition to less pain, the laser patient is able to have more comfortable bowel movements from the first day onward.

Several days after the procedure, most patients experienced some burning and irritation due to the small amount of discharge, but this was minimized by close attention to the prescribed regimen of rectal hygiene.

Occasionally, patients noticed some light bleeding after a bowel movement, but this was controlled with cotton ball pressure. In less than 1% of more than 1500 cases, electrocautery was used to fulgurate one or more small bleeding areas and only two cases required ligation.

There was an incidence of less than 2% of postoperative fissure formation, but most of these fissures were due to constipation. Eight of these patients required treatment with the CO_2 laser. Rarely, skin tags were encountered, but only two of these required further laser treatment; the remainder responded medically to sitz baths and steroid ointment. Three cases of stenosis were encountered.

Four male patients required catheterization, but there was no need for an indwelling Foley catheter.

Occasional instances of muscle spasm were relieved by levator-muscle contraction exercises, sitz baths, and ibuprofen. For the past 3 years, muscle spasm has been greatly reduced by using less Nd:YAG laser energy and introducing the grid pattern of treatment on the internal hemorrhoids.

With the dual laser procedure, there have been no cases of incontinence, abscesses, or fistulae; nor has there been any need for injectable narcotics. However, in earlier days, a rare case of stenosis was encountered with the use of higher power in the single Nd:YAG laser technique.

DISCUSSION AND SUMMARY

Nearly 20 years ago, the foundation of the present method of rectal surgery was originated by patients who desired an outpatient rectal procedure. At that time, hospitals and third-party insurers were opposed to this idea. However, concern for the patient's desires, as well as patient safety and comfort, resulted in a series of rectal surgical developments that were suitable for the oupatient surgical setting.

The stages leading up to laser surgery began with injections (2), and proceeded through the Lord dilatation (7) and associated electrocautery, rubber band ligation (3), cryosurgery (4), and infrared photocoagulation (5, 6), before eventually arriving at the use of the Nd:YAG laser for the destruction of internal and external pathology with associated cryoanalgesia.

While the Nd:YAG laser alone yielded excellent results in deep destruction of the internal hemorrhoids, the recent addition of the CO_2 laser has allowed finer definition in the eradication of all external pathology, including fissures, fistulae, pilonidal cysts, condylomata, etc. Cryoanalgesia, applied to the operative site at the end of the surgical procedure, appears to limit the extent of the trauma and give increased postoperative comfort. Burning from the rectal discharge that occurs several days postoperatively is usually well controlled with a regimen of rectal hygiene. Oral narcotics are rarely needed for pain.

Complications have been minimal, but with a vascular area such as the anorectum, bleeding is a possibility. The few cases of bleeding encountered were, with two exceptions, controlled by electrocautery. In such an event, the CSV II Bovie is an invaluable adjunct. It has the necessary type of power, in more than adequate amounts, for hemostasis—features not generally posessed by the solid-state electrosurgical units. It has the added advantage that its energy is not potentiated by blackened tissue. The CO_2 laser can also be used for superficial hemostasis.

In summary, the Nd:YAG laser is excellent for both deep tissue destruction and hemostasis as long as care is taken not to apply it to blackened tissue. The CO_2 laser, in conjunction with the Nd:YAG laser, is an instrument that gives gratifyingly precise and well-defined surgical results. The use of these two modalities together, in conjunction with liquid nitrogen cryoanalgesia, provides the safest and best form of rectal surgery with the least amount of pain.

More than 1500 anorectal operations have been performed using the Nd:YAG laser or dual laser surgery. Patients over 80 years of age and poor-risk patients have also been able to benefit from these outpatient procedures.

Villous lesions are a subject requiring a serious warning. Whether the operator is using electrocautery or the Nd:YAG laser, it is imperative that the larger tumors or encircling lesions be destroyed in segments—but only after extensive biopsies—and without using excessive power. Patience is essential and not too much tumor should be eradicated at any one time.

Training and experience are especially important for the performance of safe and accurate laser rectal surgery. Extreme complications, such as incontinence, perforation, fistula, or abscess, could occur with the use of too much power or incorrect technique. It cannot be overemphasized that the surgeon must exercise the utmost patience and caution in the use of the laser at all times.

REFERENCES

1. Kelsey CB. Treatment of haemorrhoids. Diseases of the Rectum and Anus. London: Kelsey CB, 1884.
2. Anderson HG. Injection method for the treatment of hemorrhoids. Practitioner 1924; 113:399-409.
3. Barron J. Diverse methods of managing hemorrhoids: ligation with cryotherapy. Dis Colon Rectum 1973; 16:178.
4. Lewis MI. Cryosurgical hemorrhoidectomy: A follow-up report. Dis Colon Rectum 1972; 15:128-134.
5. Nath G. New principle of infrared coagulation in medicine and its physical fundamentals. Colo-Proct 1981; 3:379-381.
6. Leicester RJ, Nicholls RJ, Mann CV. Comparison of infrared coagulation with conventional methods in the treatment of haemorrhoids. Colo-Proct 1981; 3:313-315.
7. Lord PH. A new regime for the treatment of haemorrhoids. Proc R Soc Med 1968; 61:935-936.
8. Slutzki S, Abramsohn R, Bogokowsky H. Carbon dioxide laser in the treatment of high anal fistula. Am J Surg 1981; 141:395-396.

CHAPTER

15

Contact Nd:YAG Laser Resectional Vaporization as Palliative Therapy in Esophageal Carcinoma

M. Y. Sankar

Perhaps no other tumor of mankind is so miserable and deadly as carcinoma of esophagus. Perhaps no group of cancer patients deserves palliation more than those afflicted with advanced esophageal cancer. Fifty years ago, there was no therapy for esophageal carcinoma and the patients were doomed to suffer until permanent relief came in the form of death! In 1932, Ohsawa demonstrated that esophagectomy with esophagogastrostomy was surgically feasible but the initial results were unfavorable. Most patients have large tumors, metastases are frequently present at the time of diagnosis, and the overall survival rates are very poor. (1, 2) Although the cure rate for advanced esophageal malignancy has not changed appreciably in the last 20 years, there have been significant improvements in the perioperative care, surgical techniques, and diagnostic modalities that allow earlier detection and safer palliation (3). New directions in multimodality therapy may permit the possibility of cure of this dreadful disease, marked by debilitating course, unpleasant and hazardous therapeutic options, and a dismal prognosis.

Esophageal carcinoma is a worldwide disease. The incidence of esophageal cancer in Linxian county in North China is 130/100,000 population and, by screening methods, early cancers are being detected with a high cure rate and an overall 5-year survival rate of 44% (4). In 1983, a survey in the USA showed that esophageal cancer was diagnosed in 6400 men and 2600 women, accounting for approximately 1% of all cancers in both sexes (excluding skin and in situ tumors). The risk for blacks is found to be four times higher than for whites (5). The highest incidence known is 246/100,000 population among rural black males in South Africa.

PATHOLOGY

The middle third of the esophagus is the site for 50% of esophageal carcinomas; 30% is found in the lower third, and 20% in the upper third. Adenocarcinoma of the gastric cardia invading the distal esophagus accounts for nearly 50% of all esophageal carcinomas in many series. Staging of esophageal carcinoma is by the TNM system. Intraesophageal and submucosal spread of the tumor can be extensive. Extraesophageal spread into the neighboring structures is not infrequent.

DIAGNOSIS

Dysphagia is usually the predominant and first symptom of esophageal carcinoma. But this symptom is usually not appreciated until at least two-thirds of the circumference of the esophagus is involved by tumor (6). It is the general experience that once the symptoms appear, incurable disease is almost always present. The other features include anorexia, weight loss, regurgitation of food resulting in pulmonary problems, chest pain and general pain, and hoarseness of voice, which may or may not always accompany the disease pattern. The presence of anorexia early in the disease is a poor prognostic sign. Chest pain may indicate the submucosal spread of the tumor whereas general pain may be due to metastases in the bones and mediastinal structures.

The lag time between onset of symptoms and diagnosis is 7.5 months in the United Kingdom and 3–6 months in the USA (7). Unfortunately, there is a poor correlation between tumor staging or duration of symptoms (8). A shorter history does not necessarily assure a better prognosis (9).

INVESTIGATIONS

Among the available tests, esophagogastroscopy using the flexible upper gastrointestinal endoscope seems to be a very useful and, in fact, a necessary tool. By this one test, the exact location of the tumor site and tissue diagnosis can be determined. Barium swallow is the time-honored method for diagnosing esophageal carcinoma and gives a road map. Computed tomography is the best noninvasive method to assess the local spread of the disease (10, 11). The other tests include x-rays of the chest and, perhaps, bronchoscopy and radioisotope scans for staging purposes.

THERAPY

The main objectives in the treatment are to restore swallowing and to enhance the quality of life in those patients with advanced carcinoma whose life-span is really short. Moreover, this is a disease of sixth to eighth decades of life and many patients are poor surgical candidates at the time of diagnosis. Historically, the therapeutic thrust has been surgical for a possibility of cure with the alternative being palliation when cure is not feasible. Several centers advocate aggressive surgical procedures as the most effective method of providing palliation, if not cure (4, 12–14). A critical review of surgical results concluded that, in a population with known cancer of esophagus, although 58% were subjected to surgery, only 39% had resectable lesions with a 29% operative mortality rate, an 18% 1-year survival rate, and a 4% 5-year survival rate (7). In the Cleveland Clinic experience, although the operative mortality rate seems to have dropped from 20% to 7.1%, the overall 5-year survival rate is still a disappointing 6% (15). In addition, the operative mortality for esophagogastrectomy rises with increasing age, reaching 40% for patients over 75 years of age (16). Moreover, there is considerable postoperative morbidity with a prolonged period of convalescence. Such dismal results have made others question the merits of the surgical approach to this problem (17).

The results of primary radiation therapy are slighly better than those of surgical treatment in the sense that a 5-year survival rate of 6% was found with the immediate morbidity and mortality being much lower than the surgical treatment (18). But radiotherapy is inappropriate for gastric and gastroesophageal adenocarcinoma (7, 19). Pretreatment staging by computed tomography may work better in the selection of patients for optimal and appropriate treatment toward radiotherapy or a combination of radiation and chemotherapy (20). There remains a significant number of patients suffering from incurable esophageal carcinoma who require palliation by other means. The ideal palliative technique would provide normal swallowing for the affected person's remaining days by a technique that should be quick, safe, painless, needing only a short inpatient stay, and having a low complication rate. Three main methods of palliation are (*a*) surgery, (*b*) intubation; and (*c*) laser therapy.

Intubation of the malignant stricture both endoscopically and at laporatomy has proved a useful measure, the former being preferred (21). Opinions differ as to the efficacy of such techniques because normal swallowing may not be achieved, leaving the patient confined to drinking liquids or trying the soft food (22). The *tube existence,* which forbids solid food, the care required to keep the *tube patient,* and the risk of subsequent tube migration associated with or without perforation makes the proposition a bit unattractive. Reported mortality rates vary from 2% (23) to 27% (24). Although newly designed tubes are an improvement on earlier models, recurrent growth sometimes blocks a previously well-placed tube.

In this scenario, the Nd:YAG laser therapy has been extended to manage the advanced esophageal malignant obstruction as a palliative measure.

In the early 1970s, it was shown to be possible to transmit high power laser beams down the operating channel of the flexible fiberoptic endoscopes. This made the endoscopic laser treatment a feasible proposition in the gastrointestinal tract. Early studies were directed at the control of bleeding from acute lesions in the gastrointestinal tract and enthusiastic reports claimed good success in all such cases (25). Most effective of the lasers in such situations is the Nd:YAG (neodymium: yttrium aluminum garnet) laser, which seems to have made an impact in controlling hemorrhage from peptic ulcers including stigmata of recent hemorrhage, angiodysplasias, and telangiectasias. However, several other devices are available now that may prove equally effective in the endoscopic control of hemorrhage and are much cheaper than lasers. So, perhaps the real role of lasers in the gastrointestinal field is in the management of tumors.

Laser light has several properties. It is necessary to consider the principles of interaction of laser light with biological tissue to understand how this is of value in tumor therapy. The laser light is absorbed as heat leading to thermal contraction in the immediate vicinity of the target area and, by this mechanism, the laser is able to seal the bleeding vessel walls. As more heat is dissipated, local necrosis is produced and if enough heat is delivered in a very short time, cells are vaporized. In summary, the ultimate fate of tissues exposed to intense laser beams can be from reversible effects (edema and inflammation) to destruction with reconstruction. One of the major advantages of lasers is the predictability not only of the nature, but also the extent of these changes and these can be used to good effect in the management of tumors in gastrointestinal tract in general and in esophageal tumors, in particular.

Nd:YAG laser transmission systems use a flexible quartz fiber that delivers laser energy at a distance of 0.5–2 cm from the target tissue. This noncontact system has distinct disadvantages regarding beam irradiation, backscatter, and damage to the quartz tip should it come into contact with tissue or blood.

Recently, a synthetic sapphire crystal has been developed that is easily attached to the end of the quartz fiber using a universal metal connector allowing contact irradiation. The different geometric shapes of these contact synthetic sapphire tips provide the desired effect of vaporization of the tumor or coagulation of bleeding points as well as precise incision of tissues (26, 27). Furthermore, the backscattering from the contact probes is less than 5%, the depth of tissue damage is minimal, and it is optimal to use low powers of laser energy to obtain desired effects. The power density at the tip of the contact probe is related to the distal probe diameter and the results obtained are comparable to the average power density values of different spot sizes and power levels found with CO_2 laser beam. This contact probes thus combine the coagulating and vaporizing properties of Nd:YAG laser with incising and excising capabilities previously only seen with CO_2 lasers.

Laser as Palliative Therapy in Esophageal Carcinoma

At the International Symposium held in Detroit, Michigan in 1979, the papers presented on the role of laser in the gastrointestinal tract did not discuss tumor therapy. In the Tokyo Symposium held in 1981, a number of workers discussed the use of Nd:YAG laser therapy in gastric cancers. In 1982, Fleischer and Kessler published their first account of Nd:YAG laser therapy for palliation of esophageal cancer (28). Their technique was mainly using the Nd:YAG laser transmitted through the fiber in the noncontact fashion beginning at the proximal tumor margin, treating 1–2 cm of tumor during each treatment session and working distally with repeated treatment sessions every 48 hours until the obstruction was relieved. The long lesions took more time to be opened up by this technique. A new technique was developed subsequently in 1984–1985 by Pietrafitta and Dwyer (29). In this technique, initial dilatation using Savary-Guillard dilators was done followed by laser destruction of tumor beginning at the distal tumor margin and backtracking proximally until the entire length of the tumor was treated and the lumen was reestablished. The initial dilatation allowed an upper gastrointestinal endoscope to be advanced over the same guidewire after dilatation. In this manner, the tip of the endoscope was advanced through the entire length of the tumor into the stomach along the same path as the dilators. The endoscope was then slowly withdrawn until the distal tumor margin came into view, which was then subjected to laser vaporization. By this technique, Pietrafitta and Dwyer made it possible to open up the obstructing malignant lesions of the esophagus in single session, regardless of its length. Both groups (28, 29) used the Nd:YAG laser employing the noncontact technique with the laser in high power settings (80–125 W) and a pulse duration of 0.5–1.0 sec. Coaxial gas flow was kept at a minimum to prevent gaseous distension of the stomach and small bowel. Bown (30) emphasizes that when the coaxial gas is used, some kind of venting system must be provided to prevent overdistension of the stomach. This could be done with a two-channel flexible fiberoptic scope, but it is preferable to use as thin an endoscope as possible with the optimum diameter of biopsy channel that would allow the passage of the laser fiber comfortably and, at the same time, retain maximum maneuverability. This means a separate gas escape route is required. A convenient arrangement, as suggested by Bown, is to pass a nasogastric tube alongside the endoscope. The proximal end of the nasogastric tube should be connected to an underwater drain. The use of an appropriate safety filter on the eyepiece or wearing the safety goggles is a must for the endoscopist. In addition, some authorities advise a white ceramic tip at the distal end of the endoscope instead of the usual black plastic (31). This definitely reduces the risk of the instrument damage if the laser is fired too near the endoscope but it is always a good maxim to visualize the tip of the laser fiber well outside the endoscope before firing.

Two other factors can be identified that are said to influence the technical difficulties involved. The texture of the tumor seems to play a role in the sense that if the tumor is soft, pink, and well vascularized, it is easy to vaporize even if it is a polypoid lesion. On the other hand, whitish and hard tumors reflect much of the incident light and more difficult to destroy. The former respond to a power of 50–60 W and the latter require 70–80 W when the noncontact technique is employed (30). The cancer in the middle third of the esophagus is easy to treat because, in this situation, the esophagus is straight and there is reasonable room to maneuver the endoscope. Lesions in the cervical esophagus are the most difficult from the access point of view. The risk of aspiration is equally great. Lesions at the gastroesophageal junction may, at times, cause problems especially if there is a sharp angulation as this may make identification of the way forward difficult. In addition, after the lumen is successfully cored out, food may clog in the relatively horizontal aperistaltic segment. Tumors that recur at the anastamotic site after a previous esophagogastrectomy are relatively easier to treat because the obstructed segments are found to be short and the relief, in fact, dramatic (32).

PATIENTS AND METHODS

Sankar and Joffe (Table 15.1) treated 18 consecutive patients by endoscopic contact laser resectional vaporization (ECLRV) with esophageal dilatation (ED) for advanced esophageal carcinoma from 1985–1988. Most of the patients were referred for laser therapy as the last resort because curative therapy was not considered possible anymore. This was established by computed tomography that showed distant metastases or extension beyond the esophagus or biopsy-proven metastatic disease. At least 13 patients had previous surgery and/or radiotherapy and/or chemotherapy, or a combination of multitherapy before referral. The rest were sent for laser therapy immediately by their referring physicians; their judgment was based upon the need for rapid relief of esophageal obstruction, an inability to tolerate any other type of major therapy, and/or poor nutritional status of the patient.

Before treatment, the following baseline data were obtained; (*a*) medical history; (*b*) laboratory data that included complete blood count and multichemical analysis; (*c*) endoscopic data; and (*d*) radiographic data, which included barium swallow and computed tomography of the chest and abdomen.

Even though Klass claims that among its many other virtues, doing the procedure under local anesthesia without using operating room facilities is important, the author almost always has used the operating room facilities and general anesthesia with endotracheal intubation. The majority of the patients were poor-risk cases belonging to ASA classification of 3 or, occasionally, even 4. The author strongly believes that such patients do require monitored anesthetic care (MAC) if the procedure is done under local anesthesia. Moreover, using the operating room and general anesthesia makes it possible to do the case as a single session procedure. The reflux of the stomach contents, if and when it occurs, may predispose to aspiration by the patient on the table. For these reasons, it is the author's policy to do such cases in the operating room under general anesthesia with the airway protection.

Either the left lateral or supine patient positions are used and the rigid esophagoscope or the flexible fiberoptic upper gastrointestinal endoscope (Olympus-GIF-Q1OX) may be used as the situation demands. However, all the prescribed precautions should be observed. In 1986-1987, the author used the upper gastrointestinal video endoscope system (Welch Allyn, NY) composed of a laser-treated upper gastrointestinal pediatric video endoscope and monitor, which has good optical resolution and helps in teaching as well. The additional advantage is, of course, the operating

Table 15.1. Endoscopic Contact Laser Resectional Vaporization (ECLRV) and Esophageal Dilatation (ED) for Malignant Esophageal Obstruction (Sankar and Joffe, Cincinnati, OH)—Aug, 1985-Jan, 1988

Total No.	Sex		Age in Years (Mean)	Average Duration of the Disease When First Presented (in months)	Tumor Length in cm (Mean)	Tumor Location			Mean Preoperative Luminal Diameter (in mm)	Mean Postoperative Luminal Diameter (in mm)	Histological Type of Tumor	
	Men	Women				Upper	Middle	Distal			Squamous Cell Carcinoma	Adenocarcinoma
18	14	4	62.5	7.2	7.3	2[a]	4[a]	13	1[b]	13.2	10	8

[a]One patient had tumor both at the upper and middle third of esophagus.
[b]Total obstruction was found in 50% of patients.

room personnel can dispense with the use of safety filter for the eyepiece or safety goggles.

Once the endoscope was inserted, it was important to identify the neoplastic areas causing the worst obstruction, take multiple biopsies, and then direct the main thrust of treatment toward the malignant nodules. The goal is to destroy as much exophytic, intraluminal tumor as is consistent with minimizing the risk of perforation and to slow down intraluminal recurrence. The decision has to be made whether to start at the top (proximal) and travel down (''prograde technique'') or to start at the bottom (distal) and vaporize the growth with the laser as the endoscope is being withdrawn gradually (''retrograde technique''). Generally, if the lesion cannot be passed through by the endoscope or guidewire for dilators, i.e., a situation of total or near total obstruction (Fig. 15.1), then the treatment has to start at the superior (proximal) margin. In contrast to all of the other studies (28–30, 32–35), the author has almost always used contact laser surgery using the endoprobes (SLT, Malvern, PA) for the resectional vaporization of the tumor. For vaporization, the rounded probe (Fig. 15.2) is more suitable; for resection, the chisel probe (Fig. 15.3) is the endoprobe of choice. The contact laser endoprobes enable the use of very low powers (14–18 or a maximum of 20 W), which means the chances of esophageal perforation by laser energy is remote. The duration is either on pulsed mode (1–2 sec) or CW mode. Again, the tactile feedback helps the operator to gain, literally, a ''third eye'' of what is going on, while the growth is being destroyed. Coaxial gas use is avoided but, in its place, coaxial water is used to keep the endoprobe cool and to prevent tissue adhesion. In turn, this avoids overdistension of the stomach. The low powers used plus the lack of coaxial gas reduces the production of the laser plume to low levels, providing better visualization. The effect of tumor destruction is seen in the form of blanching or superficial charring. This process is continued, literally shaving the tumor back toward the normal esophageal wall, but stopping short of normal areas (Fig. 15.4). With contact laser surgery, one may presume that further necrosis in the following 48–72 hours is unlikely; this is the time period that usually follows the noncontact technique. It may lead to further sloughing of the deeper areas, which is again a matter of concern regarding the complication of late perforation. As the tumor gets vaporized and resected using the endoprobes, the destructed tumor tissue can be removed either using the endoscopic accessories like biopsy forceps or it can be further pushed by using the tip of the endoscope itself. We also use the esophageal dilators to enlarge the lumen and to ''road-roll'' the passage created by the contact laser endoprobes. After inserting the guidewire through the biopsy channel, the endoscope is removed and graded Savary-Guillard Dilators (Wilson, Cook, Winston-Salem, NC) are passed over the guidewire under fluoroscopic control. When using the rigid esophagoscope, Jackson dilators (Pilling Co., Fort Washington, PA) are used for similar purposes. The contact laser surgery system with a special handle (SLT, Malvern, PA) can be used through the rigid esophagoscope for contact laser therapy without difficulty. Once the viable tumor is seen, this is treated and the process is repeated, if necessary, until all tumor tis-

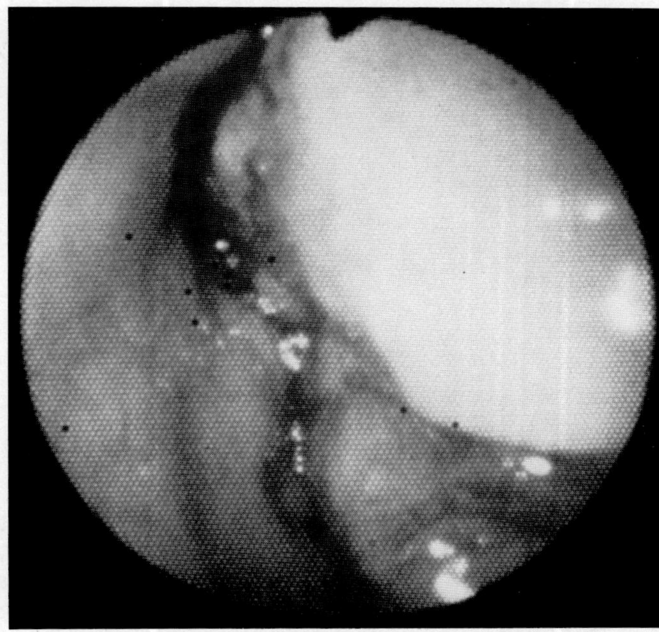

Figure 15.1. Esophageal carcinoma—middle third (total obstruction).

sue is sufficiently destroyed so that reasonable recanalization is made to permit the passage of the endoscope through and into the stomach. Once the lumen is reestablished, the whole area in the esophagus is carefully reexamined and any residual nodules may be treated by contact laser resectional vaporization. Great care, however, should be exercised in this process as overtreatment would only increase the risk of perforation. Flat malignant areas are better treated with short bursts of laser energy using the rounded endoprobe aiming to blanch the surface without resecting such areas using the chisel endoprobe. The purpose of this is to slow down intraluminal regrowth and to avoid perforation.

In treating the tumor from above downward (proximal to distal), the exposed areas that are not actually destroyed may rapidly become edematous and impair access to more distal areas especially after noncontact laser therapy. This can be avoided, when possible, by doing the retrograde technique. Again, this has not been a major problem when contact laser therapy is used as only low powers need be employed. Even though it is believed that balloon or bougie dilatation may cause considerable local tissue damage and the ensuing oozing of blood could make it difficult to see the target areas clearly (30), this problem has not been encountered by the author when esophageal dilatation has been done with the graded dilators as an adjunct to laser therapy. Through the endoscope balloon, dilators have a definite role to

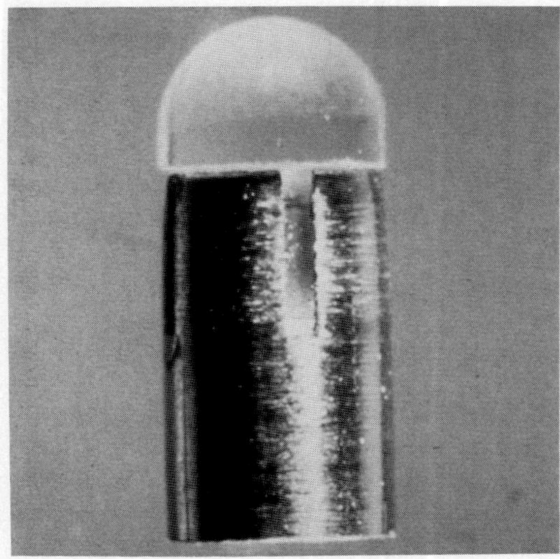

Figure 15.2. Vaporization (rounded) endoprobe (SLT Inc., Malvern, PA).

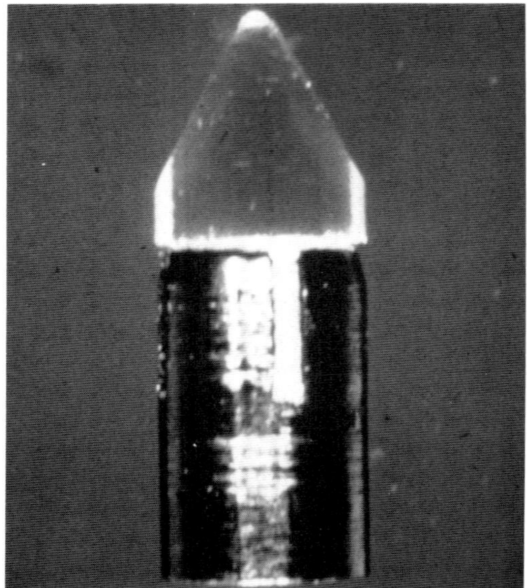

Figure 15.3. Resecting (chisel) endoprobe (SLT, Inc., Malvern, PA).

play in such situations and, when these work, it is really satisfactory; but unfortunately balloon dilators seem to have their own "good and bad days!"

It is expressed that even if the contact endoprobes help to open up a lumen, subsequent treatment in conventional method by using the noncontact technique is still necessary to produce the best long-term results (30). This is personal opinion rather than a well-proven fact. Maybe it has not yet been established whether prolonged exposure to low-power contact laser therapy can stimulate the fibrosis required for good long-term palliation without intraluminal recurrence of tumor. For that matter, it is still uncertain whether laser therapy on the whole can slow the tumor regrowth, by the fibrosis it causes (36, 37). If it is so, then such formation of fibrosis could be harnessed for the patient's benefit, but again, how to avoid the stricture formation by fibrosis is the next question. It is said that laser therapy is best limited to exophytic tumors of the esophagus. The submucosal tumors or tumors producing extrinsic compression should be treated by alternative methods such as insertion of prosthetic tube (30). Although the author agrees with this view on broad terms, there has been gratifying experience of having treated the submucosal lesions using the contact endoprobes successfully.

Energy levels are not all that important from the standpoint of safety. The amount of energy that is necessary, in joules, depends on the vol-

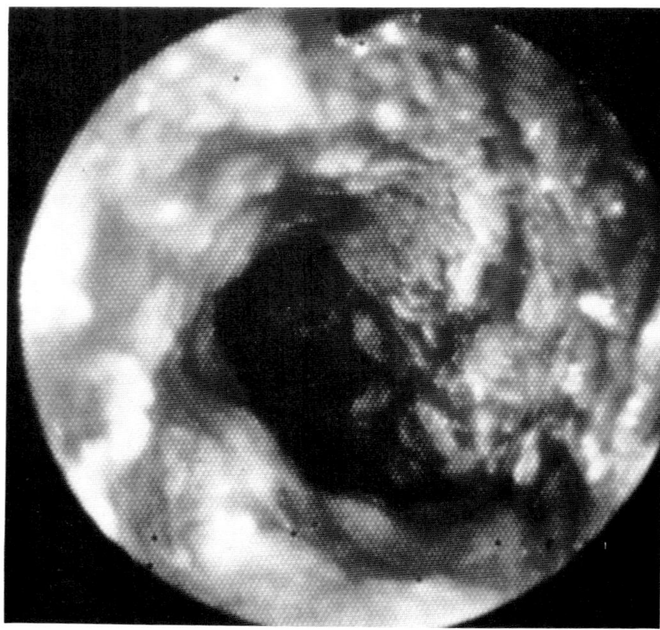

Figure 15.4. Endoscopic contact laser resectional vaporization (ECLRV) of esophageal carcinoma—appearance of esophagus toward the completion of the procedure.

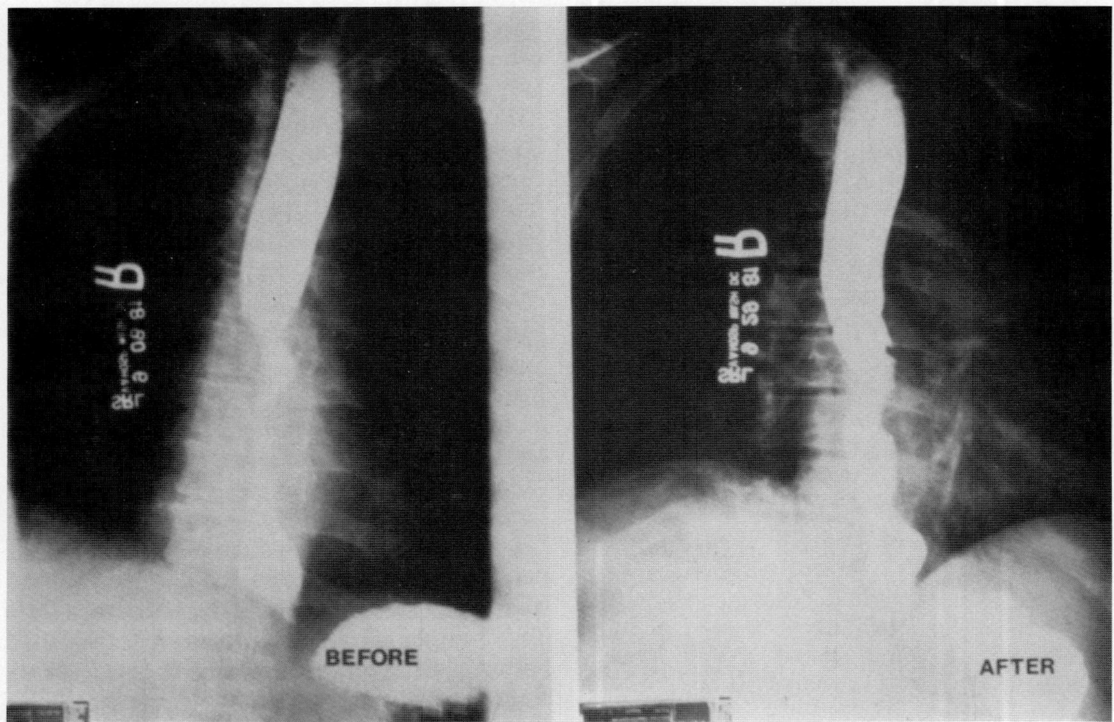

Figure 15.5. Barium swallow x-rays—before and after ECLRV of esophageal carcinoma—middle third.

ume of the tumor that had to be destroyed (29). Adenocarcinoma is more sensitive to laser light destruction because of its texture than the white, less vascular, squamous carcinoma, which reflects the incident light. Therefore, because of this, the discrepency in total energy needed per session is explained (38). Although it is difficult to match these tumors exactly not much difference has been identified between the two types of carcinoma from the expenditure of total energy (in joules) when both types of lesions have been treated using the contact laser technique.

The incidence of bacteremia associated with endoscopy varies widely for difficult endoscopic procedures. Wolf et al. (39) have found that, in patients undergoing elective endoscopic laser therapy for esophageal carcinoma, 40% developed bacteremia at some time during the procedure. However, it is believed that bacteremia appeared to be associated with the endoscopic insertion through the tumor rather than the laser treatment per se. Wolf et al. conclude that, for patients undergoing laser therapy for esophagogastric malignancy, antibiotic prophylaxis to prevent endocarditis may be indicated espeically in such high-risk patients with cardiac lesions. Broad spectrum antibiotics are given in the form of cephalosporins, half an hour before the procedure and continued every 6 hours for the first couple of days parenterally and then orally for a total period of 1 week.

To estimate the efficacy of the treatment, comparative assessments have been made before and after laser therapy and several authors (32–34, 40, 41) have reported good immediate relief of dysphagia in the large majority of cases. But there does not seem to be any uniform agreement regarding the assessment of the swallowing scale (32–34). This is important because there should not be any confusion left when one describes the results based on the swallowing scale and this is possible only when thre is general agreement among the interested "endolaser therapists" of esophageal tumors. The author's impression is that there was immediate symptomatic relief of dysphagia in the majority of cases and this was

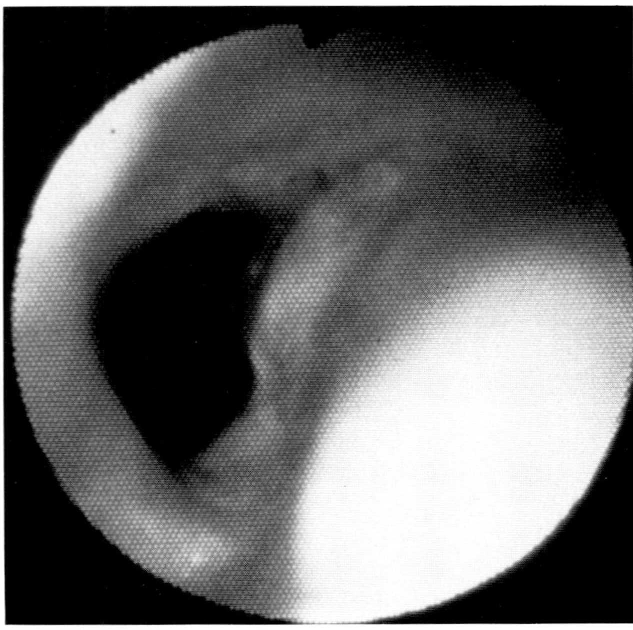

Figure 15.6. Reendoscopy at 3 weeks showing good healing of the lasered areas in the esophagus.

confirmed by postlaser barium swallow x-rays (Fig. 15.5) in agreement with other workers. Reendoscopy at 2–3 weeks showed good healing of the lasered areas in the esophagus (Fig. 15.6). All but four were able to and allowed to swallow fluids on the first postoperative day, followed by solids from postoperative day 2 onward without discomfort. Three patients were not allowed to swallow fluids due to minor perforations noted after therapy, but of these three, in two the problem was managed successfully on conservative regimen. The third patient had multiorgan failure in addition to perforation and succumbed in due course. All three patients had previous radiotherapy and it is reported that the risk of perforation is much higher in such patients (42). The fourth patient who had difficulty in swallowing was found to have carcinomatous lesions both at the upper and middle thirds of the esophagus and a mediastinal mass compressing both the esophagus and trachea from the external aspect. Even though the endolaser recanalization was a technical success, this particular patient had difficulty in swallowing and required percutaneous endoscopic gastrostomy (PEG). In fact, PEG was performed in a total of six patients after ECLRV of the malignant obstruction of esophagus. In five of these, this procedure was done mainly because of anorexia and poor nutritional status. Further, anticipating tumor recurrence, producing obstruction of the esophageal lumen, and dysphagia, which would only lead to further deterioration in the nutritional status, PEG were performed especially in these five patients with their consent. In the first five of the total six cases, the PEGs were done by using Ponsky-Gauderer 20 F gastrostomy tube (Bard Interventional Products, Billerica, MA). Although it is desirable to have a gastrostomy tube with 20 F size from feeding point of view, pulling a silicone tube through the raw surface of the intraluminal esophagus that has just been subjected to laser therapy was a cause for concern. However, there was one single case of perforation by pulling this tube along the intraluminal esophagus. In the last case the Russell gastrostomy (Wilson-Cook Medical, Inc., Winston-Salem, NC) system was used that was much better to use after esophageal intraluminal laser therapy even though the diameter of such a tube is only 16 F.

Tracheoesophageal fistulae have been reported (33, 34). In the author's initial series of 18 cases, such fistulae existed in two cases due to tumor invasion, before laser therapy but developed in one (5.5%) after multiple therapy and this was successfully treated by inserting a Celestin tube. It is worth mentioning a case, in the author's se-

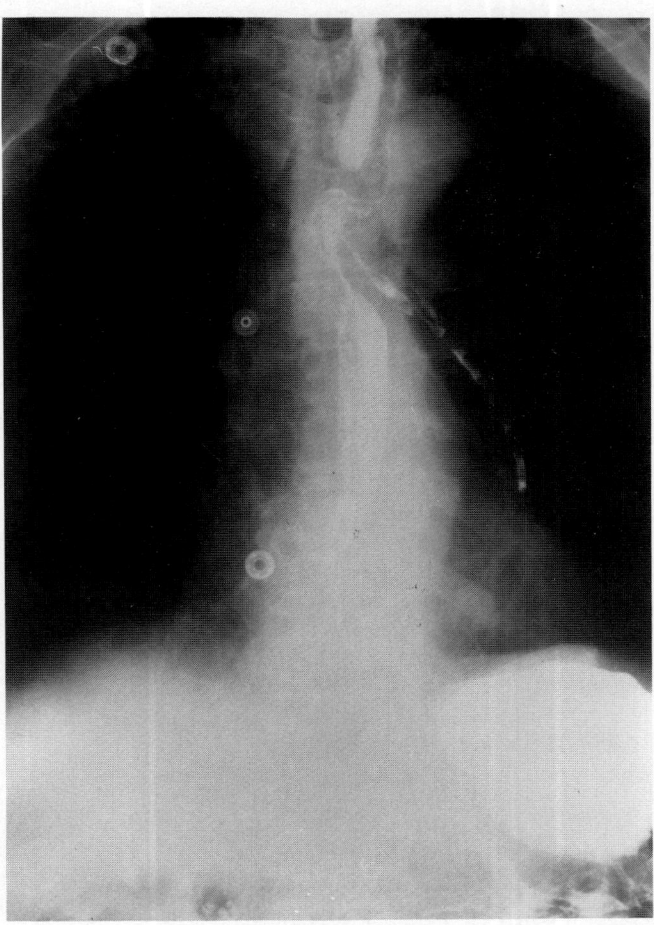

Figure 15.7. Long fistulous tract leading from the midesophagus (tracheoesophageal fistula).

ries, who had a long fistulous tract leading from the midesophagus. (Fig. 15.7) On upper endoscopy, two very narrow lumens were identified, but it was not easy to decide which orifice the endoscope should be taken down through to the stomach and so ''lasting'' the correct narrow orifice could not be carried out with certainity. Therefore, a gastrostomy through a mini-incision was performed on the anterior abdominal wall and the flexible endoscope (Olympus GIF-Q10X) was introduced through the gastroesophageal junction and advanced to the bifurcated region. Then the upper G.I. videoendoscope system (Welch Allyn, NY) was introduced per oral cavity down the upper esophagus and it was then not difficult to identify the obstructed correct orifice from above downward, thus avoiding the *pseudo tract* completely. The flexible endoscope was withdrawn and ECLRV was carried out successfully through the videoendoscope system.

A little oozing of blood is seen during these endoscopies, but significant hemorrhage is rare, probably about 1% (30). Some degree of chest pain can occur after treatment, but it is rare for this to last for more than a few hours. Such a problem is seen in patients with the tumors in the submucosal region. It is claimed that some benefit could be accrued from pretreatment injection of a local anesthetic via a sclerotherapy needle (32).

Only five groups (33, 34, 40, 41, 43) have given detailed follow-up results that are similar. After a successful initial course of treatment, about half the number of patients in each series were able to swallow satisfactorily up to the time of death from disseminated disease. The other half had recurrent dysphagia requiring further lo-

Table 15.2. Carcinoma of Esophagus

	Formal Conventional Esophagectomy	Endoscopic Laser Therapy
Length of stay (days)	18	1–2
Total cost	$11,630.00	$2150.00
Potential savings	0	$9480.00
DRG reimbursement (national average)	$7601.00	$7601.00
	$4029.00 (Loss)	$5451.00 (Profit)

cal treatment, a mean of 2–3 months after initial therapy. In the author's small series, 11 patients were retreated successfully for recurrent obstruction at a mean of 6-week interval and in fact, two were treated more than twice.

Perhaps it might be interesting to note the cost-effectiveness of using the laser through the endoscope and comparing this procedure, in a general way, to the formal conventional procedure of esophagectomy for esophageal cancer (Table 15.2). It is better to note that in those cases where it is established that the carcinoma of esophagus is definitely resectable, a formal conventional esophagectomy-type of surgery may be beneficial. But in others where such a procedure has doubtful values and in advanced cases, it is wise to pursue less commando procedures and endolaser therapy seems to be the best available at this stage.

As the sophistication of diagnostic techniques improves, so the percentage considered unsuitable for curative surgery seems to rise. One must then decide which form of palliation provides the effective symptomatic relief, both in quality and perhaps in duration as well, with minimum general disturbance to the patient. The morbidity associated with palliative surgery, radiotherapy, and/or chemotherapy is relatively extended, which makes the endoscopic options more attractive for patients with a limited life expectancy. Although endoscopic laser therapy may have just started, the results show that the majority of the affected individuals are able to return to a diet that is close to normal.

There are insufficient data available to conclude whether endoscopic laser therapy influences survival as compared with alternative forms of palliation, although one report showed that survival was increased as compared with historical controls from the same hospital (33). However, the current data suggest that the quality of palliation is good as compared with insertion of prostheses, but the incidence of serious complications is much lower. Although endoscopic laser therapy for esophageal carcinoma is technically feasible and some parameters can be defined that may help to predict the clinical outcome, more work must be done to show where laser therapy fits in the overall treatment plan so that the patient gets the maximum benefit. At least in the author's experience, laser therapy seems to have been selected as a last resort and, hence, the focus of this study was only on the immediate results rather than long-term evaluation because patients were subjected to laser therapy so late in the course of their disease. Again, it is difficult to interpret long-term results because postlaser therapy was not standardized in this series; some received radio- and/or chemotherapy, and others did not.

It is not clearly known whether a patient who has a resectable but incurable esophageal cancer is better treated by surgery or a combination of other available modes of therapies. It is unknown whether radiotherapy, chemotherapy, and/or laser therapy provide additive benefit that outweighs a potentially additive risk. The answers are not yet available to the question regarding the sequence of available therapies and about the role of peroral prosthesis placement. In an effort to answer such questions, surgeons, including therapeutic endoscopists, oncologists, and radiotherapists should collaborate and then perhaps some of the answers might be forthcoming after a planned study.

EARLY ESOPHAGEAL CANCER

It is a well-known fact that most esophageal cancers are first detected at a late stage. For those that are detected early, cure might be possible particularly if lymphatic spread has not occurred. Current developments in endoscopic ultrasound show that the depth of penetration of small neoplasms can be measured accurately (32). The depth of necrosis produced with Nd:YAG laser can be measured as well (44) and depends mainly on the energy dissipated. On an empirical basis, this has already been used in Japan to treat early esophageal, gastric, and colonic cancers (45). According to Oguro and Tajiri (45), 33 cases with superficial esophageal cancer were treated radically with laser endoscopy and, in 13 cases, biopsy results were negative for more than 1 year. However, the concern with this approach to treatment is not being certain about the true extent of the growth. It is of dubious value to ablate the tumor locally, if it has already spread to an adjacent lymph node from the viewpoint of cure. Nevertheless, lasers help to provide a means of producing local destruction with more precision than is possible with any other currently available modalities of treatment in palliative therapy. Lasers may play a role in curative therapy for early cancers in the future.

PHOTODYNAMIC THERAPY (PDT)

PDT has been the focus of considerable interest in the last few years as an approach that has potential tumor selectivity to the local treatment of malignant tumors with lasers (46). It is based on the systemic administration of sensitizing drugs, such as hematoporphyrin derivative (HpD) which are retained with some degree of selectivity in areas of severe dysplasia and/or frank malignancy. These drugs fluoresce under ultraviolet light that may be of value in localizing early lesions and can be activated by visible light of a wavelength matched to one of their absorption peaks to produce singlet oxygen which leads to local cytotoxic effect. The mechanism of PDT necrosis appears to be shut down of the tumor vasculature rather than any effect on individual malignant cells (47). It is likely that PDT may be of value in treating small, early lesions rather than advanced obstructing tumors. It has already been used in Japan with encouraging results to treat early gastric cancers in patients who were unfit for surgery (48). In addition, many kinds of hyperthermia methods are available to treat various cancers with certain efficacy (49). Based on these, PDT and laser hyperthermia using a pulsed Nd:YAG laser and pheophorbide-A have been tried on experimental brain tumors with satisfactory results (50). A new method now known as LASERTHERMIA has been tried especially in cases of depressed carcinoma of the stomach with encouraging results. A new interstitial probe and a laser attenuator have been developed and used in laserthermia on very low powers and 19 early gastric cancers, of which 17 were of depressed variety, were treated. The results suggest that endoscopic laserthermia is sufficiently effective to the depth of the upper portion of the muscularis propria without the risk of perforation, leading to disappearance of these tumors (51).

CONCLUSIONS

At present, virtually all gastrointestinal malignant tumor laser therapy is palliative. Surgery, wherever possible, still offers the good prospect of cure especially in early malignant obstruction of the esophagus with the lasting relief of dysphagia. For those who are unfit for surgery, however, endoscopic laser therapy offers simple, relatively safe and satisfactory relief of dysphagia with an added advantage of cost-effectiveness.

REFERENCES

1. Watson A. A Study of the quality and duration of survival following resection, endoscopic intubation and surgical intubation in esophageal carcinoma. Br J Surg 1982; 69:585-588.
2. Skinner DB. En bloc resection for neoplasms of the esophagus and cardia. J Thorac Cardiovasc Surg 1983; 85:59-71.
3. Stair JM, Brian JE Jr. The spectrum of esophageal carcinoma. J Arkans Med Soc 1985; 82:107-114.
4. Ying-Kai W, Chen Pao-Tien, Fang Jong-Pao: Surgical treatment of esophageal carcinoma. Am J Surg 1980; 139:805-809.
5. Cancer Statistics, 1983. Cancer 1983; 33:16.
6. Edwards DAW. Carcinoma of esophagus & fundus. Postgrad Med 1974; 50:223-227.
7. Earlam R, Cunha-Melo JR. Esophageal squamous carcinoma: I. A critical review of surgery. Br J Surg 1980; 67:381-390.
8. Younghusband JD, Alvwihare APR. Carcinoma of the esophagus: Factors influencing survival. Br J Surg 1970; 57:422-430.
9. Applequist P. Carcinoma of the esophagus and the gastric cardia: A retrospective study based on statistical and clinical material from Finland. Acta Chir Scand Suppl 1972; 430:1-92.
10. Daffner RH, Halber MD, Postlethwait RW. C.T. of the esophagus: II. carcinoma. AJR 1979; 133:1051.
11. Moss AA, Schnyder P, Thoeni RF. Esophageal carcinoma: Pretherapy staging by computed tomography. AJR 1981; 136:1051.
12. Mori S, Nakayama K. Esophageal carcinoma cases surviving for more than ten years in Japan. Semin Surg Oncol 1986; 2:45-49.
13. Akiyama H, Tsurumaru M, Kawamura T. Principles of surgical treatment for carcinoma of the esophagus: Analysis of lymph node involvement. Ann Surg 1981; 194:438-446.
14. Ellis FH Jr. Carcinoma of the esophagus and cardia: current methods of treatment. Comprehen Ther 1985; 11:10-15.
15. Galandiuk S, Hermann R, Gassman JJ, Cosgrove DM. Cancer of the esophagus: The Cleveland Clinic esperience. Ann Surg 1986; 203:101-108.

16. Leverment JN, Milne DM. Esophagogastrectomy in the treatment of malignancy of thoracic esophagus and cardia. Br J Surg 1980; 139:292-295.
17. Boyce HW Jr. Palliation of advanced esophageal cancer. Semin Oncol 1984; 11:186-195.
18. Earlham R, Cunha-Melo JR. Esophageal squamous carcinoma: II. A critical review of radiotherapy. Br J Surg 1980; 67:457-461.
19. Watson A. Carcinoma of esophagus. Surgery 1984; 1:292-295.
20. Halvorsen RA, Thompson WM. Computed tomographic evaluation of esophageal carcinoma. Semin Oncol 1984; 11:169-177.
21. Lishman AH, Dellipiani AW, Devlin HE. The insertion of esophagogastric probes in malignant strictures: Endoscopy or surgery. Br J Surg 1980; 67:257-259.
22. Belsey RHR. Palliative management of esophageal carcinoma. Am J Surg 1980; 139:292-295.
23. Den Hartog, Jager FCA, Bartlesman JFWM, Tytgat GNJ. Palliative treatment of obstructing esophagogastric malignancy by endoscopic positioning of a plastic prosthesis. Gastroenterology 1979; 77:1008-1014.
24. Diamantes T, Mannell A. Esophageal intubation for advanced esophageal cancer: The Baragwanath experience—1977-1981. Br J Surg 1983; 70:555-557.
25. Kiefhaber P, Nath G, Moritz K. Endoscopic control of massive gastrointestinal hemorrhage by irradiation with a high power Nd:YAG laser. Prog Surg 1977; 15:140.
26. Daikuzono N, Joffe SN. Artificial sapphire probe for contact photocoagulation and tissue vaporization with Nd:YAG laser. Med Instrum 1985; 19:173-178.
27. Joffe SN, Daikuzono N, Sankar MY. Contact probes for the Nd:YAG laser, SPIE (The International Society for Optical Engineering), optical fibers in medicine and biology. 1985; 576:42-50.
28. Fleischer D, Kessler F. Endoscopic Nd:YAG laser therapy for carcinoma of esophagus: A new form of palliative treatment. Gastroenterology 1983; 85:600-606.
29. Pietrafitta JJ, Dwyer RM. Endoscopic laser therapy of malignant esophageal obstruction. Arch Surg 1986; 121:395-400.
30. Bown SG. Endoscopic laser therapy for esophageal cancer. Endoscopy 1986; 18:26-31 (suppl 3).
31. Ell C, Hochberger J, Lux G. Protective tips for endoscopes used in laser therapy. Endoscopy 18:1986 (in press).
32. Fleischer D, Sivak MV Jr. Endoscopic Nd:YAG laser therapy as palliation for esophagogastric cancer: Parameters affecting initial outcome. Gastroenterology 1985; 89:827-831.
33. Mellow MH, Pinkas H. Endoscopic laser therapy for malignancies affecting the esophagus and gastroesophageal junction: Analysis of technical and functional efficacy. Arch Interm Med 1985; 145:1443-1446.
34. Krasner N, Barr H, Skidmore C, Morris AI. Palliative laser therapy for malignany dysphagia. Gut 1987; 28:792-798.
35. Klass A. Laser palliation of carcinoma of the esophagus. In Dent TC, Strodel WE, Turcotte JG, Harper MC, Eds. Surgical Endoscopy. Chicago: Year Book Medical Publ, Inc., 1985, pp. 85-98.
36. Cox J, Bennett JR. Light at the end of the tunnel? Palliation for esophageal carcinoma. Gut 1987; 28:781-785.
37. Kelly DF, Brown SG, Calder BM. Histological changes following Nd:YAG laser photocoagulation of canine gastric mucosa. Gut 1983; 24:914-920.
38. Mathus-Vliegen EMH, Tytgat GNJ. Laser photocoagulation in the palliative treatment of upper digestive tract tumors. Cancer 1986; 57:396-399.
39. Wolf D, Fleischer D, Sivak M Jr. Incidence of bacteremia with elective upper gastrointestinal endoscopic laser therapy. Gastrointest Endos 1985; 31:247-250.
40. Bown SG, Mathewson K, Swain SP, Clark CG. Follow-up of laser palliation for malignant dysphagia. Gut 1985; 26:114.
41. Rieman JF, Ell C, Lux G, Demling L. Combined therapy of malignant stenoses of the upper gastrointestinal tract by means of laser beam and bouginage. Endoscopy 1985; 17:43-50.
42. Delvaux M, Escourrou J. Complications observed during laser treatment of tumors of the upper digestive tract. Acta Endoscop 1985; 15:13-17.
43. Buset M, Dunham F, Baize M, de Toeuf J, Cremer M. Nd:YAG laser, a new palliative alternative in the management of esophageal cancer. Endoscopy 1983; 15:353-360.
44. Bown SG, Salmon PR, Storey DW. Nd:YAG laser photocoagulation in the dog stomach. Gut 1980; 21:818-822.
45. Oguro Y, Tajiri H. Present status of laser medicine and laser endoscopic treatment of gastrointestinal cancers in Japan. In Kiefhaber P, Waldelich CJ, Eds. Laser: Optoelectronics in Medicine. New York: Springer-Verlag, 1985, pp. 323-328.
46. Doiron DR, Gomer GJ. Porphyrin Localization and Treatment of Tumors. New York: Alan R. Liss, 1984.
47. Henderson BW, Waldow SM, Mang TS, Potter WR, Malone PB, Dougerty TJ. Tumor destruction and kinetics of tumor cell death in two experimental mouse tumors following photodynamic therapy. Cancer Res 1985; 45:572-579.
48. Kato H, Kawaguchi M, Konaka C. Evaluation of photodynamic therapy in gastric cancer. Lasers Med Sci 1986; 1:67-71.
49. Salman M, Samaras GM, Eng GP. Hyperthermia for brain tumors: Biophysical rationale. Neurosurgery 1981; 9:327-335.
50. Fujishima I, Sakai T, Ryu VH, Uemura K, Fujishima Y, Daikuzono N, Sekiguchi Y. PDT and laser hyperthermia using Nd:YAG laser and pheophorbide-A on experimental brain tumor. In Oguro Y, Atsumi K, Joffe SN, Eds., Nd:YAG Laser in Medicine and Surgery: Fundamental and Clinical Aspects. Tokyo: Professional Postgraduate Services, K.K., 1986, pp. 90-94.
51. Tsunekawa H, Kanemaki N, Furusawa A, Hotta M, Daikuzono N. Studies on Endoscopic local hyperthermia using Nd:YAG laser. In Oguro Y, Atsumi K, Joffe SN Eds., Nd:YAG Laser in Medicine and Surgery: Fundamental and Clinical Aspects. Tokyo: Professional Postgraduate Services, K.K., 1986, pp. 105-109.

CHAPTER
16

Applications in Gastrointestinal Bleeding

Stephen N. Joffe

In 1981, fewer than 12 medical centers in the USA were using lasers in the treatment of gastrointestinal (GI) disease. By 1984, 200 hospitals were using lasers for this purpose (1). It is projected that there will be 1000 by the end of 1986 (2). The reasons for such proliferation are several, including increased applications of the use of lasers in GI problems, the relative ease with which they can be used, and the ruling by the Food and Drug Administration that the neodymium (Nd):YAG laser is safe and effective and, therefore, is no longer considered to be an investigational device. Furthermore, lasers provide a multidisciplinary and multispecialty modality as well as therapeutic options where such choices did not exist or were limited previously (3). More importantly, they have been found to be safe, efficient, and cost-effective in most cases.

EXPERIMENTAL STUDIES

In 1979, Goodale et al. (4) first reported control of bleeding from gastric erosions using a CO_2 laser with a rigid gastroscope. In 1973, Nath et al. (5) described the transmission of a laser beam through a fiberoptic flexible gastroscope and in 1975, Dwyer and associates (6) reported laser-induced hemostasis in an animal model. Silverstein et al. (7) and Waitman et al. (8) in 1979, compared the effects of the argon laser to the Nd:YAG laser in the treatment of experimentally induced bleeding in canine gastric ulcers. Each group came to the conclusion that both types of lasers were effective in achieving hemostasis and because argon produced less tissue damage, it was considered safer. In the same year, Dixon et al. (9) published their results of the acute and chronic studies of photocoagulation, penetration, and perforation of the Nd:YAG laser in the treatment of experimental canine gastric bleeding. According to their study, Nd:YAG laser photocoagulation was an effective method of controlling experimental bleeding. Energy densities (W/cm^2) 3 times that required to achieve control of bleeding was necessary to cause the serious complication of perforation. Johnston et al. (10) compared efficacy and histological damage caused by monopolar and bipolar electrocoagulation to that of argon and Nd:YAG laser photocoagulation when applied endoscopically to control bleeding from standard canine gastric ulcers. They indicated that more energy and greater power was required with each endoscopic method than at laparotomy to treat bleeding ulcers efficiently. They concluded that each endoscopic method was 93% effective in stopping the bleeding, but the lasers were easier to use. Furthermore, the argon laser and bipolar electrocoagulation caused less tissue injury.

Laser-related tissue injury was generally predictable and correlated with total energy administered and gastric distension. A quantifiable arterial bleeding gastric ulcer was produced in dogs by McLeod et al. (11) using the splenic artery sutured to the base of the ulcer. The main artery blood flow rate varied from 50–120 ml/min. Using the Nd:YAG laser through the flexible endoscope, bleeding was successfully arrested in all dogs. It was noted that coaxial CO_2 allowed adequate visualization of the spurting blood vessel and that the helium-neon laser provided a satisfactory aiming beam.

The histological changes after Nd:YAG laser photocoagulation of canine gastric mucosa were studied by Kelly et al. (12) who concluded that exposure of the dog stomach to the Nd:YAG laser produced tissue changes varying from mild mucosal edema to cell vaporization. Thermal contraction was the primary hemostatic mechanism with thrombosis occurring only as a secondary effect.

The effect on gastric acid secretion after intragastric Nd:YAG laser application to the lesser curve and the pyloric mucosa of the stomachs of the rats has been studied. This technique of intragastric vagolysis produced a statistical reduction in acid secretion maintained over several weeks (13).

ENDOSCOPIC APPLICATIONS OF LASERS

Upper gastrointestinal (UGI) hemorrhage accounts for approximately 200,000 admissions to acute care hospitals annually, making it a major health issue. Fiberoptic endoscopes can help to determine the precise cause of the bleeding in more than 90% of cases. Duodenal ulcers (24%), gastric erosions (23%), and esophageal varices (10%) account for the bleeding in the vast majority of cases.

Therapeutic endoscopy using the laser requires a change in approach to GI bleeding. To become a therapeutic laser endoscopist requires changing from a simple diagnostic procedure into a new therapeutic arena under emergency and often adverse circumstances. By using the laser, the amount of blood transfused and the overall morbidity and mortality of GI bleeding can be decreased. It is important to have a well-trained team to achieve the goals of early endoscopic diagnosis and laser therapy, especially in the management of critically ill patients.

Application of lasers to the problem of GI bleeding was first conceived by the University of Washington group, Silverstein et al., Kiefhaber of the University of Munich, Dwyer and the Los Angeles group, and the Joffe group at the University of Glasgow. Therapeutic endoscopy developed because of a lack of any consistently effective alternate method between the extreme of ice water lavage through a nasogastric tube and laparotomy with an overall mortality rate of 10%. Widespread availability of flexible fiberoptic endoscopy in the early 1970s provided adequate visualization of the bleeding site and the door was opened for the possibility of endoscopically controlling such a situation. Many techniques were tried to achieve this goal including electrocoagulation, injection of vasoactive substances and sclerosant solutions, tissue adhesives, heater probes, and thrombotic sprays (Table 16.1). With technical advances represented by coupling lasers to flexible fiberoptic endoscopes, the next priority became the development of a technique for safe photocoagulation of the large variety and number of bleeding lesions found in the gastrointestinal tract. Of all the endoscopic modalities for treating UGI bleeding, the greatest amount of information is available about lasers. Tens of thousands of patients have now been treated. With the exception of injection sclerotherapy, the Nd:YAG laser is the only device used to treat both variceal and nonvariceal lesions (14).

Table 16.1. Endoscopic Methods of Treating Gastrointestinal Bleeding

- Injection therapy
  - Variceal sclerosants
  - Ethanol
- Topical therapy
  - Tissue adhesives
  - Clotting factors
  - Collagen
  - Ferromagnetic tamponade
- Mechanical therapy
  - Sutures
  - Balloons
  - Hemoclips
- Thermal therapy
  - Electrocoagulation
    - Monopolar
    - Electrohydrothermal
    - Bipolar (multipolar)
  - Heater probe
  - Laser
    - Argon
    - Nd:YAG
      - Noncontact (air-fiber)
      - Contact (sapphire)

The clinical applications of lasers for GI bleeding is shown on Table 16.2 and refers primarily to use of the continuous wave Nd:YAG laser with fiberoptic delivery system.

LASER FIBEROPTIC DELIVERY SYSTEMS

Present fiber delivery systems are composed of fibers with a quartz core surrounded by a silicone rubber cladding and a Teflon cover. The quartz core, cladding, and Teflon cover are enclosed within a polyethylene catheter. The catheter provides protection for the fiber, permitting gas or water to flow between the fiber and catheter to cool and clean the fiber tip and the treatment site. Fibers can range from 50–1000 μm in diameter with the production size being 400–600 μm. The divergence angle of the laser beam at the tip of the catheter is typically between 8° and 12°.

Fibers are flexible and can be used in conjunction with endoscopes or attached to microscopes.

Table 16.2. Gastrointestinal Endoscopic Applications of the Nd:YAG Laser

Coagulation
Acute hemorrhage
Active bleeding
Recent bleeding (e.g., visible vessel; fresh blood clot)
Stigmata of recent hemorrhage (SRH)
Potential bleeding
Angiodysplasia
Varices
Hemorrhoids
Vaporization
Neoplastic disease
Palliation
Curative
Ancillary (e.g., placement of esophageal prosthesis)
Benign stricture or web
Biliary disease
Strictures
Fracturing gallstones
Cutting
Tumor excision (polyps)
Sphincteroplasty
Stricture
Cyst drainage

Flexible fibers are easily inserted into commercial endoscopes. The endoscope manufacturers, such as Olympus, Fujinon, Pentax, and AOMI, provide endoscopes with biopsy channels that accept the fiber without modifications being required.

Current delivery systems have major limitations—they cannot be sterilized adequately, noncontact surgery is often difficult and imprecise, tips burn out if they touch blood or tissue, and fibers break and are expensive. If the quartz tip touches tissue or blood, it absorbs heat and melts. The delivery system then needs to be removed. the polyethylene catheter and Teflon cover cut back, the quartz fiber cleaved and polished, and a new metal tip inserted. This can take 10–30 minutes and may have to be repeated during a procedure. Contact endoscopic surgery with endoprobes made of synthetic sapphires allow direct surgery with greater precision and safety (15).

LASER ENDOSCOPY SUITE

The small examining room that is usually available for diagnostic endoscopy purposes may be inadequate. The room should be sufficiently large to house a procedure table, a cart with materials for resuscitation, cardiac monitoring devices, and suction.

The laser equipment requires proper electric supply sources with special wiring, running water facilities for cooling the high powered lasers, and space for the stretcher. The room preferably should not have multiple entry doors and a warning light with laser signs are installed outside. Patients invariably being considered for laser photocoagulation have considerable blood loss and may be actively bleeding. These patients are at risk of aspiration and may require longer periods of endoscopy. Protective glass filters can be fixed to the viewing end of the flexible endoscope to prevent eye damage when the laser is activated. Video endoscopy now allows a totally closed system for laser utilization and, with the fiber placed into the endoscope, no eye protection is required.

In patients with UGI bleeding, gastric lavage with saline or water is initially carried out with a larger bore tube until the effluent is clear. Alternatively, if not contraindicated, vasopressin is given intravenously, which assists in causing gastric emptying and may diminish the bleeding. These aid in proper visualization of the bleeding sites during endoscopy. A forward- or end-viewing endoscope with double or single channel endoscopes can be used. With the latter, it is preferable to use a separate polyethylene tube of adequate size with distal side holes attached to the endoscope for proper evacuation of coaxial gas and smoke known as "laser plume," which is produced during noncontact laser surgery. Coaxial water with the contact endoprobes avoid this problem and prevent gaseous abdominal distension. Endoscopy is done using local anesthetic and giving adequate amounts of intravenous Demerol and diazepam. General anesthesia is only required in patients who are uncooperative or in whom proper airway control is required.

The power and duration, as well as the coaxial gas or water flow, are adjusted on the laser machine and the laser fiber is inserted through the biopsy channel of the endoscope. If the laser fiber is kept 0.5–1.5 cm away from the mucosa, it is known as noncontact or air-fiber photocoagulation. Touching tissue or blood with the bare quartz fiber when the laser is activated causes damage to the tip of the fiber, which subsequently will melt. In the same way, the fiber tip should be kept well outside of the distal end of the endoscope, otherwise it will damage the endoscope when the laser is activated. There are several different methods of treating the bleeding lesion. These include peripherally, circumferentially, or Z pattern photocoagulation.

CLINICAL RESULTS IN UPPER GASTROINTESTINAL HEMORRHAGE

NonContact (Air-Fiber)

Uncontrolled Studies

In 1973 in Munich, Nath and associates (5) first described the passage of Nd:YAG laser radiation down an endoscopic wave guide. Two years later, the first patients with GI bleeding were treated by this group with the Nd:YAG laser and by 1979, Kiefhaber (16) reported treating 459 patients with 94% permanent hemostasis. Subsequently, the number of unselected patients treated by Kiefhaber has increased to 852 (17, 18). Bleeding was treated successfully in 92% of the 1092 acute bleeding episodes. In bleeding esophageal varices, the mortality was reduced from 70% to 36% by using sclerotherapy after laser photocoagulation. Comparing the results of laser treatment versus surgery, the mortality rate from bleeding acute ulcers was reduced from 58% with gastric resection to 23% using the laser and from 15% for vagotomy to 0% using the laser (18). Reasons for failure include coagulopathies, especially associated with platelet abnormalities and technical difficulties, which included a bleeding site inaccessible to the laser beam.

Many centers in the USA and Europe are now using the Nd:YAG laser for the treatment of GI bleeding. Results are variable depending on multiple factors, not the least of which is the training and learning experience in using these endoscopic methods and the ability to undertake emergency endoscopy efficiently, safely, and with accuracy in determining the bleeding lesion before the laser is even used. Use of the argon laser has been virtually discontinued for treatment of GI bleeding as it appears only adequate in stopping superficial lesions such as erosions (19–21).

Controlled Studies

The efficacy and safety of laser therapy for GI hemorrhage has been evaluated in controlled trials (22–30) and reviewed (31). Although scientific evaluation of any new modality requires a randomized and controlled study to resolve uncertainty, variations in design, size of study populations, and interpretations of data may prevent a definitive answer. Studies need to be precisely assessed with regard to which bleeding patients were included. To date, nine studies have been performed using the Nd:YAG laser with the noncontact technique, of which eight relate to nonvariceal bleeding (22–29).

Table 16.3. London Study of Nd:YAG Laser in Upper Gastrointestinal Bleeding

	Total	Rebleed	Surgery	Died
Laser	70	7	7	1
Control	68	27	24	8
		$p < 0.001$	$p < 0.005$	$p < 0.05$

The following briefly summarizes details of these controlled randomized clinical trials performed to evaluate safety and effectiveness of the Nd:YAG laser in the treatment of UGi hemorrhage. In each of these studies, patients presenting with acute UGI bleeding were allocated to either a control group or a laser-treatment group.

London Study (25, 32). In this multicenter Nd:YAG study that was completed, 527 consecutive patients were admitted with UGi hemorrhage. At emergency endoscopy, the 260 patients with peptic ulcer and the 138 cases of stigmata of recent hemorrhage (SRH) were included in the trial as being accessible to laser therapy. Twenty-six (26) patients had inaccessible lesions for laser treatment and 97 had no SRH. The laser-treated patients had a significant reduction in rebleeding ($p < 0.001$), requirement for emergency surgery ($p < 0.05$), and mortality ($p < 0.05$). It is important to note was that only 10% of the laser-treated patients required emergency surgery compared to 35% in the control group, of which 33% died postoperatively (Table 16.3).

Stratification of the different endoscopic appearances of the bleeding lesions showed the importance of treating visible vessels using the laser ($p < 0.01$) (Table 16.4).

Glasgow Study (26). The criteria for entry into this single blind controlled study were a major UGI bleed (at least 3 pints of blood, hemoglobin <10 gm/dl, shock, or postural hypotension) and, at the time of emergency endoscopy, a lesion had to be visualized. From a consecutive pool of 698 patients admitted with acute nonvariceal UGI hemorrhage, 184 patients were found to have gastric or duodenal ulceration as a cause for the bleeding. Sixteen patients were found to have a visible vessel, either bleeding or not bleeding,

Table 16.4. Lesions Found on Emergency Endoscopy

	Visible Vessel		SRH		Overlying Clots	
	No.	Rebleeding	No.	Rebleeding	No.	Rebleeding
Laser	39	6	17	0	13	1
Control	43	23	13	1	11	2
		$p < 0.01$		N.S.		N.S.

and were subsequently randomized to active laser treatment or to act as a control. Only those patients who would have been considered for emergency surgery were included.

This study, which was the first prospective randomized investigation into the therapeutic effect of the Nd:YAG laser, also showed a reduction in bleeding and the requirement for emergency surgery. No perforations were reported and the mortality rate after surgery was a high but commonly reported 25% in the nonlaser-treated patients (Table 16.5).

Belgium Study (22). In this study, 388 consecutive cases with bleeding peptic ulcers were admitted. Of these, 152 patients were included in the trial (129 ulcers). Patients were divided into two bleeding groups: patients who had active arterial bleeding and patients who had active, but nonpulsatile bleeding at the time of endoscopy. The results in the ulcer group combines recurrent and continued bleeding as rebleeding (Table 16.6).

The rebleeding rate in Group 2 was significantly reduced ($p < 0.005$) in the laser-treated group. This trial had the major disadvantage in that the ethical committee refused to allow randomization of the highest risk patients with spurting vessels to a control group.

In the first group, although the initial hemostasis using Nd:YAG laser achieved was 87%, there were episodes of rebleeding, thus lowering the figures of permanent hemostasis to 45%. In the second group, the initial hemostasis was achieved in 100% and an incidence of 5% rebleeding was noted.

In four additional studies (23, 24, 27, 28), it was concluded that the laser-treated group did no better than the control groups with regard to continued bleeding, need for surgery, or mortality. In the study of Rohde et al. (27), only active bleeders were included and the authors did not believe laser therapy was of value. In two other studies (23, 24), the features of the design may have made it difficult to ascertain a laser benefit, if one actually existed.

Krejs et al. (28) recently assessed the Nd:YAG laser in a 30-month randomized controlled trial. Actively bleeding patients (18 laser, 15 control) and patients who had recently bled and stopped but had SRH (64 laser, 69 control) were studied. The laser conferred no benefit to either group. The study must be faulted because the most severely ill patients, those that could not be transported to the laser, were excluded. Furthermore, the laser treatment was often carried out by rotating residents in training who probably did not have sufficient skill or experience.

Trudeau et al. (29) evaluated the Nd:YAG laser for patients with endoscopic SRH with visible vessels. In the 33 patients studied, the Nd:YAG laser reduced the number of rebleeding episodes, reduced the need for urgent surgery, and improved survival.

A point to be noted is that there was not a single perforation in any of these eight studies where the laser was used to treat nonvariceal bleeding in severely ill patients. Thus, the evidence is overwhelming in the truly scientifically performed studies that the Nd:YAG laser is effective in UGI bleeding and there can be no argument regarding its safety.

Fleischer's studies randomized patients with active esophageal variceal bleeding into a laser treatment group and a control group (30, 31). In this small study, initial hemostasis was significantly greater in the laser-treated group, but the

Table 16.5. Glasgow Study of Nd:YAG in Upper Gastrointestinal Bleeding

	Total	Rebleed	Surgery	Died
Laser	8	2	1	0
Control	8	8	8	2
		$p < 0.001$	$p < 0.001$	N.S.

Table 16.6. Flemish Study of Nd:YAG in Upper Gastrointestinal Bleeding

	Total	Rebleed	Surgery	Died
Group 1 Spurting				
Laser	23	14	14	7
Control		No Controls		
Group 2 Nonspurting				
Laser	38	2	1	6
Control	32	12	4	5
Group 3 Stigmation recent bleed				
Laser	14	3	2	2
Control	22	7	5	3

variceal incidence of rebleeding was high. Laser therapy may be useful for acute variceal bleeding and may be of interim benefit, but it does not represent definitive therapy. A similar conclusion was reached by Kiefhaber et al. (18) in a larger uncontrolled series. They were successful in stopping variceal herorrhage in 160 or 174 episodes of bleeding but, because of a moderately high incidence of rebleeding, recommended that sclerotherapy be performed early for more definitive treatment.

In summary, the Nd:YAG laser is effective in stopping active UGI bleeding and reduces the need for emergency surgery. The rebleeding from spurting arteries or new lesions can be managed successfully by repeated laser photocoagulation. Perforations have not been a problem. The argon laser in randomized studies has been shown to have no effect on the rate of rebleeding, necessity for operation, or mortality (19, 20).

CLINICAL RESULTS IN OTHER GASTROINTESTINAL BLEEDING CONDITIONS

Colonic Hemorrhage Due to Benign Lesions

Colonic lesions can be treated using Nd:YAG laser, bearing in mind the thinness of the distended colonic wall. Lesions such as bleeding diverticulae and arteriovenous malformations may be coagulated using 60–70 W of power and an exposure time duration of 0.1–0.3 sec with noncontact and 8–12 W with an exposure time of 2–3 sec with the contact endoprobe and coaxial water. Coaxial water avoids distension and reduces the risk of perforation and, by combining it with lower laser energy, reduces thermal damage.

Nonbleeding Benign Gastrointestinal Lesions

Osler-Weber-Rendu syndrome may exhibit as single or multiple, small or large vascular malformations. After successful laser therapy, new lesions might appear in different sites. This requires ''harvesting'' of gastric and colonic lesions on a periodic basis to prevent further bleeding episodes. Other lesions that may bleed include benign polyps in the stomach, duodenum, or colon that can be both photocoagulated and vaporized.

Malignant Lesions of the Gastrointestinal Tract

Laser therapy in such situations has been used to control bleeding; this either helps in preparing the patient for definitive surgery or obviates the need for further surgical intervention in an incurable situation.

CURRENT STATUS

Lasers are readily available in the United States, Europe, and Japan. The Food and Drug Administration no longer classifies the laser as an experimental device for any GI application. There are more controlled and uncontrolled data suggesting the safety and efficacy of the laser than is available for any other endoscopic method of treatment whether by thermal means or not.

Previously, the laser had two inherent disadvantages. One was portability and this problem is being addressed. The newer medium-powered Nd:YAG lasers require a single phase of 208–220 volts and are air cooled. This is opposed to three-phase electrical and special water hook-ups of the high-powered lasers. Mobility is now much less of a problem. Lasers cost approximately 5–20 times more than other endoscopic hemostatic methods. This means that if a physician or hospital does not plan to use the laser for purposes other than the treatment of bleeding, it is unlikely to be cost-effective unless the volume of cases to be treated is at least one per week. However, the Nd:YAG laser has other GI applications, such as recannulization of obstructing carcinomas of the esophagus, stomach, and colon, as well as treatment of polyps and other tumors. Today, more than 500 medical centers worldwide, about 300 of which are in the United States, are using lasers to treat GI disease (14).

The various methods of endoscopic therapy of UGI bleeding in humans has been reviewed by

Table 16.7. Evidence That Endoscopic Therapy Is Beneficial in Upper Gastrointestinal Bleeding[a]

	Efficacy Established							
	Bleeding from Varices				Bleeding from Ulcers			
	None	Anecdotal report	Uncontrolled series	Controlled trial	None	Anecdotal report	Uncontrolled series	Controlled trial
Topical	x			0		4		0
Injection			6	10			4	0
Mechanical	x			0			1	0
Thermal								
Monopolar	x		0	0			3	1
Bipolar	x		0	0			2	1
Heater probe	x		0	0			3	0
Laser			1	1			3	6

[a]Number indicates number of published papers (Adapted from Fleischer D. Endoscopic therapy of upper gastrointestinal bleeding. Gastroenterology 1986; 90:22–234).

Fleischer (14) (Table 16.7). The amount of information that exists from rigorously controlled scientific studies is small. Equally disturbing is the minimal information published comparing the different modalities to treat the same lesion in man. Some comparative information exists in animal models, which cannot always be translated into the clinical situation. Experimentally induced ulcers are pathologically, histologically, and hemodynamically different to those found in man.

CONTACT Nd:YAG LASER PHOTOCOAGULATION

Daikuzono and Joffe (15) developed a synthetic sapphire crystal attached to the end of the quartz fiber using a universal metal connector that allows contact Nd:YAG laser photocoagulation. The geometric shape of these synthetic sapphires provides the desired endoscopic effects of coagulation for bleeding and vaporization or excision of tumors. The power density (W/cm^2) is directly related to the distance of the probe from tissue. The contact probes prevent the backscattering of light, reduce the depth of tissue damage, and allow for much lower powers of laser energy to be used.

Several centers in Europe, Japan, and the United States (33) are currently evaluating the contact endoprobes in both upper and lower GI surgery.

Physical compression of the vessel walls allows a more effective form of closure with coagulation, known as coaptation. The noncontact Nd:YAG may be less effective than either of the other techniques, as pressure cannot be applied to tissue without burning and melting the fiber tip, making coaptation impossible. In order to stop bleeding from moderately large vessels, substantial amounts of energy must be applied to the tissue with the noncontact method causing significant damage and, occasionally, even precipitating further bleeding. Moreover, the noncontact technique produces smoke that requires special evacuation, and the coaxial gas flow creates problems of patient distension, which increases risk of perforation and gas embolization.

The conventional noncontact method is typically used for endoscopic coagulation at powers in the 60 to 100-W range. Contact laser probes safely and efficiently seal vessels 1–3 mm in diameter using powers below 10 W. Because of the low overall power and the reduction in scattered energy, there is virtually no smoke. Water irrigation applied coaxially at a low flow is adequate for cooling the fiber-to-probe junction. Contact laser probes can be applied directly to the tissue, which provides tactile feedback during YAG laser procedures, and allows tamponading of vessels for more effective hemostasis.

The *flat probe* is the instrument most often used for coagulation. The technique employed is similar to that used in the noncontact method of laser photocoagulation. Rosettes are formed around the periphery of the bleeding vessel to initiate edema. When bleeding visibly decreases, which may take up to 30–45 sec, the probe can be used mechanically to coapt and seal the vessel with short pulses of energy.

To prevent heat dissipation of the absorbed Nd:YAG laser energy in a spurting blood vessel and to create a sufficiently deep thrombosis, laser powers under 10 W administered in 0.5- to 3- sec pulses are most effective. With the power off, the flat probe can be pressed directly onto the tissue. Firing the laser in pulses produces a high temperature change in the tissue (160–250°C) which, when applied to vessel walls, induces a glue-like adhesion, providing coaptation and coagulation of the vessel.

When properly employed, the contact laser endoprobe will not melt and can be reused. However, if the laser is activated for more than 2 sec while a probe is not in contact with tissue—especially at higher powers—the probe may turn white and change shape. If this happens, the probe's optical and geometrical properties are irreversibly altered and the probe must be replaced. One should not deactivate the laser before removing the probe from the tissue or it may adhere. If sticking does occur, the probe is not pulled off, but rather a short laser pulse is given while gently withdrawing the probe from the tissue. Coaxial water irrigation further reduces the possibility of adhesion.

During the circumferential treatment of a bleeding site, one establishes a simple repetitive pattern. By setting the laser for 2- to 3-sec intervals, the probe is placed on the tissue, the foot pedal pressed, the probe lifted off, and the foot pedal released. Alternatively, the laser is set in the continuous mode and the probe is "walked" around the bleeding site, touching the tissue for 0.5- to 2.0-sec intervals at each spot. It is important when using contact endoprobes that the laser provide a stable output in a low-power range, as sudden uncontrollable power bursts will not only damage the tissue being treated but will also cause irreversible damage to the probes.

Techniques may have to be altered depending upon the type of tissue, the lesion being treated, blood flow, and numerous other factors. The only true indication of coagulation is cessation of bleeding or blanching around the treatment site. Individual users with experience develop their own methods of treatment.

Each type of bleeding lesion must be identified and evaluated independently. Before endoscopy, if the patient is actively bleeding and/or if there are blood clots in the stomach, the stomach must be emptied for adequate visualization of the bleeding site. This can be performed in one of several ways. The preferred technique is to pass a large-bore tube (Ewald) and irrigate the stomach with cold saline continuously until the effluent is minimally pink stained and there are no further blood clots. If the endoscope is passed and blood clots are still found in the stomach, the procedures should be repeated. An alternative or supplementary method is to give an intravenous injection of metoclopramide (Reglan) and a bolus of vasopressin (20 units over 10 min), provided that there are no contraindications. Endoscopy is performed in a standard manner under sedation. If the patient is actively bleeding and there is risk of aspiration occurring, then endotracheal intubation should be performed.

At the end of the procedures, all lesions are gently washed off and observed for a minimum of 3–5 min to make sure that the bleeding has stopped completely. Fresh frozen plasma and blood are given as required. Clotting defects are corrected, antacids, H_2-receptor antagonists, and cytoprotective agents are prescribed. In the event of rebleeding, the procedure can be repeated.

Bleeding Gastric and Duodenal Ulcers with a Visible Vessel

The flat probe is applied circumferentially around the rim of the ulcer. Subsequently, the probe can be applied directly to the vessel for final coagulation and coaptation. Sticking of the probe indicates that the laser power is set too high, producing vaporization of tissue. If adhesion occurs, the power is adjusted down (under 10 W), the laser is activated, and then gently disengaged from the tissue.

When there is massive bleeding from a vessel, the flat probe can be pressed directly against the vessel and the laser activated at 8–10 W for 2–3 sec. This will slow bleeding sufficiently to allow circumferential treatment.

Bleeding Erosions

Bleeding erosions have several punctate bleeding points from arteriolar and capillary vessels at the edges or in the base of the erosion. Using the flat probe, these can be directly photocoagulated. If there is a diffuse ooze, the Z-shooting technique is used. With laser power on, the probe is moved back and forth over the tissue surface in a zigzag fashion. This coagulates the vessels feeding into the bleeding area. The bleeding points within the triangular areas are then directly treated.

Bleeding Esophageal Varices

Bleeding is decreased using a vasopressin infusion and an inflated Sengstaken-Blakemore tube

Table 16.8. Comparative Endoscopic Hemostatic Techniques

	Monopolar	Bipolar	Heat Probe	Argon	Noncontact YAG	Contact YAG
Efficacy with major arterial bleeding	High	Sometimes	High	Low	Moderate	High
Tamponade during coagulation	Limited	Limited	Yes	No	No	Yes
Coagulation through dessicated tissue	No	Poor	Yes	Yes	Yes	Yes
Controlled coagulation depth	No	No	Yes	No	No	Yes
Tissue erosion potential	Yes	Yes	No	Yes	Yes	No
Risk of perforation	High	High	Low	Low	High	Low
Adjacent tissue damage	Yes	Yes	Yes	No	Yes	No
Coaxial irrigation possible	Yes	Sometimes	Yes	No	No	Yes
Gas insufflation required	No	No	No	Yes	Yes	Yes
Nonsticking probe	No	No	Yes	N/A	N/A	Yes
Large channel endoscope needed	Yes	Sometimes	Yes	No	No	No
Interference with electronic equipment	Yes	Yes	No	No	No	No
Ability to cut and vaporize	No	No	No	No	Poor	No

inserted 4 hours before the procedure. In a manner similar to the circumferential treatment, the flat probe is used to coagulate parallel lines on either side of the varix, either starting distally and working proximally or vice versa, but avoiding direct treatment of the varix. The procedure is repeated, working closer and closer to the varix until adequate vasoconstriction is obtained. Only when bleeding has decreased is the probe placed on the varix itself to coapt the vessel proximal to the bleeding site. If the varix is bleeding actively during the procedure, a gastric balloon is inflated and pulled up tightly to the cardioesophageal junction to decrease blood flow.

For a bleeding varix in the stomach, the feeding vessels around the bleeding site are coapted and waiting for 30–45 sec to allow edema and coagulation of the feeding vessels to occur.

Table 16.9. Contact vs. Noncontact Nd:YAG Characteristics

	Non-contact	Contact
Power levels		
Coagulation	60–100 W	10 W
Vaporization	70–100 W	8–15 W
Blood loss	High	Low
Smoke generation	High	Low
Width and depth of thermal damage	3–5 mm	0.2–1.0 mm
Energy lost to backscatter	30–40%	5%
Tamponading of bleeding vessels	No	Yes
Fiber maintenance requirement	Frequent	Infrequent
Tactile feedback	No	Yes
Pain to patient	Moderate	Low
Risk of perforation	High	Low

Bleeding Mallory-Weiss Lesions

The flat probe is applied around the bleeding site, which coagulates the blood vessels supplying the bleeding point. Once bleeding has diminished, the bleeding point itself can be coagulated.

Lower Gastrointestinal Bleeding

Although there are many causes of lower GI bleeding, angiodysplasia is the condition for which the Nd:YAG laser, particularly when used in conjunction with contact probes, has demonstrated the clear advantages.

Contact photocoagulation with the flat probe is performed circumferentially around the angiodysplastic lesion in an attempt to seal off the feeding vessels. Immediately upon coagulation and coaptation of the feeding vessels, bleeding stops.

More recently, we have been evaluating a *hollow cylindrical* contact probe at low power. The probe is used only with coaxial saline to prevent air embolization. The thermal effect simulates the noncontact high-powered laser regarding the effects of greater tissue depth but with the added advantage of coaptation. This endoprobe may be especially useful in the very actively bleeding visible vessels, such as arterial spurters.

The *frosted interstitial* probe provides interstitial irradiation with deep coagulation. Although primarily used in local hyperthermia and photodynamic therapy, it may have a place in GI bleeding. Pushed directly into the tissue up to its flange, adjacent to a bleeding site being either from a nonvariceal site or a varix, it delivers a power density and thermal energy in a hemispherical volume up to a 2-cm radius. With powers of 5–7 W, it coagulates and can be moved circumferentially around the bleeding site. More clinical experience is required. A comparison of endoscopic hemostatic techniques listing advantages and disadvantages is given in Table 16.8 and features of contact and noncontact laser effects are given in Table 16.9.

Currently, the endoscopic method of contact laser photocoagulation has been used in over 200 patients with a success rate of over 90% in stopping bleeding without any complications or perforation. A randomized prospective study would help in its definitive evaluation but this is most unlikely at present.

CONCLUSION

Endoscopic laser therapy for GI bleeding should be considered as one approach in the broad range of therapeutic possibilities. During emergency endoscopy for GI bleeding it is wise to anticipate that laser therapy may be required. If possible, the endoscopist should be prepared to deliver treatment, if appropriate, at the time he or she embarks on the diagnostic endoscopy. In many instances, the treatment chosen will be dictated by the availability of therapeutic modality and the skill of the operator.

For variceal bleeding, currently only schlerotherapy and Nd:YAG laser treatment are options. For nonvariceal bleeding, injection therapy, electrocoagulation, laser photocoagulation, and the heater probe are reasonable considerations. The overwhelming evidence, however, points to the success of the Nd:YAG laser in this area.

Contact laser photocoagulation combines the coagulating properties of the Nd:YAG laser with the tactile feedback and coaptive features of the contact endoprobe. It provides safe, rapid, effective hemostasis. Accurately targeted low-power Nd:YAG laser energy causes less surface damage and lateral necrosis than other thermal techniques, yet it offers a controlled penetrating thermal effect. Moreover, with a single versatile instrument, one has the ability not only to coagulate, but to cut and vaporize for other pathological conditions.

The multidisciplinary applications of the Nd:YAG laser system make it a universal tool in the armamentarium of therapeutic endoscopy and open surgery. The incorporation of minimally invasive surgery, cost-containment, and improved quality of patient care will expand its applications in the health care industry.

REFERENCES

1. Fleischer D. Endoscopic laser therapy for gastrointestinal diseases. Arch Intern Med 1984; 144:1225.
2. Joffe SN. The Nd:YAG laser—Past, present and future perspectives. Proceedings of the International Nd:YAG Laser Society, Tokyo, Japan 1986.
3. Joffe SN, Muckerheide MC, Goldman L. *Neodymium-YAG Laser in Medicine and Surgery*. New York: Elsevier, 1983.
4. Goodale R, Okaka A, Gonzales R, Bornier V, Edlich R, Wangenstern O. Rapid endoscopic control of bleeding gastric erosions by laser radiation. Arch Surg 1970; 101:211.
5. Nath G, Gorrisch W, Kiefhaber P. First laser endoscopy via a fiberoptic transmission system. Endoscopy 1973; 5:203.
6. Dwyer R, Havirback B, Bass M, Cherlow J. Laser induced hemostasis in the canine stomach. JAMA 1975; 231:486.
7. Silverstein F, Auth D, Rubin C. Argon vs. Nd:YAG laser photocoagulation and experimental canine gastric ulcers. Gastroenterology 1979; 77:491.
8. Waitman AM, Grant DZ, Debeer R, Chryssanthou C. Endoscopic laser photocoagulation: Comparison of argon and Nd:YAG. Gastrointest Endoscopy 1979; 25:52.
9. Dixon JA, Berenson MM, McCloskey DW. Nd:YAG laser treatment of experimental canine gastric bleeding. Gastroenterology 1979; 77:647.
10. Johnston JH, Jensen DM, Mautner W. Comparison of endoscopic electrocoagulation and laser photocoagulation of bleeding canine gastric ulcers. Gastroenterology 1982; 82:904.
11. MacLeod IA, Bow DR, Joffe SN. A quantifiable bleeding gastric ulcer in dogs for assessing the neodymium:YAG laser. Endoscopy 1982; 14:9.
12. Kelly DF, Bown SG, Calder BM, Pearson H, Weaver BMQ, Swain CP, Salmon PR. Histological changes following Nd:YAG laser photocoagulation of canine gastric mucosa. Gut 1983; 24:916.
13. Joffe SN, Sanker MY, Brackett K. Effect of Intragastric Vagolysis on Acid Secretion. Optoelectronics, Munich: Elsevier, 1983.
14. Fleischer D. Endoscopic therapy of upper gastrointestinal bleeding. Gastroenterology 1986; 90:222.
15. Daikuzono N, Joffe SN. Artificial sapphire probe for contact photocoagulation and tissue vaporization with the Nd:YAG laser. Med Instrum 1985; 19:173.
16. Kiefhaber P. International experience with lasers for gastrointestinal bleeding. Proceedings of the International Laser Congress, Detroit, MI, 1979.
17. Kiefhaber P, Kiefhaber K, Huber F, Nath G. (1983) Endoscopic applications of neodymium YAG laser radiation in the gastrointestinal tract. In: Joffe SN, ed.

Neodymium-YAG Laser in Medicine and Surgery. New York: Elsevier, p. 6-14.
18. Kiefhaber P, Kiefhaber K, Huber F, Nath G. Endoscopic neodymium:YAG laser coagulation in gastrointestinal hemorrhage. Endoscopy 1986; (suppl 2)18:46.
19. Vallon AG, Cotton PB, Laurence BH, Arrengolmiro JR, Salordoses SC. Randomized trial of endoscopic argon laser photocoagulation in bleeding peptic ulcers. Gut 1981; 22:228.
20. Swain CP, Storey DR, Northfield TC, et al. Controlled trial of argon laser photocoagulation in bleeding peptic ulcers. Lancet 1981; 2:1313.
21. Jensen DM, Machicado GA, Tapia JF, et al. Endoscopic argon laser photocoagulation of patients with severe gastrointestinal bleeding. Gastrointest Endoscopy 1982; 28:151.
22. Rutgeerts P, VanTrappen G, Broekhaert L. Controlled trial of neodymium:YAG laser treatment of upper digestive hemorrhage. Gastroenterology 1982; 83:410.
23. Ihre T, Johansson C, Seligsson U, et al. Endoscopic YAG laser treatment in massive UGI bleeding. Scand J Gastroenterol 1981; 16:633-640.
24. Escourrou J. Nd:YAG laser therapy for acute gastrointestinal hemorrhage. In: Atsumi R, Nimsakul N, eds. Laser. Tokyo, Tokyo Intergroup Corp., 1981.
25. Swain C, Brown S, Salmon P, et al. Controlled trial of Nd:YAG laser photocoagulation in bleeding peptic ulcers. Lasers Surg Med 1983; 3:111.
26. MacLeod IA, Mills PR, MacKenzie JF, et al. Neodymium yttrium aluminium garnet laser photocoagulation for major haemorrhage from peptic ulcers and single vessels in a single blind controlled study. Br Med J 1983; 286:345.
27. Rohde H, Thon K, Fischer M, et al. Results of a defined therapeutic concept of endoscopic neodymium-YAG-laser therapy in patients with upper gastrointestinal bleeding. Br J Surg 1980, 67:360.
28. Krejs GJ, Little KH, Westergaard M, Hamilton JK, Polter DC. Laser photocoagulation for the treatment of acute peptic ulcer bleeding: A randomized controlled clinical trial (abstr). Gastroenterology 1985; 88:1457.
29. Trudeau W, Siepler JK, Ross K, Corwisn D, Prindiville T. Endoscopic neodymium:YAG laser photocoagulation of bleeding ulcers with visible vessels. Gastrointest Endoscopy 1985; 31:138.
30. Fleischer D. Endoscopic Nd:YAG laser therapy for active esophageal variceal bleeding. A randomized controlled study. Gastrointest Endoscopy 1985; 31:4.
31. Fleischer D. Endoscopic laser therapy for upper gastrointestinal tract disease. Surv Dig Dis 1983; 1:42.
32. Swain CP, Kirkham JS, Salmon PR, Bown SG, Northfield TC. Controlled trial of Nd:YAG laser photocoagulation in bleeding peptic ulcers. Lancet 1986; 1:1113.
33. Joffe SN. Contact neodymium:YAG laser surgery in gastroenterology: A preliminary report. Lasers Surg Med 1986; 6:155.

CHAPTER

17

Endoscopic Treatment of Early Gastric Cancer

Hisao Tajiri

For many years, surgery has provided the sole chance for cure in treating gastric cancer, but the progress of laser endoscopy recently enabled the radical curative treatment on an early gastric cancer. Laser endoscopy can prove highly efficient for early phases of gastric cancer when certain conditions are met: Early gastric cancer without distant or lymph node metastasis are good indications for use of laser endoscopy. Clarifying the types of early gastric cancer is a necessary step to find whether and how laser therapy is applicable and effective. This report describes and analyzes clinicopathological and endoscopic findings of early gastric cancers resected at the National Cancer Center Hospital in Japan and, furthermore, determines the sufficient levels of the therappeutic effects by the laser treatment.

MATERIALS AND METHODS

Clinicopathological and Endoscopic Study for Indication of Endoscopic Treatment of Early Gastric Cancer

Of 1600 cases of all resected early gastric cancers at the National Cancer Center Hospital during the period between 1962 and 1985, the subjects included 1439 cases of solitary lesions. During this period, the study focused on the relationship between the presence or absence of metastasis and clinicopathological factors, such as macroscopic type, size, depth of invasion, and whether with or without ulceration in cancerous lesion. In 1262 cases, the presence or absence of metastasis and endoscopic findings, such as gross appearance, size, and histological depth of invasion with good endoscopic documentations were compared.

Table 17.1. Type of Laser and Specification of 68 Patients with Early Gastric Cancer Treated by Laser Endoscopy[a]

Type of Laser	Macroscopic Type		Total
	Elevated	Depressed	
Nd:YAG	31(3)	28(3)	59(6)
PDT[b]	2	5(2)	7(2)
Nd:YAG + PDT	2(2)	4(2)	6(4)
Total	35(5)	37(7)	72(12)

[a]Data from National Cancer Center Hospital, Tokyo, April, 1987. Numbers in parentheses: number of resected or autopsied cases.
[b]PDT: photodynamic therapy (HpD + Argon-dye laser irradiation) age: 43≈88 (mean 71 y.o.) male: female = 50:18.

Endoscopic Laser Treatment

From 1980–1987, endoscopic laser treatment was conducted on 68 cases of early gastric cancer, of which 72 lesions were diagnosed endoscopically (Table 17.1). Macroscopically, 35 of 72 cases showed elevated lesions of either IIa or IIa + IIc type, while the remaining 37 cases were found to be depressed IIc types. The mean age of these 68 cases was 71 years (range of 43–88 years), with male patients dominant over female patients in number.

Of 72 lesions, 59 were treated with Nd:YAG lasers (Medilas, MBB and SLT Model CL 60), seven with the hematoporphyrin derivative (HpD) + argon-dye laser (Lexel Model 504, photodynamic therapy) and the remaining six with the combined treatment of Nd:YAG laser and HpD + argon-dye laser. A noncontact endoprobe with a power output of 40–60 W and a duration of 0.5 sec in Nd:YAG laser, and a contact endoprobe with 15–30 W in power and 1–2 sec in duration were used (1, 2). The total number of shots varied

Table 17.2. Incidence of Lymph Node or Distant Metastasis in Solitary Early Gastric Cancer[a]

Type	Size(cm)			Total
	≤2.0	2.1–5.0	5.1≤	
Mucosal cancer				
I	0(0/18)	0(0/22)	0(0/4)	0(0/44)
IIa	0(0/32)	0(0/33)	0(0/10)	0(0/75)[b]
IIa + IIc	0(0/14)	7(2/27)	0(0/3)	5(2/44)
IIc Ul(+)	1(1/130)	6(18/292)	6(5/89)	5(24/511)
IIc Ul(−)	0(0/56)	0(0/30)	0(0/5)	0(0/91)
Submucosal cancer				
I	25(1/4)	25(10/40)	53(10/19)	33(21/63)
IIa	0(0/9)	19(3/16)	38(3/8)	18(6/33)
IIa + IIc	19(4/21)	29(17/59)	36(4/11)	27(25/91)
IIc Ul(+)	14(12/88)	18(41/228)	17(20/115)	17(73/431)
IIc Ul(−)	0(0/16)	13(3/23)	24(4/17)	13(7/56)
Total lesions				
I	5(1/22)	16(10/62)	43(10/23)	20(21/107)
IIa	0(0/41)	6(3/49)	17(3/18)	6(6/108)
IIa + IIc	11(4/35)	22(19/86)	29(4/14)	20(27/135)
IIc Ul(+)	6(13/218)	11(59/520)	12(25/204)	10(97/942)
IIc Ul(−)	0(0/72)	6(3/53)	18(4/22)	5(7/147)
			Total	11(158/1439)

[a]Data from National Cancer Center Hospital, Tokyo, May, 1962-Dec., 1985. Figures are percentages. Numbers in parentheses show positive cases/total cases.
[b]Includes 7 cases of focal cancer in adenoma.

according to the extent of mucosal spread of carcinomatous tissue.

An argon-dye laser with a 630-nm wavelength through the rhodamine B dye solution from the argon laser was used. HpD, a photosensitive agent, was administered intravenously at a dose of 2.5 mg/kg, and 60–72 hours later, when it was still highly concentrated in the cancerous lesion (3), the lesion was irradiated with the argon-dye laser for 16–48 min. By photochemical reaction, the carcinomatous tissue was destroyed selectively as far as the submucosal layer. Photodynamic therapy was notably indicated when the boundaries of lesions were ill-defined or IIb progression was suspected in early gastric cancer (4). All patients signed informed consent agreeing to participate.

RESULTS

Results of Clinicopathological and Endoscopic Study on Resected Early Gastric Cancer

Table 17.2 shows macroscopic types of resected early gastric cancer with solitary lesions and the frequency of lymph node or distant metastasis. The frequency rate in 1439 cases was 11%. The upper table shows the incidence rate of metastasis of mucosal cancers, the middle table shows submucosal cancers and the lower table shows the total number of lesions in relation to macroscopic type and size. Figures indicate percentage and numbers in parentheses show the total number of cases per positive ones. The figures with slashes show that type I and IIa with mucosal involvement in any size, regardless of the depth of invasion, have no metastasis. The focal cancer in adenoma is included in mucosal cancer of type IIa. Depressed early gastric cancer such as type IIc is divided into two groups: one with histological ulceration (ul+); and the other without ulceration (ul−). Mucosal cancers without ulceration in any size and the lesions without ulceration less than 2 cm in size, irrespective of the depth invasion, have no lymph node metastasis.

The types of early gastric cancer without metastasis are divided.

A. Type I and type IIa with mucosal involvement, including the focal cancer in adenoma;
B. Type IIa less than 2 cm in size;
C. Depressed type without ulceration less than 2 cm in size;

Table 17.3. Incidence of Lymph Node or Distant Metastasis in Solitary Early Gastric Cancer—Size and Endoscopic Appearance[a]

Type	Size (cm)			Total
	≤2.0	2.1-5.0	5.1≥	
Polypoid	4(3/67)	10(10/100)	34(12/35)	12(25/202)
Ulcerative	6(11/181)	11(48/447)	12(17/142)	10(76/770)
Gastritis-like	0(0/75)	3(2/65)	4(1/28)	2(3/168)
Advanced	33(2/6)	26(20/77)	15(6/39)	23(28/122)
			Total	10(132/1262)[b]

[a]Data from National Cancer Center Hospital, Tokyo, May, 1962 to Dec., 1985. Figures are percentages. Numbers in parentheses show positive cases/total cases.
[b]Cases with positive endoscopic documentation.

D. Depressed type without ulceration with mucosal involvement.

Endoscopically, however, these results cannot be applicable in practice, because in some cases, it is impossible to diagnose the exact depth of invasion. Moreover, in terms of accompanying ulceration, the lesion without converging folds may have histological ulceration. Thus, it will be safe to say that type IIa less than 2 cm in size and the focal cancer in adenoma may have indications for laser endoscopy.

Given these factors, the early phases of gastric cancer were classified into four groups based mainly on endoscopic appearances: *(a)* polypoid, which elevates obviously; *(b)* ulcerative, which is depressed with ulcer or converging folds like ulcer scar; *(c)* gastritis-like, which is almost flat, slightly depressed, or elevated without converging folds, namely, the cancer without ulceration endoscopically; *(d)* and advanced, which appears to be advanced but in reality is in the early phase of gastric cancer.

Table 17.3 shows the incidence of lymph node or distant metastasis of these four types of early gastric cancer and its size. Gastritis-like types less than 2 cm in size, regardless of the depth of invasion, have no metastasis. This type may be a good indication because the diagnosis of vertical invasion is not necessary.

Results of Endoscopic Laser Treatment

The clinical course of the patients is shown in Table 17.4. After the laser treatment, 11 of a total of 72 lesions had been resected. Of 61 lesions unresected, 29 had been treated for more than 1 year, 23 for less than 1 year and 8 patients with nine lesions died of other diseases within a year. Autopsy was not performed with one exception.

Table 17.5 shows specifications of 11 resected cases and one autopsied case. Of the 11 resected cases, five (cases 1–5) were operated immediately after the irradiation and the remaining six more than 1 year later. Autopsy was conducted on one case 8 months after the treatment. Histologically, the residue of cancer cells was not demonstrated in five of 12 cases, as indicated in cases 4–7 and 12. After the treatment, cancer cells were detected from the resected specimens in cases 1–3 and 8–11. Cases 1–3 were treated at the outset of the preliminary trial, while cases 2 and 3 showed minute residue of cancer cells histologicaly. Cases 8–11 were operated upon due to cancer recurrence or remnant.

The endoscopic examination was conducted on 29 of 61 lesions unresected for more than 1 year. Twenty-five of 29 lesions were negative in cancer cells by serial biopsy and the remaining four cases showed recurrence or remnant. Hence, effective rate was estimated at about 86% (25 of 29). In four lesions of cancer recurrence or remnant, two

Table 17.4. Clinical Course of Cases Treated by Laser Endoscopy for Early Gastric Cancer

Clinical Course	No. of Cases (Lesion)		
Surgery	11	(11)	
Follow-up without surgery			
Negative for cancer (more than 1 year)	23	(25)	49(52)
Positive for cancer (more than 1 year)	4	(4)	
Pending (due to less than 1 year)	22	(23)	
Died of other diseases (including one autopsied case)	8	(9)	

Table 17.5. Specification of Patients with Early Gastric Cancer Treated by Laser Endoscopy—Resected and Autopsied Cases[a]

Case no.	Age (years)	Sex	Macroscopic type	Location	Size (cm)	Type of laser	Residue of cancer cells
1	70	F	IIa	Greater antrum	2	Nd:YAG	+
2	65	M	IIa + IIc	Greater antrum	1	Nd:YAG	+
3	66	F	IIc	Anterior corpus	3	Nd:YAG	+
4	56	F	IIc	Lesser angle	1	Nd:YAG	−
5	43	F	IIc	Anterior corpus	2	PDT	−
6	71	F	IIc	Lesser corpus	3	PDT	−
7	83	M	IIa	Greater antrum	2	Nd:YAG	−
8	75	M	I	Lesser prepylorus	3	Nd:YAG + PDT	+
9	62	M	IIc	Posterior angle	2	Nd:YAG	+
10	66	M	IIa	Stomach remnant	2	Nd:YAG + PDT	+
11	63	M	IIc	Posterior corpus	4	Nd:YAG	+
12[b]	65	M	IIc	Lesser antrum	2	Nd:YAG + PDT	−

[a]Data from National Cancer Center Hospital, Tokyo, April, 1987.
[b]Autopsied case (died of esophageal cancer).

lesions were endoscopically found more than 2 cm in size and, in the remaining two, it was difficult to irradiate the spot adequately because it was located at the upper part of the corpus or prepylorus area.

The interaction between the size of lesion in maximum diameter and the number of laser irradiation in 29 unresected cases was studied in follow-up for more than 1 year. The lesions less than 2 cm in diameter were treated by one-time irradiation and were negative for cancer cells for more than 1 year. On the other hand, three of four lesions more than 2 cm in diameter received irradiation more than twice and two lesions were still cancer-recurrent or remnant.

The site distributions of 29 lesions were then studied and most of them were located at the middle and lower one-third of the stomach and could be treated one-time irradiation. In contrast, the lesions located at the upper one-third of the stomach and the prepyloric area required irradiation more than twice because oblique or tangential irradiation with lower power became unavoidable in the area.

Then the degree of vertical invasion estimated endoscopically was compared with the number of laser irradiations, but no relation was obtained because most of the lesions were endoscopically diagnosed as fundamentally mucosal cancers.

The incidence of complications in endoscopic laser treatment was only 3 of 72 lesions, and the 3 were bleeding. In all cases, bleeding occured during the treatment, but endoscopic ethanol injection stopped the bleeding. No perforation was experienced.

Two cases of well-treated early gastric cancer are now presented.

Case 1

A 58-year-old female patient had a shallow depressed lesion on the lesser curvature of the lower body, as shown in Figure 17.1. Histologically, it was diagnosed as signet ring cell carcinoma. Noncontact Nd:YAG laser irradiation was conducted on the lesion with 200 shots of 40 W for 0.5 sec. Figure 17.2 shows an endoscopic picture of the lesion taken 1 week after the treatment. The lesion turned to active ulcer. Twenty-seven days after the treatment, the patient was operated. Figure 17.3 shows a macroscopic appearance of the resected specimen, in which an open ulcer is observed on the lesser curvature of the gastric body. Histologically, the residue of cancer cells was not recognized.

Case 2

A 74-year-old male patient had a small Type IIc of early gastric cancer on the anterior wall of antrum. Because the patient had a complication of heart failure, the endoscopic Nd:YAG laser treatment was carried out. The *left half* of Figure 17.4 shows an endoscopic picture taken before the treatment. Histologically, it was diagnosed as well-differentiated adnocarcinoma. In the *right half*, taken 1 week after the treatment, a large and deep ulceration is seen on the same area of antrum.

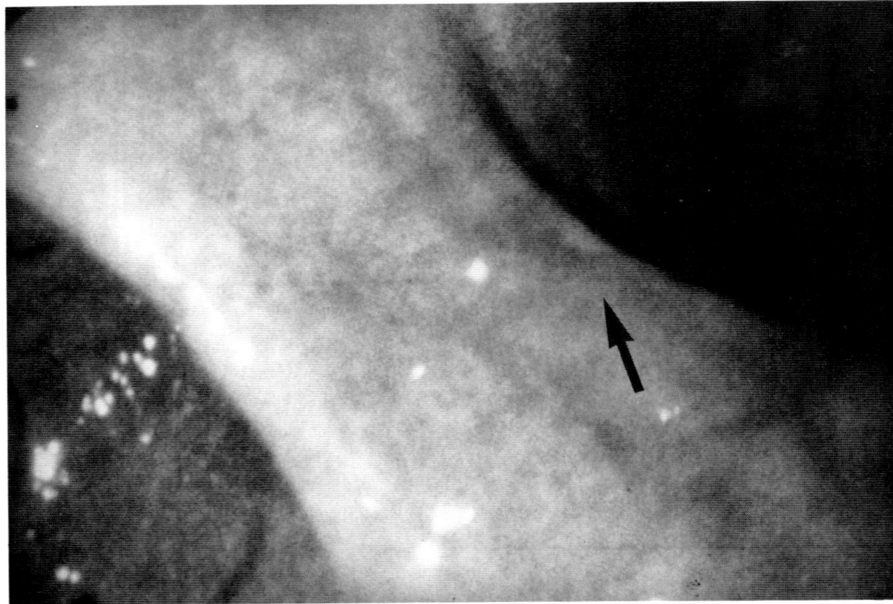

Figure 17.1. Type IIc of early gastric cancer on the lesser curvature of the lower body (case 1); before the Nd:YAG laser therapy.

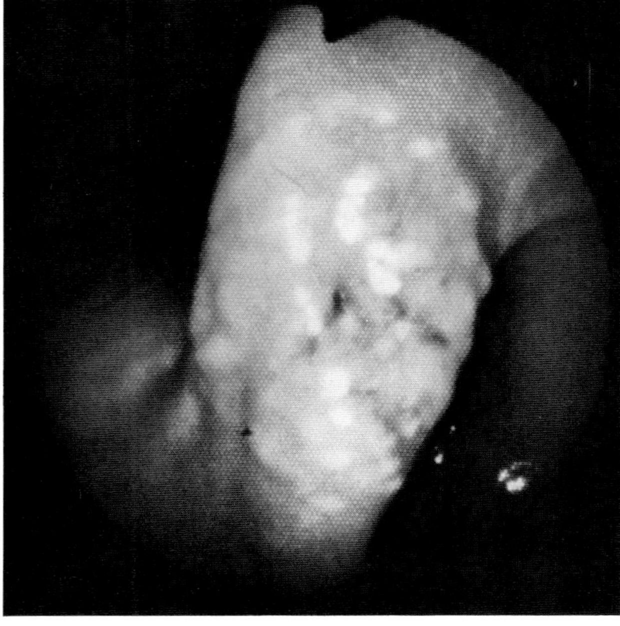

Figure 17.2. An endoscopic picture after 1 week of the treatment (case 1).

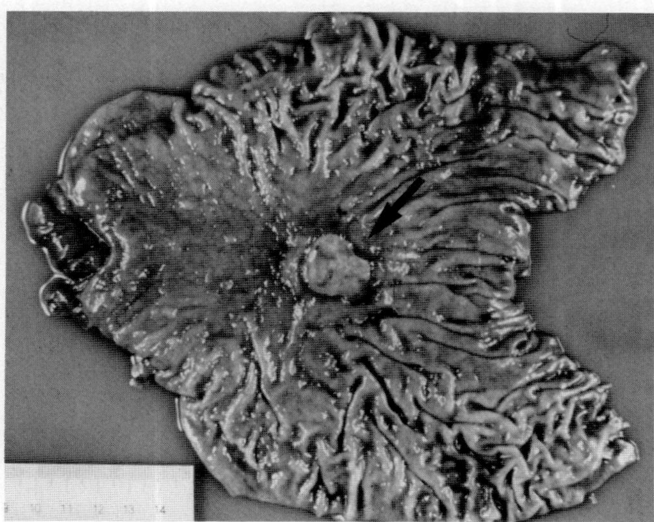

Figure 17.3. A macroscopic appearance of the resected specimen.

The *left half* of Figure 17.5 shows an endoscopic picture taken 5 months after the treatment, which shows a red scar on the antrum with marked contraction of gastric wall and converging folds. No malignancy was suggested. The *right half* shows a picture taken 3 years after the treatment. The inflammatory mucosal change has already disappeared endoscopically, and the deformity of gastric wall has notably improved.

DISCUSSION

Laser endoscopy was developed initially to be used for hematostasis of gastrointestinal hemorrhage in West Germany in 1973 (5). Since it was introduced in Japan in 1978, laser endoscopy has been used for not only gastrointestinal hemorrhage but also for the treatment of gastrointestinal cancer, with excellent results (6).

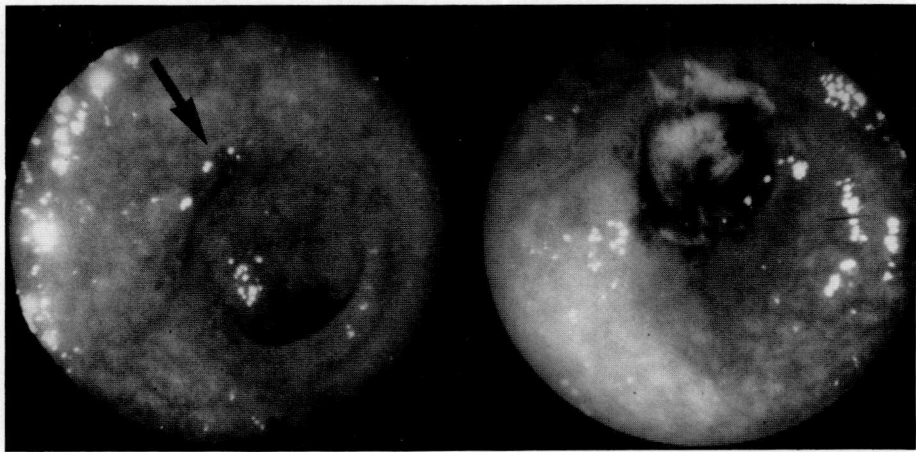

Figure 17.4. The *left half* shows a small IIc type of early gastric cancer on the anterior wall of the antrum (case 2); before the Nd:YAG laser therapy. The *right half* shows an endoscopic picture after 1 week of the treatment.

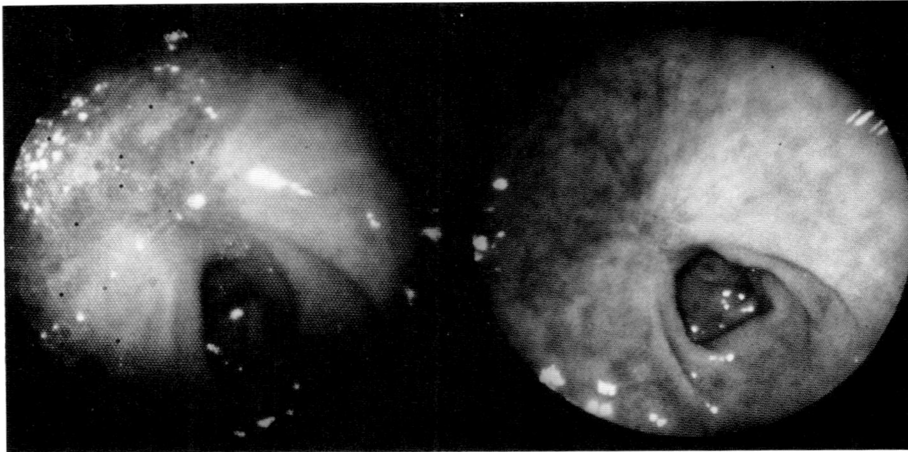

Figure 17.5. The *left half* shows an endoscopic picture after 5 months of the treatment. It shows a red scar on the antrum with marked contraction and converging folds. The *right half* shows 3 years after the treatment.

Laser irradiation has become the radial curative treatment especially for early gastric cancer, although it is allowed to be used only for inoperative cases or for the patients who refuse to undergo operation because of other problems, such as the depth of cancerous invasion and presence or absence of lymph node metastasis, affecting curability.

Recently, the progress of diagnostic techniques for early gastric cancer has enabled the laser treatment to be highly effective in the cure of minute and small gastric cancers, and in treating a number of old patients as the aging generation increases in Japan. Therefore, it is highly likely that the need of endoscopic therapy will rise further along with its indications for enahanced curability in the future.

In this paper, the indications for endoscopic laser therapy for early gastric cancer have been described, and it was found that the basic condition for conducting this therapy is that the lesion should not show metastasis. After the relationship between presence or absence of lymph node or distant metastasis and several other crucial factors clinicopathologically and endoscopically on the resected specimens of 1439 cases of early gastric cancer, suitable for endoscopic laser treatment was investigated, it was concluded that the laser treatment will be indicated for four types of early gastric cancer: *(a)* type IIa less than 2 cm in size; *(b)* focal cancer in adenoma; *(c)* gastritis-like type with less than 2 cm in size; and *(d)* polypoid type with mucosal involvement.

It was determined that the criteria of: type IIa less than 2 cm in size, focal cancer in adenoma, and gastritis-like type less than 2 cm in size were more practical indications because the depth of cancerous invasion and ulceration within cancerous lesion could not always be diagnosed accurately. Furthermore, polypoid type with mucosal involvement can be added to the indications by assistance of ultrasonographic endoscopy as the diagnosis of the depth of invasion by it for mucosal cancer is certain.

The sufficiency of treatment for the primary lesion is determined by its location and size. It should be noted that the wider the lesion is, the less likely curability becomes. The lesion more than 2 cm in diameter may not be suitable for laser therapy because it could show a metastasis in the regional lymph node. Thus, attention must be paid to the insufficiency of the treatment when a cancerous lesion is large or located at difficult areas, such as the prepylorus or the upper body, to make irradiation.

At present, any type of early gastric cancer can be an indication for laser therapy for old patients with high risk and for those who refuse operation. Additionally, even if there are no acceptable reasons for not performing surgical gastrectomy, those types presented may be indications for the laser treatment. In the future, if many cases of those types of early gastric cancer would be treated by laser irradiation and cancer cells would not be demonstrated in the lesion for a long period, they should be true absolute indications.

REFERENCES

1. Daikuzono N, Joffe SN. Artificial sapphire probe for contact photocoagulation and tissue vaporization with the Nd:YAG laser. Med Instrum 1985; 19:173-178.
2. Tajiri H, Oguro Y. Contact Nd:YAG laser treatment of gastrointestinal tract cancer. Advances in Nd:YAG Laser Surgery. New York: Springer-Verlag, 1987, p. 74-78.
3. Dougherty TJ, Kaufman JH, Goldfarb A, Weishaupt KR, Boyle DG, Mittelman A. Photoradiation therapy for the treatment of malignant tumors. Cancer Res 1978; 38:2628-2635.
4. Tajiri H, Daikuzono N, Joffe SN, Oguro Y. Photoradiation therapy in early gastrointestinal cancer. Gastrointest Endosc 1987; 33:88-90.
5. Kiefhaber P, Nath G, Moritz K. Endoscopic control of massive gastrointestinal hemorrhage with a high power Neodymium:YAG laser. Proceedings of the Symposium on Laser in Medicine and Biology. 1977, p. 21-29.
6. Oguro Y, Tajiri H. The present status of YAG laser medicine in Japan—endoscopic laser treatment for GI tract cancer. Nd:YAG Laser in Medicine and Surgery. Tokyo: Professional Postgraduate Service, 1987, p. 3-9.

CHAPTER

18

Lasers in Rectosigmoid Tumors

Jean-Marc Brunetaud, V. Maunoury, D. Cochelard, A. Cortot, J.C. Parris

Lasers were developed in gastrointestinal (GI) endoscopy for their hemostatic properties. They are now used more commonly for tumor destruction (1, 2). At the Lille Laser Center, three types of sessile rectosigmoid tumors are treated by laser photoablation: cancers (advanced and small tumors), villous adenomas and small rectal polyps in familial polyposis syndrome after total colectomy, and ileorectal anastomosis.

MATERIALS AND METHODS

Patient Preparation

Patients were treated on an outpatient basis, without anesthesia or sedative medication. Patients were prepared with a small enema at the Laser Center and no special diet was required before the treatment. Patients were treated once or twice a week until functional improvement (in cases of advanced cancers) or until complete destruction of the tumor. Then they were followed up every 2 weeks until complete reepithelialization. Then patients with an advanced cancer were retreated every month, and the other patients were followed up and retreated if a recurrence or new lesions occurred.

Material for Histology

The main disadvantage of laser protoablation is the lack of material available for a total histological study of the tumor. Before the treatment, multiple biopsies must be performed. For large tumors, a partial snare electroresection is performed when feasible. It has the advantage of debulking the tumor and decreasing the laser treatment time. New biopsies are performed during and after the treatment.

Laser Treatment Modalities

Laser photoablation can be performed in two different ways: coagulation necrosis of the tumor with a delayed slough, or vaporization with an immediate destruction. Coagulation necrosis occurs also at the frontier of the vaporized area, the amount of which depends upon the laser wavelength used.

Two types of lasers are used for GI endoscopic treatment at Lille: the argon laser and the Nd:YAG laser. The argon laser is a 770 Lasersonics (Santa Clara, CA) with a 10-W maximum power output. Its wavelength is well absorbed by the tissue. The argon laser is used for vaporization of superficial tumor (until a flat surface was obtained because delayed necrosis is negligible) at a power of 8 W, a spot size of 1 mm (power density: 1000 W/cm^2) with a continuous beam. The Nd:YAG laser is the YM 101 Cilas (Marcoussis, France) with a 80-W maximum power output. The Nd:YAG wavelength is less absorbed by the tissue than the argon wavelength. The volume of delayed necrosis occurring after Nd:YAG vaporization can be difficult to predict from the macroscopic aspect of the tissue during the treatment (3). Therefore, the Nd:YAG laser is used at Lille only for coagulation (blanching) of the tumor and an interval of 2–3 days between two treatments allows the coagulated parts of the tumor to slough off. Reproducible effects without unexpected necrosis are obtained at 70 W, 2-mm spot size (2000 W/cm^2), and exposure time of 0.7 sec.

The Laser Fibers

A 200-μm core optic fiber is used for argon laser transmission and a 600-μm fiber is used for Nd:YAG. In both cases, the fiber is protected by a Teflon catheter. Nitrogen gas is injected at a flow rate of 2 liters/min to protect the fiber tip. It also gives a neutral gas atmosphere in the rectum and avoids possible explosion when high temperature occurs during treatment. During endoscopy,

Table 18.1. Reasons for Treatment in Patients with Advanced and Small Rectosigmoid Cancers

	Advanced Lesions		Small Lesions	
Reasons for Treatment	No.	(%)	No.	(%)
Nonsurgical without metastases	85	(60)	14	(74)
Nonsurgical with metastases	22	(15)	1	(6)
Colostomy and abnormal discharge	20	(14)	0	(0)
Recurrence after surgery	11	(8)	2	(10)
Refusal of surgery	4	(3)	2	(10)
Total	142	(100)	19	(100)

care must be taken to avoid rectocolonic overdistension because it is painful and it reduces the thickness of the rectocolonic wall, thus increasing the risk of perforation. To evacuate the gas, a cannula is introduced in the rectum alongside the endoscope. The fiber tip is maintained at a distance of 5–10 mm from the tissue during the treatment.

For lesions in the lower third of the rectum, rigid anoscopy is prefered to flexible endoscopy, if the patient can tolerate the knee-chest position. A suction cannula evacuates necrotic tissue and blood with this technique. In this case the fiber is coupled to a rigid handpiece where a lens refocuses the laser beam to a 0.6-mm spot for argon laser and 1.2-mm spot for Nd:Yag laser.

PATIENTS WITH A RECTOSIGMOID CANCER

From December 1979 to August 1987 161 patients with rectosigmoid cancer were treated. The average age of the patients was 78 years (range, 47–94 years). Of the 161 patients, 142 were treated for an *advanced tumor*. Reasons for treatment, localization, and circumferential extension are given in Tables 18.1–18.3. Circumferential extension (annular size of the tumor base) was estimated by comparing the circumferential portion of the bowel lumen occupied by the tumor base to the complete luminal circumference. The main symptom at the beginning of the treatment was abnormal rectal discharge in 125 patients and occlusion symptoms in 17 patients. Ninteen patients had a *small lesion*. Small lesions were defined as a tumor that was less than 3 cm in length, with a circumferenrial extension of the base less than one-third of the circumference, without sign of infiltration, and purely exophytic without ulceration. Reasons for treatment and localization of the small lesions are given on Tables 18.1 and 18.2.

Table 18.2. Localization of Advanced and Small Rectosigmoid Cancers

	Advanced Lesions		Small Lesions	
Localization	No.	(%)	No.	(%)
Rectum	96	(68)	12	(63)
Rectosigmoid junction	26	(18)	2	(11)
Sigmoid	20	(14)	5	(26)
Total	142	(100)	19	(100)

Of the patients with an advanced cancer, 90% were improved after an average duration of 15 days for the initial treatment (average number of treatments = 2.5). The treatment was stopped in 96 patients and the average duration of improvement (ADI) was 9.3 months (range, 0.2–50.3 months). Life-table analysis shows 48% of patients surviving at 1 year, 92% of them remaining improved. The improvement rate was higher in surviving patients with initial abnormal rectal discharges (97% at 6 months) than in those with obstructive symptoms (58%). Patients with a C1 tumor did much better than the others.

Of the patients with an advanced cancer, 10% failed to improve. This was more frequent in C1 and C2 patients (11.5% failures) than in C1 patients (4%). Patients with initial obstructive symptoms were also less improved (18% failures) than patients with initial abnormal discharges (9%).

Negative biopsies were obtained without local recurrence in 6 of the 25 (24%) patients with a C1 tumor and in all of the 19 patients with a small

Table 18.3. Circumferential Extension of the Advanced Rectosigmoid Cancers[a]

	No.	(%)
C1 (< 1/3)	25	(18)
C2 (1/3-2/3)	56	(39)
C3 (> 2/3)	61	(43)
Total	142	(100)

[a]C1 indicates <1/3 circumference; C2 indicates between 1/3 and 2/3 circumference; C3 indicates >2/3 circumference.

Table 18.4. Localization and Circumferential Extension of the 247 Villous Tumors[a]

Localization	No	(%)	Circumferential Extension	No.	(%)
Lower rectum	62	(25)	C1 (< 1/3)	109	(44)
Middle rectum	89	(36)	C2 (1/3-2/3)	107	(43)
Rectosigmoid junction	54	(22)	C3 (> 2/3)	31	(13)
Sigmoid	42	(17)			
Total	247	(100)		247	(100)

[a]C1 indicates <1/3 circumference; C2 indicates between 1/3 and 2/3 circumference; C3 indicates >2/3 circumference.

rectal cancer after an average treatment duration of 5.0 months. Among the C1 patients, 1 died from lever metastsasis 3 months after the end of the treatment, 1 died from another cause after 28 months of follow-up, and the average follow-up of the 4 patients who are still followed is 4.6 months (range, 1–12.3 months). Among the patients with a small cancer, 1 patient who had a metastasis before the treatment died 8 months later, 2 patients died from another cause, and 1 was lost to follow-up. The average follow-up of the 15 patients who are still followed is 17.3 months (range, 1-51.8 months).

Five complications occurred in the group of patients with an advanced rectosigmoid carcinoma (3.7% of these patients) after 1664 sessions of laser treatment: two perforations at the rectosigmoid junction (fatal), one perirectal abscess, and two rectovaginal fistulas.

LASERS IN RECTOSIGMOID VILLOUS ADENOMA

From December 1979 to August 1987, 245 patients were treated at Lille for a rectosigmoid villous adema. The average age was 71 years (range, 32-92 years). The indications for laser treatment were *(a)* nonsurgical patients (87 patients, 36% of total), *(b)* small tumor that would require drastic surgery (98 patients, 40% of total), *(c)* recurrent tumor after a previous nonlaser treatment (57 patients, 23% of total), and *(d)* patient's refusal of surgery (3 patients, 1% of total). Localization, circumferential extension of the tumor base (from C1 to C3), and histology are presented in Table 18.4 and 18.5.

The treatment was not completed in 33 patients because 12 patients were lost to follow-up; 14 died from another cause during the treatment, and 7 are still under treatment. Results are available in the 214 remaining patients. Thirteen patients (6.1%) had positive biopsies during the treatment. However, only 9 of this latter group of 13 patients had a true adenocarcinoma (4.2%). Two patients (1%) could not be successfully treated: both had a circumferential lesion previously treated by a nonlaser procedure. The previous treatment was electrocoagulation in one patient, which resulted in a very tight stenosis making any endoscopic treatment possible. Therefore, only a diverting colostomy could be performed. The other patient had been treated by surgical transanal resection. He also developed a stenosis, but related to the laser treatment; the stenosis was not tight enough to require a colostomy, but made the endoscopic treatment impossible.

Treatment was successful for 199 patients (93% of the patients with a completed treatment). Among these 199 patients, 46 were lost to follow-up after an average follow-up after laser treatment of 12.4 months (range, 0.4-61.2 months), 6 died from another cause after a follow-up of 14.2 months (range, 1.2-37.8 months), and 147 are still being followed from the end of the treatment for an average period of 24.4 months (range, 0.9-66.6 months). Among the 199 successfully treated patients, 24 had a recurrence after an average period of 11.6 months. All of them were easily retreated except for one. The reason for laser

Table 18.5. Histology of the 247 Villous Adenomas at the Beginning of the Treatment[a]

	No.	(%)
Mild dysplasia	117	(47)
Moderate dysplasia	83	(34)
Severe dysplasia	27	(11)
Carcinoma in situ	20	(8)
Total	247	(100)

[a]A partial snare electroresection was performed in 69 patients, and forceps biopsies alone in 176.

Table 18.6. Influence of Circumferential Extension of the Tumor Base on Incidence of Cancer during Initial Treatment, Treatment Duration, Stenosis Development Requiring Dilatation and Recurrence Rate

Extension	Cancer (%)	Duration (months) of Therapy	Stenosis	Recurrence (%)
C1	1.0	2.7	0.0	10.4
C2	2.2	4.6	0.0	10.6
C3	24.0	8.5	18.8	31.3
Total	4.2	4.2	1.5	12.2

treatment in this patient was a recurrence 6 months after surgical transanal surgery. No malignancy was found on the resection specimen nor on the biopsies performed on the first recurrence. The second recurrence occurred 16 months after laser treatment and was found to be malignant.

During Nd:YAG laser treatment, some patients experienced warmth in the rectum when the tumor was close to the anus. For 2 or 3 days after a laser session, patients often had spotting with blood and evacuation of necrotic tissue. Two patients experienced fever to 38°C for 2 days unassociated with pain and this spontaneously abated. Ten patients developed a stenosis but only 3 were symptomatic and required endoscopic dilatations (1.5% of the patients). No perforations or massive hemorrhages were observed.

The circumferential extension was the main predictive factor that influenced the frequence of cancer during initial treatment, the treatment duration until reepithelialization, stenosis development requiring dilatation, and recurrence rate (Table 18.6).

LASERS IN RECTAL POLYPOSIS

Seventeen patients were treated for rectal polyposis. The average age was 29 years (range 11–48 years). Twelve patients had familial polyposis and 5 had Gardner's syndrome. All of them had surgery with an ileorectal anastomosis before rectal treatment with the lasers. No rectal carcinoma was observed in the 12 patients with familial polyposis. Eleven patients were regularly treated at the Laser Center with an average follow-up of 8.5 years (range, 1-15 years) after the colectomy. One patient was lost to follow-up 10 years after the colectomy. Among the 5 patients with Gardner's syndrome, 2 were lost to follow-up at 1.0 and 1.5 years after colectomy, 2 were regularly followed for 2 years, and the last patient required a rectal amputation 5 years after the colectomy for an adenocarcinoma. No complications occurred in this group of patients.

DISCUSSION

The technique of using both argon and Nd:YAG lasers is rather original. The use of the argon laser in GI endoscopy is not widespread, probably because the purchase of a second laser is found too expensive by most gastroenterologists. The multidisciplinary use of the lasers (4) is a good solution to share the expenses with other specialities, and to have the appropriate laser wavelength for each particular lesion. In fact, those who have access to an argon laser (5) prefer the absence of delayed effects, risk of perforation, and thermal stenosis for treatment of some tumors compared with higher risks with Nd:YAG laser treatment.

The way of using the Nd:YAG laser is also controversial. Some vaporize the tissue with a very high power density (over 10,000 W/cm^2) (6), or they coagulate with the Nd:YAG the small lesions and vaporize the larger ones (7, 8). The authors prefer to coagulate with a lower power density (between 1500 and 2000 W/cm^2) and wait until the coagulated areas slough off (3, 9).

The treatment of ambulatory patients without special diet or medication is well adapted to the elderly population. The treatment technique of using both argon and Nd:YAG lasers and limitating the Nd:YAG laser effects to coagulation is also safe. No complications occurred in the patients with small cancers or rectal polyposis. The complication rate for advanced rectosigmoid cancers (3.7%) or villous adenomas (1.5%) is significantly lower than the 10% of Mathus-Vliegen and Tytgat (7, 8) who use high power Nd:YAG for vaporization and coagulation.

The 90% immediate success rate in palliation of advanced rectosigmoid cancers was not significantly dependent upon the initial symptomatology. However, at 6 months, 95% of the surviving patients with abnormal rectal discharge and 60% of those with obstructive symptoms remained improved. Mathus-Vliegen and Tylgat (7) and Escourrou et al. (10) have immediate success rates of 93% and 100% for hematochezia, and 83% and 67% for obstructive symptoms, respectively. The benefit from laser treatment appears to be better for patients with predominant hematochezia than with obstructive symptoms.

Complete local destruction of C1 cancers or small rectosigmoid cancers with negative biopsies can be achieved by endoscopic laser treatment. This result was obtained in 24% of the patients with C1 tumors and all of the 19 patients with small tumors. Similar results were reported by others (8, 10). However, possible local or regional diffusion of these tumors cannot be detected and their endoscopic treatment must be limited to nonsurgical patients.

A large proportion of the patients with villous adenomas were difficult cases: 56% of the patients with a villous adenoma had a large lesion (C2 and C3) and 23% had a recurrence after a previous nonlaser treatment. However, 198 of the 214 (93%) patients with a completed treatment were cured by the laser therapy. These results are better than those of Mathus-Vliegen who has only a 40% cure rate in almost the same type of lesion and Tytgat (8). The recurrence rate after laser treatment in this study was 12.2%, which is much lower than for other treatments like transanal surgery where it is higher than 20% in most series. In this series, recurrences occurred after an average period of 12.4 months after the end of the treatment. Therefore, these patients are followed-up every 3 months during the first 18 months after treatment and every 6 months thereafter. The treatment of C3 villous adenomas takes longer than for C1 and C2 tumors. C3 tumors have also a higher rate of recurrence and stenosis. However, laser photoablation is probably the only conservative treatment available at present for these tumors.

Nine malignancies (4.2%) occurred during the initial treatment in this series of villous adenoma patients. The malignancy rate was higher in C3 lesions (24.0%) than in C1 (1.0%) and C2 (2.2%) tumors. This is in accordance with the natural history of the villous adenoma where the malignancy rate increases with the tumor size. Mathus-Vliegen and Tytgat (8) reported a higher rate, 20% of malignant degeneration. Therefore, the authors think that it is very important to get the best histological aspect from the tumor before the treatment, with large snare resections when feasible. Patients are selected and the indications are limited to nonsurgical, previously operated patients or to those with small tumors that would require drastic surgery.

The management of patients with an ileorectal anastomosis for a familial polyposis is not easy. The risk of malignancy, even in patients regularly treated, is not negligible. One of the patients in this study developed a carcinoma 5 years after the colectomy. Therefore, the laser treatment has the same limitations as electrocoagulation in this type of treatment. But its main advantages over electrocoagulation are the rapidity (5) and the good healing quality without scarring, as demonstrated by Mathus-Vliegen and Tytgat (8).

In conclusion, endoscopic laser treatment is a safe and effective technique for the treatment of benign sessile rectosigmoid tumors and for palliation of symptoms from malignant tumors. The two main disadvantages of the lasers are their high cost and the lack of total histology, particularly with villous adenoma and familial polyposis. The first problem can be solved by a multidisciplinary use (4). The solution for the second problem is a very careful histological investigation before, during, and after the treatment, and a good selection of the patients where the risk of malignancy has to balanced with the risk of surgery. Patients with biopsy-proven adenocarcinoma should be selected for palliation only if they are not candidates for surgery.

REFERENCES

1. Fleischer D. Lasers and colon polyps. Technology and pathology. The Courtship Continues. Gastroenterology 1986; 90:2024-2025.
2. Jensen DM. Lasers in the GI cancer war and on other fronts. Gastroenterology 1984; 87:974-976.
3. Brunetaud JM, Mosquet L, Houcke M, et al. Villous adenomas of the rectum: Results of endoscopic treatment with argon and Nd:Yag lasers. Gastroenterology 1985; 89:832-837.
4. Brunetaud JM, Mosquet L, Bourez J, et al. Organization of a multidisciplinary laser center. In Fleischer D, Jensen D, Bright-Asare P, eds. Therapeutic Laser Endoscopy in Gastrointestinal Disease. Boston: Martinus Nijhoff, 1983, pp. 167-72.
5. Dixon JA, Burt RW, Roetering RH, McCloskey DW: Endoscopic argon laser photocoagulation of sessile polyps. Gastrointest Endosc 1982; 28:162-165.
6. Lambert R, Sabben G. Photodestruction par laser des tumeurs colorectales: résultats précoces (Abstr). Gastroenterol Clin Biol 1983; 7:59A.
7. Mathus-Vliegen EM, Tytgat GN. Nd:YAG laser photocoagulation in gastroenterology: Its role in palliation of colorectal cancer. Laser Med Sci 1986; 1:75-80.
8. Mathus-Vliegen EM, Tytgat GN. Nd:YAG laser photocoagulation in colorectal adenoma. Evaluation of its

safety, usefulness, and efficacy. Gastroenterology 1986; 90:1865-1873.

9. Brunetaud JM, Maunoury V, Ducrote P, Cochelard D, Cortot A, Paris JC. Palliative treatment of rectosigmoid carcinoma by endoscopic laser photoablation. Gastroenterology 1987; 92:663-668.

10. Escourrou J, Delvaux M, Frexinos J, et al. Traitement du cancer du rectum par le laser neodyme YAG. Gastroenterol Clin Biol 1986; 10:152-157.

CHAPTER

19

Laparoscopic Surgery

Jack M. Lomano

HISTORICAL BACKGROUND

Puncture of the peritoneal cavity with the subsequent introduction of a lens system to visualize the intraabdominal viscera was first practiced in the early 1900s to diagnose diseases of the abdominal cavity. Peritoneoscopy or laparoscopy is a common procedure practiced today by gynecologists, internists, and general surgeons. In 1944, Decker was the first to describe incision of the posterior cul-de-sac to create a pneumoperitoneum for the visualization of the pelvic viscera. Palmer later described the same procedure accomplished through a transabdominal incision using the Trendelenburg position for visualization of the abdominal viscera. These procedures became quite popular because of the ability to make a diagnosis without an open laparotomy. At the same time, there was an intense interest in the development of endoscopic instrumentation in order to make the procedures more effective. The introduction of fiberoptic light cables allowed a better illumination of the abdominal cavity while, at the same time, providing a cool light and avoiding the potential complication of inadvertent burning of the abdominal contents. Steptoe first demonstrated that forceps could be introduced through the laparoscopic puncture in order to sterilize patients using an electrical current applied to the fallopian tubes. The potential for sterilization became quite popular because of the intense interest and concern regarding the overall world population in the 1960s and 1970s.

The American Association of Gynecologic Laparoscopists was first organized by Phillips to provide a scientific meeting ground for those physicians interested in laparoscopic techniques. This association became the forum for the introduction of new laparoscopic techniques and the presentation of data supporting the success or failure of surgical procedures done through the laparoscope. Nonelectric sterilization procedures using Silastic bands or clips were introduced in response to a growing number of complications using electrosurgical sterilization tecniques. Laparoscopic sterilization has now become the most popular means of birth control in the United States. The procedure of diagnostic laparoscopy expanded tremendously as the techniques of laparoscopy became more sophisticated and safe for the patient. Therapeutic laparoscopy has become a common procedure to replace open laparotomy for procedures of lysis of adhesions, aspiration of cysts, in vitro fertilization, biopsy, as well as removal of pelvic endometriosis. Initial investigations by Bruhat, Tadir, and Daniell led to the introduction of the carbon dioxide (CO_2) laser coupled with the laparoscope to treat intraabdominal pathology. Keye first introduced the argon laser for the treatment of pelvic endometriosis and Lomano introduced the use of the neodymium Nd:YAG laser in the treatment of pelvic endometriosis.

INDICATIONS AND CONTRAINDICATIONS

The presence of acute pelvic pain with an unclear definitive diagnosis has perplexed surgical specialists for years. The option of continued observation and testing is not ideal because of the tremendous amount of economic hardship that goes with hospitalization, as well as the potential of continuing a disease process that could have been interrupted through more prompt surgical or medical management. Prompt laparoscopic diagnosis can distinguish between a variety of clinical entities (Table 19.1) when the diagnosis is not apparent from the intitial history, physical, and laboratory examination. Chronic abdominal pain is another clinical entity that can be frustrating to the clinician who has treated patients with medical therapy and has seen no significant improve-

Table 19.1. Differential Diagnosis of Acute Abdominal Pain

Acute salpingitis
Appendicitis
Colicystitis
Diverticulitis
Ectopic pregnancy
Normal pelvis
Ovarian cysts
Pelvic endometriosis
Regional enteritis
Ruptured corpus luteum cyst

ment over a 6-month period of time. Before diagnostic laparoscopy, many of these pateints ended up in an "exploratory laparotomy" to diagnose the etiology of their chronic pain. Laparoscopy accomplished on a same-day surgical basis can distinguish between the various diseases that can present themselves as chronic refractory abdominal pain (Table 19.2).

Sterilization is the most common indication for laparoscopy today. This procedure is accomplished on an outpatient basis with a minimum of pain and discomfort to the patient. It is important that the patient receive thorough counseling before sterilization so that she understands the permanent nature of the operation as well as the remote failure rate if the fallopian tubes should recannulize. Risk of subsequent pregnancy (less than 1/100 women sterilized), as well as the alternatives and potential complications, are precisely outlined in a pamphlet published by the American College of Obstetrics and Gynecology (1).

Infertility in couples who have had unprotected intercourse for a period of 12 months without contraception is an indication for diagnostic laparoscopy. Patients with an abnormal hysterosalpingogram and patients with significant pelvic pain associated with infertility should undergo laparoscopy early in the infertility work-up. Diagnostic laparoscopy for infertility should be scheduled in the luteal phase of the cycle to document the presence or absence of ovulation, as well as thorough evaluation of the uterus, fallopian tubes, and ovaries. Indigo carmine dye is introduced through a cervical cannula to determine the patency of the fallopian tubes. Tubal and periovarian adhesions are a common cause of female sterility. Dr. Hulka has described a classification system for pelvic adhesions that should be utilized when doing diagnostic laparoscopy (2). Pelvic endometriosis affects 1/10 adult women and is also a common cause of infertility. Laparoscopy to determine the extent of pelvic endometriosis has become the accepted standard for the diagnosis and management of the disease. The American Fertility Society has devised a diagnostic classification system for pelvic endometriosis (3). Proper recording and staging of pelvic pathology becomes important when comparing various methods of therapy and determining the recurrence rates after medical or surgical therapy (4).

Table 19.2. Differential Diagnosis of Chronic Pelvic Pain

Abdominal malignancy
Chronic pelvic inflammatory disease
Colicystitis
Diverticulitis
Ovarian cysts
Pelvic adhesions
Pelvic endometriosis
Regional enteritis

COMPLICATIONS

Complications from laparoscopy are relatively rare because of the safety factors that have been incorporated into the modern techniques of laparoscopy. Mortality from laparoscopy is in the range of 4–6/100,000 procedures performed. Approximately one-half of these deaths are anesthetic complications. Bowel burns are seen in approximately 1/2000 cases performed, but many of these heal spontaneously and do not require recurrent laparotomy and prolonged hospitalization. Bowel perforation should be considered in those patients who have continued abdominal pain after the laparoscopy. Many patients will complain of slight shoulder pain secondary to diaphragmatic irritation from the gases introduced during the procedure. Recongized laparoscopic lacterations of bowel during the procedure should be promptly treated by open laparotomy and suture of the defect. Unrecognized lacerations will present with acute abdominal pain and signs of pelvic peritonitis 12–24 hours after the surgery. These patients must be treated with open laparotomy and often require bowel resection at the time of their surgery.

The most common complication of laparoscopy is bleeding, usually secondary to inadvertent laceration of the broad ligament during laparoscopic sterilization. This bleeding is usually controlled with bipolar or unipolar coagulation. Occasionally, a small Pfannenstiel incision is necessary to control the bleeding vessel directly. Perforations of the bladder are often a result of introduction of the laparoscopic trocar when the bladder is full. Cystitis is a minor complication usually caused by the improper cleansing of the instruments after soaking in a bacteriostatic solution.

The procedure of laparoscopy has very few contraindications. These contraindications must always be weighed in light of the indications for the surgery. Certainly, patients who have had multiple previous laparotomies run the potential of significant anterior abdominal wall adhesive disease, thus putting them at greater risk for bowel perforation. Patients with severe cardiac disease may not be able to tolerate a general anesthetic as well as the steep Trendelenburg position that is required for the procedure. Patients who are on anticoagulative drugs run the increased potential of bleeding during the procedure. Patients on Coumadin are best managed by converting them to short-term anticoagulative drugs before the surgery. Some morbidly obese patients are difficult to laparoscope because of the large dead space between the fascia and the abdominal pertoneum. If the indications are appropriate, these problems can be minimized by using longer trocars or using the "open laparoscopy technique" (5).

EQUIPMENT AND INSTRUMENTATION

Modern techniques of laparoscopy require a high intensity light source that is introduced into the instrument through fiberoptic bundles. These light sources will provide adequate illumination for 35 mm slides or videotape documentation of the laparoscopic findings. Many companies supply laparoscopes in various lengths and diameters to provide the operating surgeon with equipment that is suitable to the surgical goals. A 10-mm diagnostic laparoscope with a 5-mm operating channel is a common laparoscope that is capable of carrying out most laparoscopic techniques. There should be at least on 3-mm or 5-mm "second-puncture trocar" through which probes can be used for manipulation, coagulation, laser application, or excision. A cervical cannula attached to a uterine elevator is often helpful in manipulating the pelvic structures for sterilization as well as visualization. This same system can then be used for the introduction of dye to determine the patency of fallopian tubes. The elevator is introduced into the uterine cavity and then attached to a tenaculum that is placed on the anterior lip of the cervix. After their use, these instruments should be thoroughly washed and rinsed in clear water. Before the next use, they should be soaked in a disinfectant or gas sterilized. Occasionally, condensation will appear on the distal lens. This problem can be minimized by warming the instrument before introduction or by placing the lens gently on an abdominal viscus to warm the lens before visualization. Condensation on the eyepiece of the endoscope can be avoided by using various antifogging solutions or by placing a small amount of pHisoHex on the eyepiece as the problem occurs.

Because the introduction of a large trocar into the free peritoneal space carries an increased risk of perforation of the bowel, it is important that one create a "gas work space" before introduction of the laparoscopic trocar. Both CO_2 and nitrous oxide have been used for this purpose. CO_2 is rapidly absorbed and is most ideal for creating a pneumoperitoneum. Nitrous oxide, on the other hand, is not absorbed as well as CO_2 and will support combustion, thus making it a less ideal insufflating gas. A Veress needle is the most ideal instrument for the introduction of the gas because it has a blunt end making viscous perforation less likely. It is important that one have a well-maintained gas insufflator that will supply the gas at a rate of 1 liter/min. This instrument should provide the appropriate gauges that will measure the pressure of the gas in the insufflator, as well as the pressure of the gas as it is inflated into the abdomen. The insufflator should also indicate the volumes of gas that are transferred to the patient. Most surgeons prefer the introduction of 2–4 liters of CO_2 gas before puncture with the 10-mm laparoscopic trocar. The intraabdominal pressure should remain betwen 10 and 20 mm Hg at volumes of less than 4 liters. Certainly, pressures greater than 30 mm Hg would indicate the possibility of insufflation into a confined abdominal viscera or the preperitoneal space.

TECHNIQUE

Because the abdomen must be completely relaxed for the surgeon to create an adequate pneumoperitoneum, a general anesthetic is most ideal. The procedure can, however, be accomplished using local anesthesia provided the patient is informed and reassured during the procedure. Preoperative medications have been largely eliminated because of the outpatient status of the procedure. Patients are brought directly to the operating room and then returned to a postanesthesia holding area until they are stable and have metabolized their anesthetic agents. Patients are preoxygenated before paralysis and introduction of the endotracheal tube that has become mandatory for safe laparoscopic technique. The endotracheal tube not only assures adequate oxygenation of the patient, but also avoids gastric distention, which can be a potential target for the laparoscopic trocar. Trendelenburg position is helpful in temporarily relocating the abdominal viscera above the point of entry of the abdominal trocar.

A small infraumbilical incision is made after anesthesia is established. The subcutaneous fat is then pushed away with the blunt end of the scalpel. The abdominal wall is elevated at the level of the umbilicus and the Veress needle is placed against the anterior rectus fascia. The Veress needle is then thrust through the fascia, preperitoneal fat, and abdominal peritoneum is an attempt to locate the end of the needle in the free peritoneal space. It is important that the Veress needle be directed into the center of the true pelvis, thus avoiding potential contact with the sacral promontory and the iliac vessels. The proper intraperitoneal location of the Veress needle tip can then be checked by introducing 10 ml of sterile saline through the hub of the Veress needle. This fluid should flow through the needle with minimal resistance. A syringe is then placed on the needle and negative pressure is applied. If there is a significant amount of fluid return, one should consider the possibility that the needle is in a confined space, such as the preperitoneal fat. If, on the other hand, bowel contents or blood returns, the surgeon most likely has placed the needle into the intestine or an abdominal blood vessel. A small drop of saline should be placed on the Veress needle hub and the anterior abdominal wall pulled in an upward direction to create a negative pressure in the peritoneal space. The droplet of saline on the Veress hub should then rapidly disappear into the shaft of the needle if the instrument has been properly placed. The abdominal trocar (Fig. 19.1) is introduced into the pneumoperitoneum by directing the sharp trocar into the center of the true pelvis, thus avoiding the potential perforation of the iliac vessels. It is also

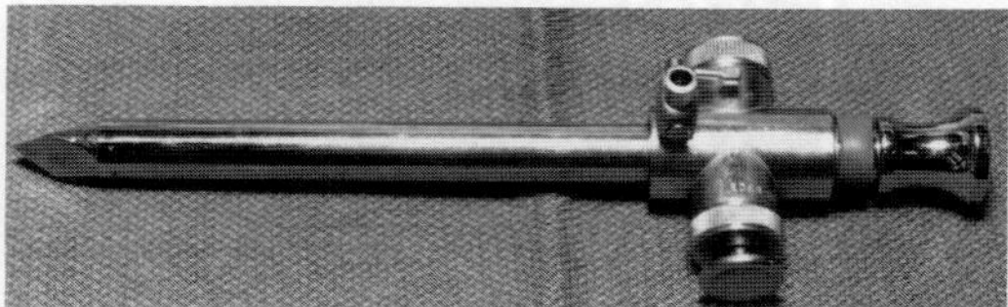

Figure 19.1. Laparoscopic trocar.

helpful to grasp the skin and subcutaneous fat and pull it in an upward direction as the trocar is introduced through the fascia. This maneuver provides stabilization of the anterior abdominal wall, as well as elevation of the anterior abdomen from the loops of bowel in the more posterior portions of the abdominal peritoneum.

Dr. Hasson (5) introduced a technique of "open laparoscopy" which is ideally used for those patients where the surgeon expects a difficult pneumoperitoneum. Using the open laparoscopy technique, the surgeon sharply dissects the skin, subcutaneous fat, and the anterior abdominal wall fascia. The peritoneum is then grasped with hemostats and brought into the visual field. The peritoneum is opened using sharp dissection under direct visualization. A blunt laparoscopic trocar is then introduced into the free peritoneal space. It is important that the surgeon seal the peritoneum around the laparoscopic trocar to prevent the inadvertent leakage of carbon dioxide gas from the abdomen.

After proper creation of the pneumoperitoneum and introduction of the sharp trocar, the laparoscope is then introduced for visualization of the abdominal cavity (Fig. 19.2). A steep Trendelenburg position will allow one to adequately visualize the lower one-half of the abdomen, whereas a reverse Trendelenburg position will allow better visualization of the upper abdominal structures. It is often helpful to place a second puncture just above the pubic hairline in the midline to permit the introduction of other instruments to manipulate intraabdominal structures. The surgeon should then begin a systematic inspection of the entire abdominal contents. The pelvic structures should be thoroughly evaluated and described in the operative note. One should then proceed along the ascending transverse and descending colon and describe any abnormalities that are found. The appendix and gallbladder can be visualized with a standard single puncture technique provided the appendix is not retrocecal

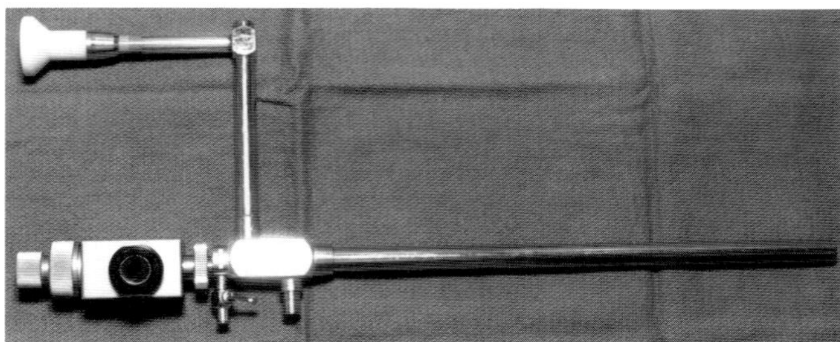

Figure 19.2. Laparoscope introduced through an infraumbilical incision.

and there is no significant intraabdominal adhesive disease. The entire anterior and lateral peritoneal surface should be inspected for potential malignant disease. The posterior peritoneum is difficult to observe with standard laparoscopic technique. The right and left lobes of the liver should be thoroughly inspected to rule out intrahepatic mass. Parenchymal disease can often be diagnosed with the laparoscope by recognizing architectural patterns common to the disease process. If an inflammatory process is suspected during initial diagnostic laparoscopy, appropriate bacterial cultures can be taken from the right and left colic gutters as well as the posterior cul-de-sac. Specific therapeutic procedures, such as tubal sterilization, chromotubation, lysis of adhesions, peritoneal biopsy, liver biopsy, and drainage of cysts can be accomplished after thorough diagnostic laparoscopy.

LASER LAPAROSCOPY

The laser has been a feature of intraabdominal surgery since 1969 and has been combined with laparoscopy since 1979 (6, 7). By combining the techniques of endoscopy and laser surgery, one is able to avoid laparotomy and benefit with greater patient convenience, better hemostasis, and less cost because of the outpatient requirement for the procedures. The CO_2 laser can be coupled to the laparoscope by using a combination of mirrors and articulated arms to reflect the laser energy down the operating channel of the laparoscope. The CO_2 laser can be discharged in a prefocused, focused, or defocused zone (Fig. 19.3), so that the spot size can be varied. The surgeon controls the laser energy by manipulating the power, duration of exposure, and the spot size of the laser beam. The maximum power density is obtained when the impact on the tissue is at the beam's focal point. Exposures can be set for single, repeat, or continuous pulses. A laparoscopic operating instrument has been designed with a special metal backdrop that prevents the laser beam from penetrating surface adhesions onto vital structures of the abdominal cavity. Adhesiolysis can be accomplished with this instrument by trapping the adhesion between the metal backdrop and the focused beam of the CO_2 laser (Fig. 19.4). Solutions of saline or Ringer's lactate can be placed into the abdominal cavity in order to provide a backstop when vital structures can be covered with these solutions.

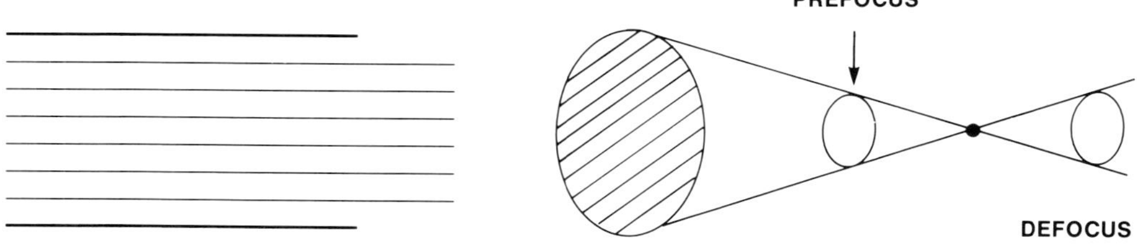

Figure 19.3. Adjustment of spot size.

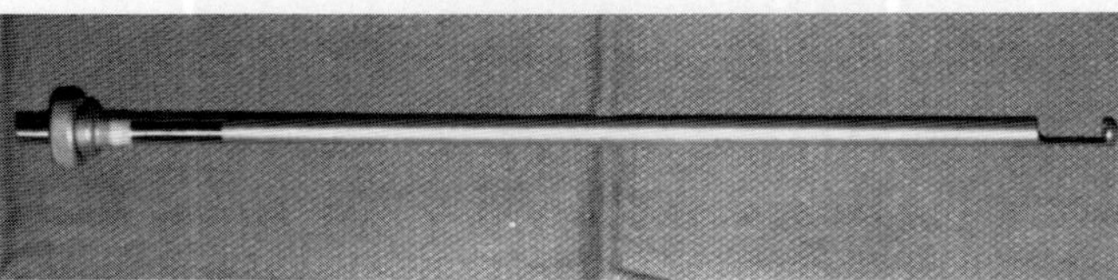

Figure 19.4. Laser attachment with metal backdrop.

A common problem with the CO_2 laser is that of removing smoke as tissues are vaporized in the abdominal space. Rapid insufflation equipment (30-80 liters of CO_2 per procedure) will allow for a rapid turnover of the insufflating gas and thus a more clear operating field. Suction devices can be placed near the operating field to remove the plume as it is created with vaporization. These suction apparatuses do, however, remove the gas creating the pneumoperitoneum and will require high flows of replacement gas to maintain an adequate work space.

There are three basic surgical techniques that can be accomplished using laser laparoscopy (Fig. 19.5). Tissue coagulation is accomplished by raising the tissue temperature until protein coagulation takes place. Coagulation is a destructive process and can be used for the destruction of pelvic endometriosis and small tumors of the peritoneal cavity. By raising the power density, one increases the temperature of the tissue to greater than 100°C and a process of tissue vaporization is accomplished as the cells are individually vaporized as they explode from the target tissue. Actual excision of abdominal lesions can be carried out by using the CO_2 laser in a focused mode that will result in tissue incision. The specimens are removed with the laparoscopic grasping forceps. Dr. Feste has described the use of the carbon dioxide laser in the treatment of pelvic endometriosis and pelvic adhesive disease with results comparable to open laparotomy (8).

The CO_2 laser has the distinct disadvantage of creation of plume, which obscures the operative field. In addition, the CO_2 laser will not follow fiberoptic bundles and, therefore, must be delivered with lenses that are outside the abdominal cavity. The argon laser for the treatment of pelvic endometriosis was first described by Keye et al. (9). The Nd:YAG laser for vaporization and coagulation of endometriosis was first described by Lomano (10). Dr. Daniell (11) has described the use of the KPT twin crystal laser for the laparoscopic ablation of pelvic endometriosis. All three of these lasers offer the distinct advantage of being coagulating rather than cutting tools, thus they avoid the problem of accumulation of plume within the peritoneal space. In addition, all three lasers will follow fiberoptic bundles and, thus, provide a distinct advantage for the operating surgeon. Laser energy can be directed through fiberoptic bundles directly onto the tissue that is to be destroyed. This author has had personal experience with the use of the sapphire tips attached to the quartz fiber carrying the Nd:YAG laser energy. The "contact technique" for delivery allows one to use the Nd:YAG laser as a cutting as well as a vaporizing tool. The use of the sapphire tips with the Nd:YAG laser is a new horizon in laser surgery that is currently being investigated throughout the United States and Europe. Techniques are currently being developed for a laser laparoscopic cholecystectomy.

FUTURE LASER LAPAROSCOPY

Newer lasers are currently being developed that will provide a variety of tissue effects. One promising area is that of a pulsed dye laser which,

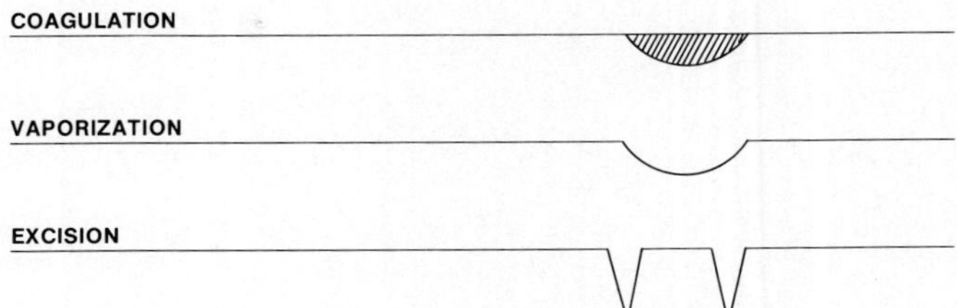

Figure 19.5. Laser techniques.

when applied to tissue, results in a tremendous burst of laser energy capable of fracturing stones. This technology has already been applied to the removal of ureteral stones by introducing the laser energy onto the stone through a small fiberoptic bundle introduced cystocopically. This technology is continuing to develop and many researchers are investigating the possibility of the fracture of gallstones using the same pulsed dye laser introduced through an endoscopic delivery system.

Photodynamic therapy (PDT) is a recent technique that has been developed to treat cancer. Hematoporphyrin derivative (HPD) is injected into the patient 3 days before exposure of the cancer cells to a red light at 630 nm. Cancer cells will selectively hold the HPD while normal cells will excrete the HPD during this 3-day interval. Exposure of the cells containing the HPD to red light results in selective tissue death at the same time there is a release of singlet oxygen. The pathophysiology has not been well established, but it appears as though there is a collapse in the vasculature leading to the tumor cells and subsequent necrosis secondary to loss of blood supply. The entire concept of photodynamic therapy is particularly important to the laparoscopist because of the ability to deliver light energy into the abdominal cavity. Although this treatment is currently reserved for terminal cancer patients who have exhausted all other medical and surgical modalities of therapy, the true future of photodynamic therapy will be the treatment of early cancers that can be treated before metastases.

REFERENCES

1. Diagnostic Laparoscopy: A patient education pamphlet. ACOG, 1985.
2. Hulka JF. Adnexal adhesions: A prognostic staging and classification system based on a five-year survey of fertility surgery results at Chapel Hill, North Carolina. Am J Obstet Gynecol 1982; 144:141-148.
3. American Fertility Society: Classification of endometriosis. Fertil Steril 1979; 32:633-634.
4. Wheeler JM, Malinak LR. Recurrent endometriosis: Incidence, management, and prognosis. Am J Obstet Gynecol 1983; 146:247-253.
5. Hasson, HM. Open laparoscopy: A modified instrument and method for laparoscopy. Am J Obstet Gynecol 1971; 110:886.
6. Fox JL. The use of laser radiation as a surgical light knife. J Surg Res 1969;9:199.
7. Bruhat MA, Mage G, Manhes M. Use of CO_2 laser via laparoscopy. In Kaplan I: Proceedings of the Third International Congress of Laser Surgery. Tel Aviv, OT-PAZ, 1979, p. 274.
8. Feste JR. Laser laparoscopy: A new modality. J Reprod Med 1985; 30:413-417.
9. Keye WR, Abbott T, Bowers J, et al. Feasibility studies of the argon laser in the treatment of endometriosis. Fertil Steril 1983;39:429.
10. Lomano JM. Photocoagulation of early pelvic endometriosis with the Nd:YAG laser through the laparoscope. J Reprod Med 1985; 30: 77-81.
11. Daniell JF. Initial evaluation of the use of KTP twin crystal laser in gynecologic laparoscopy. Fertil Steril In press.

CHAPTER

20

Laser Angioplasty of Peripheral Arteries

Johannes Lammer, Ernst Pilger, Peter-Wolf Ascher

In the last decade, the treatment of peripheral vascular disease has changed completely. Invasive but "nonsurgical" procedures like balloon angioplasty (1) and intraarterial fibrinolysis (2–4) have become well-established methods of treatment for limiting claudication due to arterial stenosis or obstruction. Because neither of these methods is able to remove obstructing plaque material, laser angioplasty has opened a new dimension in the field of invasive but nonsurgical recanalization procedures.

The initial experimental work on the recanalization of obstructed arteries by laser energy was done in the early 1980s by G. Lee and D.S.J. Choy and associates (5, 6). Clinical pilot studies demonstrated the feasibility of percutaneous laser recanalization of arterial stenosis and obstruction in peripheral (7, 8), coronary (9), and carotid arteries (10). These led to further experimental and clinical research studies and technical development. At the Departments of Radiology and Neurosurgery of the Karl-Franzens-University in Graz, Austria, a research program on laser angioplasty has been underway since 1984.

TECHNICAL HARDWARE

Lasers

For vascular applications, three lasers are currently under experimental and clinical investigation: the excimer, argon ion, and neodymium (Nd): Yttrium-aluminum-garnet (YAG) lasers.

Excimer Lasers (Excited Dimer)

Excimer lasers are gas lasers. The active medium contains halides of noble gases. Helium, added as a buffer gas, acts as a collision partner and is essential for stabilizing the discharge. Excimer lasers operate in the ultraviolet spectrum (ArF at 193 nm, KrF at 248 nm, XeCl at 308 nm, and XeF at 351 nm). The power output ranges between 5 and 100 W. In vascular work, energies of 10 mJ per pulse with a pulse duration of 10–30 nsec and repetition rates of 10–30 Hz have been used.

Argon Ion Laser

The argon ion laser is a gas laser that operates in the blue-green spectrum at 488 and 514.5 nm. Argon ion lasers are very inefficient and have a power output of only 20 W. In vascular work, the argon ion laser is used in a continuous wave (CW) mode. The average power setting is between 5 and 15 W.

Nd:YAG Laser

The Nd:YAG laser is a crystal laser that operates in the near-infrared spectrum at 1064 and 1318 nm. The power output ranges 1–110 W. In vascular work only, the wavelength of 1064 nm is used in a CW mode. The power setting is between 10 and 20 W. The effect of Q-switched pulsed Nd:YAG lasers on atheromatous plaques and normal vessel wall is in an early stage of investigation.

FIBEROPTIC CONDUCTORS

A flexible optical fiber consists of a silica glass core with a high refraction index coated by a glass or plastic cladding with a lower index of refraction. Internal reflection due to the higher refraction index of the inner core keeps the light beam within the flexible fiber until it emerges relatively unchanged from the distal end. Therefore, light can escape only if the fiber is bent beyond a critical radius (about 1 cm), so that total reflection will not occur and light will be refracted through the cladding. Currently, depending on the wavelengths, a transmission with a loss of less than 1 db/km is possible.

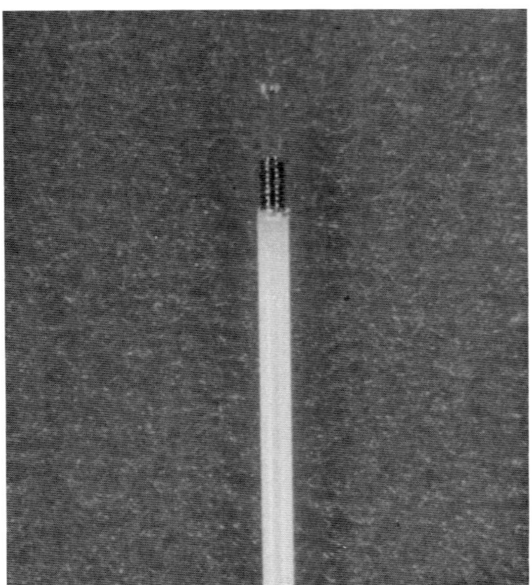

Figure 20.1. A 600-μm silica fiber for bare fiber recanalization.

Fiberoptic transmission of the laser light is a presupposition for intravascular applications. Argon and Nd:YAG laser light can be transmitted in a pulsed and CW mode, through glass fibers. Excimer lasers work in a pulse mode with high peak pulse powers that can destroy glass fibers. Therefore, the short wavelengths of excimer lasers cannot be transmitted effectively through glass fibers. Only the longer wavelengths of 308 and 351 nm can be transmitted through a fiberoptic conductor and intravascular work has been examined recently (11, 12). The CO_2 infrared laser, which is very attractive for medical applications can be transmitted only through fibers that are too toxic for medical work (e.g., thallium bromoiodide).

The connections of the optic conductors are a further problem of light transmitting systems. Any discontinuity due to an irregular or unclean surface will cause reflection, scattering, and power loss that will instantly cause temperatures that destroy the fiber at the connection. This has become of increasing importance with the development of contact probes for laser angioplasty that have to be connected with the fiber.

LASER CATHETERS

Bare Fiber

Initial work in laser angioplasty was done with bare silica fibers, 200–600 μm in diameter (Fig. 20.1). The 200-μm fibers are flexible enough to be guided into the coronary arteries via a transfemoral route. For laser angioplasty of peripheral or carotid arteries, the stiffer 600-μm fibers can be used safely. Bare fibers have shown some disadvantages for intravascular usage.

Decreased Power Density

Because a simple polished fiber disperses the light in an angle of 10°, the power density decreases with the distance between the target tissue and the fiber tip according to a logarithmic function (13). Therefore, the power density 5 mm from the fiber tip will be only 10% of that at the tip if there is no additional absorption of the medium between fiber and target tissue. If the light is dispersed in a 90° angle, the power density is attenuated to 10% at a distance of 0.5 mm from the tip. Because of the absorption characteristics of blood, further energy attenuation will occur. Therefore, the fiber tip has to be as close as possible to the tissue—ideally in direct contact.

High Perforation Rate

A glass fiber, 200–600 μm in diameter, which has to be maneuvered as close as possible to the obstructing lesion tends strongly to mechanical or laser-dependent perforation (14). Perforation of peripheral vessels with such a small fiber does not cause serious complications, but further attempts to find the right lumen usually remain unsuccessful.

Recurrent Fiber Damage

If the fiber is directly in contact with the tissue, or if a layer of coagulated blood surrounds the fiber tip, the temperature of the tip increases during laser irradiation. Because the melting point of quartz glass is about 1000°C, melting or backburning of the fiber is a common complication during intravascular application.

Insufficient Diameter of the Recanalized Segment

With a 600-μm fiber, a channel with a maximum diameter of 800 μm can be lased through the obstructed segment. The reduction of a stenotic plaque is a time-consuming procedure.

Therefore, subsequent mechanical dilatation has to be done in every patient.

Ball-tipped Fiber

The tip of a 600-μm silica fiber is melted and shaped to a ball or drop-like configuration. This ball-tip is meant to prevent inadvertant perforations, to increase the diameter of the recanalized segment, and to achieve some focus characteristics of the distal end of the silica fiber (15). The relatively low melting point of quartz glass (1000°C) limits the suitability for contact irradiation.

Balloon Laser Catheter (Lastac, GV Medical, Inc.)

This is a combination of an angioplasty balloon catheter and a silica fiber for laser irradiation. The laser fiber is located within the central catheter lumen that is normally used for contrast material injections and guide wires. The purpose of the balloon, which is inflated proximal to the obstructing lesion, is to center the laser fiber in order to prevent an inadvertant perforation of the vessel wall (16). Additionally, the inflated balloon prevents blood flow around the laser fiber so that under continuous perfusion with saline, premature absorption of the laser beam can be minimized. After successful traversion of the obstruction, the balloon catheter can be used for dilatation of the lumen of the recanalized segment.

Metal-probe (Hot-Tip, Trimedyne, Inc., Tustin, CA)

This is an olive-shaped metal cap, 1.5–3.0 mm in diameter, attached around the end of the 600-μm silica fiber (Fig. 20.2). The metallic tip is heated by absorption of photons of laser light and distributes thermal energy circumferentially (17, 18). Due to a special alloy of the cap, the probe heats up and cools down very rapidly. Experiments with thermocouples have shown a temperature increase and decrease of 120–150° C/sec using an argon laser with 10 W at the fiber tip (19). If the tip is in direct contact with the target tissue, heat conduction leads to coagulation and vaporization of tissue. A layer of coagulated and carbonized blood and tissue elements acts as a thermal insulation and reduces heat conduction during therapy. Currently, a hybrid form has been developed. A window at the tip of the metal probe allows beaming 40–80% of the laser light directly into the tissue. The remaining energy heats the metallic probe, so that a combined effect can be achieved.

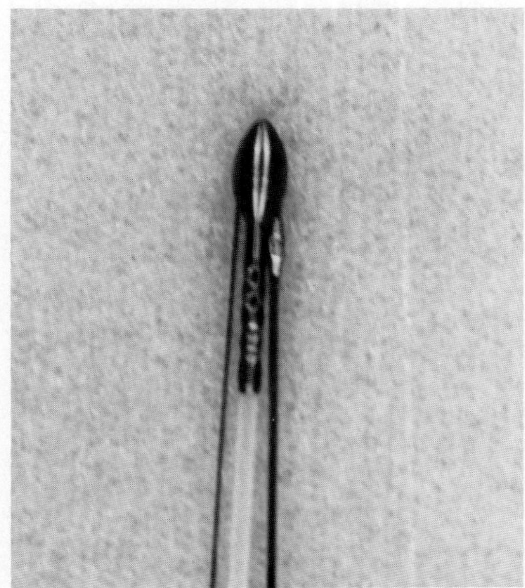

Figure 20.2. A metal probe (Hot-Tip) that is 2 mm in diameter.

Sapphire Probe (Surgical Laser Technologies, Inc., Malvern, PA)

A spherical sapphire is attached to the end of the silica fiber (Fig. 20.3). This sapphire is 1.8–3.0 mm in diameter, melts at 2030°C, and has 90% transmittance and a refraction index of 1.77. Due to the spherical configuration of the sapphire, the laser beam will be focused. The focus area with an increased power density is about 0.5 mm from the surface of the sapphire. In saline, the sapphire itself shows only a minimal temperature rise (5°C after 10 W CW Nd:YAG laser). Back scattering of laser light at the connection between the fiber tip and the sapphire leads to a temperature increase of the metallic connector, which has to be cooled actively by saline perfusion. During laser therapy, a layer of coagulated blood and tissue elements around the sapphire probe leads to an accumulation of heat at the surface of the sapphire so that an increase of the temperature of the sapphire can be observed during therapy (250°C after 10 sec of CW Nd:YAG laser with 10 W). The sapphire probe allows direct contact with the target tissue, an increase of the power density due

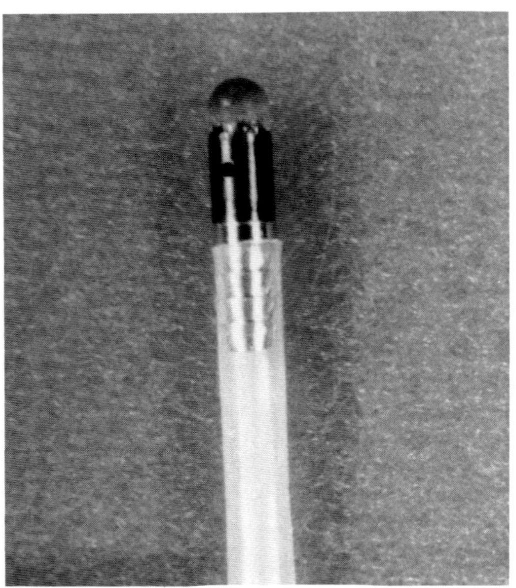

Figure 20.3. A sapphire probe that is 2.2 mm in diameter.

to the optical characteristics, and prevents perforation and fiber damage that occurred with the bare silica fiber, and increases the diameter of the recanalized segment (20). The basic differences between the metal probe and the sapphire probe are that within the metal probe the photons of the laser light are absorbed and converted to heat that conducts into the tissue, whereas the sapphire probe has a 90% transmittance for laser light and absorption occurs in the target tissue.

Multifiber Catheter

This catheter consists of a bundle of silica fibers. Initially, a laser pulse in the mJ range is emitted through all fibers for spectroscopic analysis of the tissue in front of each fiber. Because plaque tissue, normal vessel wall, and blood or blood clot have different characteristics during fluorescence spectrometry, the tissue in front of each fiber can be identified (21). The purpose of this spectroscopic analysis is to irradiate only through those fibers that are in front of the plaque. This should prevent perforations of the arterial wall (22, 23). After initial laser therapy the coagulated surface of plaque and normal vessel wall has similar spectroscopic characteristics, so that differentiation becomes difficult. This fact is a serious limitation.

LASER-TISSUE INTERACTION

If the photons of the laser light strike on the inner surface of the arterial wall, four things can occur:

absorption,
reflection at the surface,
scattering into the tissue, and
transmission.

The predominant factor in laser-tissue interaction is absorption. The absorbed energy can be converted into heat: the so-called *photothermal effect*. If the temperature rises within the tissue, coagulation of cell proteins and melting of elastic fibers occurs at 70°C. Cell water is converted to steam at 100°C causing vacuolization, cell rupture, and tissue dehydration. Dehydration causes a plateau of the temperature increase during laser irradiation. After dehydration, a rapid increase of the tissue temperature can be observed, which finally leads to tissue ablation. Solid components of the tissue over 250°C are directly vaporized. Vaporization of obstructing thrombi and plaques is the aim of laser angioplasty.

Pulsed lasers with a high pulse energy and a low-pulse duration (<150 ns) cause two further effects. The *photoablative effect* is observed at short ultraviolet wavelengths of excimer lasers (193 nm, 248 nm). It is not completely understood but similar to the photoacustic effect molecular bonds are disrupted without thermal reaction (24, 25). The *photoacustic effect* can be observed, for instance, with pulsed Q-switched Nd:YAG lasers in liquids. A plasma of free electrons is produced in the focal spot of the high peak power laser beam. This electron plasma pulsates due to recurrent rapid expansion, breakdown and reexpansion—causing acoustic shock waves that can destroy tissue without thermal reactions.

The argon and Nd:YAG lasers in the CW mode cause predominantly a thermal ablation of tissue. Characteristically, a laser mark consists of a central crater where tissue has been vaporized with temperatures of more than 250°C (Figs. 20.4 and 20.5). This tissue defect is surrounded by a zone of thermal necrosis. The necrosis zone is caused by absorption of laser light that has been scattered into deeper tissue layers and by heat conduction. Corresponding to the heat distribution, a superfi-

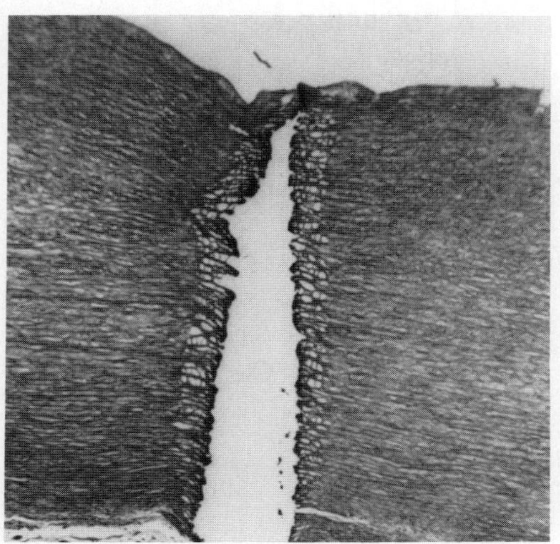

Figure 20.4. A laser crater in the aortic wall after irradiation through bare silica fiber.

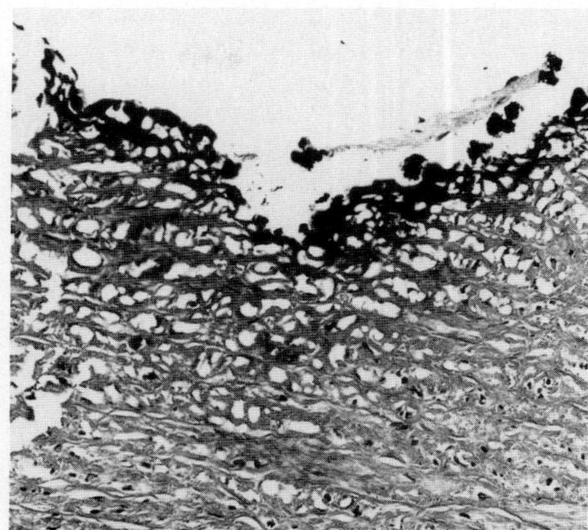

Figure 20.6. A magnification view of the necrosis zone with superficial carbonization and cell rupture under the laser crater.

cial zone of carbonization and deeper zones of vacuolization, cell rupture, and coagulation necrosis can be observed (Fig. 20.6) (26, 27). The depth of this zone of thermal necrosis depends on the duration of laser irradiation and the wavelength. Longer irradiation times cause an accumulation of heat under the surface layers of the tissue and, thus, a deeper zone of thermal necrosis (20). The argon laser is well absorbed at the surface of plaques and only minimally scattered into deeper layers. Nd:YAG laser light is poorly absorbed in plaque tissue and shows more than 30% scattering into deeper layers, causing thermal damage under the surface of the target tissue. Consequently, the Nd:YAG laser used in a CW mode causes a deeper zone of thermal necrosis under the ablation crater, followed by a CW argon laser, pulsed Nd:YAG laser, and pulsed excimer lasers in the longer wavelength spectrum (308 nm, 351 nm). After application of 10 J, the depth of the necrosis ranged between 200 and 10 μm in normal vessel wall and fibrofatty plaques (20).

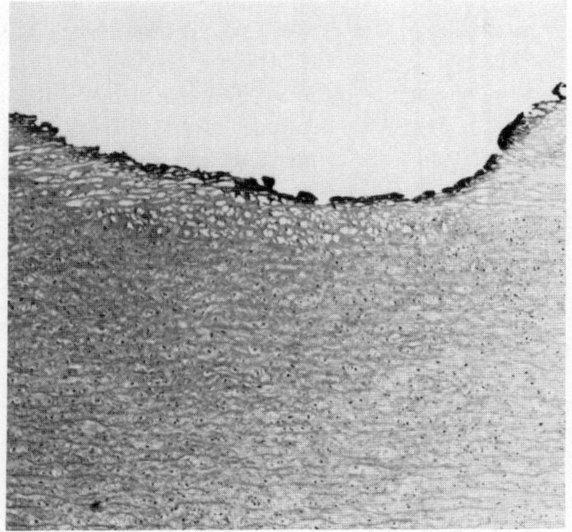

Figure 20.5. A laser crater in the aortic wall after irradiation through a sapphire probe.

For intravascular laser application, the absorption characteristics of blood have to be considered. These are mainly determined by the hemoglobin and the water content. The absorption curve of hemoglobin has a maximum of between 500 and 600 nm with absorbent peaks at 414, 531, 543, and 569 nm (28). Thus, the argon laser is strongly absorbed by hemoglobin. This is an advantage for laser recanalization of obstructing thrombi, but a big problem for intravascular work. Water absorbs the long wavelengths of the infrared spectrum. Therefore, CO_2 lasers cannot be used for intravascular laser angioplasty. Absorption of the Nd:YAG laser (1064 nm) in water is low, the argon laser shows almost no absorption in water. Therefore, the Nd:YAG laser at 1064 nm has the lowest absorption in blood, an advantage for intravascular application (29).

The absorption characteristics of atheromatous plaques are determined by the content of fatty substances like cholesterol, by collagen within fibrous tissue, calcium, blood components, and water (30). The argon laser is well absorbed by the yellowish lipids (cholesterol, cholesterol esters, phospholipids, glycerol esters, lipoproteins) and by blood components attached to the surface of the plaque or within the plaque. The absorption in fibrous tissue is poor. The Nd:YAG laser is poorly absorbed by all components of an atheromatous plaque. Ablation of calcium by the low energy densities of CW argon and Nd:YAG lasers used for laser angioplasty is not possible because the low absorption coefficient of calcium salts does not allow a sufficient increase of the temperature for ablation (1800°C). The short wavelengths of excimer lasers have a high surface absorption on tissue, so that these short wavelengths could be ideal for laser angioplasty.

During ablation with the excimer, argon, and Nd:YAG lasers, an almost linear relation exists between the irradiation dose (J/mm^2) and the volume of the ablated tissue (20, 28, 29, 31). The ablated tissue is mainly converted to gas. Analysis of these gases revealed a composition of low molecular weight hydrocarbons, CO_2, hydrogen, and nitrogen (32). A few debris particles that could cause embolic occlusion of small vessels distal to the recanalized segment were observed (33). Of the particles, 90–95% tended to be in the 10- to 20-μm range. Particles larger than 50 μm in diameter, which could cause embolic occlusions of clinical importance, were observed in less than 3% of all particles. None of the particles or gaseous products exhibited cytotoxic properties (32).

After photothermal laser recanalization of an artery, an irregular surface denuded of the intimal layer remains. This endovascular segment has an increased thrombogenicity, probably similar to a mechanically deendothelialized segment. The denuded area is immediately covered by platelets, macrophages, and loosely packed fibrin. After 2 weeks, partial reendothelialization with cuboidal, bulgy, and randomly oriented endothelial cells can be observed. By 8 weeks after the recanalization, reendothelialization is completed and fibrous scarring of subintimal layers can be observed (34).

CLINICAL EXPERIENCE

Since 1985, clinical series of laser recanalizations of peripheral artery occlusions have been performed using argon lasers with a bare fiber (35), the metal contact probe (36–38), and the Nd:YAG laser with a sapphire contact probe (39, 40).

Indications

Established indications for laser recanalization are obstructions of femoropopliteal arteries that cause limiting claudication (stage IIb), rest pain (stage III), or gangrene (stage IV). Experience in recanalization of iliac arteries is very limited. Tibial vessels have been recanalized successfully but the clinical value of treatment of small distal vessel disease is not established.

Contraindications

Absolute contraindications for peripheral laser angioplasty currently do not exist; however, relative contraindications do.

1. Acute thrombosis, which can be recanalized by means of intraarterial fibrinolytic therapy;
2. Tortuous vessels like iliac arteries, which pose a higher risk for perforation;
3. Occlusions of the popliteal artery including the trifurcation because of a higher perforation risk at the trifurcation of the tibial arteries;
4. Obstructions longer than 15 cm have been recanalized but the complication and reocclusion rate seems to be higher;
5. Highly calcified plaques that cannot be ablated by means of low power CW argon or Nd:YAG lasers;
6. Stenoses at the common femoral artery bifurcation, because steerable laser delivery systems do not exist and stenoses in this location can be treated easily by vascular surgery.

Technique

Intravascular laser recanalization can be done under endoscopic visualization and under roentgenographic fluoroscopy. Because vascular endoscopes are still at an early stage of development, and endoscopy can be done only in a blood-free field, the majority of laser angioplasties have been done under fluoroscopic visualization. The puncture of the ipsilateral femoral artery is done under local anesthesia using the Seldinger technique. For femoropopliteal and for iliac recanalizations antegrade and retrograde punctures, re-

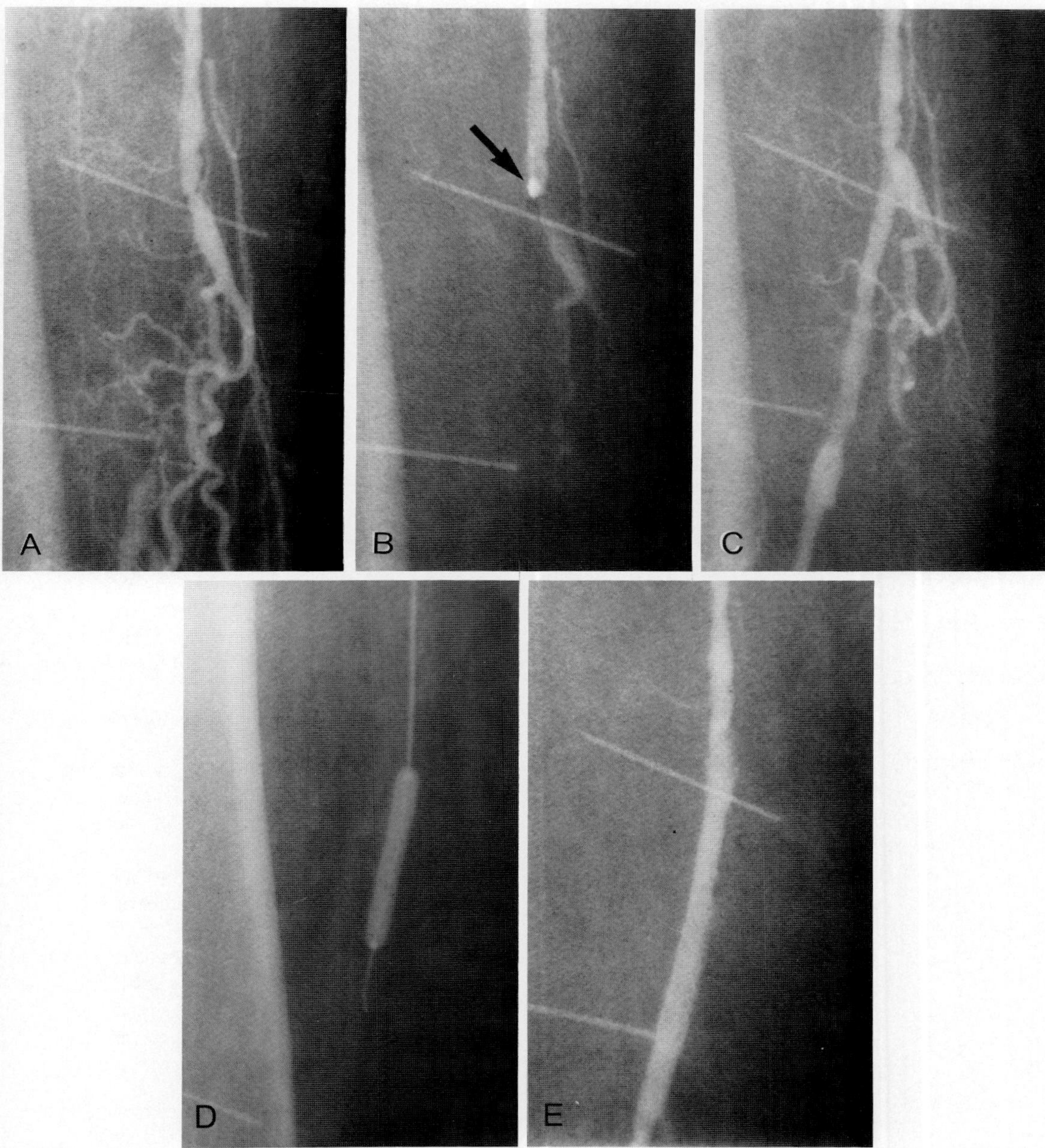

Figure 20.7. Recanalization of a 5-cm occlusion of the superficial femoral artery. **A**, Angiogram before recanalization. **B**, Hot-Tip *(arrow)* in place. **C**, Control angiogram after recanalization. **D**, Dilatation balloon in place. **E**, Recanalized segment after balloon dilatation.

spectively, are done. A 7-French catheter introducer sheath is inserted and a baseline angiogram can be obtained (Figs. 20.7 & 20.8). Intraarterial injection of 2500–5000 IU of heparin for low-dose heparinization during the entire procedure is recommended. The laser catheter system should

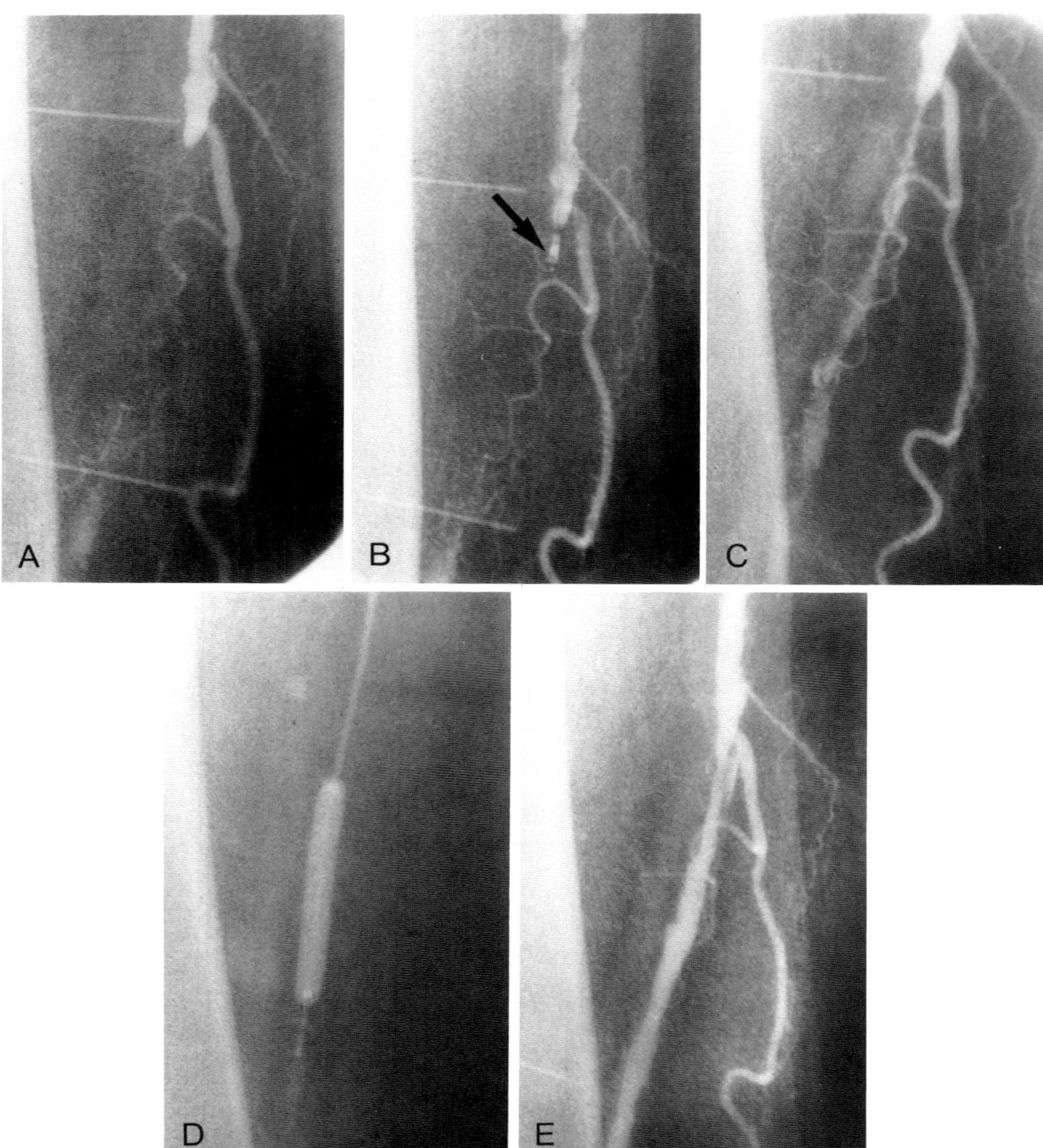

Figure 20.8. Recanalization of a 7-cm occlusion of the superficial femoral artery. **A**, Angiogram before recanalization. **B**, Sapphire probe during recanalization *(arrow)*. **C**, Partial recanalization of the occluded segment. **D**, Balloon dilatation after successful recanalization. **E**, Control angiogram after percutaneous transluminal angioplasty.

be cooled continuously at the tip to reduce thermal damage of the normal vessel wall and to dilute the blood that minimizes premature absorption of the laser beam. To avoid loss of energy density with distance to the target, and because of the absorption in blood, the laser catheter should be in contact with the obstructing lesion. A bare fiber should be centered by a balloon catheter, contact probes (metal tip sapphire tip) are self-centering due to their outer diameter of 2–3 mm. The power setting for the argon laser was 6–12 W with a continuous exposure for 5–20 sec. The power setting for heating the metal-tipped probe was 10 W of argon laser for 5–20 sec. For laser recanalization with Nd:YAG laser through the sapphire contact probe, the power setting was 10–20 W of 1-sec bursts every 2 secs. After successful recanalization, a control angiogram should be performed for estimation of the diameter of the recanalized segment and for documentation of the antegrade flow (Figs. 20.7 and 20.8). On the basis of this angiogram the decision can be made whether or not to complete the procedure by a balloon angioplasty.

If perforation or subintimal dissection occurs (both causing warning pain during the procedure), further attempts to recanalize the obstructed segment should be omitted. The nonperfused segment and the perforation undergo a rapid rethrombosis so that complications requiring emergency surgery are unusual.

Immediate and Long-term Results

The immediate success of laser recanalization by means of a bare silica fiber, 400–600 μm in diameter, is limited by the high perforation rate of 15–25% and a dissection rate of 25% (20, 35, 36). Therefore, the initial recanalization rate was only 50–66%. Contact probes have proven to have a lower perforation rate. Cumberland reported a successful recanalization with the metal-tipped probe in 88% of 86 patients with peripheral artery occlusion. Perforations occurred in only 5% and the patency rate after 1 year was 72% (37). Motarjeme has a 78% success rate with the metal-tipped probe in 59 patients suffering from femoropopliteal occlusions that were 3–31 cm in length. The perforation rate was 9% (38). In the authors' own clinical series of the initial 50 patients who underwent femoropopliteal recanalization with the Nd:YAG laser irradiated through a sapphire contact probe, the primary success rate was 80%. Perforations occurred in 11%. The long-term patency rate after 1 year was 83% (39, 40). Reocclusions occurred in 17% of the patients, restenoses causing recurrent claudication occurred in 13%.

CONCLUSION

Obstructing thrombi and atheromatous plaques have been ablated successfully by laser irradiation in experimental and clinical series. Experimentally, the argon laser has been shown to have a higher absorption in plaques and thrombi than the Nd:YAG laser. Clinically both lasers can be utilized equally for laser angioplasty. The development of contact probes (metal tip, sapphire tip) has increased the success rates of arterial laser recanalizations to 80–85%. This improvement is based on a much lower perforation rate (5–10% with contact probes versus 25% with bare fibers) and an increased diameter of the recanalized segment. Nevertheless, balloon dilatation of the laser channel has to be done in the majority of cases. Therefore, the preliminary long-term patency rates of 70–80% 1 year after recanalization are the result of two different procedures: thermal laser recanalization and mechanical balloon dilatation. Technical improvement of laser catheters will enable recanalization of larger channels, so that balloon dilatation will be come unnecessary.

Despite these improvements, the ideal laser for removal of arteriosclerotic obstructions has not been found. The properties of this laser should be:

a high absorption in plaques;
a low absorption in blood and normal arterial wall;
a high surface absorption with thermal or nonthermal ablation properties without damage to surrounding tissue.

None of the three lasers currently under clinical investigation has shown a selective absorption by plaque. Selective staining with hematopophyrins or tetracyclines has not been successful. Research is now directed to reduce thermal damage of the arterial wall adjacent to the obstructing lesion. This can be achieved by using high-energy densities with short emission times at low repetition rates, so that heat accumulation in the adjacent tissue does not occur. Pulsed lasers probably could fulfill this goal, when transmission of high energies through small fibers becomes possible. Future research should follow two main directions.

1. Improvement of delivery systems to enable CW laser thermal recanalization without balloon angioplasty, so that clinical data about

thermal injury to arteries and their long-term consequences become obtainable.
2. Technical improvement of delivery systems for pulsed excimer and Nd:YAG lasers, so that clinical application becomes possible.

REFERENCES

1. Grüntzig A, Hopff H. Perkutane Rekanalisation arterieller Verschlüsse mit einem neuen Dilatationskatheter. Dtsch Med Wschr 1974; 99:2502.
2. Hess H, Ingrisch H, Mietaschk A, Rath H. Local low-dose thrombolytic therapy of peripheral arterial occlusions. N Engl J Med 1982; 307:1627-1630.
3. Lammer J, Pilger E, Justich E, Neumayer K, Schreyer H. Fibrinolysis in chronic arteriosclerotic occlusions: Intrathrombotic injections of streptokinase. Radiology 1985; 157:45.
4. Lammer J, Pilger E, Neumayer K, Schreyer H. Intraarterial fibrinolysis: Long-term results. Radiology 1986; 161:159.
5. Lee G, Ikeda RM, Kozina J, Mason DT. Laser dissolution of coronary atherosclerotic obstruction. Am Heart J 1981; 102:1074-1075.
6. Choy DSJ, Sterzer SH, Rotterdam HZ, Sharrock N, Kaminow IP. Transluminal laser catheter angioplasty. Am J Cardiol 1982; 50:1206-1208.
7. Geschwind H, Boussignac G, Teisseire B, et al: Percutaneous transluminal laser angioplasty in man (letter). Lancet 1984; 1:844.
8. Ginsburg R, Kim DS, Guthaner D, Toth J, Mitchell RS. Salvage of an ischemic limb by laser angioplasty: Description of a new technique. Clin Cardiol 1984; 7:54-58.
9. Choy DSJ, Sterzer SH, Myler RK, Marco J, Fournial G. Human coronary laser recanalization. Clin Cardiol 1984; 7:377-381.
10. Lammer J, Ascher PW, Choy DSJ: Transfemorale katheter-laser-thrombendarterektomie (TEA) der arteria carotis. Dtsch Med Wschr 1986; 11:607-610.
11. Mohr FW, Lenz W, von Kusserow S, et al. Excimer laser for angioplasty and cardiac valve repair. Laser 1987; 3:93-97.
12. Schwarten DE, Cutchiff W. Excimer laser angioplasty—the use of the excimer in peripheral vascular disease. Proceedings of the European and American Society of Cardiovascular and Interventional Radiology, Sardinia, 1987; p. 59.
13. Choy DSJ. Vascular recanalization with the laser catheter. IEEE J Quant Electron 1984; 12:1420-1426.
14. Crea F, Abela GS, Fanech A. Transluminal laser irradiation of coronary arteries in live dogs: Angiographic and morphologic study of acute effects. Radiology 1986; 161:286.
5. Ramee SR, White C. Argon laser ablation with a new silica ball-tip device. Proceedings of the European Laser Association, Amsterdam, 1986.
16. Nordstrom LA, Castañeda-Zuniga WR, Grewe DD, Schoster JV. Laser-enhanced transluminal angioplasty: The role of coaxial fiber placement. Sem Intervent Radiol 1986; 3:47-52.
17. Lee G, Ikeda RM, Chan ML. Dissolution of human atherosclerotic disease by fiberoptic laser-heated metal coutery cap. Am Heart J 1984; 107:777-778.
18. Sanborn TA, Haudenschild CC, Faxon DP, Ryan TJ. Experimental angioplasty: Circumferential distribution of laser thermal energy with a laser probe. J Am Coll Cardiol 1985; 5:934-938.
19. Pashazadeh M, Crea F, Davis G, McKenna WJ, Kidner P. In vitro study in a simulated artery of temperatures generated by a metal-capped optical fiber coupled to an argon laser. Proceedings of the 1st International Symposion on Lasers in Cardiovascular Diseases, Vienna 1986. Laser 1986; 2(A): 7 (abstr).
20. Lammer J, Pilger E, Kleinert R, Ascher PW. Laserangioplastie peripherer arterieller Verschlüsse. Experimentelle und klinische Ergebnisse. Fortschr Roentgenstr 1987; 147:1-5.
21. Rickards AF, Bowker TJ, Edwards P. Differential transmission spectrometry of normal and atheromatous arterial wall. Br Heart J 1985; 53(A): 101.
22. Kittrell C, Cothren RM, Hayes GB, et al. Laser angiosurgery and special diagnostics. Proceedings of 1st Symposion on Lasers in Cardiovascular Diseases, Vienna 1986. Laser 1986; 2(A):4(abstr).
23. Kittrell C, Willell RL, de los Santos-Pacheco C. Diagnosis of fibrous arterial atherosclerosis using fluorescence. Appl Optics (in press).
24. Grundfest W, Litvak F, Forrester J. Pulsed ultraviolet lasers provide precise control of atheroma ablation (abstr). Circulation 1984; 70(Suppl. II):35.
25. Grundfest W, Litvak F, Forrester J. Laser injury of human atherosclerotic plaque without adjacent tissue injury. J Am Coll Cardiol 1985; 5:929-933.
26. Abela GS, Normann S, Cohen D, Feldman RL, Geiser EA, Conti CR. Effects of carbon dioxide, Nd:YAG, and Argon laser radiation on coronary atheromatous plaques. Am J Cardiol 1982; 50:1199-1205.
27. Lee G, Ikeda RM, Herman I, et al. The qualitative effects of laser irradiation on human arteriosclerotic disease. Am Heart J 1983; 105:885-889.
28. Lee G, Ikeda RM, Stobbe D, Ogata C, Chan MC, Mason DT. Effects of laser irradiation on human thrombus: Demonstration of a linear dissolution-dose relation between clot length and energy density. Am J Cardiol 1983; 52:876-877.
29. vanGemert MJC, Welch AJ, Bonnier JJM, Valvano JW, Yoon G, Rastegar S. Some physical concepts in laser angioplasty. Sem Intervent Radiol 1986; 3:27-38.
30. vanGemert MJC, Verdaasdonk R, Stassen EG, Schets G, Gijsbers GHM, Bonnier JJ: Optical properties of human blood vessel wall and plaque. Lasers Surg Med 1985; 5:235-237.
31. Frank F, Beck OJ, Keiditsch E, Schönberger JL, Unsöld E, Wondrazek F. Investigations under neurosurgical aspects with the 1.32 μm Nd:YAG Laser. Laser 1987; 3:40-44.
32. Grewe DD, Castañeda-Zuniga WR, Nordstrom LA, et al: Debris analysis after laser photorecanalization of atherosclerotic plaque. Sem Intervent Radiol 1986; 3:53-60.
33. Vielledent Ch, Geschwind HJ, Boussignac G, Goujour, B, Teisseire BP. Debris after laser arterial recanalization. Laser 1986; 2:31-34.

34. Gerrity RG, Loop FD, Golding LAR, Ehrhart LA, Argenyi ZB. Arterial response to laser operation for removal of atherosclerotic plaques. J Thorac Cardiovasc Surg 1983; 85:409-421.
35. Ginsburg R, Wexler L, Mitchell RS, Profitt D. Percutaneous transluminal laser angioplasty for treatment of peripheral vascular disease. Radiology 1985; 156:619-624.
36. Cumberland DC, Taylor DI, Procter AE: Use of lasers in percutaneous peripheral angioplasty. Sem Intervent Radiol 1986; 3:65-68.
37. Cumberland DC: Laser-assisted angioplasty—clinical experience. Proceedings of the American and European Society of Cardiovascular and Interventional Radiology, Sardinia, 1987; p. 60.
38. Motarjeme A. Percutaneous laser angioplasty. Proceedings of the American and European Society of Cardiovascular and Interventional Radiology, Sardinia, 1987; p. 58.
39. Lammer J, Pilger E. Laser angioplasty by sapphire contact probe. Experimental and clinical results. J Intervent Radiol 1988; 3:53-58.
40. Lammer J, Karnel, F. Percutaneous transluminal laser angioplasty with contact probes. Radiology 1988; 168:733-737.

CHAPTER

21

Lasers in Cardiothoracic Surgery[a]

Mahmood Mirhoseini, Mary M. Cayton

Early pioneers in the field of cardiovascular surgery accomplished magnificent and daring feats in developing techniques to treat congenital and acquired diseases of the circulatory system. The groundwork was firmly established for those who came later to build on and further develop the surgical concepts of these imaginative investigators. In the last 25 years, cardiovascular surgical techniques have reached a high level of sophistication. Concurrent development of surgical skills as well as materials and instrumentation to accomplish delicate procedures has produced a reasonable probability of a positive outcome with a relatively low level of risk.

The advances made in treatment methods and increased efforts to advocate prevention and moderation of risk factors have contributed to declining death and disability rates. In spite of accomplishments in this area cardiovascular disease is the leading cause of death in the United States; approximately one-quarter of the population suffers from some form of this disease. The implications of these disorders are life-threatening, limb-threatening, or seriously compromise the quality of life for those afflicted. Economic expenditures are estimated to exceed 80 billion dollars per year (1).

Additional areas of interest to the cardiothoracic surgeon are lesions of the tracheobronchial tree and of the esophagus. Some tracheobronchial lesions and lesions of the esophagus, while not as prevalent as cardiovascular diseases, are eminently suited to laser therapy. The incidence of carcinoma of the lung is estimated to be 117,000 new cases diagnosed each year. This number is increasing. Carcinoma of the lung is the most common cause of death from cancer in men, and ranks second in women to carcinoma of the breast. Fifty percent of cases are deemed to be inoperable at the time of diagnosis (2). Obstructions of the trachea or major bronchi can be life-threatening and, in the absence of immediate danger, these conditions can be extremely debilitating and can adversely affect the quality of life. Laser ablation of these lesions can be palliative and, in some cases, curative. Esophageal obstructions and stenosis also respond to laser irradiation.

Although the interest and involvement of cardiothoracic surgeons in laser applications has lagged behind those in other disciplines, there has been a trend toward active involvement in this specialty. Early development in techniques for the treatment of cardiovascular disease has been spearheaded by colleagues in cardiology. Techniques for the treatment of tracheobronchial lesions has largely been developed by otolaryngologists and those in pulmonary medicine, and techniques for treatment of esophageal lesions has been developed by gastroenterologists. As in other areas of medicine and surgery, the multidisciplinary approach can use the perspective and experience of all those who have unique contributions to make.

A review of the current status of invetigational and clinical applications of lasers in cardiothoracic surgery, including cardiac, intravascular, vascular, and tracheobronchial techniques will be discussed.

[a] Support for research activities is provided through a generous grant from St. Luke's Foundation, Milwaukee, WI. The authors would like to thank John Kampline, M.D., Ph.D. for his invaluable assistance and to thank Jack Tomlinson and Edward Murray for technical assistance.

CARDIOVASCULAR SURGERY

Direct Laser Revascularization of the Myocardium

The development of cine coronary angiography by Sones et al. (3) to diagnose the location and extent of coronary arterial lesions, and coronary artery bypass surgery (4) opened a new era in the treatment of ischemic heart disease. Refinement and increasing sophistication of techniques enable patients who formerly had no alternative to be treated by surgery. In spite of the advances in this field in the last two decades there are patients who are not candidates for coronary artery bypass, angioplasty, or thrombolysis procedures, and who do not respond to medical management. Included in this group are those with diffuse disease, diabetics with attendant small vessel disease, and those who have had previous surgery with poor results.

Direct revascularization of the myocardium by the CO_2 laser may be a method of treatment for these patients. Channels created by the CO_2 laser between the epicardium and the endocardium take advantage of the heart's ability to perfuse itself. Studies of myocardial circulation by Wearn et al. (5) demonstrated arterioluminal connections between the coronary arteries, myocardial sinusoids, and the ventricular chambers. Myocardial perfusion occurs directly through this interconnecting network in the embryo, and continues to provide perfusion to a lesser degree in later developmental stages. In response to stress, such as acute cononary occlusion, Pina and Pina (6) demonstrated increased flow through the sinusoidal network. Early investigators seeking a means to revascularize the ischemic myocardium directly attempted to create channels by a variety of methods. This included T-tubes inserted directly into the ventricular cavity and myocardial tissue (7), free arterial grafts (8), needle acupuncture (9), and mechanically boring transventricular plugs (10). Similar experimental results were reported by all of these investigators (7-10). In the acute period, perfusion occurred through the channels, followed by closure at about 3 months. This was attributed to fibrosis and scarring caused by mechanical trauma. Internal mammary artery implants (11) achieved a degree of clinical success, but were largely replaced by coronary artery bypass.

Long-term follow-up on patients who have undergone coronary artery bypass procedures has shown that, in addition to poor results in patients with diffuse disease, the atherosclerotic process also affects vein grafts. Restenosis remains a concern (12). The current conduit of choice, the internal mammary artery, has achieved higher long-term patency rates (13) but, obviously, the supply is limited. These patients as well as those refractory to medical management are candidates for direct CO_2 laser revascularization of the myocardium.

Advantages of laser revascularization in the absence of a suitable coronary artery to bypass are that revascularization can still be achieved, and the myocardial tissue is vaporized with little damaged to cells surrounding the channels. Investigational studies show that survival is increased, the channels perfuse the myocardium, and that the channels remain patent (14, 15) (Figs. 21.1–21.3). Lack of a suitable vascular conduit, vein, or internal mammary artery is not a consideration in recommending surgery (16–18).

Technique

Investigational studies were performed through a left thoracotomy incision, on the beating heart, with a 400-W laser (17). Clinical application of the technique has been performed with a readily available 80- to 100-W CO_2 (Sharplan 743, Laser Industries, Tel Aviv, Israel) laser as an adjunct to coronary artery bypass. The initial clinical protocol was designed to assess the results in a series of 12 patients.

Patients selected were those in whom, because of the location of the pathology, revascularization would have been incomplete. Selection criteria included those with total occlusion of one vessel, diffuse disease, hypokenesia or dyskenesia of the left ventricle, viable muscle in the area selected for laser channels, and at least one coronary artery suitable for bypass. Thallium stress test, cardiac enzyme studies, pyrophosphate scan, and echocardiography was required for each patient.

After institution of cardiopulmonary bypass and 30°C hypothermia, the anastomosis of distal coronary artery grafts were performed. The aorta was then again cross-clamped and 4°C cardioplegia solution injected through an aortic root cannula. Laser channels were then made in the area of left ventricle prevously selected for direct revascularization (Figs. 21.4 and 21.5).

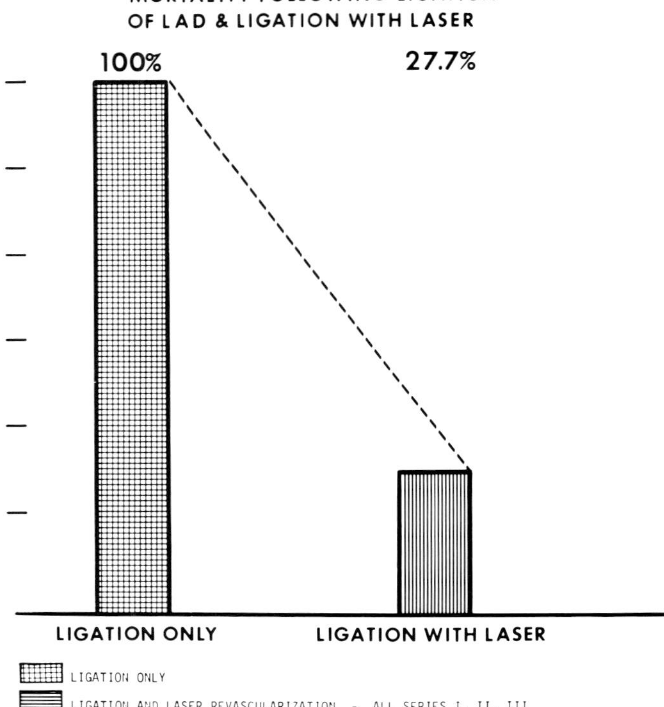

Figure 21.1. In animal studies, after high ligation of the left anterior descending coronary artery (LAD) all animals suffered irreversible cardiac arrest. When the laser was used to revascularize the ischemic area, either before or after ligation, mortality was greatly reduced.

On the cooled and arrested heart, channels are made that penetrate from the epicardium through to the endocardium. Continuous wave laser energy of 80 W with a 0.17-mm spot size and 125-mm focal distance is used. The number of channels is determined by the pathology involved and the size of the ischemic area. In general, about 10-12 channels are needed in the area of an occluded artery, however, further studies are needed to actually determine the optimum number of channels required. It was initially thought that 20-30 channels per cm^2 would have to be made, it was later determined that this was probably not necessary. After the use of the laser, the left ventricle is vigorously flushed with cardioplegic solution. Once the heparin is reversed, the epicardial component of the channel seals itself, bleeding from the channels has not been a problem.

Results

In the immediate postoperative period, cardiac enzymes are elevated: levels return to normal by the third or fourth postoperative day (Figs. 21.6 and 21.7). In general, this rise is comparable to the elevation seen in patients undergoing other myocardial procedures. Pyrophosphate scans of the myocardium taken during this period have not shown perfusion deficits that would indicate perioperative infarction.

Patients follow-up is from 3 months to almost 3 years with zero mortality. In all patients there has been clinical improvement. A consistent postoperative finding at the time of thallium stress testing is increased uptake of radionucleides in the area of laser channels, indicating perfusion occurs (Fig. 21.8). Left ventriculography shows improved left ventricular wall motion, improved ejection fraction, and improved left ventricular end-diastolic pressure. On left ventriculography, patent channels have been visualized in 6 of 10 patients (Fig. 21.9). In the absence of perfusion the channels would close; as with any vessel there must be suitable runoff for patency to be maintained.

Endocardial Procedures

There are exciting areas of surgical application and investigation currently underway. Intraopera-

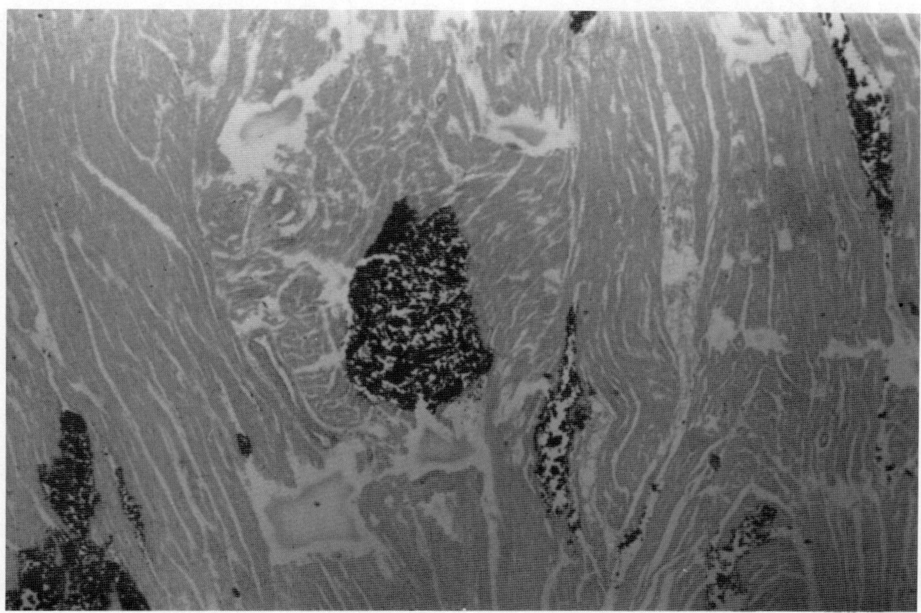

Figure 21.2. Permeation of charcoal particles from the left ventricular cavity into the myocardial tissue via laser channels is illustrated on this photomicrograph.

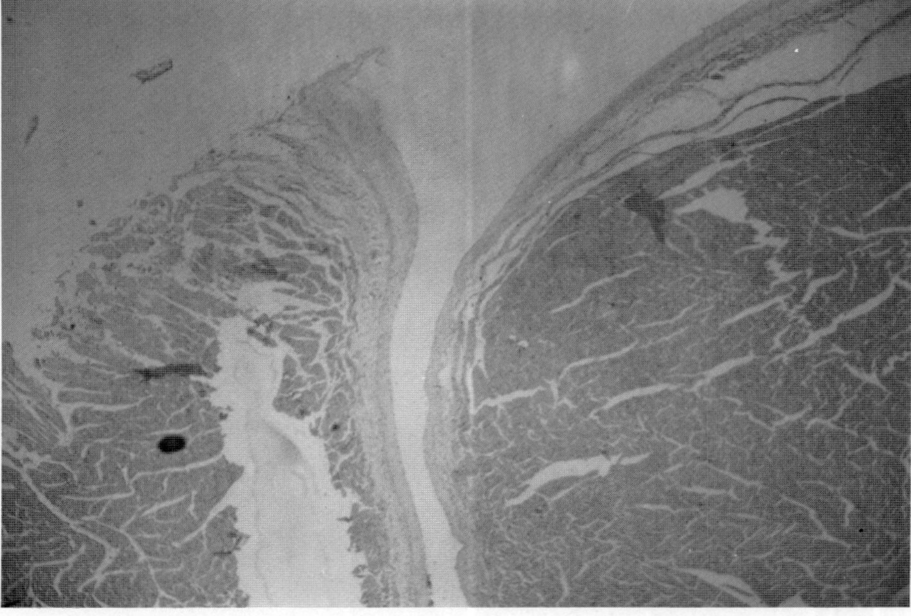

Figure 21.3. Photomicrograph of myocardial tissue showing a healed laser channel in an animal sacrificed 4 months after laser revascularization (hematoxylin and eosin stain, 100×).

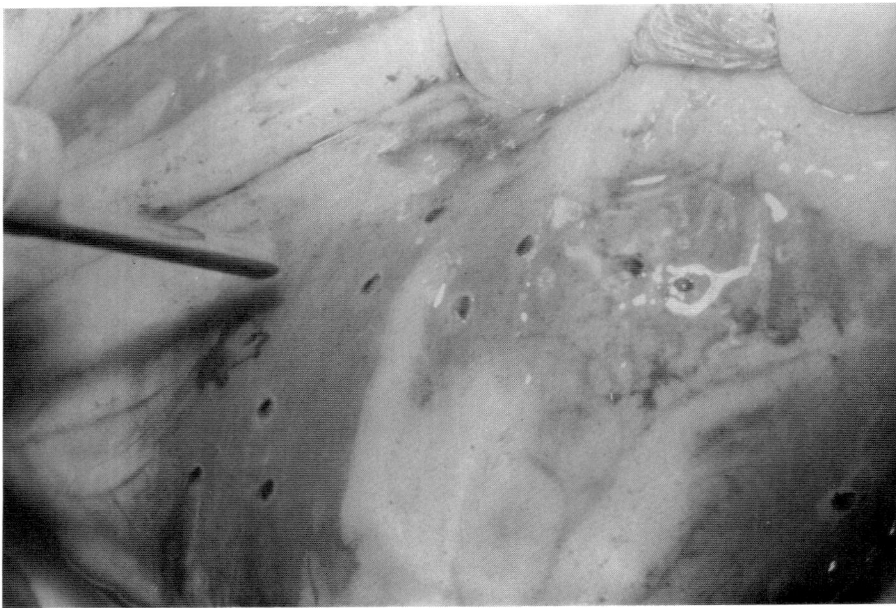

Figure 21.4. Clinical procedure showing CO_2 laser channels being vaporized in the inferior wall of the left ventricle.

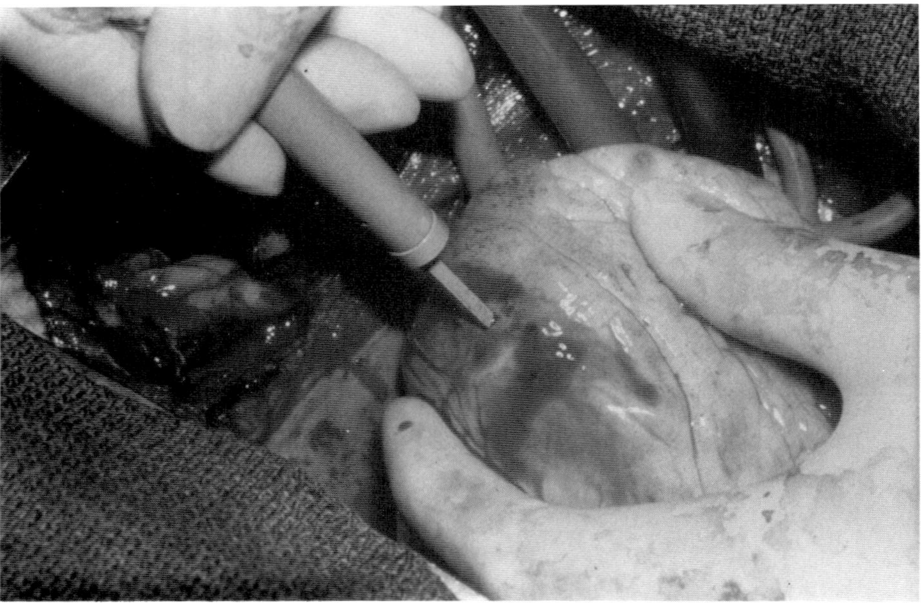

Figure 21.5. The apex and anterolateral wall of the left ventricle during revascularization by laser. The patient is on cardiopulmonary bypass.

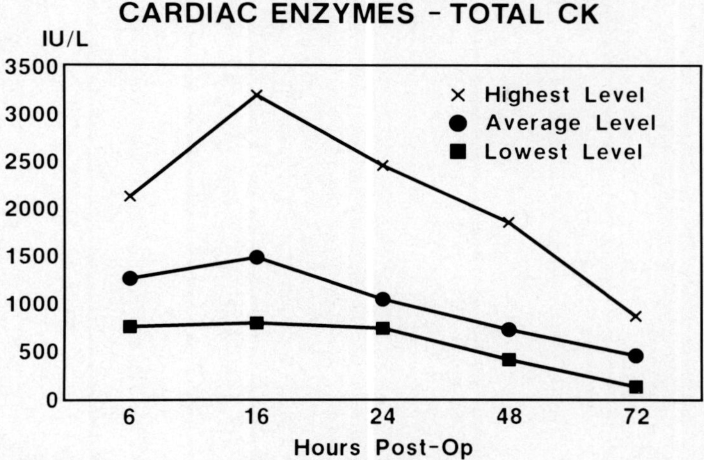

Figure 21.6. Total creatine kinase (CK) rises after direct laser revascularization of the myocardium.

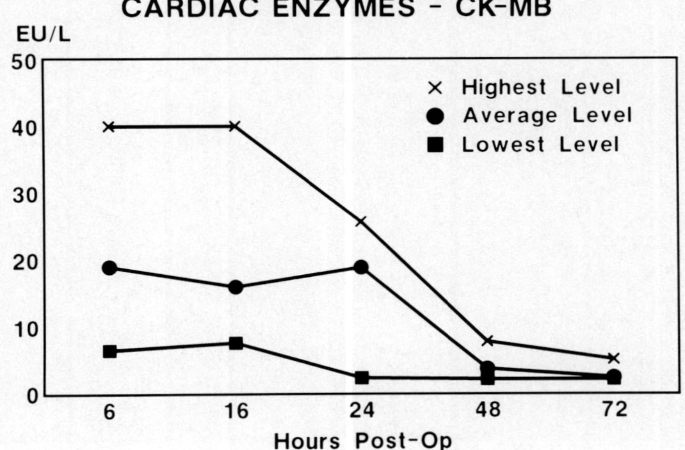

Figure 21.7. Results of cardiac enzymes after direct laser revascularization of the myocardium. There is a rapid increase in enzyme levels in the immediate postoperative period. Enzyme levels return to normal within 48-72 hours.

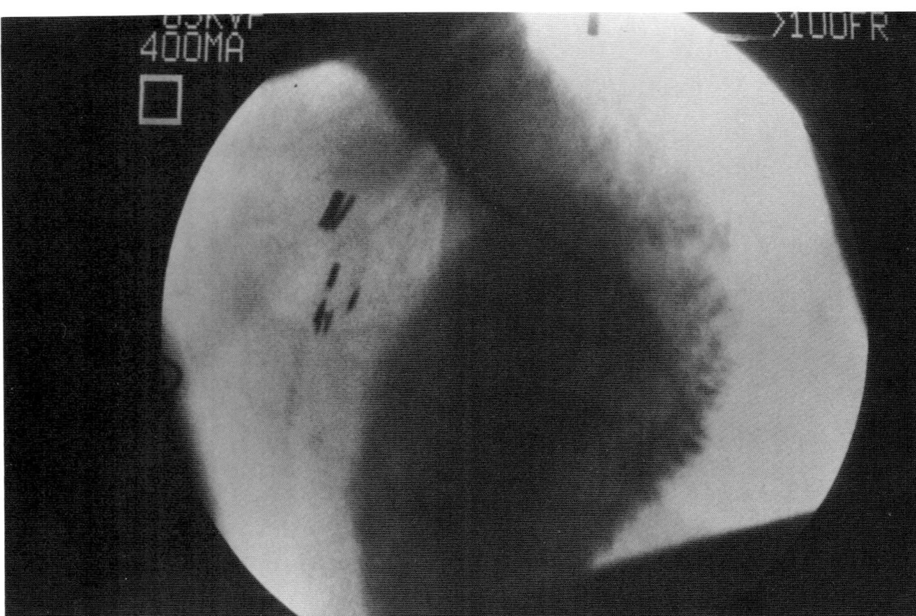

Figure 21.8. Left ventriculography in a patient 2 years after direct laser revascularization of the myocardium. Contrast material can be seen beginning to fill laser channels in the inferior wall.

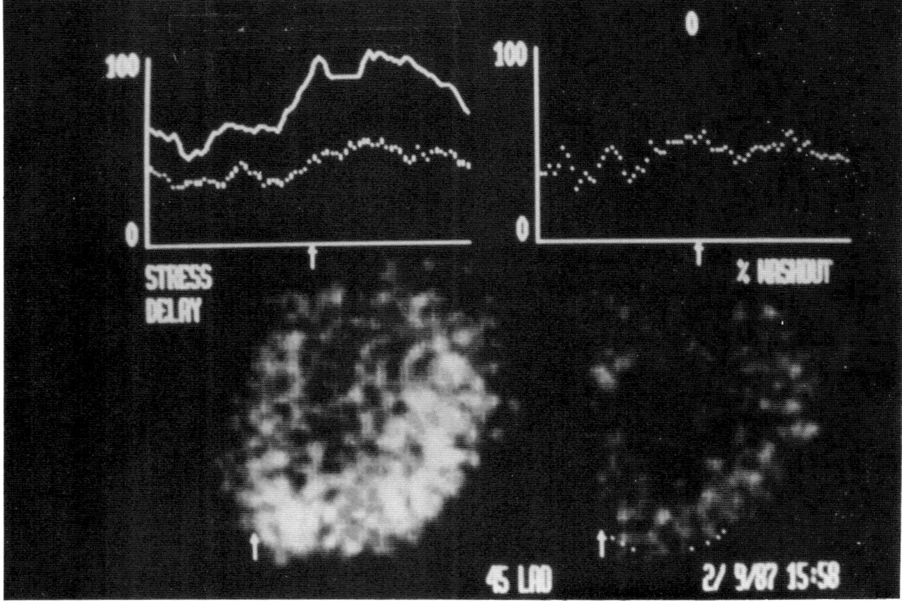

Figure 21.9. After stress test, increased uptake of thallium isotope can be seen in the area of laser recanalization. The follow-up time was 2 years.

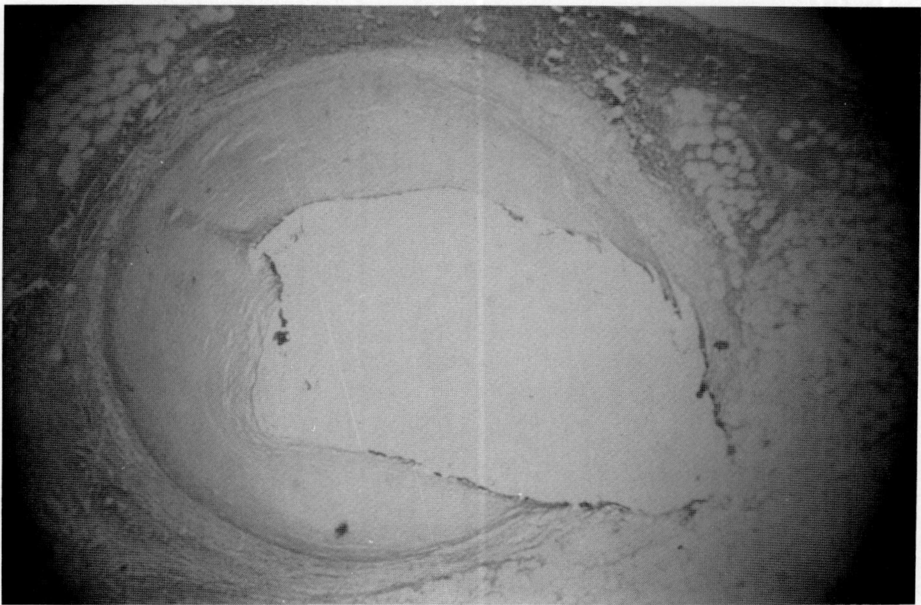

Figure 21.10. Photomicrograph showing evaporation of atherosclerotic plaque by CO_2 laser. The investigational study was performed in 1970.

tive, perhaps to be followed by percutaneous transluminal methods, ablation of calcific lesions of cardiac valves, valvuloplasty, resection of hypertrophic myocardium, and ablation of aberrant conduction pathways are procedures that are in investigational stages. Developments are promising in these studies, although clinical application has been limited at this time, and will perhaps revolutionize the approach to the treatment of valvular stenoses, myocardial hypertrophies, and conduction disorders (19, 20). There are certainly areas that are open to further in-depth research followed by clinical investigations. In particular, the implication for the treatment of calcific valvular stenosis, ablation rather than replacement, is significant.

Intravascular Recanalization

Intravascular plaque ablation appears to be a natural extension of the evolution of laser techniques and of techniques acquired with experience in ballooon angioplasty for application to diseases of the peripheral vascular tree. Considerable attention has been given to this method of arterial recanalization recently.

McGuff (21) was the first to suggest that plaque ablation, with the Ruby laser, was feasible. The authors experimented with this technique in this laboratory in 1970 using the CO_2 laser (Fig. 21.10). The conclusion reached was that the CO_2 laser was an excellent wavelength for ablating or vaporizing plaque but, because of limitations with the delivery system, was not a practical method of treatment. Accessible lesions could be ablated under direct vision but it was impossible to traverse the length of the vessel.

The development of the argon and Nd:YAG laser for clinical use and the development of flexible fiber delivery systems rekindled interest in intravascular applications. The feasibility of intraarterial plaque ablation became more attractive and a new generation of studies was initiated.

Experimental studies by Macruz et al. (22) and Lee et al. (23) explored the possibility of using the argon laser. Ablea and associates (24) compared the effects of the CO_2, argon, and Nd:YAG energy on atherosclerotic plaque. Choy et al. (25) reported intracoronary ablation of plaque in the clinical setting. Livesay and Cooley (26) described experience with a CO_2 probe to ablate intracoronary plaque directly. Ginsburg et al. (27)

and Geschwind et al. (28) reported clinical success recanalization in the peripheral arteries with the Nd:YAG laser. Studies by Linsker et al. (29) and Grundfest and associates (30) explored the possibility of using the excimer laser for ablation of plaque. Photosensitization of atheromas before laser application, designed to achieve complete vaporization of plaque without extension of injury to the vessel wall, has been another area of investigation (31).

Limitations in available equipment and delivery systems still exist. Definition of the optimum wavelength remains to be determined. Problems to be overcome include ways to avoid vessel perforation, postoperative aneurysm formation, and a method to achieve a channel size of sufficient diameter to effect complete revascularization. Studies are needed to define the energy required for ablation, a method to predetermine the variable composition of atherosclerotic plaque, and how to avoid necrosis of the elastic intimal and medial vessel lining. Further investigations are needed to assess the long-term effects on atherogenesis, to continue to evaluate the effects of the products of vaporization within the vascular system, and to further quantify the possibilities of distal embolization.

Developments of the future will perhaps define the wavelength and delivery system of choice, as well as the long-term effects of clinical application of lasers to the circulatory system. The excimer laser, contact sapphire tips with the Nd:YAG laser, and laser-assisted angioplasty with a thermal probe heated by the argon laser are the current choices. Experiments in this laboratory indicate contact tips show promise, the advantages are that a larger size channel can be made, the ablated surface is smooth, and the thermal energy required is reduced. Current clinical experience is with the steel-tipped Laserprobe (Trimedyne, Inc., Santa Ana, CA) argon laser-assisted angioplasty of the peripheral arteries.

Technique

An advantage of laser recanalization is that less invasive intervention is required to restore circulation to ischemic extremities. Either a percutaneous transluminal approach or surgical exposure of the femoral artery through a small incision can be used.

Careful patient selection is required to achieve the best results. Those with stenosis or short, 3–4 cm, arterial segments, or two or three small areas of occlusive disease of the iliac, femoral, or popliteal system are the ideal candidates. Preoperative preparation includes careful clinical evaluation of symptoms as well as arteriography and noninvasive vascular studies. A regimen of aspirin and persantine is started before intervention.

A percutaneous or intraoperative approach can be used. In the intraoperative technique a small arteriotomy is made in the femoral artery, and a sheath introduced through which all required instrumentation can be passed. Angiosocopy can be performed at this time (32) and will, at times, illuminate intraluminal flaps or areas of disease that are not perceived or delineated with arteriography. After this comparative visual assessment, the steel-tipped laser catheter is introduced. Sites of obstruction are delineated by intraoperative arteriography and fluoroscopy, comparison with arteriograms, and tactile sensation (Fig. 21.11).

The argon laser activation heats the steel tip that is attached to a flexible laser fiber and thermal energy is used to recanalize the obstructed area. Power settings and time required to traverse the obstructions depend on the composition of the plaque, length of obstruction, the size of the vessel, and the size of the probe used.

Intraluminal channels made by this procedure are limited by the size of the probe tip, usually 1.5–2 mm, but this is sufficient to allow a guidewire to be introduced for enlargement of the lumen by balloon dilatation.

Immediate verification of recanalization is made by intraoperative arteriography, measurement of pressure gradients, and measurement of flow with arterial flow probes (Fig. 21.12 and 21.13) Follow-up angioscopy should be approached with care at this point because of the danger of lifting a flap of intraluminal plaque, which causes a check valve effect and then may prevent downward flow.

In the immediate postoperative period, patients are put on a drip of Rheomacrodex 40 at 15 me/hour for the first 24 hours to inhibit platelet aggregation. An important consideration in management is prevention of platelet aggregation at the recanalization site until reendothelialization of the vessel lining occurs. This normally occurs within 4-6 weeks. The regime of persantine and aspirin is reinstituted as soon as possible. Follow-up includes clinical evaluation, brachial-ankle index at

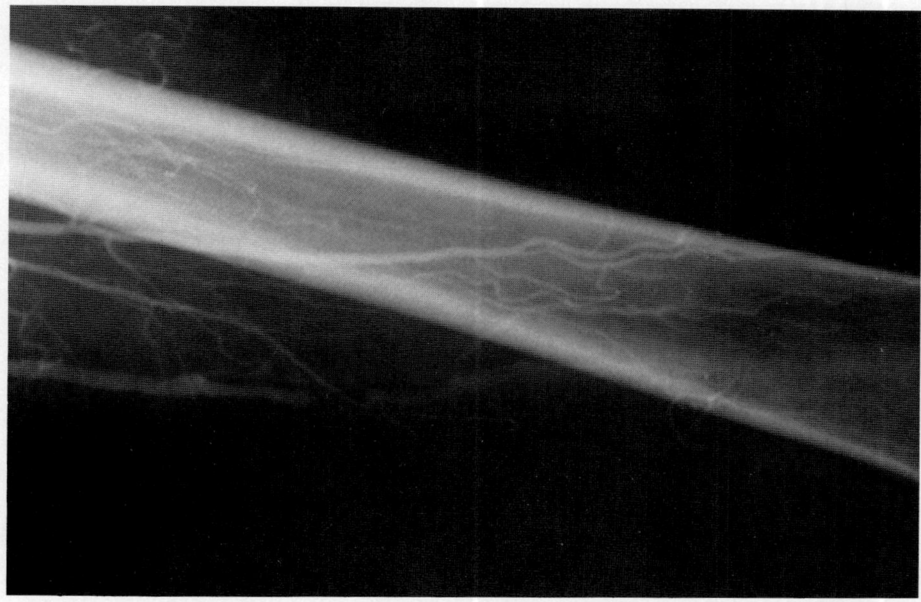

Figure 21.11. Intraoperative arteriogram in a patient with total occlusion of the superficial femoral artery.

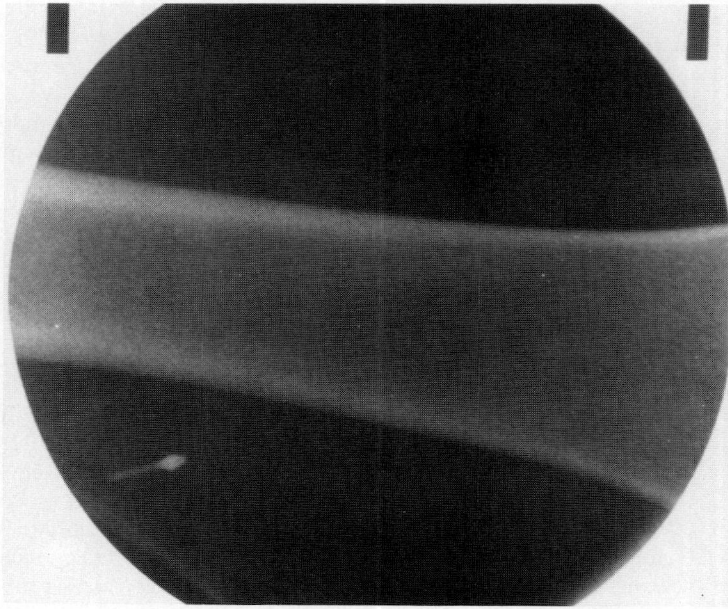

Figure 21.12. Fluoroscopic view of steel-tipped laser probe traversing the area of superficial femoral occlusion.

2 weeks, noninvasive vascular studies every 3 months, and repeat arteriography as indicated.

Results

Complications that have been reported include immediate closure of the channel, vessel perforation, dissection of an intimal flap, and aneurysm formation. In this series of 114 patients, overall patency at 1 year is 85%. Some of the complications occur because of the technical problems encountered in working with the blood-filled cardiovascular system, the small size of tortuosity of some of the arteries involved, the presence of diffuse disease, and the condition of the distal vascular bed. If there is resistance to flow there is a high probability of early closure. Perforations of the vessel wall can be mechanical or thermal, careful technique and experience is required to avoid this complication. The advantage of the intraoperative approach is that complications of this nature, if they do occur, can be handled immediately.

The potential for laser recanalization has been established. Refinement of technique, determination of optimum wavelength, further study of the mechanisms involved are evolving through the efforts of several investigators in this field. The immediate goal, recanalization of vascular obstructions, is being achieved. The procedures are less invasive than conventional reconstructive procedures, with the attendant reduction in the length of procedures and required length of hospitalization. Further goals to be achieved include exceeding patency rates achieved by conventional reconstruction procedures and to have the ability to recanalize arteries not amenable to conventional bypass.

Conventional saphenous vein bypass has a patency rate of 60–75% at 5 years. Patency rates for synthetic grafts range from 50–70% at 5 years depending on the conduit used. Factors influencing graft patency include atherogenesis, occlusive disease distal to the graft, and technical failures. The same factors will also be a consideration in evaluating laser procedures. Patency rates for laser recanalization have not been established at this time. Cumberland and Sanborn (33) have reported a series of 26 patients followed for 10 months with two reocclusions. It is, however, too early to draw any meaningful conclusions. Further experience, longer follow-up times, and larger numbers of patients studied are needed.

Vascular Anastamosis and Vessel Welding

Laser welding or vascular anastamoses by laser bonding of arteriotomy has been reported using the CO_2, Nd:YAG, and argon lasers. The advantages are that microvascular structures, as well as larger arteries, can be anastamosed with less cross-clamping time than conventional suture techniques, the potential for vessel trauma caused by placing sutures and manipulation of the vessel is reduced, and, potentially, patency rates are superior to those of conventionally sutured arteries.

Early studies reported that an initial coagulum bond was responsible for anastamosis and repair. Histology studies showed a decrease in elastic and collagen fibers. Quigly (34) and his coworkers reported similar results using the mW CO_2 laser. Wukasch et al. (35) reported 250 cases of laser-assisted microvascular anastomosis in vessels 2.5–3.0 mm in size. Patency rates in the laser group was 96% at 6 months compared to 94% for sutured arteries. Late aneurysm formation, a complication that has concerned many, was 7% for the laser anastomoses and 13% for suture anastomoses in this series.

Okada and his associates (36) confirmed patency in 109 vessels studies at 1 week to 2.5 months, pressure tolerances of up to 300 mm Hg, and tensile strength of the bond exceeding that of sutured vessels. Microscopic examination showed collagen bonding with excellent healing. In this study, results of mW CO_2 laser anastomoses in 35 clinical cases are reported. Vessels anastomosed by this method included femeral-popliteal bypass vein grafts and internal mammary artery to coronary artery grafts without complications.

The technique is suitable for end-to-end, end-to-side, and side-to-side anastomosis. Stay sutures are used to coapt the vessel edges and to provide a means for exerting gentle traction. The number of stay sutures required depends on the size of the vessel to be welded. The focused beam of the low-energy CO_2 laser is moved slowly along the suture line until bonding occurs. This is subjective and requires practice to accomplish. Energy levels of 20–80 mW have been reported, with exposure times ranging from 30–150 sec. Continuous wave and pulsed energy has been used. The authors prefer continuous wave energy with power settings ranging from 50–80 mW. Certainly, parameters must be determined by the spot size, the laser system in use, and the luminal

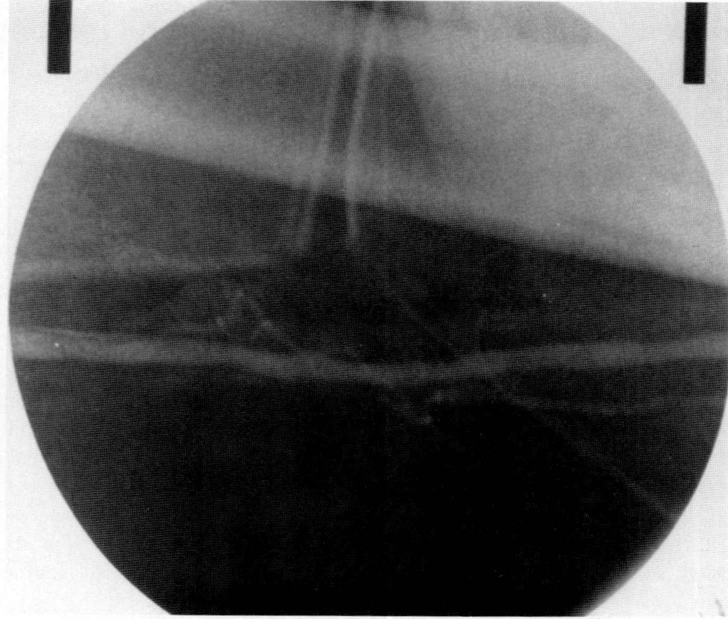

Figure 21.13. Postoperative arteriogram in this patient after laser-assisted recanalization of the femoral artery. Six months after the procedure, the patient continues to do well.

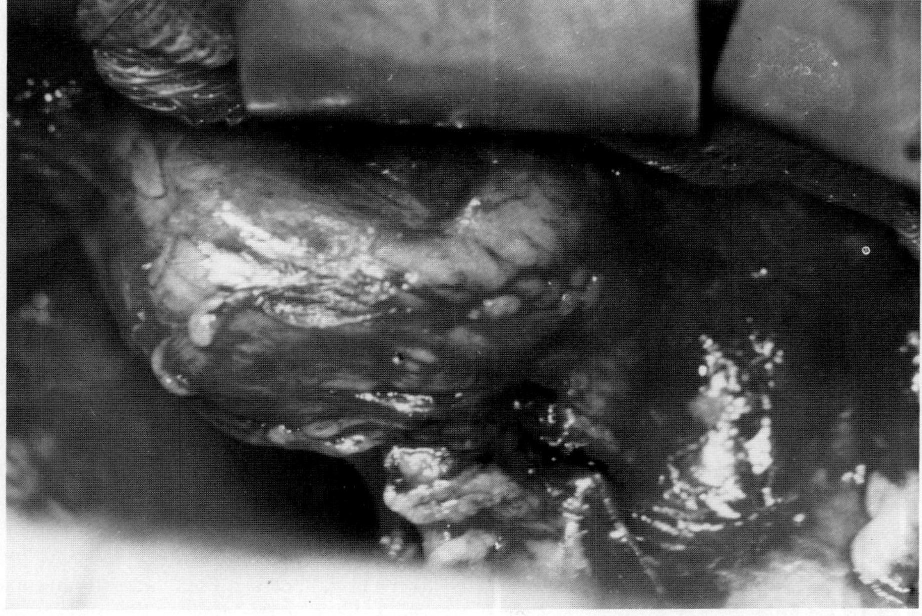

Figure 21.14. Large malignant thymoma invading the chest wall with extensive vascular connections.

size as well as the thickness of the vessel to be anastomosed.

Experimental studies in this laboratory support this concept. The authors have found that experience with the technical aspects of vessel anastamosis dramatically affect the results. A disadvantage is that if the bond is not secure during the initial laser application it is then difficult to achieve anastomosis due to adventitial thermal damage, which causes contraction of this layer. It is a matter of operator choice, and equipment available, whether to use free hand or microscopic techniques. The microscope is an added advantage if the vessels one is working with are extremely small.

Internal Mammary Artery Dissection for Coronary Artery Bypass

Dissection of the left internal mammary artery from the chest wall using the CO_2 laser is a possible future application. Experience to date is anecdotal in one patient. An impression is that vessel spasm was significantly less in the laser-dissected artery than in arteries dissected using electrocautery. In the absence of spasm, the vessel wall had more substance and seemed easier to suture. A small pedicle was required surrounding the mammary artery, possibly reducing chest wall pain after surgery. The concept of laser dissection of internal mammary artery for coronary bypass has potential merit.

THORACIC SURGERY

The CO_2 laser can be used effectively for resection or ablation of pancoast or mediastinal tumors involving the chest wall. Precise excision of tumors involving vital structures allows debulking of large tumor masses. Although the mumber of candidates for combined approach, surgical resection, and laser excision is not large, it can be effective when used before postoperative radiation therapy. For example, a patient with malignant thymoma of the mediastinum has remained free of evidence of recurrence of disease for more than 5 years after laser excision of the tumor. This mass was 3 × 7 cm, and attached to the right anterior chest wall (Fig. 21.14). The CO_2 laser was used to excise the tumor from the chest wall structures, which then enabled it to be shelled out easily. Although this is an extremely vascular area, this was accomplished with minimal blood loss and without the need for transfusion. Similar techniques have been used for resection of peripheral lung masses invading the chest wall.

Endobronchial Lesions

Important uses of the laser in the airway are the ablation of tracheal and bronchial obstructions to improve ventilation, relieve the obstruction, and to treat hemoptysis. The laser can be used effectively before, after, or in combination with other intervential measures such as surgery, all forms of radiation therapy, or chemotherapy. Objectives are to open the airway, ablate or vaporize malignant or benign tumors, or hemostasis.

The lasers most frequently used are contact and noncontact Nd:YAG laser, CO_2 laser, and photodynamic therapy with the argon dye laser. Each system has specific advantages. Selection is determined by the pathology of the lesion involved, delivery system or laser tissue interaction desired, and operator experience. Familiarity, versatility, and experience with both rigid and flexible bronchoscopy is necessary. There are issues existing regarding the advantages and criteria for flexible versus rigid bronchoscopy; both techniques are indicated for laser applications. Flexible bronchoscopy techniques allow treatment of distal lesions not accessible with the rigid scopes and are less stressful to the patient, particularly those who are very ill. The rigid bronchoscope allows ease of removal of larger tissue samples and thick or copius secretions, is required for CO_2 laser energy delivery, is effective in the larger airway segments, and, at times, is required as an emergency measure. Proper precautionary laser safety measures must, of course, be observed.

Clinical application and bias in treating endobronchial lesions is weighted toward Nd:YAG laser techniques, due to part to flexibility of the delivery system. Following the lead of early investigators (37–39), the efficacy and safety of the procedures were ascertained and newer techniques were developed and are practiced in several centers.

Indications for use of the laser in the airway are inoperative endotracheal or endobronchial obstructing tumors causing dyspnea, inoperable tumors of uncertain prognosis, obstructing lesions in those who have refused surgery, benign tumors that do not extend beyond the extramuscular layer, bronchial stenoses, and granulomas. The goal of treatment is measurable improved ventilation of the airway and lung parenchyma as well as

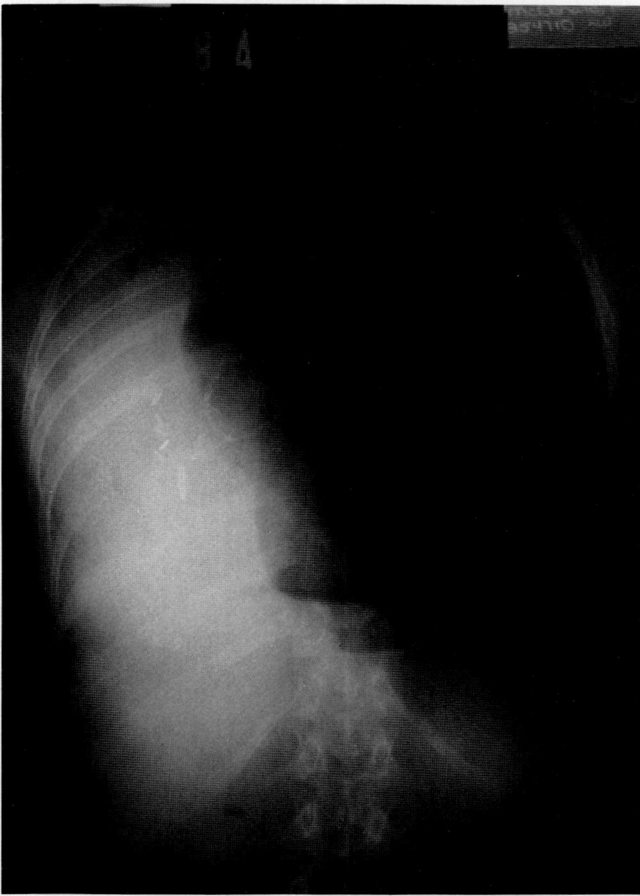

Figure 21.15. Total collapse of the left lung before Nd:YAG resection of obstructing lesion of the left mainstem bronchus. Mediastinal structures are shifted to the right.

removal of the offending obstruction. Objectives are ventilatory improvement noted on chest x-ray, improvement in pulmonary function as measured by flow volume loop studies, and improved blood gas measurements. In patient selection functional lung capacity and reversible perfusion deficit potential is a consideration. Due to the nature of these lesions results are difficult to assess, treatment is, in most instances, palliative. Therapeutic effectiveness rather than length of survival is a measure of success at this time (Figs. 21.15 and 21.16).

Contraindications to endobronchial laser therapy are tracheal bronchial cartilage involvement, compression of the trachea from outside the lumen, extension of tumor mass into vital structures, or bleeding sites that cannot be identified.

Resection of endobronchial lesions with the Nd:YAG laser can be performed with local anesthesia or in conjunction with general anesthesia. When local anesthesia is used, it is advisable to have anesthesia on a standby basis to monitor the patient and to be ready to intervene with general anesthesia or other resuscitative measures should this become necessary. Flexible or rigid bronchoscopy is selected as indicated by the anatomy and pathology of the lesion involved. Maintaining adequate ventilation during the procedure is of prime importance to avoid hypoxemia and its sometimes irreversible sequlae.

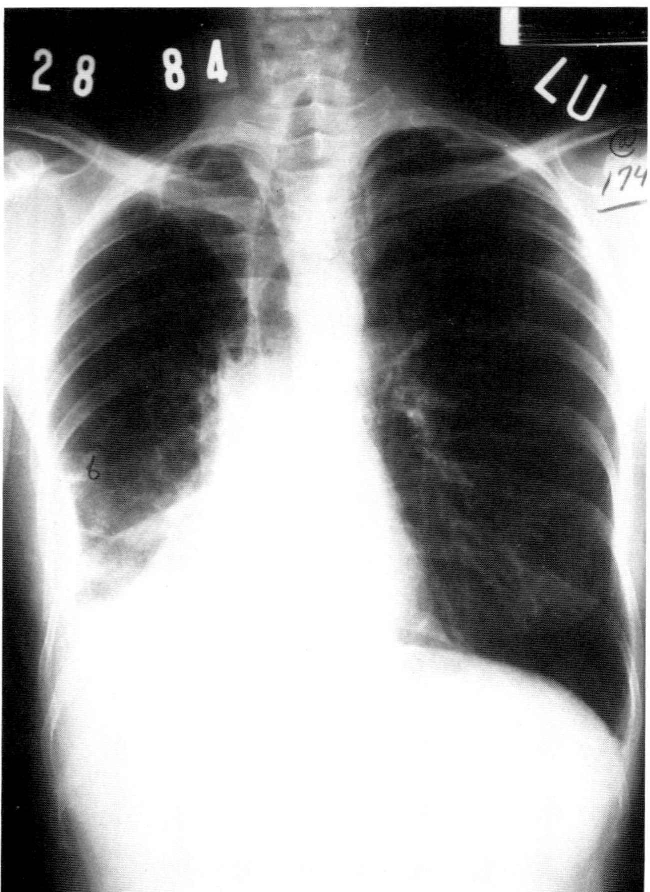

Figure 21.16. Chest x-ray 24 hours after Nd:YAG laser therapy shows reexpansion of the lung.

Specific techniques for treatment are dictated by the location, size, and pathology of the obstructing lesion. It is safer to err on the side of caution rather than overzealous removal of tumor and possible complications. With the Nd:YAG tissue is heated to a friable state, sloughing and necrosis continue after treatment. Retreatment in the immediate period or during the follow-up period is not uncommon.

Laser resection alone or in conjunction with surgical resection, radiation therapy, or brachytherapy can play a major role in treating patients with endobronchial lesions. Photodynamic therapy(PDT) (40, 41) as an alternative treatment can also be used alone, or as an adjunct to Nd:YAG laser therapy, or as an adunct to radiation or other therapy. The investigational protocols and treatment methodologies for PDT are well defined. The results with both Nd:YAG and PDT indicate that these treatment modalities are effective palliative measures to treat patients with endobronchial carcinomas. As development continues, efforts are likely to be made toward early detection and treatment to affect the overall outcome of bronchial carcinoma.

DISCUSSION

With all laser applications, meticulous attention to details and safety policies and procedures are required. All those involved in treatment need to be aware of the hazards for each laser and precautions to take. Protective eyewear of the appropriate optical density for the patient and the operating team is needed for use with the Nd:YAG, argon, and CO_2 lasers. Windows need to be covered and warning signs indicating the laser is being used posted at entry points to the operating room.

Appropriate filters placed over the eyepieces of endoscopes are used to protect the operators' eyes during laser procedures. The tip of the laser fiber must be fully extended and in full view before the laser is activated. Backscattering of Nd:YAG laser energy could possibly ignite the flexible endoscope; flexible endoscopes clad in a light color material are not available and their advantage, if available, has not been determined. When working in the airway with general anesthesia, treatment may have to be interrupted to ventilate the patient properly. The use of the pulse oximeter allows continuous monitoring of oxygen saturation. Dual channel flexible endoscopes are available for constant suctioning during laser procedures, the disadvantage is that they are of larger diameter than the usual flexible endoscopes used and, therefore, less manueverable. The dual chanel scope is most frequently used during PDT. When using the flexible bronchoscope the rigid bronchoscope should be set up and availabe for immediate use to handle urgent situations. Safety in the upper airway requires additional precautions.

During CO_2 laser procedures, the immediate operative area and drapes need to be covered with saline-soaked towels. The smoke evacuator is helpful during open procedures when a large amount of tissue is being vaporized.

There are many other factors to consider in laser safety. Each institution and those involved with laser procedures needs to evaluate the lasers being used, and the procedures the lasers are used for, to set up procedures for the safe conduct of laser surgery.

The current applications of lasers in cardiothoracic surgery are many. Further refinement of present techniques will continue as will the development of new applications and procedures. The nature of this specialty requires familiarity with the most frequently used clinical lasers, the CO_2, Nd:YAG and argon, as well as with the present and evolving laser technology that is changing methods of treatment.

REFERENCES

1. American Heart Association: Heart Facts, 1986. Dallas, TX.
2. Sabiston DC Jr, Spencer FC. Carcinoma of the lung. In Gibbons FC, ed. Surgery of the Chest. Philadelphia, W.B. Saunders, 1983, Vol 1, p.453-498.
3. Sones FM Jr, Shirey EK, Proudfit WL. Cine-coronary arteriography. Circulation 1959; 20:773.
4. Favaloro RG. Saphenous vein graft in the surgical treatment of coronary artery disease. J Thorac Cardiovasc Surg 1969; 58:178-185.
5. Wearn JT, Mettier SR, Klump TG, Zschiesche AB. The nature of vascular communications between the coronary arteries and the chambers of the heart. Am Heart J 1933; 9:143-164.
6. Pina JARE, Pina JG. The vascular anastomoses of the human heart. Prog Clin Biol Res 1981; 59B:89-99.
7. Massimo C, Boffi L. Myocardial revascularization by a new method of carrying blood directly from the left ventricular cavity into the coronary circulation. J Thorac Surg 1956; 14:257-264.
8. Goldman A, Greenstone SM, Preuss FS, et al. Experimental methods for producing a collateral circulation to the heart directly from the left ventricle. J Thorac Surg 1956; 11:364-373.
9. Sen PK, Udwadia TE, Kinare SG, et al. Transmyocardial acupuncture. J Thorac Cardiovasc Surg 1965; 50:181-189.
10. Walter P. Hundeshagen H, Borst HG. Treatment of acute myocardial infarction by transmural blood supply from the ventricular cavity. Eur Surg Res 1971; 3:130-138.
11. Vineberg AM, Walker J. Development of an anastomosis between the coronary vessels and a transplanted internal mammary artery. J Can Med Assoc 1946; 55:117-119.
12. Loop FC, Bruce WL, Carl CG, et al. Trends in selection and results of coronary artery reoperations. Ann Thorac Surg 1983; 36:380-388.
13. Jones EL, Lattouf O, Lutz JF, King SB III. Important anatomical and physiological considerations in performance of complex mammary-coronary artery operations. Ann Thorac Surg 1987; 43:469-477.
14. Mirhoseini M. Revascularization of the myocardium with laser. In Second Henry Ford Hospital International Symposium on Cardiac Surgery. New York: Appleton-Century Crofts, 1977, pp. 595-597.
15. Mirhoseini M, Cayton MM. Revascularization of the heart by laser. J Micro surg 1981; 2:253-260.
16. Mirhoseini M, Shelgikar S, Cayton MM. New concepts in revascularization of the myocardium. Abstract. 21st Annual Meeting Society of Thoracic Surgeons. Sept 20-23, 1987.
17. Skobelkin OK. Laser revascularization of the myocardium. Surgery (Soviet) 1984; 10:99-102.
18. Okada M, Nakamura K. Laser application in the field of cardiovascular surgery. In Oguro Y, Atsumi K, Joffe SN, Eds., Nd:YAG Laser in Medicine and Surgery. Tokyo: Professional Postgraduate Services. 1986. pp. 319-323.
19. Isner JM, Michlewitz H, Clark RH, et al. Laser-assisted debridement of aortic valve calcium. Am Heart J 1985; 109:448-452.

20. Hunter JG, Dixon JA. Lasers in cardiovascular surgery—Current status. West J Med 1985; 4:506-509.
21. McGuff PE. Surgical Applications of Lasers, Springfield, IL, Charles C Thomas, 1966.
22. Macruz R, Armelin E, Gomes OM. Aplicacao do laser no sistema cardiovascular. Arq Bras Card 1982; 39:5-10.
23. Lee G, Ireda R, Herman I, et al. The qualitative effects of laser irradiation on human arteriosclerotic disease. Am Heart J 1983; 105:885-889.
24. Abela GS, Normann S, Cohen D, et al. Effects of carbon dioxide, Nd:YAG, and argon laser radiation on coronary atehromatous plaques. Am J Cardiol 1982; 50:1199-1205.
25. Choy DSJ, Stertzer SH, Myler RK, Marco J, Fournial G. Human coronary laser recanalization. Clin Cardiol 1984; 7:377-381.
26. Livesay JJ, Cooley DA. Laser coronary endarterectomy: Proposed treatment for diffuse coronary arteriosclerosis. Tex Heart Inst J 1984; 11:276-279.
27. Ginsburg R, Kim DI, Guthaner D, et al. Salvage of an ischemic limb by laser angioplasty: Description of a new technique. Clin Cardiol 1984; 7:54-58.
28. Geschwind HG, Boussignac G, Teisseire B, et al. Conditions for effective Nd:YAG laser angioplasty. Br Heart J 1984; 52:484-489.
29. Linsker R, Srinivasan R, Wynne JJ, Alonso DR. Far-Ultraviolet laser ablation of atherosclerotic lesions. Lasers Surg Med 1984; 4:201-206.
30. Grundfest WS, Litvack F, Forrester JS, et al. Laser ablation of human atherosclerotic plaque without adjacent tissue injury. J Am Coll Cardiol 1985; 4:929-933.
31. Spears JR, Serur J, Shropshie D, et al. Fluorescence of experimental atheromatous plaques with hematoporphyrin derivative. J Clin Invest 1983; 61:395-399.
32. Mirhoseini M. Laser applications in thoracic and cardiovascular surgery. Med Instrum 1983; 6:401-403.
33. Cumberland DC, Sanborn TA, Tayler DI, Moore DJ, et al. Lancet 1986; 1:1457-1459.
34. Quigley MR, Bailes JE, Kwaan HC, et al. Microvascular anastomosis using the milliwatt CO_2 laser. Lasers Surg Med 1985; 5:3357-365.
35. Wukasch DC, Morris JR, Mueller JA, et al. Laser vessel welding. Abstract. 21st Annual Meeting Society of Thoracic Surgeons. Sept 20-23, 1987.
36. Okada M, Shimizu K, Ikuta H, et al. An alternative method of vascular anastomosis by laser: Experimental and clinical study. Lasers Surg Med 1987; 7:240-248.
37. Toty L, Personne C, Colchen A, Vourch G. Bronchoscopic management of tracheal lesions using the neodymium yttrium aluminum garnet laser. Thorax 1981; 36:175-178.
38. Dumon JF, Reboud E, Garbe L, et al. Treatment of tracheobronchial lesions by laser photoresection. Chest 1982; 81:278-284.
39. McDougall JC, Cortese DA. YAG laser therapy of malignant airway obstruction. Mayo Clinic Proc 1983; 58:35-39.
40. Dougherty TJ, Kaufman JH, Goldfarb A. Photoradiation therapy for the treatment of malignant tumor. Cancer Res 1978; 38:2628-2635.
41. Hayata Y, Kato H, Konaka C, et al. Hematoporphyrin derivative and laser photoradiataion in the treatment of lung cancer. Chest 1982; 81:269-277.

CHAPTER

22

Contact Nd:YAG Lasers in Head and Neck Reconstructive Surgery

Goro Mogi, Yuichi Kurono, Issei Ichimiya

Laser technology in medical science has developed remarkably. The application of laser power in surgery—using both carbon dioxide (CO_2) and neodymium (Nd):yttrium-aluminum-garnet (YAG) lasers—to the field of head and neck surgery has grown within the last decades. The CO_2 laser is generally used in laryngomicroscopic surgery. Because the Nd:YAG laser is able to pass through optical fibers, it is mainly used in flexible endoscopic treatment of the tracea and of the bronchus. Although Nd:YAG laser treatment has a beneficial effect on coagulation and vaporization, the use of noncontact Nd:YAG lasers is limited because of their inability to cut tissue. The contact laser probe, made of ceramics, is a new form of Nd:YAG laser delivery system that, by contact irradiation, can be used in coagulation, vaporization, and cutting.

Reconstructive procedures using a pedicle flap have improved the cure rate of head and neck cancer because such procedures make it possible to resect a large part of the dissected lesion, including an adequate safety margin, and to provide acceptable, functional, and cosmetic rehabilitation. Particularly, it has been proven that a myocutaneous (MC) island flap is an invaluable reconstructive material for head and neck cancer patients (1–4). The one-stage operation—which consists of composite resection of the primary tumor, radical neck dissection (RND), and subsequent reconstructive surgery using a MC island flap—causes a large volume of blood loss requiring a blood transfusion because of the highly vascularized operation fields. Postoperative hematoma sometimes causes major flap necrosis (4).

In order to compensate for the disadvantage of this procedure, contact Nd:YAG laser surgery using a new ceramic laser probe was applied. Its efficacy in head and neck reconstructive surgery is discussed.

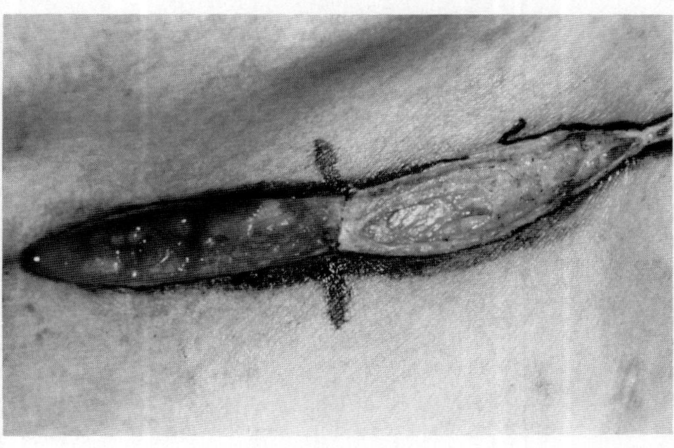

Figure 22.1. Skin incision made by contact Nd:YAG laser (*right half*) and by a conventional surgical scalpel (*left half*).

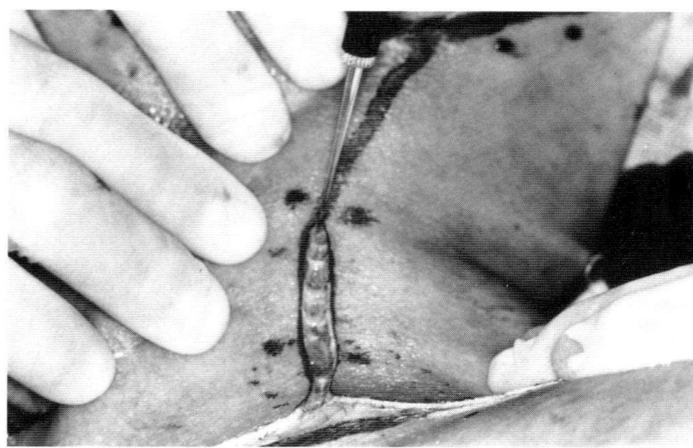

Figure 22.2. Skin incision without bleeding can be made by the contact Nd:YAG laser.

PATIENTS AND TECHNIQUES

Contact Nd:YAG laser surgery was used to treat 76 patients. Of these, 23 patients had a cancer lesion in the oral cavity, tongue, or palatopharynx; 17 had pharyngoesophageal cancer; and the remaining 36 had cancer of the larynx, maxillary sinus, or thyroid gland. Sixty-three patients underwent RND. Of them, 37 had reconstructive surgery using the MC flap immediately after the composite resection of the tumor lesion. A pectoralis major MC flap was prepared as reported by Ariyan (5), and a latissimus dorsi MC flap was made according to the method described by Morris et al. (6). The latissimus dorsi MC flap was used in a female patient with pharyngoesophageal cancer.

Model 130 YZ (Nippon Infrared Industries Co., Ltd. Tokyo, Japan), which is able to irradiate both Nd:YAG and CO_2 lasers, was employed. Two ceramic scalpels (SLT Japan Co., Ltd. Tokyo, Japan), one with a 0.4-mm diameter tip (small) and the other with a 0.6-mm diameter tip (large), were used. The small scalpel was used for skin incision at 12 W; the large scalpel was employed for dissection fo the subcutaneous tissues, resection of muscle, and the other procedures at 15 W. The larger the diameter of the tip, the greater the coagulation effect; but the more thermal damage is caused to adjacent tissue.

RESULTS

Skin Incision

Incision of the skin could be made without bleeding. Figure 22.1 shows a skin incision, half of which was made by the contact Nd:YAG laser (*right half* of incision) and half made by a conventional surgical scalpel (*left half* of incision). No bleeding is seen in the right half, whereas the left half is moistened by blood. As shown in Figure 22.2, skin incision and dissection of the subcutaneous tissue could be performed more effectively by producing adequate tension on the tissue either manually or with forceps. Skin incision in the preparation of a MC island flap was also performed by contact Nd:YAG laser. However, the cut surface of the MC island flap was slightly resected by scissors to avoid a suture insufficiency attributable to its thermal damage (Fig. 22.3).

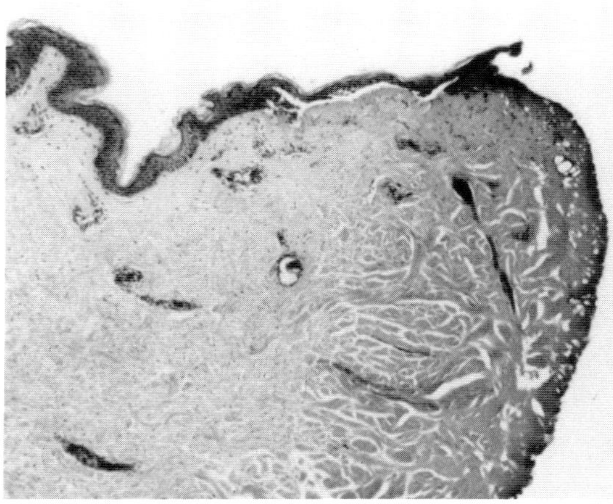

Figure 22.3. Thermal damage of the skin by contact Nd:YAG laser irradiation.

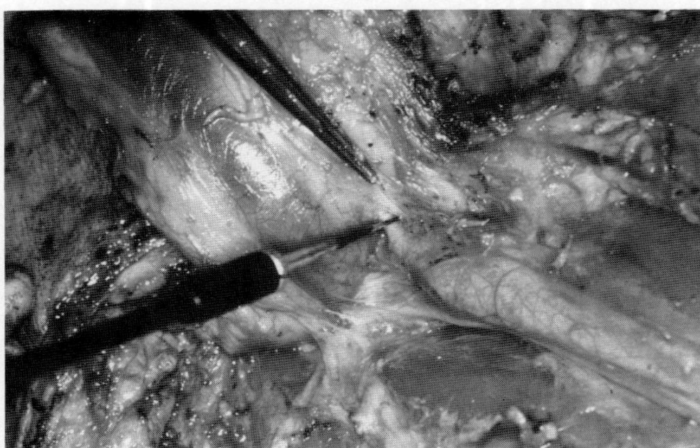

Figure 22.4. Dissection of the tissue close to the jugular vein and carotid artery.

Radical Neck Dissection and Composite Operation

Dissection of the subcutaneous tissues and the procedures of RND were completed safely. This was because tactile impression, provided by use of conventional steel scalpels but not by noncontact laser surgical procedures, can also be obtained by use of ceramic scalpels, and because the identification of blood vessels, nerve fibers, and other parts is easier in contact Nd:YAG laser surgery than in conventional operating methods because of less bleeding (Fig. 22.4). Because the contact laser scalpel differs from the electric knife, large muscle bundles, such as the sternocleidomastoid muscle, and the tongue, were transsected without muscular constriction (Fig. 22.5). Moreover, the resection area of primary tumor, including the safety margin, could be accurately and easily found, as almost no bleeding occurred while cutting the pharyngeal mucosa and tongue.

Blood Loss

The mean volume of blood loss during the composite operation, including RND, performed on 63 patients by use of the contact Nd:YAG laser was 98 ± 23 ml; whereas that of 110 patients operated on in the Department of Otolaryngology, Medical College of Oita, by conventional procedures was 730 ± 351 ml. The preparation of the MC flap caused an average blood loss of 76 ± 38 ml in 37 cases using the contact Nd:YAG laser; whereas conventional procedures caused an average blood loss of 280 ± 134 ml in operations. The mean volume of blood and exudate from neg-

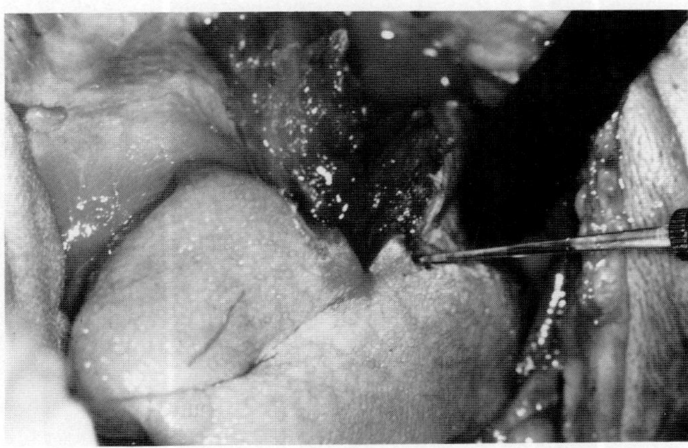

Figure 22.5. Transsection of the tongue.

Table 22.1. Mean Volume of Blood Loss in Laser Surgery and Conventional Surgery

	No.	During Surgery (mean ± SD, ml)	24 hours after Surgery (mean ± SD, ml)
Conventional surgery			
Composite operation	110	730 ± 351	206 ± 104
Preparation of MC flap	28	280 ± 134	124 ± 39
Nd:YAG laser			
Composite operation	63	98 ± 23	95 ± 31
Preparation of MC flap	37	76 ± 38	64 ± 45

ative pressure drainage after contact laser surgery was 95 ± 31 ml from the RND incision; 64 ± 45 ml from the donor's site of the MC flap. By use of conventional surgery it was 206 ± 104 ml from the RND incision; and 124 ± 39 ml from the donor's site of the MC flap (Table 22.1). Of 37 patients who had reconstructive surgery, 24 received no blood transfusion. Patients who received blood transfusions suffered anemia preoperatively.

Results of Reconstructive Surgery

In 6 of the 11 patients who underwent pharyngoesophageal reconstruction with the contact Nd:YAG laser, fistulas occurred at the lower attachment between the flap and recipient mucosa. Stenosis occurred in three cases. All of them were cured by conservative treatment. The average period until taking food orally was no different in laser surgery than in conventional surgery (Table 22.2). Of 18 patients who had reconstruction of the tongue and oral cavity, 9 had a dehiscence between the flap and donor's mucosa. However, this was probably due to insufficient remaining oral mucosa. In 8 of 37 patients who had RND and reconstructive surgery, slight suture insufficiency occurred in the skin incision of the neck, although all of them were cured without surgical treatment.

COMMENT

The results of the present study demonstrate that contact Nd:YAG laser surgery using ceramic scalpels is very useful in head and neck tumor surgery and reconstruction. Because contact laser surgery offers precise, controlled cutting and hemostasis, the surgeon is not troubled by bleeding from small vessels. Moreover, as the thermal effect is extremely localized, and it is easy to identify blood vessels, nerve fibers, and other parts, the operation can be carried out very safely. From the experience of the authors, vessels as large as 1 mm in diameter can be cut and sealed simply by moving the laser scalpel slowly across them. If bleeding occurs, it can be stopped by use of the side of the ceramic scalpel. Cutting speed is slow with contact laser scalpels when compared to conventional surgery using steel scalpels. However, operation time is not prolonged in contact laser surgery because of the advantage of hemostatic capability.

The most notable merit of contact Nd:YAG laser surgery for one-stage operations of head and neck cancer is the remarkable reduction in blood loss. Thus, the one-stage operation can be carried out without blood transfusion, which sometimes causes hepatic disorders or other problems.

Based on this research, the authors believe that contact Nd:YAG laser techniques are revolutionary in the field of head and neck surgery.

Table 22.2. Number of Complications After Pharygoesophageal Reconstructive Surgery

		Fistula		Stenosis		
	No.	+	−	+	−	Period Until Taking Nutrient Orally
Conventional surgery	21	15	6	15	6	39 days
Nd:YAG laser	11	6	5	3	8	40 days

REFERENCES

1. Biller MF, Baek S, Lawson W, et al. Pectoralis major myocutaneous island flap in head and neck surgery. Analysis of complications in 42 cases. Arch Otolaryngol 1981; 107:23-36.
2. Schuller DE. Pectoralis myocutaneous flap in head and neck cancer reconstruction. Arch Otolaryngol 1983; 109:185-189.
3. Mogi G, Fujiyoshi T, Kurono Y, et al. Latissimus dorsi myocutaneous-iliac bone flap for massive defects of mandible and oral basis. Laryngoscope 1986; 96:171-177.
4. Mogi G, Fujiyoshi T, Kurono Y, et al. Reconstructive surgery of head and neck cancer using various pedicle flaps. Auris-Nasus Larynx 1986; 12(Suppl. II) S:24-29.
5. Ariyan S. The pectoralis myocutaneous flap. Plast Reconstr Surg 1979; 63:73-81.
6. Morris RL, Given KS, McCabe JS. Repair of head and neck defects with the latissimus dorsi myocutaneous flap. Am Surg 1981; 47:167-173.

CHAPTER
23

Application of Lasers in Plastic Surgery and Dermatology

David B. Apfelberg

Pioneering work was performed by Kaplan and Ger (1) with the carbon dioxide (CO_2) laser in the 1960s, and Apfelberg et al. (2) and Goldman et al. (3) with the argon laser in the 1970s. Since that time, lasers have assumed a definitive place in the treatment of various cutaneous and subcutaneous disorders in plastic surgery and dermatology. The skin and its underlying components are uniquely accessible to lasers due to their superficial location. This renders the treatment quite simple and easy without resorting to cumbersome delivery systems such as in endoscopic treatment. It also lends itself to outpatient treatment, often under local anesthesia. Lasers have improved the treatment of several very ordinary disorders with marked diminution in pain, edema, and healing time, and have allowed treatment of lesions that were previously thought to be untreatable.

REVIEW OF LASER PHYSIOLOGY APPLICABLE TO PLASTIC SURGERY AND DERMATOLOGY

The argon laser produces intense blue-green light between 488 and 514 nm. This laser light is selectively absorbed by hemoglobin, which has a coefficient of light absorption at approximately 500 nm or by pigment particles suspended in the upper dermis (decorative tattoo, melanin). The argon laser light is able to penetrate intact the overlying skin and is absorbed by the hemoglobin-laden abnormal blood vessels on the pigment particles. Light absorption is then converted to heat, which coagulates the abnormal vessels or vaporizes the pigment, sparing skin appendages such as sweat glands and pilosebaceous glands that aid in the rapid healing of the laser wound. Thus, photocoagulation is the mechanism of action. The spot or aperture size used in this series varied between 0.2 and 2nm. The power range varies from 0.6–2.5 W, depending on the lightness or darkness of the lesions. The pulse duration most frequently used is a continuous mode. The laser stylus is handheld perpendicular to the skin at a distance of 1-2 cm and is slowly advanced according to the clinical blanching (vascular lesions) or vaporization effect. Total laser exposure averaged between 25 and 125 J/cm^2 of treatment area. Histopathology of laser wounds after treatment for hemangiomas has demonstrated obliteration of the large ectatic vesseis or pigment particles to a depth of the upper 1 mm of the dermis with replacement by a diffuse collagenous deposit that contains only sparse, slit-like vessels and reconstruction of a normal epidermis. These changes have been permanent and stable over an 8-year period (4).

The CO_2 laser produces intense light in the invisible infrared spectrum (10,600 nm), which is capable of being absorbed by water. Because biological tissue contains 75-90% water, the laser acts by vaporizing tissues at its focal point, leaving adjacent tissue practically unaffected and thus enabling a fine hemostatic incision. The primary advantage of the CO_2 laser in hemangioma surgery is its ability to cut like a knife and seal small blood vessels at the same time. Larger vessels do require clamping, but defocusing the laser beam accomplished cautery, thus reducing blood loss during surgery. A defocused CO_2 laser can accomplish precise surface vaporization or ablation of superficial lesions with precision. Laser dermabrasion (''laserbrasion'') can selectively and precisely remove superficial skin layers to any desired depth in the dermis with excellent subsequent wound healing. CO_2 laser spot or aperture size varies between 0.2 and 1.0 mm, power

Table 23.1. Lesions Amenable to Argon Laser Therapy

Vascular
Port-wine hemangioma
Capillary hemangioma
Cavernous hemangioma
Telangiectasia (face, neck)
Rosacea
Venous lake
Postrhinoplasty red nose
Cherry (senile) angioma
Angiokeratoma
Inflammatory
Pyogenic granuloma
Granuloma faciale
Acne rosacea
Miscellaneous
Decorative tattoo
Nevus of Ota
Lentigo
Cafe-au-lait spots
Adenoma sebaceum
Trichoepithelioma

varies from 5-15 W, and focusing the laser to its point of maximum power density accomplishes cutting while defocusing accomplishes cauterization or vaporization. Postoperative scarring is similar to that seen with conventional techniques, and postoperative pain and edema are significantly reduced.

The Nd:YAG laser produces light in the near-infrared spectrum at 1064 nm. Such light has the ability to be transmitted through fiberoptics and can penetrate to a tissue depth of 5–7 mm in the dermis (5, 6). This laser light is relatively impervious to either water or hemoglobin pigment. Thus, deeper photoablation than the argon laser is produced, suggesting use of the Nd:YAG laser for deeper or thicker lesions. The usefulness of the Nd:YAG laser has recently been greatly extended by the use of ingenious peripheral devices based on synthetic sapphire technology. Due to the geometry and optic design of the synthetic sapphire probes that can be fitted to the end of fiberoptics, the laser scalpel combines excellent cutting with the coagulative hemostatic ability of the Nd:YAG laser (7). Nd:YAG laser energy is sharply concentrated near the tip of the scalpel for cutting and vaporization, while rounded or flattened tips give more diffuse energy distribution for greater hemostatic effect. These products are used with direct tissue contact, as opposed to noncontact with other lasers.

LESIONS AMENABLE TO ARGON LASER (TABLE 23.1)

The mechanism of the argon laser, photocoagulation or superficial vaporization, suggests its benefits are mainly for superficial or cutaneous vascular lesions. Hemangiomas deep in the dermis, those with large vascular channels or spaces, arteriovenous fistulae, and the like are not amenable to the argon laser. Categories of lesions that are preferentially treated by the argon laser include hemangiomas and related vascular tumors, certain inflammatory superficial lesions, and lesions characterized by upper dermal pigmentation. Hemangiomas and related vascular tumors include port-wine hemangiomas, telangiectases, capillary/cavernous hemangiomas, strawberry marks of infancy, venous lakes, and Campbell de Morgan hemangiomas (8-12). Inflammatory lesions include granuloma faciale, acne rosacea, and pyogenic granuloma. Miscellaneous lesions with superficial pigmentation include decorative tattoo, nevus of Ota, trichoepithelioma, and adenoma sebaceum (13-18).

The argon laser has two separate and distinct benefits for port-wine hemangiomas. A 50-80% blanching or lightening of the color of the hemangioma has been estimated to occur in over two-thirds of the cases (Figs. 23.1 and 23.2). In addition, the hypertrophic growth and thickening that these lesions exhibit can be smoothed with elimination of the elevation down to normal skin level (Figs. 23.3 and 23.4). Complications of port-wine hemangioma treatment include hypopigmentation in 28% of cases, skin texture change in 22%, and hypertrophic scarring in 5-10% (19). Port-wine stains on the trunk and extremities and those in patients under 12 years of age are excluded from treatment due to minimal fading and increased risk of scarring.

Small capillary/cavernous hemangiomas are also readily amenable to argon laser treatment. Other superficial vascular lesions such as venous lakes, which are dark blue blobs composed of markedly dilated blood vessels commonly located in the face, ears, and lips are easily blanched with the argon laser. Strawberry hemangiomas (capillary hemangiomas) of infancy have been treated with the argon laser (20). In each instance, the involution was instigated by the laser treatment

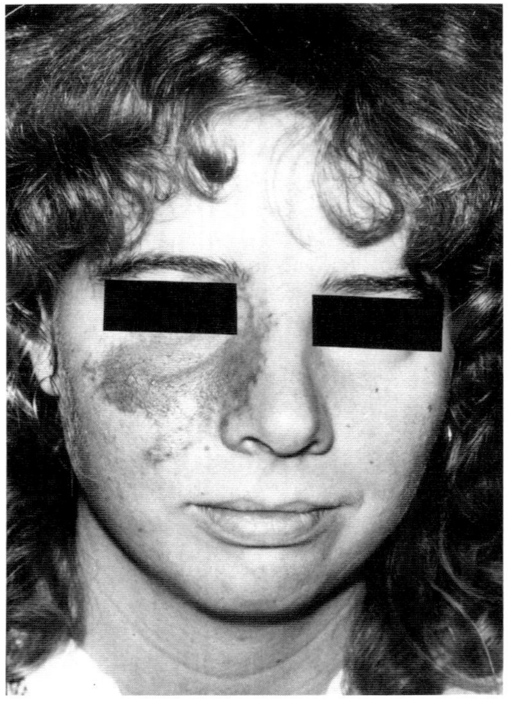

Figure 23.1. Port-wine hemangioma on the right cheek of a 25-year-old patient before laser treatment.

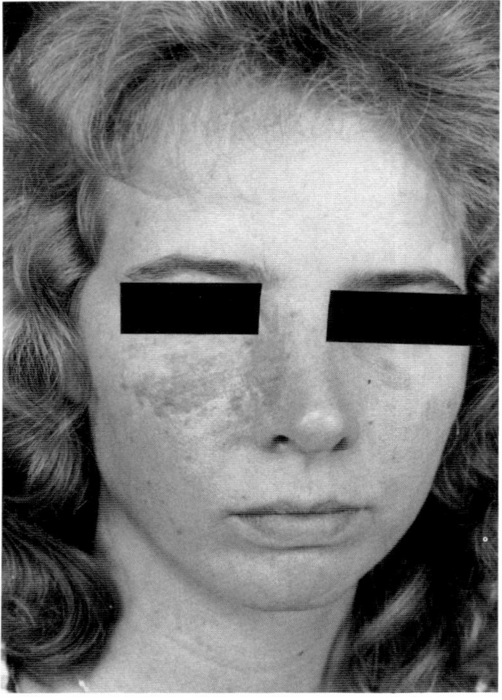

Figure 23.2. Subtotal blanching and obliteration of port-wine hemangioma of the right cheek 12 months after argon laser treatment.

with subsequent spontaneous involution and shrinkage of the lesion over the ensuing 3-4 months. Residual surface texture change but no hypertrophic scarring has resulted. Because the argon laser penetrates only to the upper 1 mm of dermis, a superficial thrombogenesis which then incites further spontaneous natural involution is postulated as the mechanism of action.

Telangiectasia of the face, scalp, and neck are uniquely amenable to argon laser treatment either as isolated lesions, part of a generalized hereditary hemorrhagic telangiectasia, or in the case of adult-onset multiple telangiectasis (Figs. 23.5 and 23.6). Superficial varicosities or telangiectasia of the lower extremities are *not* benefited by laser treatment.

Inflammatory lesions contain numerous dilated vascular components and ectatic vessels. Granuloma faciale, a granulomatous inflammatory infiltrate in the upper dermis presenting as single or multiple red-purple plaques on the face, has been satisfactorily and permanently treated with the argon laser. The rosacea component of acne rosacea can be totally blanched and eliminated by laser treatment, but the acneiform component of irregular, oily, uneven skin cannot be improved.

Nevus of Ota (oculodermal melanocytosis), found in the trigeminal nerve distribution in the face of Oriental patients, can be moderately improved with argon laser treatment. The beneficial effects may be partial obliteration of the dermal melanocyte and partial camouflage of the melanocytes by a diffuse dermal collagen deposition.

LESIONS AMENABLE TO CO_2 LASER (TABLE 23.2)

The CO_2 laser is uniquely suitable and useful for excision of highly vascular lesions or bodily areas and treatment for patients with coagulation disorders due to the hemostatic properties of the cutting light. Similarly, it is indicated for excision or debridement of inflammatory or infectious lesions because the heat of the laser sterilizes both viral and bacterial particles. The CO_2 laser seals adjacent lymphatics, thus limiting spread of ma-

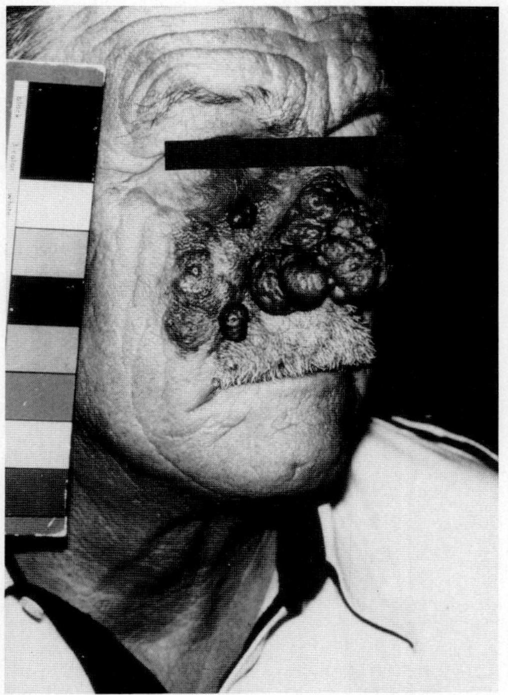

Figure 23.3. Bulky hypertrophic and deforming port-wine hemangioma of the nose and cheek. (Reprinted from *Vascular Diagnosis and Therapy*, 4:3, 21 May-June, 1983, with permission of Brentwood Publishing Corp., a Prentice-Hall/Simon & Schuster Unit of Gulf & Western, Inc.).

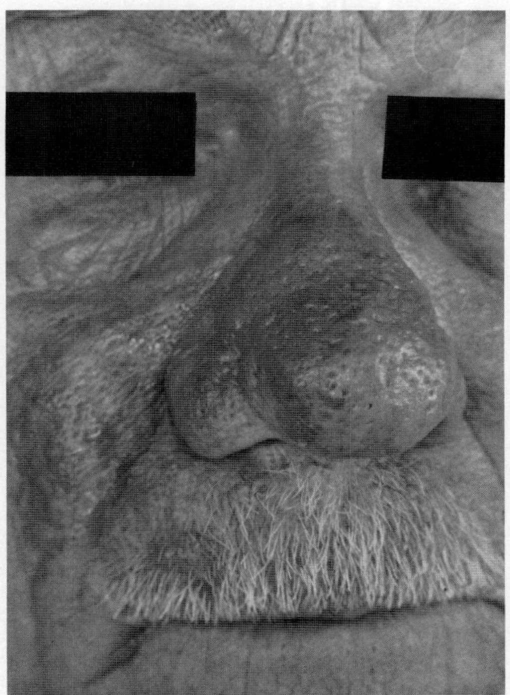

Figure 23.4. Marked improvement of hypertrophy and deformity of cheek and nose following argon laser photocoagulation.

lignant cells, and also sterilizes cancer cells by its heat.

Oral hemangiomas and hemangiomatous hypertrophy are uniquely amenable to CO_2 laser surgery (21). In fact, the CO_2 laser has been able to convert inpatient general anesthesia procedures that may necessitate blood replacement to local anesthesia outpatient procedures without blood replacement. Capillary/cavernous hemangiomas of the lips, tongue, and buccal mucosa have been easily resected with minimal blood loss, mainly as outpatients (Figs. 23.7 and 23.8). Hemangiomatous hypertrophy that accompanies port-wine hemangiomas can be readily sculpted under local anesthesia with minimal bleeding by the CO_2 laser.

Large or deep capillary/cavernous hemangiomas can be resected with the aid of the CO_2 laser with limited blood loss (22). In this instance, the laser dissection at the periphery of the hemangioma in low-flow areas is relatively bloodless; however, brisk hemorrhage requiring either cautery or ligation is still encountered with high flow or large vascular channels.

Hand and foot surgery offers numerous opportunities to take advantage of the CO_2 laser's capability for vaporization (23). Plantar or hand warts can be vaporized with comfortable healing and minimal recurrence (Figs. 23.9 and 23.10) (24). Sterilization of fungal infections by the heat of the laser with normal uninfected regrowth of the nail can be affected (25). Nail matrixectomy for ingrown nails (onychocryptosis) is readily done with the CO_2 laser.

Numerous miscellaneous superficial lesions can be treated with the CO_2 laser (26-29). Nevi and lentigo can be superficially vaporized down to the dermal elements with CO_2 "laserbrasion." Xanthelasma palpebrarum of the eyelid has been vaporized without recurrence in over 2 years of observation with the laser (Figs. 23.11 and 23.12) (30). Any lesion that is ablated by the CO_2 laser

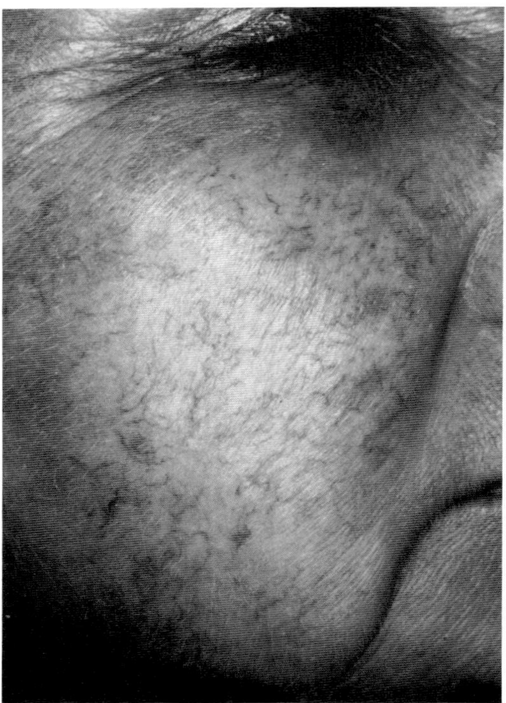

Figure 23.5. Multiple adult-onset telangiectasia of the cheek.

Table 23.2. Lesions Amenable to CO_2 Laser Therapy

Excisional
Capillary/cavernous hemangioma
Rhinophyma
Keloids
Malignancies
Patients with coagulation problems
Burn eschars
Decubitus ulcers
Vaporization
Trichoepithelioma
Adenoma sebaceum
Xanthelasma palpebarum
Cherry (senile) angioma
Leukoplakia
Keratoses (actinic, seborrheic)
Syringoma
Pyogenic granuloma
Edpidermal nevi
Verruca (hand, foot, condyloma)
Granuloma faciale
Laserbrasion
Acne scars
Rhytids
Decorative tattoo
Traumatic tattoo
Ablative
Digital mucous cyst
Matrixectomy
Fungus nails

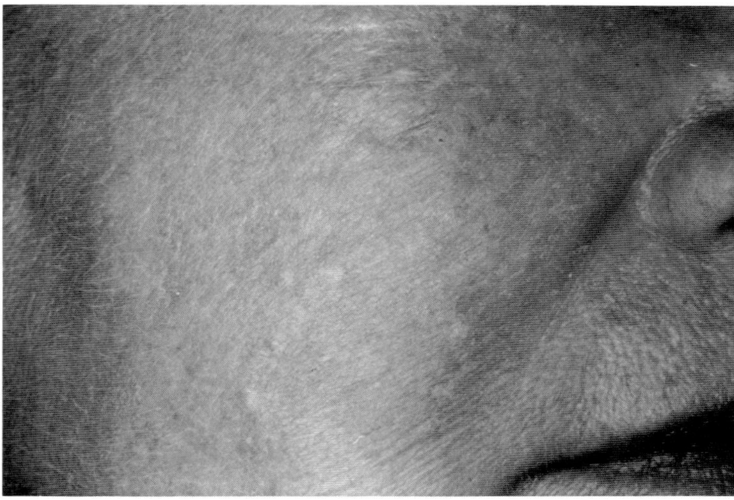

Figure 23.6. Satisfactory blanching and obliteration of telangiectasia of the cheek without recurrence or scarring after 6 months.

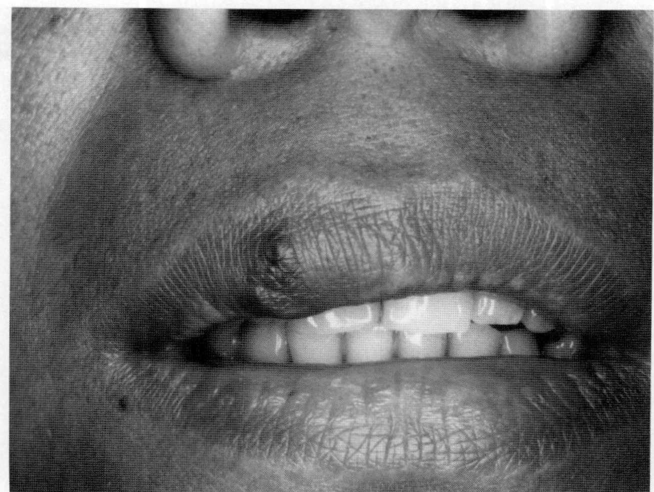

Figure 23.7. Capillary/cavernous hemangioma of right upper lip margin.

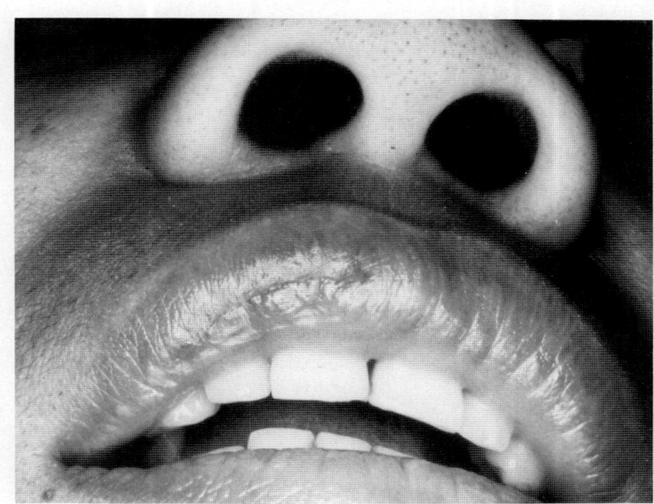

Figure 23.8. Appearance after CO_2 laser resection of cavernous hemangioma of upper lip demonstrating excellent lip contour, minimal scarring, and no recurrence.

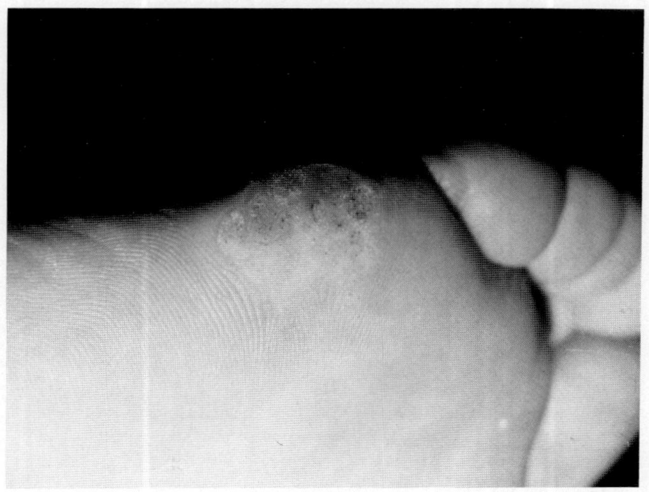

Figure 23.9. Plantar wart of lateral aspect of the foot.

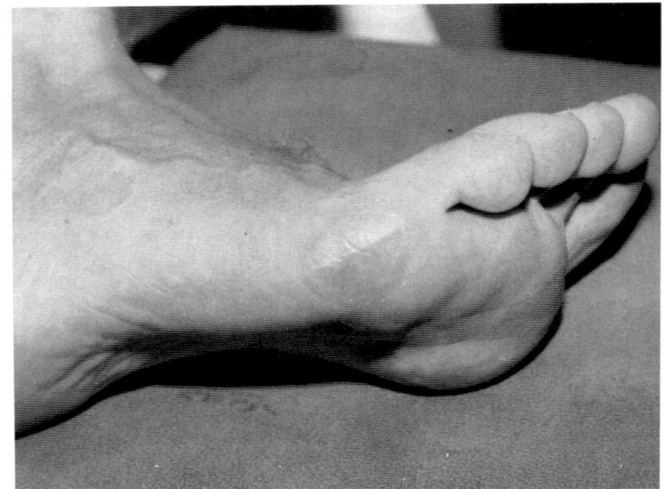

Figure 23.10. Complete resolution of plantar wart 12 months after CO_2 laser treatment.

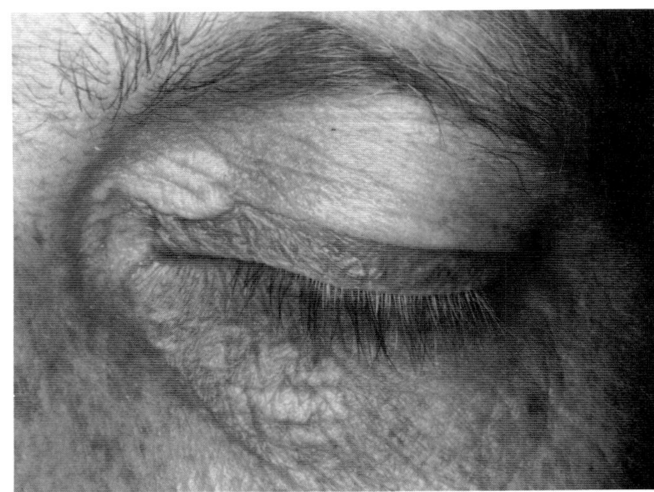

Figure 23.11. Xanthelasma palpebarum of the eyelid. (Reproduced with permission from Apfelberg DB, Maser MR, Lash H, White DN: Treatment of xanthelasma palpebarum with the carbon dioxide laser. J Dermatol Surg Oncol 1987; 13:149-156. Copyright 1987, The Journal of Dermatologic Surgery and Oncology, Inc.)

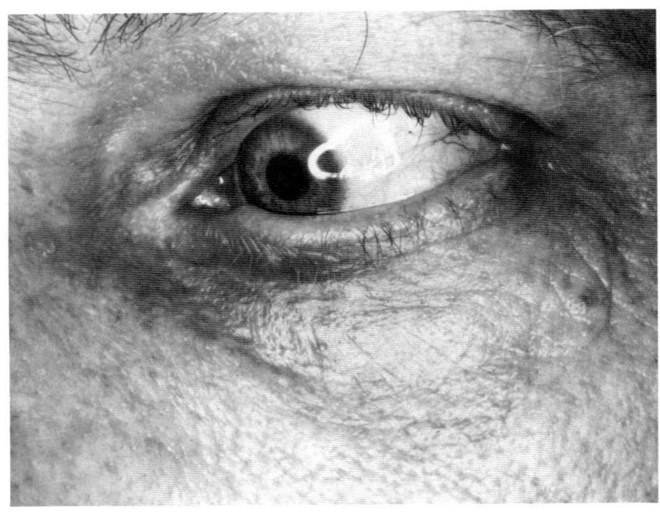

Figure 23.12. Removal by vaporization with the CO_2 laser of xanthelasma of the eyelid with minimal texture or color change of the skin and no recurrence after 2½ years. (Reproduced with permission from Apfelberg DB, Maser MR, Lash H, White DN: Treatment of xanthelasma palpebarum with the carbon dioxide laser. J Dermatol Surg Oncol 1987; 13:149-156. Copyright 1987, The Journal of Dermatologic Surgery and Oncology, Inc.)

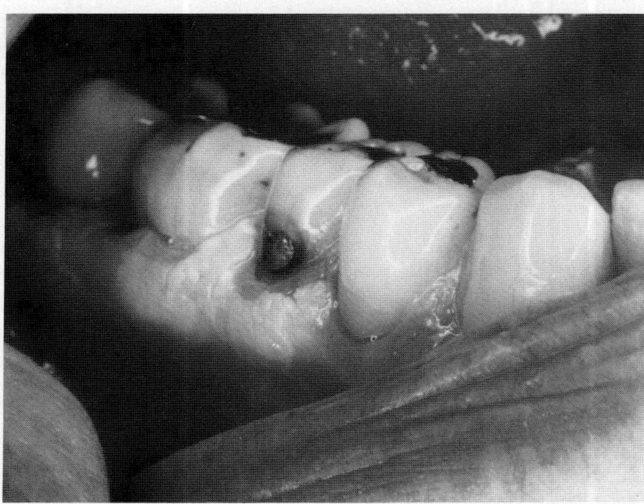

Figure 23.13. Leukoplakia of gingiva.

should be biopsied first to determine the exact pathology (Figs. 23.13 and 23.14).

LESIONS AMENABLE TO BOTH ARGON AND CO_2 LASER (TABLE 23.3)

Most extremely superficial lesions will readily absorb the energy of either the argon or CO_2 laser. Adenoma sebaceum of the facial skin is present in 85-90% of patients' tuberous sclerosis. These angiofibromatous lesions are distributed symmetrically in the midfacial area, appearing as single or multiple red or purpole papules or plaques. The argon laser is attracted by the hemoglobin pigment and vaporizes these lesions, as does the CO_2 laser. Trichoepithelioma may be similarly treated. Pyogenic granuloma, superficial polypoid lesions consisting of inflammatory capillaries, may be vaporized down to their base with the laser and resultant sterilization of the infectious component by the laser's heat. Campbell de Morgan (''cherry'' or ''senile'') hemangiomas may be superficially vaporized. These lesions occur in multiple waves on the trunks of middle-aged patients. Angiokeratomas, which often accompany Klippel-Trenauney syndrome, present as superficial black-blue wavy mass of thin-

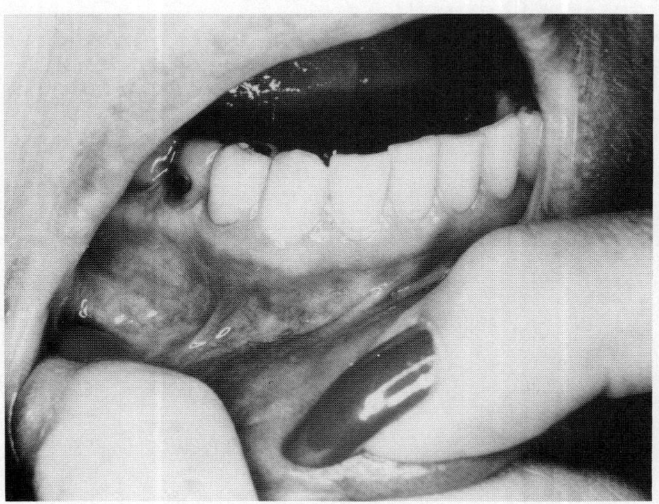

Figure 23.14. Resolution of leukoplakia after CO_2 laser vaporization.

Table 23.3. Lesions Amenable to Both Argon and CO_2 Laser Therapy

Vascular
Capillary/cavernous hemangioma
Angiokeratoma
Cherry (senile) angioma
Port-wine hemangioma
Telangiectasia
Inflammatory
Pyogenic granuloma
Granuloma faciale
Neoplastic
Trichoepithelioma
Adenoma sebaceum
Miscellaneous
Decorative tattoo
Verruca
Lentigo

walled endothelial lined vascular spaces. Either laser can superficially vaporize these lesions flush with normal skin level.

Decorative tattoo may be treated with satisfactory results (Figs. 23.15 and 23.16) (17, 26). The argon laser light is absorbed by the pigment particles in the upper dermis that are vaporized out of the skin. Subsequent inflammatory reaction with phagocytosis of pigment cells leaches residual pigmentation from the skin. The CO_2 laser may be used to "laserbrade" the skin and upper dermis with enclosed pigment particles layer by layer. As each layer is vaporized, the carbonized residue is debrided with saline or peroxide, exposing ever deeper layers of pigmentation. Laser wounds heal by epithelialization from adjacent skin and undamaged dermal appendages, such as hair follicles and pilosebaceous glands. Complications of laser treatment of decorative tattoo include skin texture change in over 75% of the cases, residual pigment particles in 25-35% of the cases, and hypertrophic scarring in 20-25% of the cases. Results of removal of the majority of the pigmentation without hypertrophic scarring occurs in 50–60% of patients.

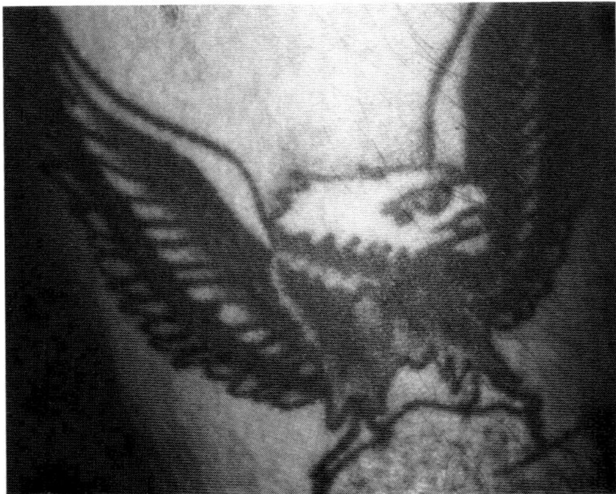

Figure 23.15. Decorative professional tattoo of forearm.

LESIONS NOT AMENABLE TO ARGON OR CO_2 LASER

Despite numerous attempts at treatment of hypertrophic scars or keloids by various laser modalities, no uniformly permanent improvement had been demonstrated. Henderson el al. (31) have published a series showing a beneficial effect from either argon or CO_2 laser treatment of scars in some instances. Bailin (32) has used the CO_2 laser to shave keloids of the head and neck with resultant improvement. On the other hand, Apfelberg et al. (33), in a carefully controlled clinical study, applied the exact techniques of these authors and were unable to reproduce their results. Abergel et al. (34) have reported in vitro and limited clinical reports that have described the benefits of the Nd:YAG laser in relationship to collagen sythesis and degradation.

Although telangiectasia of the face, scalp, and neck are uniquely amenable to treatment, mainly by the argon laser, Apfelberg and associates (35, 36) have been unable to duplicate a similar success in superficial telangiectasia or varicosities of the lower extremities. A study of patients treated with both the CO_2 and argon lasers failed to demonstrate satisfactory results in over two-thirds of the patients. Hydrostatic pressure, numerous anastomotic connections, and general poor wound healing of the lower extremity are postulated as explanations for such failure.

LESIONS AMENABLE TO Nd:YAG LASER (TABLE 23.4)

Apfelberg et al. (37) have reported on 34 patients with 57 cutaneous lesions that have been treated with the Nd:YAG laser and studied over a period of 2 years. The majority of the patients were done as outpatients. Main categories of treatment areas were capillary/cavernous heman-

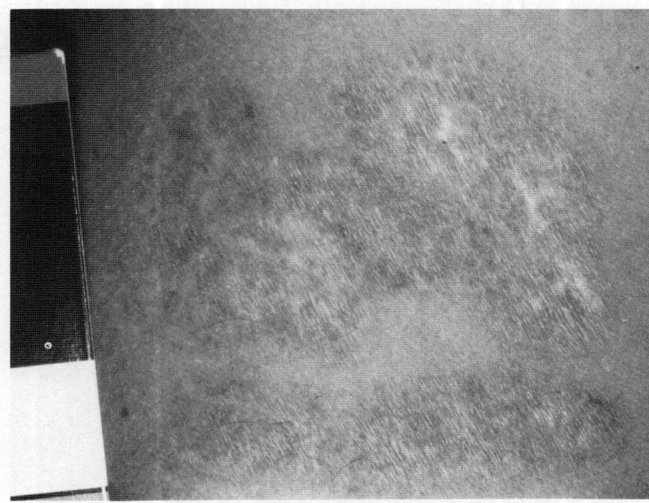

Figure 23.16. Appearance after laser vaporization of tattoo, demonstrating disappearance of tattoo pigment but some change in skin color and texture (this result can be achieved with either the argon or the CO_2 laser).

giomas of the oral cavity which responded well. Hypertrophic scars and keloids were treated with the Nd:YAG laser in conjunction with steroid injections and results were fair to poor in most cases.

Capillary/cavernous hemangiomas of infancy were photocoagulated with the addition of steroid injections with beneficial improvement in most cases (Figs. 23.17 and 23.18). Epistaxis in patients with hereditary hemorrhagic telangiectasia responded well for 4–5 months with marked diminution in bleeding episodes. Repeated treatments were necessary in order to control the nasal bleeding every 6 months. Superficial skin cancers and keratosis were quite amenable to Nd:YAG laser treatment. Major excisions (lymphangiomas, hemangiomas) have been facilitated by sapphire tip technology (Figs. 23.19 and 23.20)

Table 23.4. Lesions Amenable to Nd:YAG Laser Therapy

Noncontact
Capillary/cavernous hemangioma
Keloid (minimal result)
Superficial malignancies
Epistaxis (hereditary hemorrhagic telangiectasis)
Contact
Hemangioma
Rhinophyma
Malignancies
Breast surgery
Patients with coagulation problems
Epistaxis
Lymphangioma

CONCLUSIONS

The argon, CO_2, and Nd:YAG lasers have assumed a definitive role in the treatment of various plastic surgery and dermatological disorders. Each has a separate mechanism of action that suggests its indications. Vascular abnormalities with hemoglobin that are quite superficial are very amenable to the argon laser, which is readily ab-

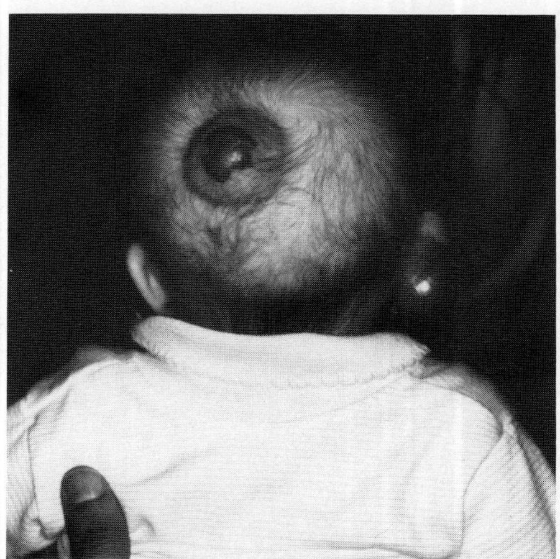

Figure 23.17. Strawberry hemangioma of infancy occurring on occipital scalp.

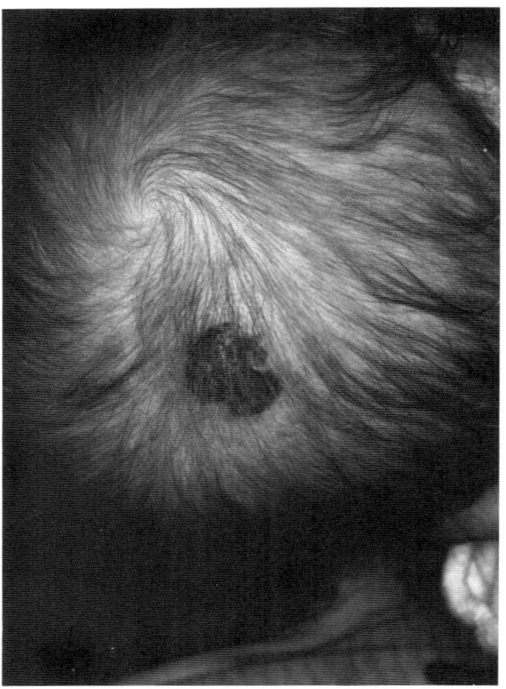

Figure 23.18. Resolution and shrinkage of hemangioma after Nd:YAG laser photocoagulation in conjunction with direction injection of steroids.

sorbed by hemoglobin with satisfactory photocoagulation. Excision of highly vascular lesions

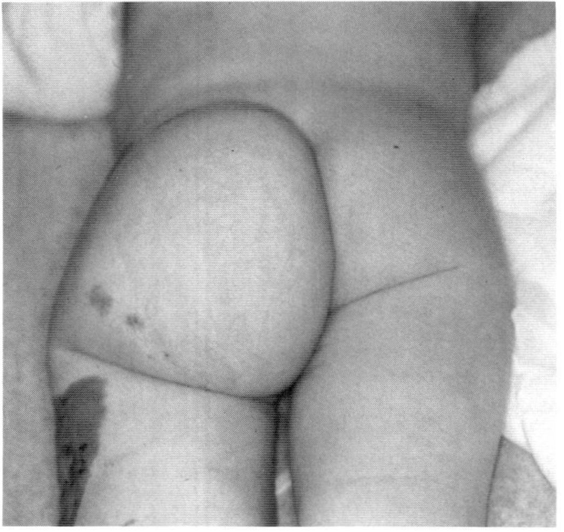

Figure 23.19. Lymphangioma of the left buttock.

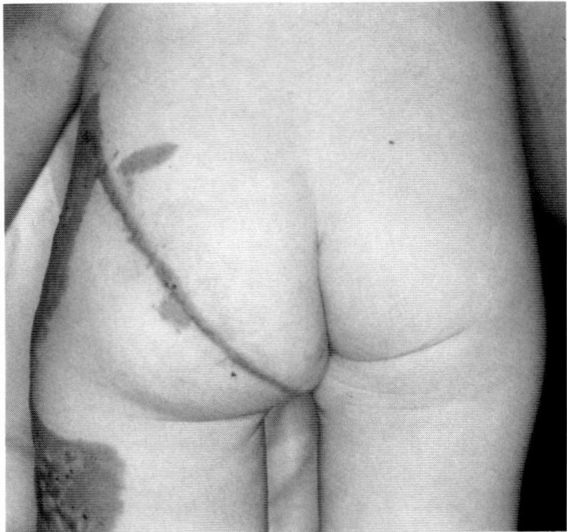

Figure 23.20. Appearance after Nd:YAG laser with sapphire tip resection of lymphangioma of the left buttock, demonstrating greatly improved symmetry. Surgery was accomplished with minimal blood loss.

may be accomplished with the CO_2 laser or with the Nd:YAG laser equipped with sapphire tips. Superficial ablation or vaporization of many lesions can be achieved with the CO_2 laser. Deeper thicker lesions require the Nd:YAG laser for destruction. These lasers have allowed treatment of a variety of cutaneous and subcutaneous disorders that were difficult to treat in the past and have markedly improved treatment of other lesions as well.

REFERENCES

1. Kaplan I, Ger R. The carbon dioxide laser in clinical surgery. Isr J Med Sci 1973; 9:79-83.
2. Apfelberg DB, Maser MR, Lash H. Argon laser management of cutaneous vascular deformities: A preliminary report. West J Med 1976; 124:99.
3. Goldman L, et al. Treatment of port wine marks by an argon laser. J Dermatol Surg 1976; 2:385-388.
4. Apfelberg DB, Kosek J, Maser MR, Laub D. Histology of port wine stains following argon laser treatment. Br J Plast Surg 1979; 32:232-237.
5. Brunner R, Landthaler M, Haina D, Waidelich W, Braun-Falco O. Treatment of benign, semimalignant, and malignant skin tumors with the Nd:YAG laser. Lasers Surg Med 1985; 5:105-111.
6. Landthaler M, Haina D, Brunner R, Waidelich W, Braun-Falco O. Neodymium-YAG laser therapy for vascular lesions. J Am Acad Dermatol 1986; 14:107-117.

7. Suzuki S, Aoki J, Shiina Y, Nomiyama T, Miwa T. New ceramic endoprobes for endoscopic irradition with Nd:YAG laser: Experimental studies and clinical applications. Gastrointest Endoscop 1986; 32:282-286.
8. Apfelberg DB, Maser MR, Lash H. Treatment of cutaneous vascular abnormalities with the argon laser—progress report. Ann Plast Surg 1978; 1:14-19.
9. Apfelberg DB. Summary of argon laser usage in plastic surgery. Scand J Plast Reconstr Surg 1986; 20:13-18.
10. Apfelberg DB. Discussion of congenital port wine stains. JAMA (Questions and answers) 1980; 244:288.
11. Apfelberg DB, Maser MR, Lash H. Treatment of nevi aranei by means of an argon laser. J Dermatol Surg Oncol 1978; 4:172-174.
12. Apfelberg DB, Maser MR, Lash H, Rivers J. The role of the argon laser in the management of hemangiomas. Int J Dermatol 1982; 21:579-589.
13. Apfelberg DB, Maser MR, Lash H. Extended use of the argon laser for cutaneous lesions. Arch Dermatol 1979; 115:719-721.
14. Apfelberg DB, Maser MR, Lash H, Flores J. Expanded role of the argon laser in plastic surgery. J Dermatol Surg Oncol 1983; 9:145-151.
15. Apfelberg DB, Druker D, Maser MR, Lash H, Spence B, Deneau D. Granuloma fasciale—treatment with argon laser. Arch Dermatol 1983; 119:573-576.
16. Flores JT, Apfelberg DB, Maser MR, Lash H. Trichoepithelioma: Successful treatment with the argon laser. Plast Reconstr Surg 1984; 74:694-698.
17. Apfelberg DB, Maser MR, Lash H, White D, Flores JT. Comparison of argon and carbon dioxide laser treatment of decorative tattoos: A preliminary report. Ann Plast Surg 1985; 14:6-15.
18. Apfelberg DB, Lash H, Maser MR, White DN. Comparison of the efficacy of argon and CO_2 lasers in the treatment of adenoma sebaceum in tuberous sclerosis. Ann Plast Surg 1985; 15:132-138.
19. Apfelberg DB, Flores JT, Maser MR, Lash H. Analysis of complications of argon laser treatment for port wine hemangiomas with reference to stripe treatment. Lasers Surg Med 1983; 2:357-372.
20. Apfelberg DB, Greene RA, Maser MR, Lash H, Rivers JL, Laub DR. Results of argon laser exposure of capillary hemangiomas of infancy—preliminary report. Plast Reconstr Surg 1981; 67:188-193.
21. Apfelberg DB, Lash H, Maser MR, White DN. Benefits of the CO_2 laser for oral hemangioma excision. Plast Reconstr Surg 1985; 75:46-50.
22. Apfelberg DB, Maser MR, Lash H. Review of usage of argon and carbon dioxide lasers for pediatric hemangiomas. Ann Plast Surg 1984; 12:353-361.
23. Apfelberg DB, Maser MR, Lash H, White DN. Efficacy of the carbon dioxide laser in hand surgery. Ann Plast Surg 1984; 13:320-327.
24. Apfelberg DB, Rothermel E, Widtfeldt A, Maser MR, Lash H. Preliminary report on the use of carbon dioxide laser in podiatry. J Am Podiatr Med Assoc 1984; 74:509-513.
25. Apfelberg DB, Rothermel E, Widtfeldt A, Maser MR, Lash H. Progress report on use of carbon dioxide laser for nail disorders. Curr Podiatr 1983; 32:29-32.
26. Bailin P, Ratz J, Levine H. Removal of tattoos by CO_2 laser. J Dermatol Surg Oncol 1980; 6:997-1001.
27. Bailin P, Kantor GR, Wheeland RG. Carbon dioxide laser vaporization of lymphangioma circumscriptum. J Am Acad Dermatol 1986; 14:257-262.
28. Wheeland RG, Bailin PL, Reynolds OD, Ratz JL. Carbon dioxide laser vaporization for the treatment of multiple trichoepithelioma. J Dermatol Surg Oncol 1985; 11:861-864.
29. Ratz JL, Bailin PL. The case for use of the carbon dioxide laser in the treatment of port-wine stains. Arch Dermatol 1987; 123:74-75.
30. Apfelberg DB, Maser MR, Lash H, White DN. Treatment of xanthelasma palpebarum with the carbon dioxide laser. J Dermatol Surg Oncol 1987; 13:149-156.
31. Henderson D, Cromwell T, Mes L. Argon and carbon dioxide laser treatment of hypertrophic and keloid scars. Lasers Surg Med 1984; 3:271-277.
32. Bailin P. Use of the CO_2 laser for non-PWS cutaneous lesions. In Arndt KA, Noe JM, Rose S, Eds. Cutaneous Laser Therapy: Principles and Methods. New York: John Wiley & Sons, 1983, pp. 187-200.
33. Apfelberg DB, Maser MR, Lash H, White DN, Weston J. Preliminary results of argon and carbon dioxide laser treatment of keloid scars. Lasers Surg Med 1984; 4:283-291.
34. Abergel RP, Meeker CA, Dwyer RM, Lesavoy MA, Uitto J. Nonthermal effects of Nd:YAG laser on biological functions of human skin fibroblasts in culture. Lasers Surg Med 1984; 3:279-284.
35. Apfelberg DB, Maser MR, Lash H, White DN, Flores JT. Use of the argon and carbon dioxide lasers for treatment of superficial venous varicosities of the lower extremity. Lasers Surg Med 1984; 4:221-232.
36. Apfelberg DB, Maser MR, Lash H, White DN, Smith T. Study of three laser systems for treatment of superficial varicosities of the lower extremity. Lasers Surg Med 1987; 7:219-224.
37. Apfelberg DB, Smith T, Lash H, Maser MR, White DN. Preliminary report on use of the neodymium:YAG laser in plastic surgery. Lasers Surg Med 1987; 7:189-198.

CHAPTER

24

Superficial Blood Vessels and Lasers

Leon Goldman

The lack of bleeding is a characteristic of many types of lasers that has been known for many years. Despite that, research on basic vascular mechanisms, originally of interest and concern, has not been continued in great detail. Usually, direct laser relief of the blockage of superficial arteries and even coronaries is accomplished without a detailed understanding of many of the basic mechanisms. An example of this is the relatively little research, and the development of platelet aggregation and changes in the endothelial cell structure and function after laser impacts. Work is progressing on this by Glueck of the Coagulation Laboratory of the University of Cincinnati.

The superficial blood vessels of man, or perhaps in a more practical sense, of woman, offer much as a test model for basic studies on the effect of extra- and intravascular impacts of laser systems on the vessels of humans. The practical side is mentioned because, especially in women, those "gorgeous" sunbursts on the thighs are usually not appreciated by the wearer, especially in view of the current fashions, and by active tennis players. So, without interpolating from the veins of the ear of rabbits, it is possible now to study in a more striking and dynamic fashion, the patterns of superficial vessels of humans, especially on the thighs and lower extremities.

As indicated, very little is still known and very few modern studies are done to examine the minute structure and detailed function of many of these blood vessels on the lower extremity. Disruption of valves, thickening of the blood vessel wall, increased intravascular pressure in vessels of the lower extremities with leakage, hemorrhage, and hemosiderotic tattooing are only mentioned.

With the interest of Doppler effects in recent cardiovascular research, it would be interesting to study the Doppler changes in the superficial blood vessels in different areas under different stresses. Nicotinamide adenosine dehydrogenase (NADH) studies are also of interest in determining the function of enzymes in the vessels of the lower extremities. Also, this NADH fluorometry would do much to show the basic physiological mechanisms. With these functional studies and with detailed transmission and scanning electron microscopy (TEM and SEM) studies, some ideas of what is happening in these vessels when walking and standing around, especially in the erect posture, could be discovered. Wokalek et al. (1) have recently done TEM studies and call the sunburst vessels "sunburst varicosities."

CLASSIFICATION OF THE SUPERFICIAL VEINS

It is evident that there are different types of superficial veins, with regard volume, blood flow, color, width, depth, especially in the lower extremities. These should be qualified in describing and treating types of these superficial vessels. For example, in the treatment procedures it is recommended that a local group of superficial veins be treated so that the individual vessels (all of the same classification in this group) could be treated with the control instruments at the same time. This would assure a more controlled study in the patient. So the individual vessels in this group have a specific classification number to be compared with the other vessels of this same group and treated with different modalities. A rough and rather crude clinical classification was made up to attempt greater control for these studies. So the individual vessels are qualified by color and mass size. This arbitrary classification has been developed in previous articles (2, 3).

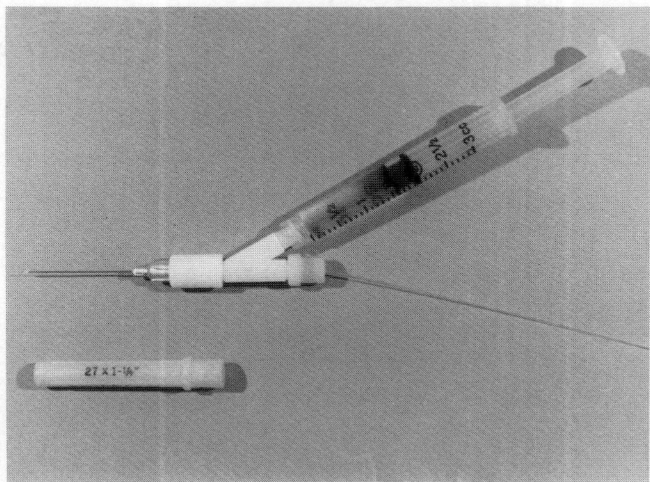

Figure 24.1. The argon intravascular miniprobe (Pat.) attached to the head of the argon laser. The attached saline syringe is to purge the needle. This probe may be used also paravenously.

Class 1
  Superficial vessels
  Either pink or red, diameter approximately 0.5–0.75 mm

Class 2
  Bluish vessels
    A. 0.75–1.0 mm
    B. 1.50 mm
    C. 2.0–2.5 mm
    D. 3.0-mm elevation, 3.0–4.0 mm
    E. 3.5 to 5.0-mm elevation, 3.0–4.0 mm

Class 3
  Varicosities greater than 5.0 mm in diameter and of varying depths in tissue

These measurements of superficial vessels can be made with a small flexible millimeter rule. Therefore, there is now a clinical classification.

The next laser instrument used after the ruby laser was the argon (3). Today, the preferred factors for argon laser treatment of the superficial blood vessels are the 100-μ spots; 0.01–0.02 sec of the laser's duration depending on the class of the superficial telangiectasia, especially in classes 2 and 3. Because of the poor results in earlier days by using large spots of the argon, the 100-μ size spots follow the studies of Adrian Scheibner of Sydney, Australia for the port-wine mark (personal communication).

Therefore, it is the small spot and short pulse for one of the programs being used today in the therapy of the superficial telangiectasia.

The other argon laser used was the argon intravascular miniprobe (Fig. 24.1); a 100-μ fiber inserted into a small intravascular needle. This may be used intravascularly or even perivascularly. The intravascular and perivascular argon miniprobe was developed to obtain better cosmetic results and to avoid surface skin damage. With the skin surface chilled, a requirement in all superficial vein treatments, the instruments can be used intravascularly or even perivascularly with heat radiation to the adjacent blood vessel. All these caveats would make for minimal epidermal disturbances with decreased scarring.

Some experiments have been done with the 532-nm laser. It was believed that it had no particular advantage over the argon laser, especially the small spot argon laser.

The other laser system offered in recent times was the 577-nm and 585-nm flash pumped-dye lasers. The 12-14 J/cm^2 is necessary with this laser to become effective, especially for classes 2 and 3 blood vessels. The number of impacts depends upon the classification of the blood vessel. It was found that 6–8 J/cm^2 is not adequate for most of the superficial telangiectasia of the lower extremity. The pulse duration is 350 μsec; the spot size is 1 mm. As with all treatments of the superficial vessels on the lower extremities, pretreatment and posttreatment chilling is done with

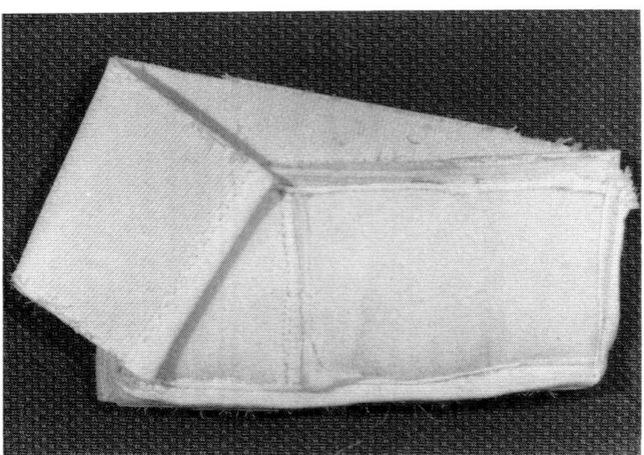

Figure 24.2. The postoperative Velcro pressure bandage.

chemical chilling packs. Also, postoperative pressure packs are used with Velcro pressure bandages for 2–3 weeks after therapy (Fig. 24.2).

For facial telangiectasia, this is done with the slit lamp, for easy visability and flexibility of the "joy stick." With the argon ophthalmology laser, streaking is done over the entire length of the superficial blood vessel; this is done with minimum pain and discomfort to the patient.

As yet, there has been no clinical experience in humans with the use of excimer lasers for superficial telangiectasia. CO_2 lasers have been used in clinical applications for telangiectasia but often results in scarring. No information is available as yet on the Erbium (ER)-YAG laser for such clinical applications.

Contact sapphire tips have been tried but they have been too large and the Nd:YAG lasers used are too strong (4). It would be of considerable interest to use other laser systems with short pulses and tiny contact areas on chilled surfaces.

In the latter part of the 1960s, these superficial vessels were treated with the ruby laser. These tests were done on patients and animals, especially in the heparinized rat, after sectioning of the tail. Ruby laser treatments were ordinarily used at 10 J/cm^2 for 20 μsec. With Q-switched ruby of 20 nsec the results were excellent. No funding was available to continue this interesting experiment.

Two other nonlaser controls are important in this program. One is the intravascular and perivascular electrogalvanic needle. In this set-up, the instrumentation is simple; an electrogalvanic apparatus with a special insulated needle, 30-31 gauge. The factors were 0.8-1 + ma, with a time duration of 1 sec. Here, too, the needle may be inserted, properly insulated for avoidance of surface sparking, intravascularly or perivascularly. As indicated previously, pre- and posttreatment skin chilling was done and posttreatment Velcro pressure bandages were used. The fourth control was the sclerotherapy. In the author's experiments, 20% and 23.4% saline were the preferred agents (4). These treatments took more time than the much more expensive laser treatments and were usually more painful. Chilling did help to some extent for paravenous infiltration. There is no doubt (5–7) that, at present, sclerotherapy is the most popular therapy. A special issue of the *Journal of Dermatologic Surgery and Oncology* has been devoted to this (8). However, the individual patient with multiple lesions of the same color and mass still needs adjacent control treatments (9).

As shown in all of these treatment procedures, an effort is made with more pulsed treatments to localize the thermal energy produced. This can be done easily with dry chemical chilling packs put on the skin before with the use of the intravascular laser procedures or the electrogalvanic procedures. The chemical chilling pack does cover up the skin; therefore, the need of eye protection during the use of the laser system is lessened.

At the conclusion of the treatment, irrespective of whatever control is used, chilling of the skin is continued for 5–10 min afterwards. This persistent chilling reduces the heat transmission to the skin surface and also aids any pain. Then it is necessary that a pressure bandage be kept on the area to further continue the thrombogenesis. These Velcro pressure bandages are changed daily. This is continued for 2–3 weeks. This bandage is more comfortable than an Ace bandage or heavy adhesive bandages. The application of 20% urea in distilled water is sponged on first, then the gauze and Velcro pressure bandage are put on top. The urea is a nonirritating, nonsensitizing, mild antiseptic material. Standard color photography is taken at intervals so that the persistency or fading of the color of the superficial vessels can be followed very easily. Instruments are under development to measure sharply localized hue, value, and chroma of a specific area.

In order to detect early development of collateral circulation that can occur around the ends of the area treated, infrared photography may be used for early detection of these new vessels. The

585-nm flash pumped-dye laser is effective for those tiny red vessels for which sclerotherapy is not possible. Infrared photography can detect other veins and deep vessels. The use of various forms of pressure stockings is also recommended for the treatment of the rest of the areas that are not part of the early treatment procedures.

With the short pulses and especially the 100-μ spots with the argon laser and the flash pumped-dye laser, these appear to be the effective treatment procedures. With new concern over the control areas, there has been a rare development with less frequent hemosiderotic tattooing and superficial scarring (10, 11). Over the past 4 years there has been no evidence of any embolism developing and no reactions of patients on aspirin or on contraceptives (the "Pill"). Histological studies, so far, have been limited to routine sections (4) with thickening of the blood vessel wall. These have shown minimal evidence of epidermal damage. Perivascular lymphocytic infiltration, and thrombosis were found in the superficial vessels. Again, a plea is made for SEM and continued TEM, and for detailed histochemical studies of all types of superficial telangiectasia.

CONCLUSION

It is difficult to determine, at present, the ideal for the diffuse group called superficial telangiectasia. With preliminary results of tests in the past 3 years of the argon and other lasers, and for 8 months' observation only for the flash pumped 5-nnm dye laser, these are the two laser systems recommended at present. As suggested in class 1 and early parts of class 2 (2A and B), the flash pumped-dye lasers (577- and 585-m), and 100-μ spot argon laser 1 W at 0.1–0.01 sec followed by the chilling and the continued use of pressure bandage has made for an effective program. There still remains the great need for continued basic studies as has been mentioned. Repeated biopsies, not easy to take at present time, will show the effect of these continued treatment procedures on the superficial telangiectasia. There should also be concerns for prevention programs. This can be made effective in families in whom there is an increase in the early age development of the superficial telangiectasia. The correlations of new vessels with the onset of the Pill should also be of concern.

It is believed that the great needs for basic laser angioplasty, the expansion of the laser programs for the therapy of that group with superficial telangiectasia is of great need and value.

REFERENCES

1. Wokalek H, Vanschuat W, Martay K, Leder V. Morphology and localization of sunburst varecusities: An electron and morphometric study. J Dermatol Surg Oncol 1989; 15:149-154.
2. Goldman L, Gregory O, Stefanovsky D. Accessories for laser dermatology and plastic surgery. Fifth International Congress of Laser Medicine and Surgery. Detroit, October 7, 1983.
3. Goldman L. Laser dermatology, 1985. Lasers Surg Med 1986; 6:387-388.
4. Bodian E. Techniques for sun burst venous blemishes. J Dermatol Surg Oncol July 1985; 11:7.
5. Zugerman C. Sclerotherapy of "starburst" veins. Thirtieth Annual Meeting Rancho has Palmas Rancho Mirage, March 26, 1987, Noah Worcester Dermatological Society.
6. Smith, T. 537 nm for telangiectasia. Skin Allergy News 1987; 18:7.
7. Goldman P. Significant improvement in telangiectasias seen with sclerotherapy. Cosmet Dermatol 1989; 2:41-44.
8. Bodian E, Goldman M. Special Issue, Sclerotherapy. J Dermatol Surg Oncol 1989; 15:(No. 2).
9. Goldman L. The need for controlled treatments for telangiectasia. Noah Worcester Dermatologic Society, March 13, 1989, Tucson, AZ.
10. Apfelberg DB, Maser MR, Lash H. Treatment of nevi aranei by means of the argon laser. Dermatolo Surg Oncol 1981; Nov:172-174.
11. Shields JL, Jansen GT. Therapy for superficial telangectasias of the lower extremities. J Dermatol Surg Oncol 1982; 8:857-860.
12. Kirchner RA. Nd:YAG with sapphire tip. Skin Allergy News 1987; 18:7.

CHAPTER
25

Photodynamic Therapy of Malignancies

James S. McCaughan, Jr.

Photodynamic therapy (PDT) is now being evaluated at many centers worldwide both for use in diagnosis and treatment of malignancy. When external light energy is absorbed by an atom of some dyes (or sensitizers), its energy level is raised and it becomes unstable. If the energy level drops back to its stable or "ground state," the added energy is given off as a quantum of energy with a specific wavelength. Because all of the energy is not given off, the wavelength of that given off will be longer than the initiating light wavelength (Stokes' rule). If this longer wavelength is in the visible range, visible fluorescence is created. Therefore, by radiating hematoporphyrin derivative (HpD) with near ultraviolet light (wavelength in the 405-nm range), such as a Wood's lamp, a red-orange fluorescence (670-nm range) is seen. This is the basis for the diagnostic use of this sensitizer and its fractionated mixture, dihematoporphyrin either (DHE), to detect malignancy.

The therapeutic use of HpD or DHE is based on the absorption of the light energy by the sensitizer in the presence of oxygen. This increased energy is then transferred from the sensitizer to the oxygen to produce an "excited" state of oxygen called "singlet oxygen," which then oxidizes adjacent cell components.

Thus, PDT requires sensitizer, oxygen, and light, which must be able to reach the tumor cells containing the sensitizer. The use of chemotherapy, ionizing irradiation, or surgery does not preclude the use of PDT and, unlike ionizing irradiation, repeated injections and treatments can be made almost indefinitely.

By far, the majority of clinical research being conducted today is in the realm of therapy; however, the development of this modality has been intertwined with the study of the fluorescence.

HISTORICAL REVIEW

In 1900, while working as a medical student in the laboratory of Hermann von Tappenier, Raab (1) showed that paramecia swimming in solutions with acridine dye were killed when exposed to sun rays but lived for a long time in the sunlight when there was no dye present. Four years later, Tappenier and Jodlbauer (2) coined the term "photodynamic therapy" to describe the process by which a biological system becomes sensitized to light after exposure to a substance that absorbs the light to produce a photochemical reaction in conjunction with oxygen.

During the next 20 years, several investigators described various reactions to hematoporphyrin dye. Haussman (3), in 1910, reported that white mice injected with hematoporphyrin, and then exposed to light, developed reactions that varied directly with the amount of sensitizer or the amount of light. Three years later, Meyer-Betz (4) injected himself with hematoporphyrin dye and demonstrated solar photosensitivity that lasted for 2 months and was associated with edema and hyperpigmentation. Finally, Policard (5) observed in 1924 that some tumors produced a red-orange fluorescence when exposed to near-ultraviolet light. This was thought to be due to the presence of endogenous porphyrins.

In 1941, Blum (6) published a thorough monograph detailing the research on PDT to that time. Interestingly, much of the current work has rediscovered those observations made by Blum almost 50 years ago.

In 1942, Auler and Banzer (7) observed that hematoporphyrin injected into rats accumulated in neoplastic tissue. Six years later, Figge and coworkers (8) noted an increased fluorescence in lymph nodes, tumors (sarcomas and mammary tumors), previously incised or traumatized tissue, the placenta of pregnant mice, and the necrotic centers of tumors. Likewise, in 1955, Rassmussen-Taxdall and coworkers (9) reported the fluorescence of tumors in patients injected with hematoporphyrin including cancer of the penis, breast, mesenteric, and axillary nodes.

In 1960, Lipson and Baldes (10), using a derivative of hematoporphyrin (HpD) prepared by Schwartz, demonstrated that the reaction in white mice exposed to light varied with the amount of HpD, the amount of light exposure, and the time of exposure to the light from the time of injection. A year later, Lipson and coworkers (11) reported their studies of endoscopic fluorescence observed in 15 patients with endobronchial tumors using HpD as the sensitizer. Lipson and coworkers (12) investigated the use of HpD for the detection and management of cancer and treated the first patient with breast cancer. Gregorie and coworkers (13) reported a study of 226 patients injected with intravenous HpD. They reported a 75–85% correlation of fluorescence with positive biopsies of squamous and adenocarcinoma, as well as a 23% false-positive result in 53 benign lesions.

Several investigators have reported on their experience using HpD to treat tumors. Diamond and coworkers (14) reported destruction of experimental tumors in rats by exposure to white light after injection with hematoporphyrin. In 1976, Kelly and Snell (15) used HpD to treat a patient with bladder cancer and reported that 48 hours after treatment the superficial recurrent bladder carcinoma showed necrosis of several papillary tumors but the rest of bladder appeared undamaged. In that same year, Weishaupt and coworkers (16) demonstrated that the destruction of the tumors was initiated when singlet oxygen was produced by the absorption of the light energy by the HpD.

Dougherty and coworkers (17) reported complete or partial response in 111 of 113 cutaneous or subcutaneous malignant lesions treated with PDT using HpD as the sensitizer. Hayata and coworkers (18) reported on using fiberoptic bronchoscopic laser photoradiation for endobronchial tumors. Since then, numerous worldwide reports have suggested the validity of this form of therapy to treat malignancies (19-28).

In 1984, Dougherty and coworkers (29) reported that he had created a new dye by the fractionation of HpD and separation of a submixture that was designated DHEs and contained the active component of the HpD mixture. This product is now commercially known as Photofrin. Two years later, Dougherty's review of the world literature (30) stated that more than 3000 patients had been treated with PDT.

Beginning in 1986, phase III clinical trials were begun to establish the efficacy of PDT with DHE in treating lung and bladder cancers.

MECHANISM OF ACTION

Current research indicates that intravenously injected HpD or DHE disseminates to all cells and then is preferentially retained by tumor cells, reticuloendothelial cells, liver, spleen, kidney, and inflammatory tissue. After a varying period of time, more sensitizer remains in these tissues than in the adjacent normal tissue. The reason that the dye remains longer in tumor cells has not been established; it may be that the sensitizer cannot escape because tumors have no lymphatic mechanism.

Singlet oxygen is formed when the sensitizer is exposed to light energy. The singlet oxygen then oxidizes adjacent proteins in the cell. The site of action has been found at least on the mitochondria, cell wall, and endothelial cells in the tumor vasculature (31-34).

CLINICAL STUDIES

From April 1982 to July 1987, 222 patients were treated with PDT at this center. All patients have been followed until their death or until the time of this report. All had already received, refused, or were medically ineligible for surgery, ionizing radiation, and/or chemotherapy. The time from injection to treatment varied from 1–7 days, and the maximum number of injections to one patient was 10. A total of 355 injections were given, 172 with HpD and 183 with DHE. Patients experienced very few adverse effects from these injections. One patient experienced vomiting. Five experienced photosensitivity requiring treatment; four of these patients received corticosteroids and one required hospitalization. A total of 814 treatments were delivered; the maximum number of treatments to one patient was 16. Table 25.1 shows the breakdown of patients by tumor site.

Sensitizer

Initially, HpD was used (Photofrin I, PI) (Photofrin Medical, Inc., Cheektowaga, NY). Since 1984, dihematoporphyrin ether (DHE,

Table 25.1. Number of Patients Treated at Different Tumor Sites

Site	No. of Patients
Bile ducts	2
Bladder (urinary)	1
Colon metastasis	1
Breast	22
Chondrosarcoma	1
Colon	8
Rectum	2
Rectal stump	2
Perineal metastases	3
Pelvic metastases	1
Choroid	42
Melanoma	41
Oat cell	1
Esophagus	40
Adenocarcinoma	9
Melanoma	2
Squamous	24
Esophagus-stomach-adenocarcinoma	5
Gynecological	6
Head and neck	27
Adenocystic	1
Nasopharynx	1
Squamous	25
Lung	45
Adenocarcinoma	4
Cylindroma	1
Large cell	1
Oat cell	1
Poorly differentiated	1
Squamous	26
Undifferentiated	3
Metastatic	6
Pleura	1
Liposarcoma	2
Arm	1
Retroperitoneal	1
Skin	23
Basal cell	11
Bowen's	1
Melanoma	4
Squamous	7
Stomach	1

Photofrin II) has been used from Photomedica (Johnson & Johnson, Raritan, NJ).

Sensitizer dose has varied worldwide from 2.5–5.0 mg/kg of HpD. Most investigators are now using 2 mg/kg of DHE. Dougherty (personal communication, 1987) is currently investigating the use of 1 mg/kg of DHE with higher light doses to decrease the reaction in adjacent normal skin and decrease the solar photosensitivity, both of which occur in all patients. Standard doses for IV HpD of 3 mg/kg of body weight for all patients have been used, except those with melanoma of the choroid where 2.5 mg/kg was used. When using DHE, the dose is 2 mg/kg of body weight i.v. for all patients. Doses were calculated on a body surface area basis and found to be an average of 74 mg DHE/m^2 of body surface. However, the doses ranged from 59–91 mg/m^2, a twofold difference for the same amount of DHE given on a weight basis.

Technique

DHE is injected as a single bolus through a running IV of 5% glucose in Ringer's lactate, and the tumor area is treated with 630 ± 2 nm light from the dye laser 2–5 days after the injection. Although HpD and DHE absorb more light energy in the near-ultraviolet wavelengths (405 nm) than the red wavelength (630 nm), the latter penetrates tissue deeper and a biological effect can be obtained to a depth of 5–15 mm, depending on the color and density of the tissue (35).

Light

A Kodak projector with a red filter (Corning 2418) was used as the light source for the first five patients treated (21, 22). Since then, a 20-W argon (Spectra Physics, model 171) tunable dye (Spectra Physics, model 375) laser system has been used to generate 630 ± 2 nm light. Rhodamine-B dye was used initially (Exciton, Dayton, OH) without the tuning wedge, but since 1984, kiton red (Exciton Dayton, Ohio) has been used with a single plate birefrigent filter because the latter is more stable and does not have to be changed as often as the rhodamine-B.

Light is delivered through 200- to 600-μ quartz fibers from the dye laser to the treated area. For the reaction to occur, the light must reach the target. The ends of the fibers are modified in accordance with the treated area. A straight-cleaved fiber delivers a nonhomogeneous light with a Gaussian type of curve, resulting in higher power densities centrally and, therefore, nonuniform light delivery. A lens on the end of the fiber is used to smooth out the light distribution for surface irradiation. A cylinder-diffusing fiber delivers the light 360° perpendicular to the axis of the fiber and can be made in lengths varying up to 3 cm. These fibers are used for interstitial treatments (inserted directly into the tumor) or for treating intraluminal tumors as in the bronchus, esophagus, biliary tree, colon, vagina, etc. A re-

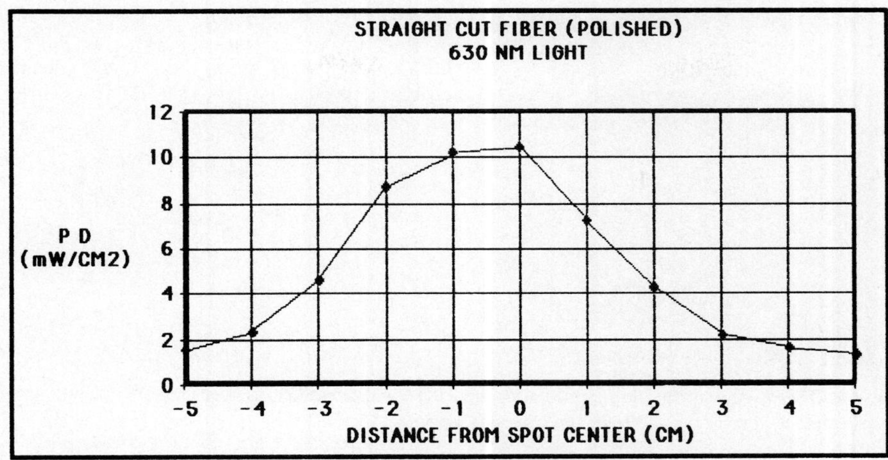

Figure 25.1. Nonhomogenous power densities across the light spot from a straight-cleaved fiber.

trobubar lens is used to irradiate the posterior wall of the choroid. This directs the light backward. Bulb tips that deliver the light spherically are used to treat hollow cavities, such as the bladder or excised hollow tumor beds.

The photodynamic effect is a function of the amount of sensitizer present in the target atoms and the amount of light energy absorbed by the sensitizer. For the same amount of sensitizer, the reaction is initially reciprocal when power densities are used below a thermal damage threshold and is dependent on the product of the power density and the length of exposure (Bunsen-Roscoe law). Biological systems, however, will undergo changes as the light exposure continues and the absorption and light transmission characteristics will change during therapy.

Several factors determine the correct and standardized measurement of the power output and the power density. These must be understood because such a determination is critical for effective therapy.

1. Homogeneity of the light source: The light delivered from an unmodified quartz tip fiber, even when polished, has a Gaussian type of distribution with a higher power in the center of the spot than the periphery. Figure 25.1 shows the power density across such a spot. This causes overtreatment to the center and undertreatment to the periphery. The clinical effect is seen in Figure 25.2, which shows a central area of necrosis. This type of light distribution also occurs with projectors. The light distribution can be greatly smoothed out by putting a small lens on the end of the quartz fiber as shown in Figure 25.3.
2. Distance from the light source: The light from the quartz fiber tip and lens radiates as a cone. Therefore, the power density increases with distance, and the top of a tumor or curved body surface receives more energy over a given time than that further away. Figure 25.3 shows the change in power density that occurs when the distance of the light source is altered by only a few centimeters.
3. Angle of incidence of the light to the tissue: The light from the quartz fiber tip diverges from a point source so that the tissue directly under the source is perpendicular (normal) to the light rays, whereas that in the periphery receives light at an angle. Thus, even with a homogenous lens light source, the peripheral tissue still does not receive the same amount of light as does the center of the treatment spot.
4. Radiometer and technique for measuring power: The different techniques used to measure power densities are not equivalent and can vary by up to 20%. Therefore, reports of response to specific light doses cannot be compared unless the exact technique of measurement is known. In fact, most of the research so far has involved a nonhomogeneous light source, which is a particularly inadequate method.

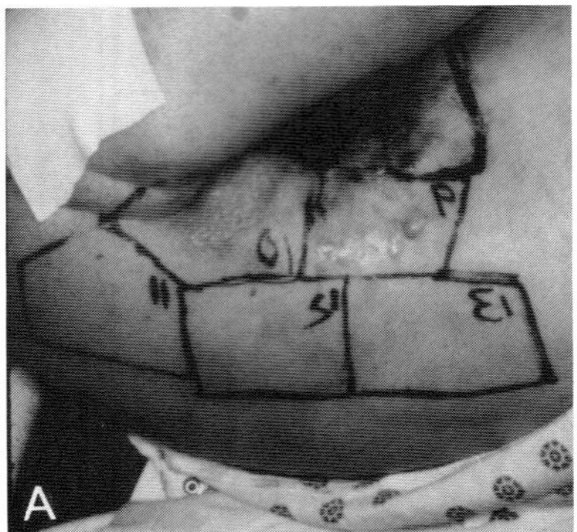

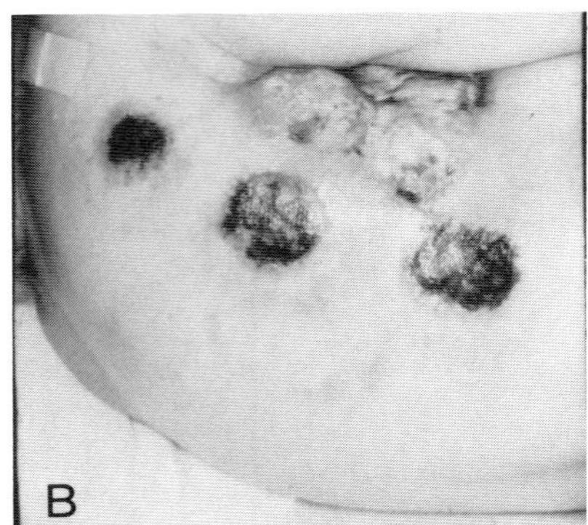

Figure 25.2. **A**, The reaction of the skin immediately after PDT with a straight-cleaved fiber. **B**, Nonhomogenous fiber results in overtreatment in center of the light spot, causing necrosis.

Radiometer Techniques

Surface Irradiation with Lens Fibers. The equation for this type of irradiation is as follows:

Power density = power/unit area (mW/cm^2)
Light dosage = power density × exposure time = Joules (J)/cm^2
Joules = number of W × number of sec
Reciprocity = power density × time

The photochemical reaction for a given amount of sensitizer depends on the number of J delivered/cm^2. The thermal changes in the tissue are mainly a function of the power density of mW/cm^2. The total power output of the tip is measured with an integrating sphere radiometer or a Coherent 210 radiometer. This is divided by the spot size to give the average power density, assuming the light is homogeneous. An alternative method is to measure the power density directly at the surface being treated with either a Yellow Springs radiometer or the Coherent 210 radiometer.

Cylinder Diffusing Fibers. The total power output of the fiber tip is measured with an integrating sphere radiometer. This measurement is divided by the length of the diffuser to provide the

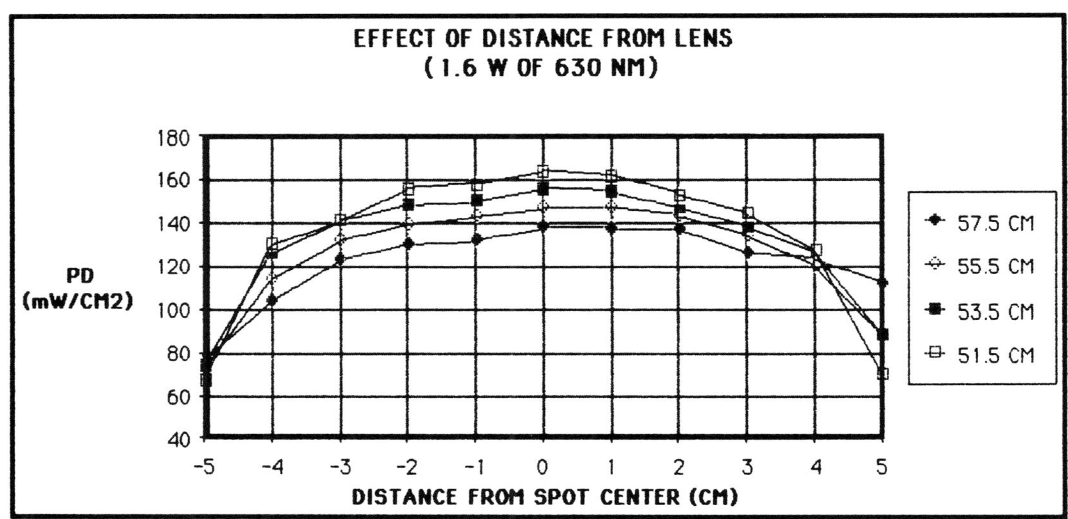

Figure 25.3. Power density across the light spot with lens on the end of the fiber and the effect of varying the distance from the fiber tip to the target.

power/cm length of diffuser. The number of J delivered/cm of diffuser length is calculated from the length of exposure time.

Bulb Fibers. The total power output is measured with the integrating sphere radiometer. The volume of the area being treated is measured and the total number of J delivered/cm^2 of surface is calculated making the assumptions that the bulb is held in the center of the hollow area, the area is spherical, and the light distribution from the bulb fiber is homogeneous.

Skin and Subcutaneous Tumor Treatments

The first 27 consecutive patients with skin or subcutaneous tumors treated with PDT after sensitization of the tumors with i.v. HPD or DHE were evaluated. Fifteen had metastatic breast cancer, three had melanoma, one had liposarcoma, and 14 and 25 basal or squamous skin cancers. All had failed on, refused, or were inelligible for conventional surgery, chemotherapy, and/or ionizing radiation therapy. Forty-five injections and 72 treatment sessions were used to treat 248 separate areas. A treatment session might involve treating up to 13 separate areas, and each area could be up to 10 × 10 cm with multiple tumors.

Tumors response was assessed according to the following categories: complete response (CR)—no visible abnormality, negative biopsy and cytology; partial response (PR)—degree of obstruction or size of tumor reduced over 50%; some response (SR)—degree of obstruction or size of tumor reduced 20–50%; and progression (PROG)—degree of obstruction or size of tumor reduced by less than 20%. One month after a treatment session, 67% of the areas were rated as CR and 26% were rated PR. Fifteen patients who had CR were followed for more than 1 year. Of 31 lesions rated as CR at 1 month, 15 (48%) continued as a CR with no evidence of new or residual tumor in the treated area. Two patients who received adjuvant PDT at the time of surgical excision of their tumors has histologically proven tumor at the margins of resection (one liposarcoma, one melanoma). Twelve and 24 months after PDT they had no evidence of recurrence. CR have lasted in some patients for as long as 48 months.

The selectivity of the therapy can be best seen on patients with skin cancers. Figure 25.4 shows a patient with metastatic breast cancer. Figure 25.5 shows the light exposure and Figure 25.6 shows the reaction to PDT. All areas in the rectangles received the same amount of light dosage and only the tumors have become reddish brown. Figure 25.7 shows the reaction of the same tumor 6 months after PDT.

Shown in Figure 25.8 is a patient with squamous cell cancer of the eyelid. Two years after treatment with external surface PDT, there was no evidence of disease (Fig. 25.9). The patient is alive with no recurrence of disease 4 years after treatment.

Metastatic basal cell cancer is shown in Figure 25.10. The tumor was treated with interstitial irradiation (Fig. 25.11), which resulted in complete absence of the tumor 3 months later (Fig. 25.12).

Esophageal Tumors

From a review of the first 25 patients treated for tumors of the esophagus, it was established that PDT entails essentially a prolonged flexible esophagoscopy, which can be performed with minimal risk to the patient who is placed under IV sedation (Fig. 25.13) (36). One month after the first treatment of all 25 patients, there was an average increase of the esophageal grade of 18 points (after Stoller et al. [37]), the Karnofsky Performance Scale (KPS) increased an average of 10 points, and patients' weights remained stable. The average minimum opening increased from 5–11 mm.

Completely obstructed patients who were otherwise active were able to eat popcorn, toast, steak, etc. until just before their deaths. The average survival of all patients was 6.8 months. All except two with preexisting tracheoesophageal fistulaes and one who received a cervical esophagostomy were able to swallow at least liquids before they died. Three patients with a KPS of 30 or less never left the hospital. However, they were able to swallow at least liquids until their deaths. Figure 25.14 shows complete esophageal obstruction, which was relieved 2 days after PDT, and the result 2 months after PDT. At this time, the patient was able to eat a regular diet. Figure 25.15 shows the results of a barium swallow before and 2 months after PDT for squamous cancer of the esophagus. The patient progressed from taking clear liquids to a regular diet.

Lung Tumors

Forty-nine tumor sites in the first 31 consecutive patients with tracheobronchial malignant neoplasms treated with PDT were analyzed. After

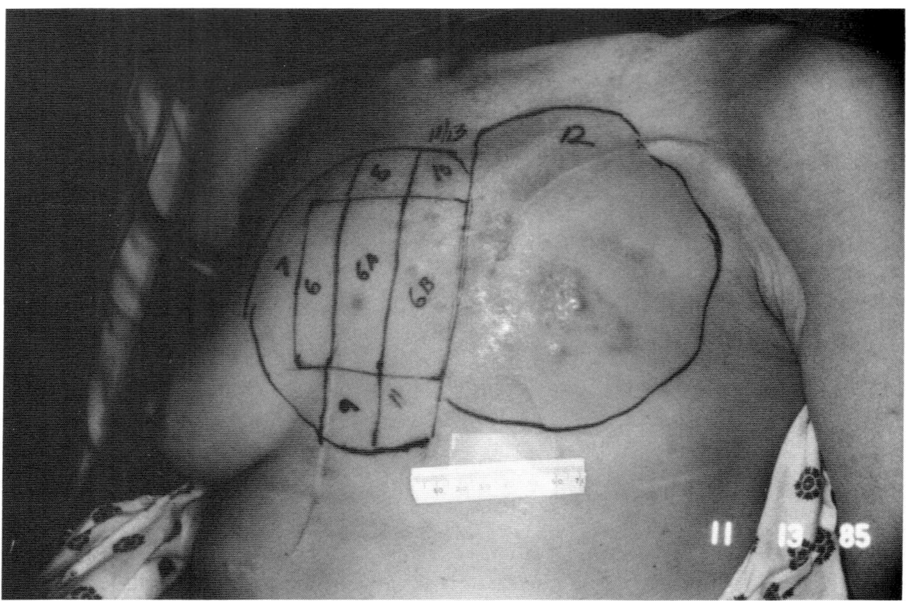

Figure 25.4. Metastatic cutaneous and subcutaneous breast cancer.

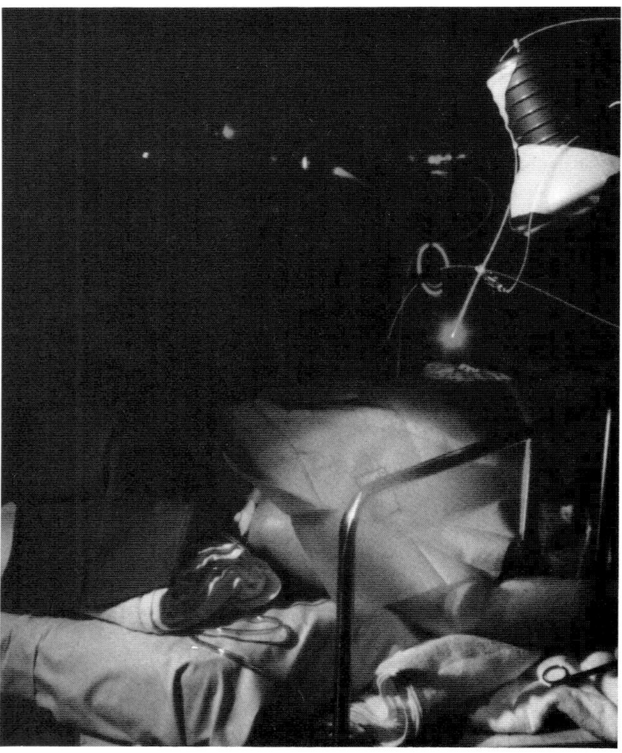

Figure 25.5. The technique of external irradiation.

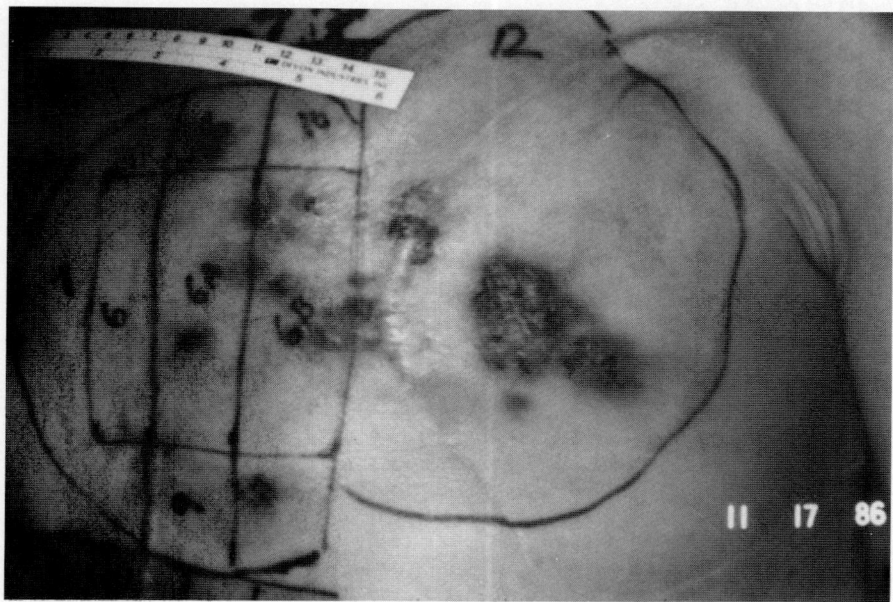

Figure 25.6. Three days post-PDT.

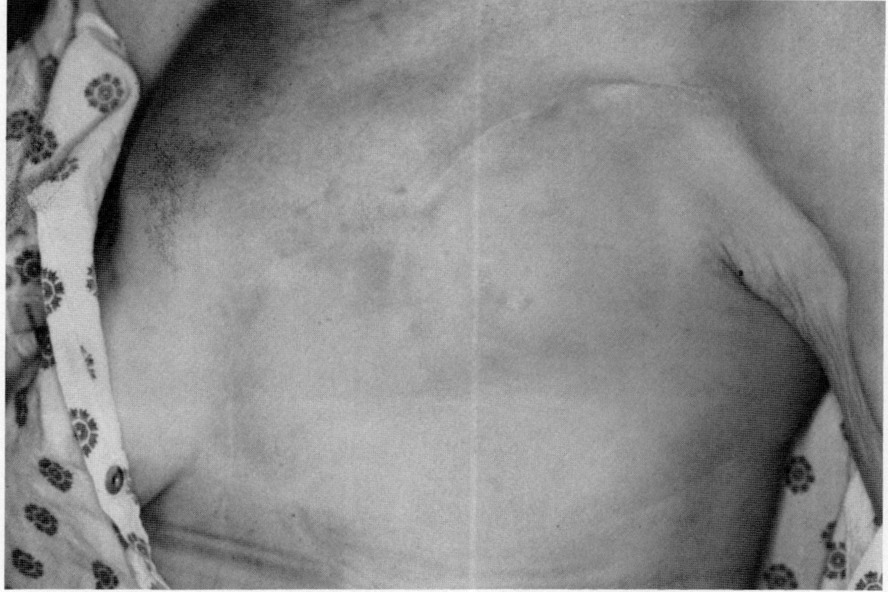

Figure 25.7. Six months post-PDT.

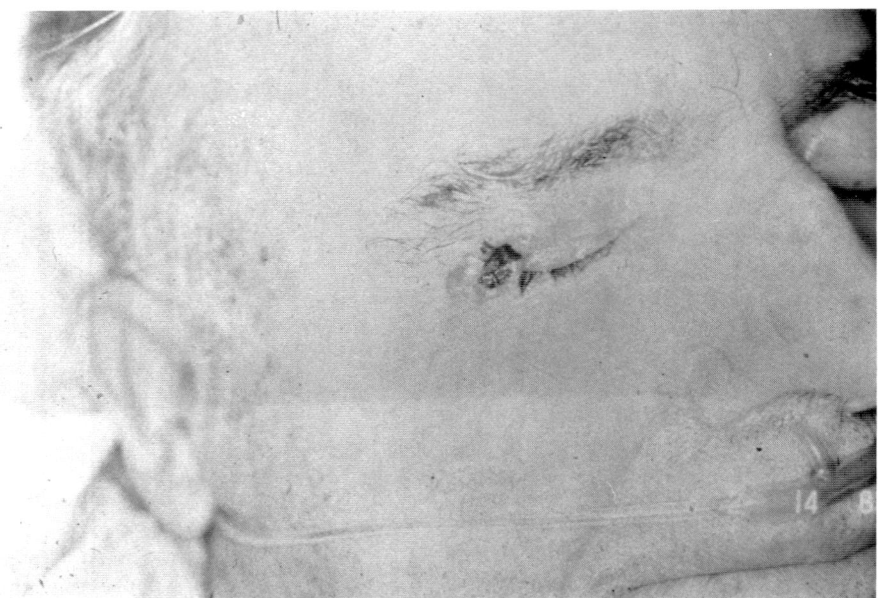

Figure 25.8. Squamous cell cancer of the eyelid before treatment.

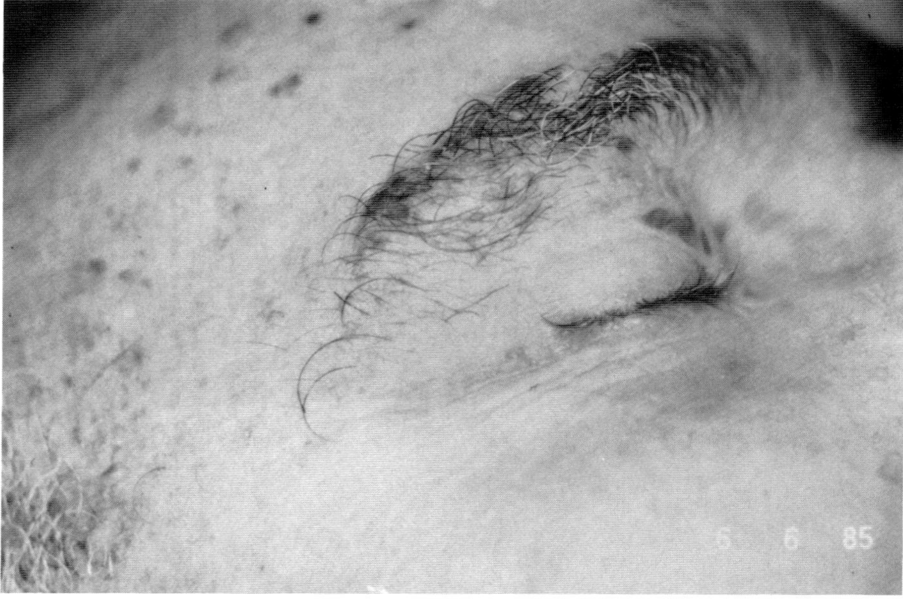

Figure 25.9. No evidence of disease 2 years after treatment. The patients is now 5 years posttreatment with no evidence of recurrence.

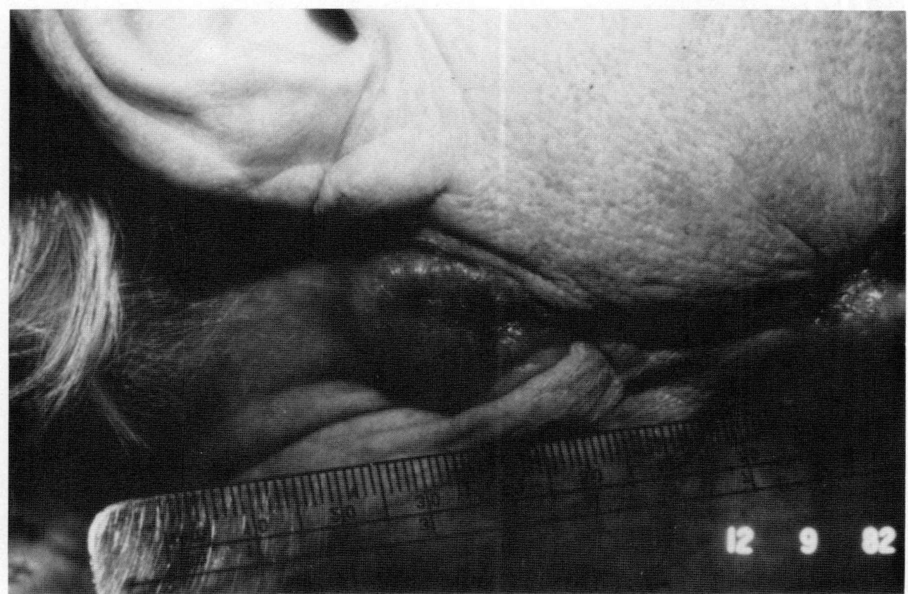

Figure 25.10. Metastatic basal cell cancer.

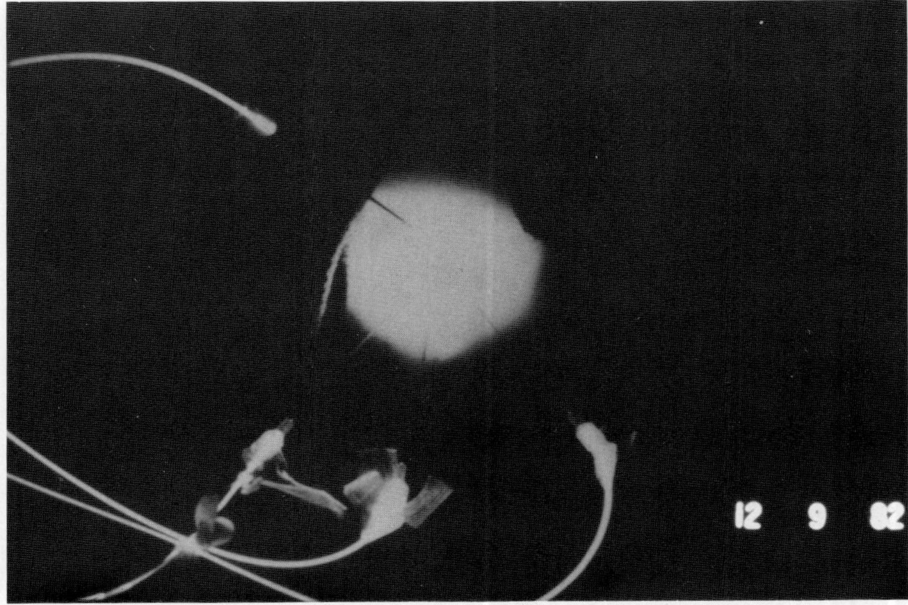

Figure 25.11. Technique of interstitial irradiation with fibers inserted into tumor.

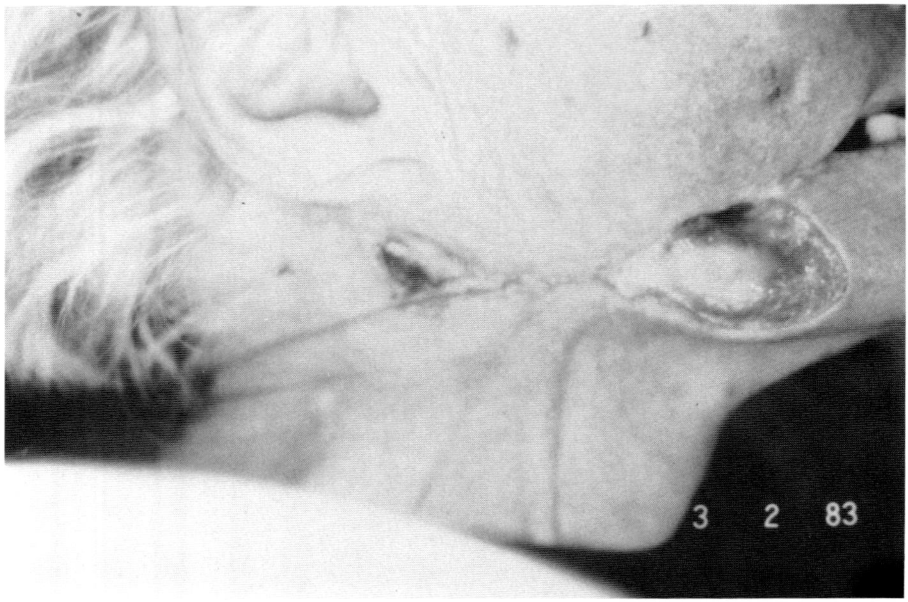

Figure 25.12. Complete absence of tumor 3 months after treatment.

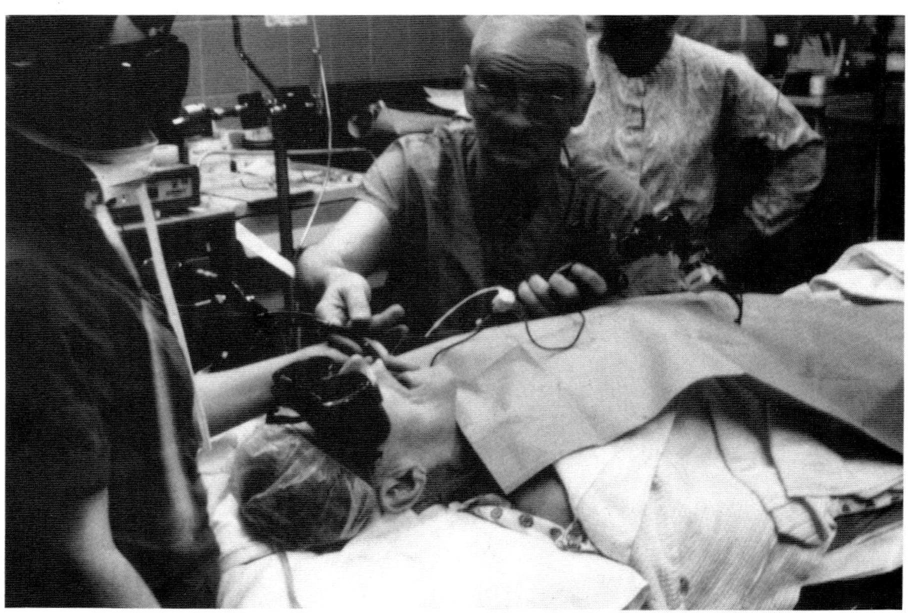

Figure 25.13. A fiber is passed through the esophagoscope to treat an intralumenal tumor.

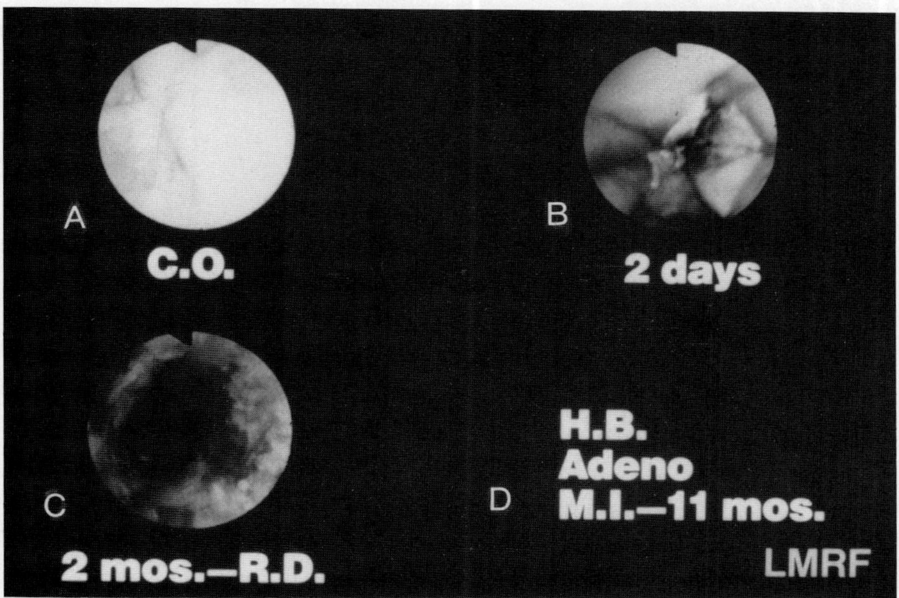

Figure 25.14. **A**, Complete obstruction *(C.O.)* of the esophagus by adenocarcinoma. **B**, The reaction 2 days after PDT. **C**, Reaction 2 months after PDT, at which time the patient was eating a regular diet and maintaining his weight. **D**, The patient was treated three times over the ensuing 11 months and died of a myocardial infarction.

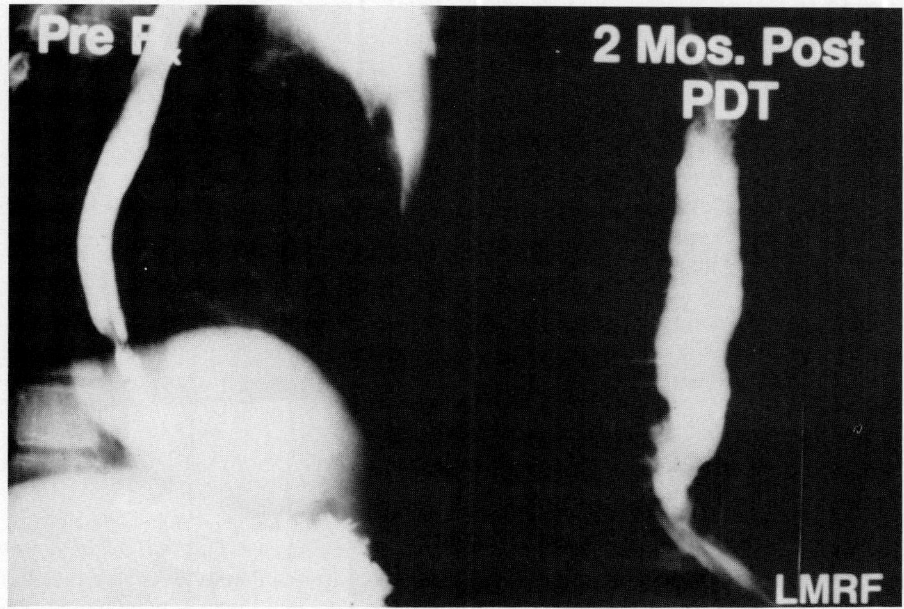

Figure 25.15. *Left*, Barium swallow before treatment in a patient with squamous cell cancer of the esophagus. *Right*, Barium swallow 2 months after PDT.

Table 25.2. Outcome of Endobronchial Sites with Complete Response[a]

Histology	Site	1 Month after PDT Recurrence (Months)	Last seen (Months)	Comment
Squamous	RUL	0	13	Expired—COPD (NED)
Squamous (TIS)	RUL	0	34	Alive—NED
Colon	LUL	9-12	13	Expired—Liver metastases
Squamous	RLL; TR	0	4	Expired—Aspir pneumonia
Breast	RIB; RUL	0	7	Expired—metastases
Undifferentiated	RIB; RUL	6	17	Expired—disease

[a]Abbreviations used: Aspir—aspiration; COPD—chronic obstructive pulmonary disease; LMB—left main bronchus; LUL—left upper lobe bronchus; NED—no evidence of disease; RIB—right intermediate bronchus; RLL—right lower lobe bronchus; RUL—right upper lobe bronchus; TIS—carcinoma in situ; TR—trachea.

sensitization with i.v. HpD or DHE 630 nm of light from a tunable sensitizer argon light system was delivered to the tumor site through the biopsy channel of a flexible bronchoscope using topical anesthesia and i.v. sedation.

Depending on the length of the tumor or number of sites treated and the light dose delivered, the endoscopic treatment lasted 20–45 min.

Before or at 1 month after each treatment, tumor response was evaluated with the following results: 37% of tumors treated achieved CR, 55% achieved PR, 4% achieved SR, and 4% of tumors were categorized as PROG. Complete follow-up was achieved in all patients. Follow-up of at least 3 months of eight patients with 11 sites that resulted in CR after treatment is presented in Table 25.2. Five patients, with seven treated sites achieving a status of CR, were followed more than 6 months. Two tumors recurred in one patient at 6 months, and one tumor recurred in another patient between 9 and 12 months after treatment. One patient with carcinoma in situ had no recurrence at 34 months. Figure 25.16 shows the tumor before treatment and 2 days later. Four other CR sites in three patients who were followed from 3–6 months have not recurred. All patients who died had been bronchoscoped within 1 month of their deaths.

Clinical effect was evaluated 1 month after treatment by comparing KPS, dyspnea level, oxygen requirement, and presence of symptoms. Of the 31 patients, 68% had clinical improvement in at least one parameter and 48% in two or more parameters. Five severely disabled patients with a KPS of 40 or less (average, 30) benefited substantially from PDT because a major component of their disability was related to the endobronchial disease. At 1 month after treatment, these individuals had an average KPS of 80. One patient's status improved from bedrest with continuous oxygen to ambulatory without oxygen for 12 months. Figure 25.17 shows metastatic colon cancer protruding from the left upper lobe and the reaction 2 days after PDT. The resulting fibrinous plug must be removed. The lower photographs show the staples in the patient's left upper lobe from a resection performed 2 years earlier. Figure 25.18 shows metastatic breast cancer completely obstructing the right upper lobe and causing hemoptysis and cough. After two PDT treatments, both the right upper lobe and right inferior bronchus appeared completely normal and were negative on biopsy and bronchoscopy.

There were no instances of pulmonary hemorrhage during treatment or toilet bronchoscopy. Nor did any patients experience performations or fistula formation. However, several patients did develop strictures when PDT encompassed normal bronchus. Two patients became completely obstructed with scar tissue, which was negative for tumor on biopsy, brushing, and washings for cytology. Both patients improved symptomatically. Coughing stopped, and one patient is now alive 16 months posttreatment. Perhaps in patients where tumor is already compromising a lobe, PDT may be seen as a way to isolate the tumor to that lobe, thus preventing endobronchial spread and ensuing obstruction of other bronchi, as well as the symptoms of cough and hemoptysis.

Gynecological Tumors

Five patients with various gynecological neoplasms were treated with PDT using 630-nm light delivered from an argon dye laser system (38). A patient with multifocal squamous cell cancer of the vagina had no evidence of disease 15 months after her first PDT treatment. Autopsy 9 months

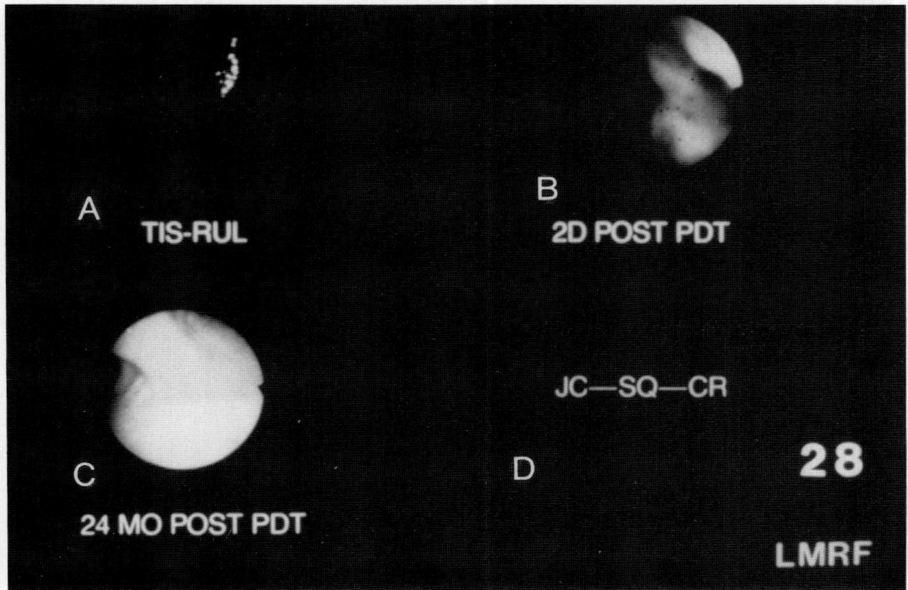

Figure 25.16. **A**, Carcinoma in situ of the right upper lobe *(RUL)*. **B**, Reaction 2 days after PDT. **C**, The bronchus 2 years after PDT showing complete response *(CR)*. **D**, The patient *(JC)* maintained this status for 34 months.

after the first treatment of another patient with multifocal invasive cancer of the vagina and parametrium showed no evidence of tumor on the surface of the vagina. Eight months after treatment of an 8 × 12 cm area of Bowen's disease of the vulva and thigh, there was no evidence of disease. Bowen's disease of the vulva with exophytic squamous cancer just above the rectum is shown in Figure 25.19; the same lesion is depicted with negative biopsies 8 months post-PDT (Fig. 25.20).

Vaginal bleeding from breast cancer metastatic to the endometrium was controlled by one treatment until the patient expired 5 months later from her disease. Adenocarcinoma metastatic to the vaginal cuff showed partial response when vaginectomy was performed 5 weeks after PDT.

Melanomas of the Choroid

Twenty-five patients were treated with PDT with follow-up of 6–48 months. There was a 60% CR; 24% PR; 12% PROG; and 4% had no response (metastatic oat cell). There have been four deaths due to metastases and one death from a ruptured aneurysm (23).

Head and Neck Tumors

Twenty-four patients with recurrent and/or metastatic cancers were treated with PDT using HpD or DHE to study the feasibility of this technique. This demonstrated that PDT is a viable treatment for head and neck cancer and that the toxic reactions and complications are minimal (28).

DISCUSSION

Behavior of Sensitizer

Based on this clinical experience with PDT, several observations can be made. First, no absolute time frame has been established in which all of the sensitizer will be cleared from normal tissue. The author's clinical experience has demonstrated the presence of sensitizer in normal tissue several days after injection. In addition, sensitizer remains in the tumor tissue for many days after treatment. CR was achieved in a patient up to 7 days after one injection. Thus, it must be concluded that retreatment can be performed at least up to 7 days after injection of DHE.

Hyperthermia Combined with HpD

From temperature measurements made at the skin at the time of treatment of that area in pa-

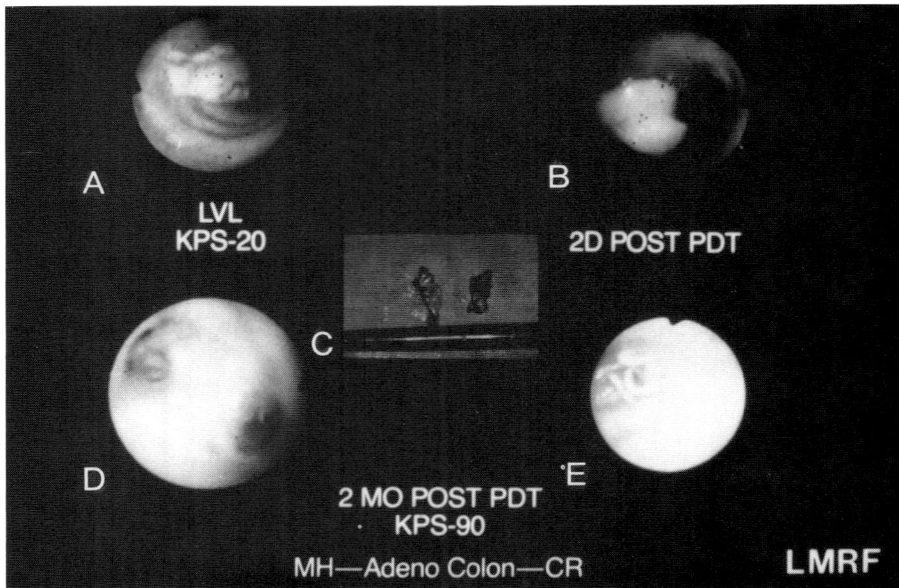

Figure 25.17. **A**, Metastatic colon cancer protruding from left upper lobe occluding the left main bronchus. **B**, Reaction 2 days after PDT. **C**, Fibrinous plug that must be removed at toilet bronchoscopy. **D**, Bifurcation of the left main bronchus showing the left upper lobe and lower lobe. **E**, Left upper lobe showing visible staples from previous left upper lobectomy with no evidence of tumor 2 months after PDT. Patient was originally on continuous oxygen at bedrest and survived for 13 months when she expired from liver metastases. Most of this time, she was ambulatory and asymptomatic.

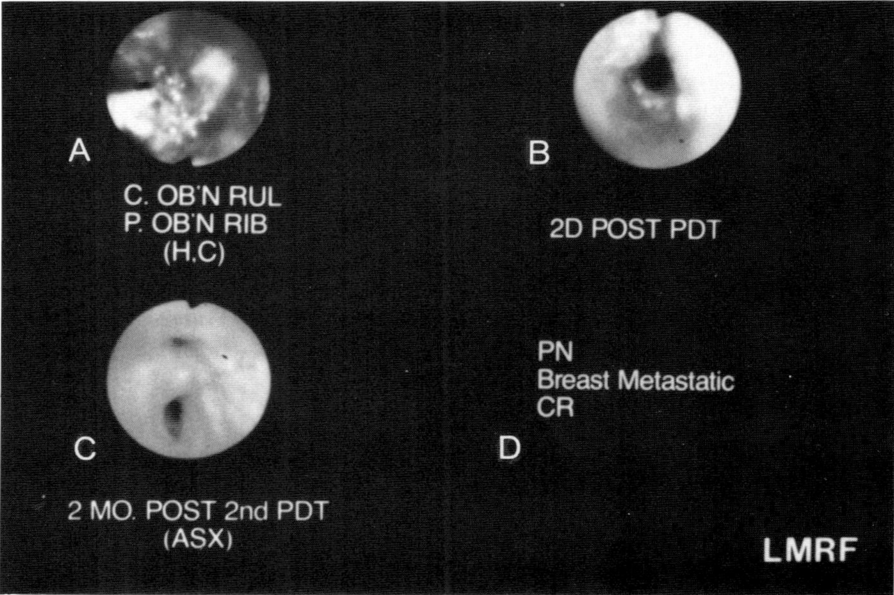

Figure 25.18. **A**, A fiber in the right intermediate bronchus *(RIB)* of a patient with metastatic breast cancer with a complete occlusion of the right upper lobe *(RUL)* and hemoptysis and cough. **B**, Reaction 2 days after PDT. Patient was retreated. **C**, Right upper lobe and right intermediate bronchus completely open 2 months after second PDT treatment. **D**, Patient was asymptomatic.

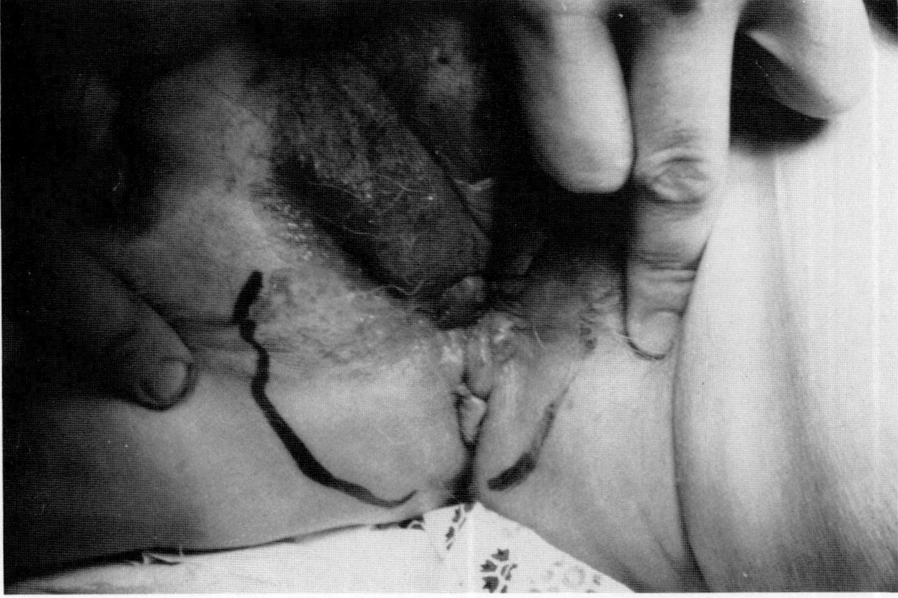

Figure 25.19. A 76-year-old patient with Bowen's disease of vulva and exophytic lesion just above the anus, shown just before PDT.

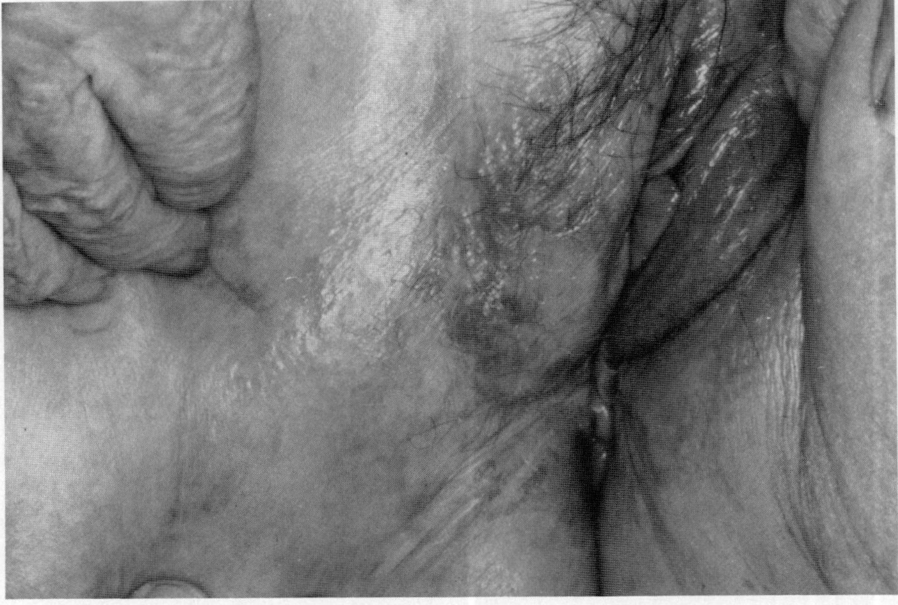

Figure 25.20. Eight months after PDT, exophytic lesion is absent and biopsies are negative.

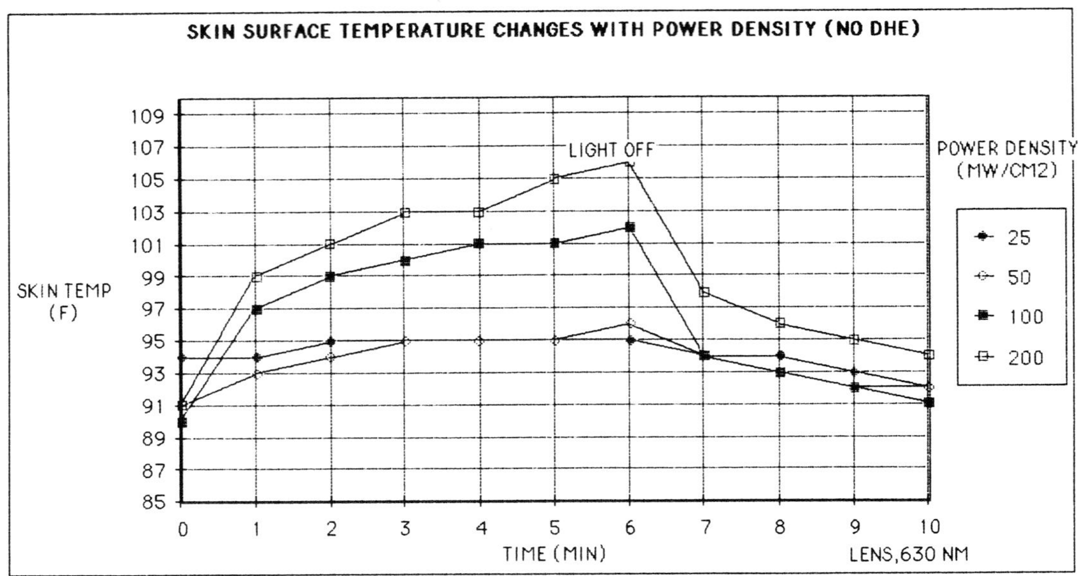

Figure 25.21. Temperature rise in normal skin without sensitizer and subjected to various power densities.

tients with skin tumors, a direct relationship of temperature rise with power density was found. Figure 25.21 shows the temperature rise in normal skin that has not been injected with DHE. An immediate rise in temperature occurs when the skin is subjected to light. The temperature then levels off and immediately falls when the light is turned off.

In 1960, Lipson and Baldes (39) found that heat combined with PDT using HpD as the sensitizer in white mice produced a higher mortality than heat or PDT alone. They established that the heat must be given after the PDT and not the reverse. They also showed the reaction to PDT was greater when the PDT was given 3 hours after the injection than when performed immediately after the injection. Waldow and coworkers (40) reported the effects of hyperthermia combined with PDT in tumors of mice. They found a 5° C rise at the tumor base with 150 mW/cm^2 of 630-nm light. In addition, more damage in terms of tumor necrosis occurred when hyperthermia induced by a microwave system was given immediately after PDT than with PDT or hyperthermia alone.

The power density ranges in which surface PDT (20–100 mW/cm^2) is usually performed do not contribute much to the thermal effect. Figure 25.22 shows skin temperature changes at different power densities in patients injected with DHE. Thus, the concerns of Lipson and Baldes (39) and Waldow and coworkers (40) do not seem relevant. During or near the end of some treatments, patients receiving power densities of 25–75 mW/cm^2 have complained of a burning sensation. However, the temperature remained stable and below 99° F. Apparently, this sensation is due to the photodynamic reaction and not to the thermal effect. Power densities above 20–100 mW/cm^2 do increase the temperature (107°F for 200 mW/cm^2), and patients are uncomfortable if the density is above 300 mW/cm^2.

Light Transmission

The transmission of 630-nm light through various tumors and tissues was measured. Freshly obtained operative specimens were collected at surgery and placed in iced saline and within 2 hours the color of the tissue was measured with a Munsell color chart and the density of the tissue was measured. The light was generated by an argon dye laser system and transmitted through a quartz fiber modified with a cylindrical diffusing tip. A leakage meter was attached to the fiber and calibrated to the power output from the cylindrical fiber measured by an integrating sphere radiometer (35). The cylindrical diffusing fiber was then inserted into a core of tissue that was placed in the glass test tube in the integrating sphere. The total

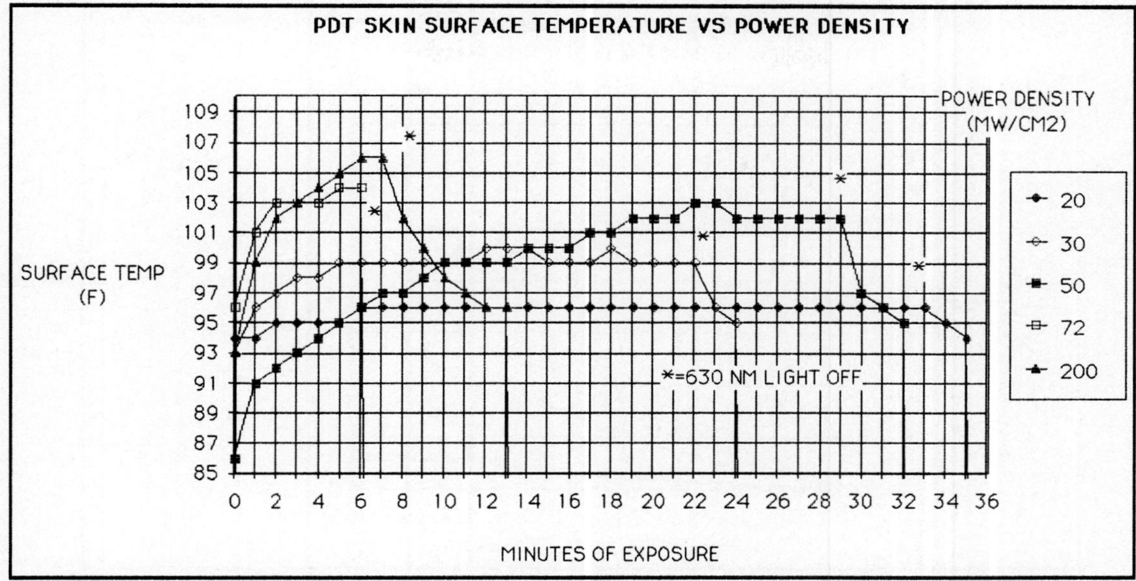

Figure 25.22. Skin temperature measurements of patients with DHE, showing the effect of different power densities.

power transmitted through the tissue was then measured with the integrating sphere at varying leakage meter readings. From this information, the transmission through a fixed thickness and volume of various tissues for known fiber output powers was compared with the type, color, and density of the tissue. Figures 25.23 and 25.24 show light transmission through different tissues from a cylinder fiber set at different power densities.

PDT as an Intraoperative Adjuvant

If reasonable precautions are taken, no serious adverse effects should result from the operating room environment during adjuvant PDT performed when the subcutaneous tissue, abdomen, and thoracic cavity have been exposed to the operating room lights for periods of several hours. Care should be taken not to use the high intensity lights before the exposed skin, including the face, is draped. Normal operating room draping suffices except for the laser light, which can penetrate through two thicknesses of standard operating room towels. Concern about liver exposure to the operating room lights appears unjustified because the penetration of even high intensity 630-nm light through liver is very limited.

The following observations can be made about the effects of sensitizer given before or after other procedures.

1. Scars and incisions made up to at least 6 months before the injection of sensitizer will have a greater reaction to light treatment than the adjacent normal skin.
2. Wounds made and closed either with a CO_2 laser or scalpel 2–5 days after the injection of the sensitizer heal no differently than wounds made when sensitizer has not been injected. This observation applies even to skin grafts.
3. Tumors treated with the Nd:YAG laser 2–20 days after injection with sensitizer react no differently than tumors not injected with sensitizer.
4. Incisions and exposed tissue made after the injection of the sensitizer and then treated with PDT do not react as violently as do open ulcerations that were present before the injection of the sensitizer.
5. Incisions in the skin made at the time of PDT treatment do not react differently from the adajcent normal skin.

Comparison of PDT to Nd:YAG and CO_2 Lasers

PDT has both advantages and disadvantages over Nd:YAG and CO_2 laser therapies. The major

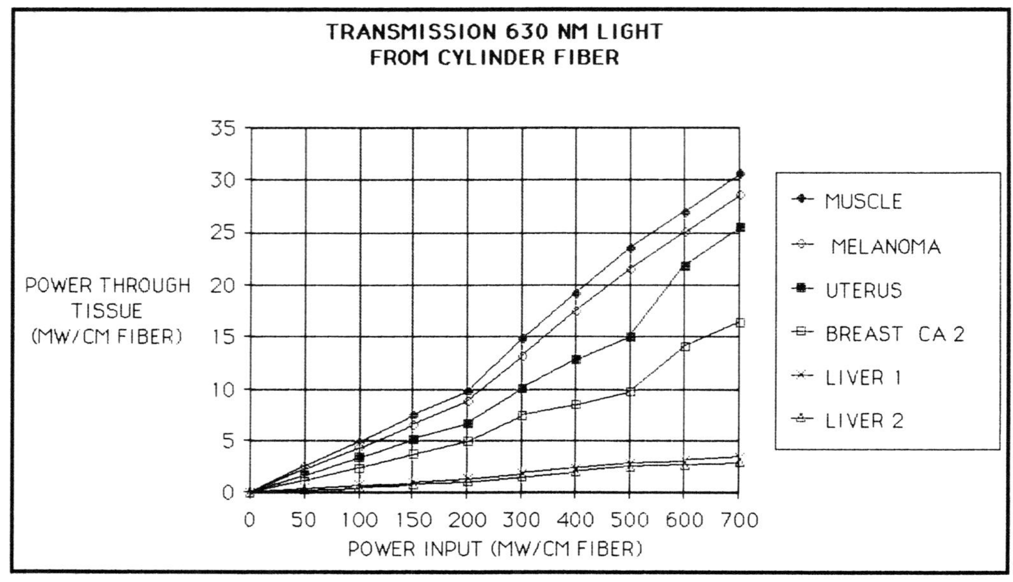

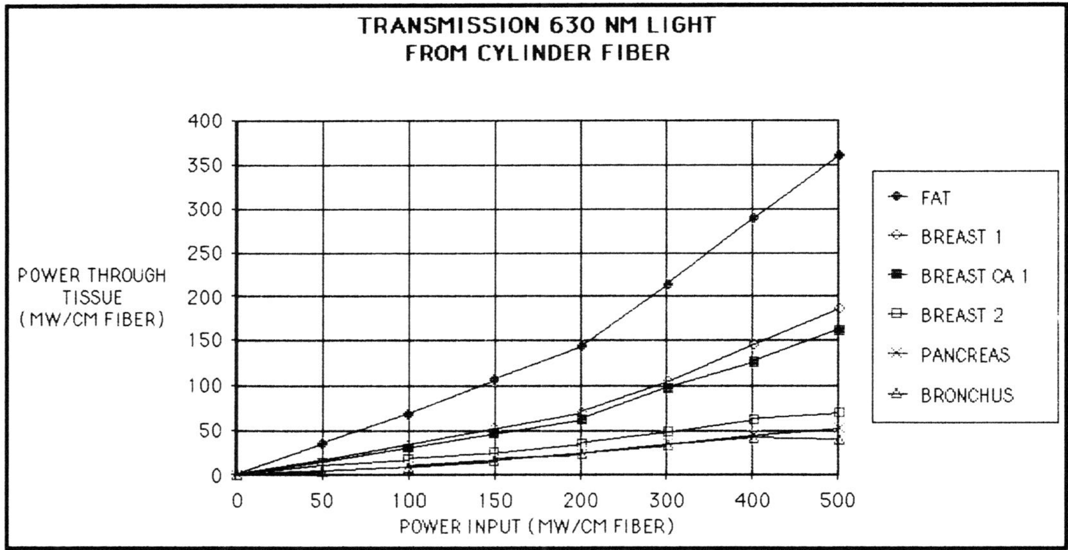

Figures 25.23 and 25.24. Light transmission from cylinder fiber inserted into freshly obtained tissue placed into a glass test tube, which was then inserted into an integrating sphere radiometer. Transmission obviously depends greatly on the color and density of the tissue with very little penetrating the dark, dense liver.

disadvantage of PDT is that it is inappropriate as a first treatment for patients with acute conditions, such those in repiratory distress, since a minimum of 2 days is required between injection of the dye and treatment. Moreover, PDT may produce edema, which in some patients, would be life-threatening. Advantages of PDT include the following points.

1. Some investigators (41–43) have reported pulmonary hemorrhage to be a major complication during the use of the Nd:YAG laser. The author has encountered no such complication with PDT.
2. PDT creates a fibrinous plug that often can be lifted easily off the bronchus in large pieces at toilet bronchoscopy a few days after treat-

ment. The Nd:YAG laser typically produces a burn with charred and coagulated tissue that is difficult to tease out piecemeal.

3. Unlike the fiber used with the Nd:YAG laser, the fiber for PDT can be inserted blindly into the tumor for treatment without fear of burning a hole into an adjacent vessel.
4. Unlike both CO_2 and Nd:YAG lasers, PDT does not produce endobronchial smoke, which, when combined with the decreased PO_2 and pH and increased PCO_2 may contribute to the complications of myocardial infarction as reported by Dumon et al. (44).

REFERENCES

1. Raab O. Uber die wirkung fluorescierendes stoffe and infusorien. Z Biol 1900; 39:524.
2. Tappeiner H, Jodlbauer A. Die sensibilizierende wirkung fluorescierender substanzen. In FCW Vogel, Ed. Gesammelte Untersuchungen uber die photodynamische. Leipzig: Erscheinung, 1907.
3. Haussman W. The sensitizing action of hematoporphyrin. Biochem Z 1911; 30:176.
4. Meyer-Betz F. Untersuchungen uber die biologische (photodynamische) wirkung des hematoporphyrins and ander derivate des blut-and gallen-farbstoffe. Dtsch Arch Clin Med 1913; 112:476.
5. Policard A. Etudes sur les aspects offerts par des tumerurs experimentales examinees a la luminere de Woods. Compt Rend Soc Biol 1924; 91:1423-1428.
6. Blum HF. Photodynamic Action and Diseases Caused by Light. New York: Rhineholt Publishing Corp., 1941.
7. Auler H, Banzer G. Untersuchungen uber die rolle der porphyrine bei geschwul stranken menschen and tieren. Z Krebsforsch 1942; 53:65.
8. Figge FHJ, Weiland GS, Manganiello LOJ. Cancer detection and therapy. Affinity of neoplastic, embryonic, and traumatized tissues for porphyrins and metalloporphyrins. Proc Soc Exp Biol Med 1948; 68:181-188.
9. Rassmussen-Taxdal DS, Ward GE, Figge FHJ. Fluorescence of human lymphatic and cancer tissues following high doses of intravenous hematoporphyrin. Cancer 1955; 1:78-81.
10. Lipson RL, Baldes EJ. The photodynamic properties of a particular hematoporphyrin derivative. Arch Dermatol 1960; 82:517-520.
11. Lipson RL, Baldes EJ, Olsen AM. Hematoporphyrin derivative: A new aid for endoscopic detection of malignant disease. J Thorac Cardiovasc Surg 1961; 42:623-629.
12. Lipson RL, Gray MJ, Baldes EJ. Hematoporphyrin derivative for detection and management of cancer. Proceedings of the Ninth International Cancer Congress, 1966, p. 323.
13. Gregorie HB Jr, Horger EO, Ward JL, Green JF, Richards T, Robertson HC Jr, Stevenson TB: Hematoporphyrin-derivative fluorescence in malignant neoplasms. Ann Surg 1968; 167:820-828.
14. Diamond I, McDonagh AF, Wilson CB, Granelli SG, Nielsen S, Jaenicke R. Photodynamic therapy of malignant tumours. Lancet 1972; 2:1175-1177.
15. Kelly JF, Snell ME. Hematoporphyrin derivative: A possible aid in the diagnosis and therapy of carcinoma of the bladder. J Urol 1976; 115:150-151.
16. Weishaupt KR, Gomer CJ, Dougherty TJ. Identification of singlet oxygen as the cytotoxic agent in photoinactivation of a murine tumor. Cancer Res 1976; 36:2326-2329.
17. Dougherty TJ, Kaufman JE, Goldfarb A, Weishaupt KR, Boyle D, Mittleman A. Photoradiation therapy for the treatment of malignant tumors. Cancer Res 1978; 38:2628-2635.
18. Hayata Y, Kato H, Konaka C, Ono J, Takizawa N. Hematoporphyrin derivative and laser photoradiation in the treatment of lung cancer. Chest 1982; 81:269-277.
19. Ward BG, Forbes IJ, Cowled PA, McEvoy NM, Cox LW. The treatment of vaginal recurrences of gynecologic malignancy with phototherapy following hematoporphyrin derivative pretreatment. Am J Obstet Gynecol 1982; 142:356-357.
20. Wile AG, Dahlman A, Burns RG, Mason GR, Johnson FM, Berns MW. Laser photoradiation therapy of recurrent human breast cancer and cancer of the head and neck. In: Kessel D, Dougherty TJ, Eds. Porphyrin Photosensitization. New York: Plenum Press, 1983, pp. 47-52.
21. McCaughan JS Jr. Photoradiation of malignant tumors presensitized with hematoporphyrin derivative. In: Dorion DR, Gomer CJ, Eds. Porphyrin Localization and Treatment of Tumors. New York: Alan R. Liss, 1984, pp. 805-827.
22. McCaughan JS Jr, Guy JT, Hawley P, et al. Hematoporphyrin derivative and photoradiation therapy of malignant tumors. Lasers Surg Med 1983; 3:199-209.
23. Bruce RA Jr. Evaluation of hematoporphyrin photoradiation therapy to treat choroidal melanomas. Lasers Surg Med 1984; 4:59-64.
24. Kennedy JC, Oswald K. Hematoporphyrin derivative photoradiation therapy, in theory and in practice. In: Andreoni A, Cubeddu R, Eds. Porphyrins in Tumor Phototherapy. New York: Plenum Press, 1984, pp. 365-374.
25. Balchum OJ, Doiron DR. Photoradiation therapy of endobronchial lung cancer. Clin Chest Med 1985; 6:255-275.
26. Balchum OJ, Doiron DR, Huth, GC. HpD photodynamic therapy for obstructing lung cancer. In: Dorion DR, Gomer CJ, Eds. Porphyrin Localization and Treatment of Tumors. New York: Alan R. Liss, 1984, pp. 727-745.
27. Benson RC. The use of hematoporphyrin derivative (HpD) in the localization and treatment of transitional cell carcinoma (TCC) of the bladder. In: Dorion DR, Gomer CJ, Eds. Porphyrin Localization and Treatment of Tumors. New York: Alan R. Liss, 1984, pp. 795-804.

28. Schuller DE, McCaughan JS Jr, Rock RP. Photodynamic therapy in head and neck cancer. Arch Otolaryngol 1985; 111:351-355.
29. Dougherty TJ, Potter WR, Weishaupt KR. The structure of the active component of hematoporphyrin derivative. In: Dorion DR, Gomer CJ, Eds. Porphyrin Localization and Treatment of Tumors. New York: Alan R. Liss, 1984, pp. 301-314.
30. Dougherty TJ. Photosensitization of malignant tumors. Semin Surg Oncol 1986; 2:24-37.
31. Selman SH, Kreimer-Birnbaum M, Goldblatt PJ, Anderson TS, Keck RW, Britton SL. Jejunal blood flow after exposure to light in rats injected with hematoporphyrin. Cancer Res 1985; 45:6425-6427.
32. Star WM, Marijnissen HP, Vandenberg Blok AE, Versteeg JAC, Franken KAP, Reinhold HS. Destruction of rat mammary tumor and normal microcirculation by hematoporphyrin derivative photoradiation observed in vivo in sandwich observation chambers. Cancer Res 1986; 46:2532-2540.
33. Valenzeno DP, Pooler JP. Photodynamic action. Bioscience 1987; 37:270-276.
34. Allison AC, Magnus IA, Young MR. Role of lysosomes and of cell membrane in photosensitization. Nature 1966; 209:874-878.
35. Walker J. McCaughan JS Jr. Transmission of 630 nm light through human tumors and tissues (abstract). Lasers Surg Med 1986; 6:232.
36. McCaughan JS Jr, Hicks W, Laufman L, May E, Roach R. Palliation of esophageal malignancy with photoradiation therapy. Cancer 1984; 54:2905-2910.
37. Stoller JL, Samer KJ, Toppin DI, Flores AD. Carcinoma of the esophagus: A new proposal for the evaluation of treatment. Can J Surg 1977; 26:454-459.
38. McCaughan JS Jr, Schellhaas HF, Lomano J, Bethel BH. Photodynamic therapy of gynecologic neoplasms after presensitization with hematoporphyrin derivative. Lasers Surg Med 1985; 5:491-498.
39. Lipson RL, Baldes EJ. Photosensitivity and heat. Arch Dermatol 1960; 82:517-520.
40. Waldow SM, Henderson BW, Dougherty TJ. Hyperthermic potentiation of photodynamic therapy employing photofrin I and II: Comparison of results using three animal tumor models. Lasers Surg Med 1987; 7:12-22.
41. Hetzel MR, Millard FJC, Ayesh R, et al. Laser treatment for carcinoma of the bronchus. Br Med J (Clin Res) 1983; 286:12-16.
42. McCaughan JS Jr, Williams TE Jr, Bethel BH. Photodynamic therapy of endobronchial tumors. Lasers Surg Med 1986; 6:336-345.
43. McElvein RB, Zorn GL Jr. Carbon dioxide laser therapy. Clin Chest Med 1985; 6:291-295.
44. Dumon JF, Shapshay S, Bourcereau J, et al. Principles for safety in application of Nd:YAG laser in bronchology. Chest 1984; 86:163-167.

CHAPTER

26

Laser Biostimulation in Wound-Healing[a]

Andrew F. Mester, Adam Mester

BASIC RESEARCH

Since the first ruby laser was made in 1960, multiple applications of lasers have been identified. The special burning, coagulating, and vaporizing effects of high output lasers, together with their easy manipulation using optical systems, have resulted in extensive medical use. Additionally, there is much interest in the nonthermic effects of lasers in photodynamic tumor therapy and in biostimulation.

Early research suggested that several biological systems and physiological processes are influenced by a variety of low-output lasers. The biophysical law of Arndt-Schultz was found applicable to the laser: stimulation by low incident energy density (IED) and inhibition by high IED of radiation (1-21).

Carcinogenicity was not observed after repeated ruby laser irradiation of the skin (9, 21), but hair growth increased in depilated mice by an IED of 1 J/cm^2 applied twice weekly for 3-5 weeks. After the 10th irradiation, hair loss occurred (1, 3).

Phagocytosis of bacteria by human and rat leukocytes increased with an IED of 0.05 J/cm^2, while it decreased with 2-4 J/cm^2 (2, 4). These effects were increased with methylene blue and Janus B green staining and decreased with acridine orange staining (12). When the supernatant of the laser-irradiated leukocyte suspension was added to fresh normal leukocytes, a significant increase in phagocytosis was observed within 1 hour, followed by a rapid decrease after 2 hours, with inhibition occurring between 3 and 4 hours. This suggests the involvement of an active extracellular and transferable substance (22, 23).

Small bowel activity is sensitive to laser irradiation (9). The spontaneous movement of jejunal villi in dogs increased with IEDs of 1-3 J/cm^2 and decreased with IEDs of 4-7 J/cm^2 (13). Aminoethyl-thiouronium (AET), an x-ray protective substance, administered before laser irradiation, prevented both stimulation and inhibition of bacteriophagocytosis by leukocytes as well as intestinal mucosal micromotility (19, 20).

DNA and RNA content (as measured by labeled thymidine and uridine incoroporation) and cell counts increased in 1 J/cm^2 ruby laser-irradiated *Escherichia coli* CR54 cultures in the presence of the exogenic light stabilizer, methylene blue, when compared to the control. Higher IEDs decreased cell counts (24).

Retinal pigment epithelium cultured on chorioallantoic membrane and irradiated with the helium-neon (He-Ne) laser was observed to increase mitosis (25), and thymidine uptake and incorporation (26).

Body weight of mice inoculated with laser-irradiated Ehrlich's ascites tumor cells increased 10-16%, and the number of tumor cells increased 19-30% compared to controls. Survival time after inoculation with laser-irradiated cells was shorter than that of the control group (6). Electron microscopic subcellular changes observed in the laser-irradiated Ehrlich's tumor cells were not observed after acridine orange staining (15). The biostimu-

[a] The authors express deepest gratitude to Dr. Endre Mester, late father and mentor. The authors also thank Mr. Jozsef Toth for his technical help in research and his humane attitude in patient treatment; and Mrs. Gyorgyi Csiki, Mrs. Agota Mester, Ms. Vera Selmeczi, Mrs. Kati Szaller, Mrs. Zita Kakossy, and Mrs. Judit Forgacs for their generous and heartfelt work. Finally, thanks to Dr. James B. Snow, Jr., for his invaluable personal help and comments on the manuscript. This work was supported by the Central Research Institute of Physics of the Hungarian Academy of Sciences, the Hungarian Optical Works, and the U.S. National Institute of Neurological and Communicative Disorders and Stroke (NS 16365).

lating effect of argon-ion laser irradiation on human squamous carcinoma cells was reported recently (27).

The remote effect of laser irradiation on vessel formation in the rabbit cornea was observed. The angiogenesis-promoting effect of adrenal gland total extract decreased with 1-3 J/cm^2 IED (He-NE laser) and increased with 5 J/cm^2 IED. The latter effect was also observed in the contralateral cornea, which received adrenal gland total extract only (14,28).

Low-output laser irradiation has been reported to stimulate wound healing (3-11, 15-18, 22-23, 28-42). Granulation tissue and collagen production in fibroblasts were studied with electron microscopy (31, 41, 42). There was no significant effect on 2C-glycine incorporation, but the 3H-proline incorporation of the purified collagen exceeded the control by 50% (29). Incorporation of 3H-thymidine in human fibroblast culture, irradiated with ruby laser, increased reproduction by 53%, compared to the control (43). A stimulating effect on procollagen production was observed recently after low-output Nd:YAG laser (44) and after He-Ne and GaAs laser irradiation (45-47).

Enzymatic events in the early stages of wound healing have been studied. Activity of succinic acid dehydrogenase was significantly greater 8-48 hours after wounding in the basal epithelial cells within the sound tissue zone next to the wound lips compared to control wounds. Additionally, activity of the lactic acid dehydrogenase and nonspecific esterase was higher in laser-irradiated fibroblast tissue than in the control tissue (48).

Regeneration of microcirculation in rabbit ears is significantly affected by laser irradiation, inasmuch as a significant increase in revascularization has been observed in He-Ne laser-irradiated wounds compared to controls (49). A similar effect was demonstrated in the regeneration of the lymphatic circulation (50).

Regeneration of muscle fiber (posterior great adductor of the rat), injured through open skin, healed faster when irradiated by 1 J/cm^2 IED ruby laser every third day through the sutured skin compared to control animals (51). He-Ne laser has been found to stimulate revascularization and regeneration of osseus tissue using direct radiation in rabbits and transcutane radiation in mice (39, 52).

Few studies dealing with the effects of low-intensity laser irradiation have been performed on neural tissue. Increased acetylcholine release was demonstrated on guinea pig ileum after ruby laser exposure, suggesting possible effects on neurotransmitter release (53). Prevention of neural degeneration and enhancement of neural regeneration following crush injury have been demonstrated with daily He-Ne laser irradiation resulted in maintenance of the continuity of the injured optic nerve of the rabbit (54). Reduced scar tissue formation and an increase in the amplitude of the action potential of the sciatic nerve of the rat following He-Ne laser irradiation was reported (55). He-Ne laser irradiation increased the development of neuritic outgrowth of olfactory bipolar receptor cells in neuroepithelial explants from rat fetuses (56).

Tensile strength (TS) of He-Ne laser-irradiated wounds in rat skin was studied. TS of clipped wounds was not different on the 3rd postoperative day. On the 8th postoperative day, the laser-irradiated wounds were 47% stronger, and on the 12th postoperative day, they were 21% stronger compared to the control animals (57). Similar results have been obtained by Abergel et al (58).

An immunosuppressive effect of laser irradiation has been reported. The mean survival time (MST) of skin allotransplant in mice treated with antithymocyte serum (ATS) rose by 56.2% compared with that of the control animals. Treatment with ATS and He-Ne laser irradiation resulted in a 84.7% MST increase (59), while laser irradiation alone had no significant effect.

In phytohemagglutine (PHA)-stimulated lymphocyte cultures, 60-80% of the cells went through blast formation, while in cultures stimulated with PHA and irradiated with 1 J/cm^2 ruby laser, blast formation increased 20% when compared to unlased but PHA-stimulated cells (60, 61).

The model experiment of the immunosuppressive effect of low-output laser irradiation (He-Ne, ruby, and argon-ion laser) on T- and B-lymphocytes (62, 63) was applied to study the effect of noncoherent light sources. The monochromatic light had no effect, but with planopolarization, 80% of the effect produced by low-output lasers was found (64). Both mitogenic proliferation in response to phytohemagglutinin and spontaneous cell proliferation were inhibited in cultured human lymphocytes after gallium-arsenide laser irradiation (65), thus supporting the hypothesis of the immunosuppressive effect.

Prostaglandin (PG) content in wounded dorsal skin of the rat was studied. Both PGs tested showed an increase in 4-day-old wounds. After 8 days, the value of PGE_2 dropped below the level observed with the control group, while that of PFG_{2a} continued to rise (66).

Biostimulatory effects of low-output laser irradiation have been demonstrated at a variety of molecular and cellular levels, as well as at whole organ and tissue levels. Under certain circumstances, synergistic effects with laser irradiation have been demonstrated; e.g., an effect on the immune system. Evidence exists that indicates that effects remote to the irradiated site occur, suggesting the presence of a circulatory active substance. Furthermore, the biostimulatory effects of low-output laser irradiation are dose-dependent and, with sufficient intensity, the stimulatory effect disappears and inhibition occurs.

CLINICAL STUDY

Materials and Methods

In 1971, Mester and his group began treating patients (67, 68). The hypothesis of the experimental trial was that since low-output laser irradiation has been found to stimulate biological processes, it may stimulate the healing of ulcers with refractory nature to therapies. The strategy of the study was to select patients suffering with chronic and nonhealing ulcers who had been subject to unsuccessful conservative and surgical treatments. Patients with healing wounds were not eligible to participate in the study. The reasons for this selection and exclusion were (*a*) the ethical issue, because it was not certain whether laser irradiation has adverse side effects (i.e., carcinogenic), and (*b*) the possible benefit of self-control in patients declared incurable. Because of the successful results, the study developed into a sequential trial, and new patients were admitted to the program having acute ulcers with life-threatening characteristics.

The standard protocol included medical examination, routine laboratory, and complementary tests searching for the independent variables, namely, the factors that influence the disease generally, resulting in nonhealing ulcers. The data of 2167 patients with cutaneous and mucosal ulcers, regardless of the etiology, were computer analyzed. The total number of 1361 laser-treated patients from 1971-1985 comprised four groups: leg ulcers, other wounds and ulcers, nonulcer laser biostimulation, and laser coagulation. This study focused on the first two groups. The data of the nonulcer biostimulation and laser coagulation groups will not be mentioned here.

Treatment Protocol of Ulcers

Patients had received various therapies before entering the study. However, all patients were resubjected to conventional medical treatment according to the protocol. The largest population of the laser-treated experimental group had leg ulcers (1018 cases, 75%). Its control group included 806 patients treated only with the conservative therapy (within the period of 2 years, from 1984-1985). Once patients were or had been recruited, the compression therapy began, in order to treat primary or secondary edema. Each patient was asked to elevate the end of his/her bed at the leg to 15-20 cm (6-8 inches), using two or three bricks as props. The purpose was to assure a smooth slope from the leg to the heart and not only to the hip. One pillow was allowed under the head, but not under the legs. The ulcer was cleaned twice a day by placing a sterile gauze impregnated with antiseptic solution on the wound every 2 min for a total of 15 min. After this procedure, the wound was dressed with local antibiotics, according to the sensitivity in cultures. Compression bandages were applied forcibly during the day, and the patient was told to increase walking activity. This protocol was carried out for 2-3 months.

Patients with improved or healed ulcers made up the control group and the conservative treatment continued until total healing. Those who (*a*) did not improve at all for 3 months; (*b*) did not show further improvement, or (*c*) declined (for an additional period of 2 months), formed the experimental group.

The study protocol of the ulcers not on the leg group (230 cases, 16.4%) was similar to the leg ulcer group, without the antiedema treatment. In come cases, laser irradiation started forthwith, because of life-threating problems, i.e., coumarin-caused skin necrosis (69) or sepsis. Patients did not get medication to help granulation and proliferation of the wounds. Antibiotics were given locally, as part of the treatment since 1978, when it was discovered that the IED of 4 J/cm^2 does not influence the bacteria remarkably, and septic ulcers become sterile as a result of wound healing and better immune protection. Medication of associated systemic illnesses (i.e., diabetes, hypertension) continued.

Protocol of Laser Therapy

Patients early in the study were treated with ruby laser (694.3 nm) and later, with He-Ne (632.8 nm. 5–50 mW), argon-ion (457–514 nm, 100–150 mW), and GaAlAs diode lasers (820 nm, 15 mW). The IED of 4 J/cm^2 was identical for all patients and lasers. The outcoming laser beam was controlled by a photodensitometer passing through the refractive mediums, and the treatment time was calculated correlating to the diameter of the laser spot at the target:

$$\mathrm{IED} = \frac{\mathrm{I} \times \mathrm{t}}{\mathrm{S}}$$

IED = Incident Energy Density (J/cm^2), I = intensity of laser (W), t = time of exposure (sec), S = surface of the laser spot at target (cm^2).

The output of the He-Ne lasers were in the range of 5–50 mW. Lens was not in use, but a prism or mirror directed the unfocused beam to the wound surface. The treatment time of 1 cm^2 wound surface was about 2 min, using the 50 mW output He-Ne laser, but if the output was only 5 mW, the time increased to 15 minutes. Extensive ulcers were irradiated with 3-W output argon-ion laser. The higher the output of the laser, the shorter the treatment time. The laser beam was spread by a divergent lens and halved by a dividing mirror. The two beams were directed with mirrors or prisms independently to afford the possibility of simultaneous laser treatment of two patients. The spot area on the wound surface was 3 cm^2, and the output was 150 mW on 1 cm^2 (450 mW on 3 cm^2). The length of irradiation of 3 cm^2 wound was around 30 sec. GaAlAs diode laser was used in the treatment of small and deep ulcers, in the immediate vicinity of the treated area.

The choice of laser type to be used dependent mainly on the dimension of the ulcers and not on the absorption differences of the wavelengths. Fiberoptics were used for laser endoscopy (He-Ne and argonion lasers) and the loss of energy was measured and equalized with the time factor. w571 After the irradiation of a laser spot area, the beam was directed forward manually, until all of the wound surface became irradiated. Laser treatments were carried out twice a week (Tuesday and Friday), then once a week, and in acute septic cases, daily. Most of the patients were outpatients.

Results

The mean age of the patients was 55.2 years, with 55% women and 45% men. The most frequent anatomical locations of ulcers were the lower extremities (87.9%), followed by the mouth and oral cavity (3.1%), the abdominal wall (1.1%), and the genitalia (1.0%). The most frequently associated secondary diseases were: diabetes (8.5%), varicose veins (8.2%), obesity (8.1%), previous fracture of the lower extremity (6.4%), high blood pressure (5.8%), locomotor diseases (4.3%), superficial phlebitis (4.3%), and heart failure (3.8%). The incidence of different ulcers in diabetic patients was analyzed: all patients with lypoid necrobiosis ulceration were diabetic; mal perforans foot (78.8%), neurotrophic (58.8%), occlusive arterial (21.2%), decubitus (11.1%), radionecrosis (9.7%), mixed occlusive and stasis (9.5%), stasis (6.3%), postthrombotic (4.8%), other ulcers (3.8%).

The number of leg ulcers in the study totalled 1824. Wounds were more often on the left leg (51.7%) than on the right (36.2%), whereas 12.1% were bilateral. The most frequent location of leg ulcers was on the medial surface (58.0%), compared to the lateral (13.7%), anterior (9.9%), nearly circumferential (6.6%), both medial and lateral (5.8%), posterior (3.4%), circumferential (1.9%), and amputation stump (0.7%). Referring to the vertical position, 52.4% of the leg ulcers were on the distal crus; followed by the ankle (36.3%), foot (7.1%), proximal crus (2.9%), thigh and knee (0.8%), and heel (0.5%).

The average duration of persistent leg ulcers was 5.1 years; according to the etiology: amputation stump (12.8 years), mixed occlusive and stasis (6.4) years), after deep venous thrombosis (6.1 years), stasis ulcer (4.2 years), lymphatic obstruction (4.0 years), posttraumatic (3.1 years), occlusive arterial (3.0 years), infectious (2.9 years), neurotrophic (2.7 years), ulceration of necrobiosis lypoidica (2.7 years), and mal perforans foot ulcers (1.6 years).

One, two, and three or more bacterial species have been idenfied in 69.9% (617 cases), 22.3% (197 cases), and 7.8% (69 cases) of the wound cultures, respectively. *Staphylococcus aureus* turned out to be the most frequent (37.4%), followed by *Pseudomonas* (14.5%), *Escherichia coli*

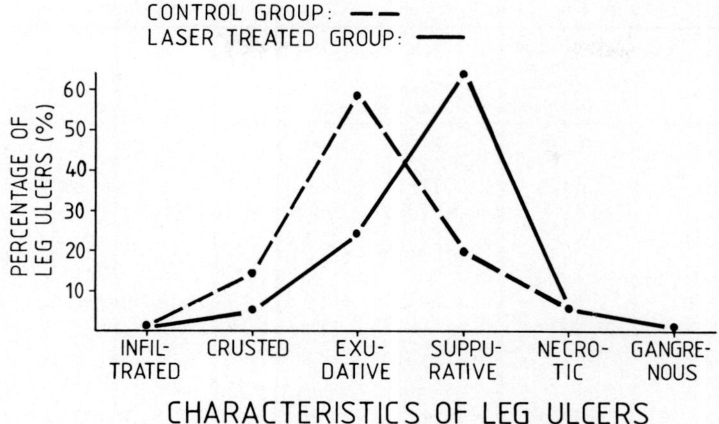

Figure 26.1. Characteristics of leg ulcers in the conservatively treated control group (n = 761), and in the laser-irradiated experimental group (n = 903). Ulcers of the experimental patient population were more severe than those of the control group.

(10.7%), and *Proteus* (9.1%). Because of the bacteria combinations *S. aureus* was treated locally in 54.4% of the cases with trimethoprim sulfa, or with gentamycin (19.2%), erythromycin (13.1%), chloramphenicol (11.6%), neomycin (11.2%), and polymyxin (7.1%); *Pseudomonas* was treated with polymyxin (45.3%), gentamycin (33.3%), trimethoprim sulfa (28.3%), neomycin (18.9%), and chloramphenicol (6.9%); *E. coli* was treated with trimethoprim sulfa (56.0%), gentamycin (24.8%), polymyxin (12.8%), chloramphenicol (11.2%), and neomycin (8.8%); *Proteus* was treated with trimethoprim sulfa (47.2%), gentamycin (34.3%), polymyxin (17.6%), chloramphenicol (12.0%), and neomycin (11.1%).

In the control group, the conservative therapy continued until the patient healed or improved. Surprisingly, 73.9% of the patients visiting this center because of nonhealing leg ulcers, healed with conservative therapy, and only 22.4% made up the experimental group and became subjects for laser treatment. There is no further information on the remaining 3.7% who did not show up for control. One-third of the patients (33.1%) in the control group healed completely during the 3-month period; 22.4% healed in 2 months, 21.7% in 4 months, 12.1% in 5 months, 4.8% in 6 months, 2.4% in 7 months, and 3.5% in 8 or more months.

Characteristics of leg ulcers were analyzed according to seriousness: infiltrated, crusted, exudative, suppurative, necrotic, and gangrenous. Data exemplified that the more serious the nature of the ulcer, the greater the number of patients who had to be added to the laser treated experimental group (Fig. 26.1).

Laser Treatment of Leg Ulcers

The majority of laser treated patients constituted the leg ulcer group. Table 26.1 demonstrates the classificiation of the principal diseases, the average number of laser treatments, and the healing rates. Patients with history of deep venous thrombosis were put in the category of postthrombotic ulcers, whereas others without such history, but with evidence of chronic venous insuficiency, were rated into the stasis ulcer group. The best healing rates were found in the groups of necrobiosis lypoidica ulcers (100%), stasis ulcers (91.0%), postthrombotic ulcers (82.2%), infectious ulcers (92.3%), and posttraumatic ulcers (83.3%). The healing rate of the most resistent ulcers on the amputation stump proved to be 50.0%, while it was 58.7% with the mal perforans foot, 51.5% with the occlusive arterial ulcers, 57.4% with the mixed arterial and stasis ulcers, 62.5% with the neurotrophic ulcers.

Laser Treatment of Ulcers Not on the Leg

Patients in this group, just like in the experimental group of leg ulcers, had nonhealing ulcers with refractory nature to therapy. Table 26.2 illustrates the etiology of principal disease, the av-

Table 26.1. Number of Laser Treatments and Patients' Conditions with Leg Ulcers

Etiology	Average No. of Laser Treatments	Complete Healing	Improved	No Change	Under Treatment	Unknown	No. of Patients
Postthrombotic	31	352 (82.2%)	31 (7.2%)	7 (1.6%)	24 (5.6%)	14 (3.2%)	428 (42.0%)
Stasis	23	322 (91.0%)	14 (4.0%)	5 (1.4%)	3 (0.8%)	10 (2.8%)	354 (34.8%)
Occlusive arterial	21	17 (51.5%)	5 (15.2%)	3 (9.1%)	4 (12.1%)	4 (12.1%)	33 (3.3%)
Mixed occlusive and stasis	34	31 (57.4%)	6 (11.1%)	4 (7.4%)	10 (18.5%)	3 (5.6%)	54 (5.3%)
Lymphatic obstruction	12	1			1		2 (0.2%)
Posttraumatic	22	35 (83.3%)	4 (9.5%)		1 (2.4%)	2 (4.8%)	42 (4.1%)
Neurotrophic	21	30 (62.5%)	8 (16.7%)	3 (6.3%)	4 (8.3%)	3 (6.3%)	48 (4.7%)
Infectious	18	12 (92.3%)		1 (7.7%)			13 (1.3%)
Amputation stump	22	3 (50.0%)	2 (33.3%)		1 (16.7%)		6 (0.6%)
Necrobiosis lypoidica	16	9 (100%)					9 (0.9%)
Mal perforans foot	32	17 (58.7%)			9 (31.0%)	3 (10.3%)	29 (2.8%)
Total	23	829 (81.4%)	70 (6.9%)	23 (2.3%)	57 (5.6%)	39 (3.8%)	1018 (100%)

erage number of laser treatments, and the healing rate.

The x-ray ulcers are confirmed diseases, because of decreased cell division and microvascularization. The healing rate with laser irradiation proved to be 67.9%; but with the longest healing period in the study (average laser treatment: 38). In addition to the high healing rates of perilous cases like coumarin-caused extensive skin necrosis (90.9%), decubital ulcer (73.1%), burn ulcer (82.4%), and sepsis-caused ulcerations (100%), a remarkable phenomenon was observed, namely, minimal scarring and special cosmetic results. The healing rate of postoperative skin ulcers was 73.9%; the rate for cervical erosions in the vagina was 75.0%; and for anal fissures, the rate was 100%.

Common labial herpes and stomatitis were not involved in the study. The healing period of the laser irradiated recurrent labial herpes and ulcerous stomatitis (causing drinking inability in children) was two-thirds of the time measured in the control group. But the important result is not only the quick recovery, but the significant decrease of recurrency. Female patients with monthly recurrence of labial herpes (accompanying their period) became symptom-free for the average term of 1 year.

The key to osteomyelitis and to the fistula problem is mostly behind the aperture; however, laser was helpful occasionally. Nevertheless, it was not unlikely that the fistula closed, but a few days or weeks later the area had to be exposed with surgical intervention because of retention (i.e., retroauricular fistulae).

Endoscopy was applied to patients with long existing ulcers in the urinary bladder, causing painful pollakiuria and disturbing nycturia. Two-thirds of the patients' ulcers healed, one-third improved, and the urinary bladder capacity increased by 25–200%. The pain ceased and the pollakiuria and nycturia decreased (70). The theoretical importance of this experiment is the biostimulative effect of nonpolarized He-Ne and argon-ion lasers.

The average length of healing of the total laser treated experimental group was 5.5 months, excluding the previously applied 3 months of fruitless conservative therapy. About one-half of the healed patients (52.5%) were treated with He-Ne

Table 26.2. Laser Treatments and Patients' Conditions with Ulcers not on the Leg

Etiology	Average No. of Laser Treatments	Complete Healing	Improved	No Change	Under Treatment	Unknown	No. of Patients
Radionecrosis	38	19 (67.9%)	5 (17.9%)	3 (10.7%)	1 (3.6%)		28 (12.2%)
Decubitus	18	19 (73.1%)	4 (15.4%)	2 (7.7%)		1 (3.8%)	26 (11.3%)
Postoperative skin ulcer	13	17 (73.9%)	4 (17.4%)			2 (8.7%)	23 (10.0%)
Burn ulcer	15	14 (82.4%)	1 (5.9%)		1 (5.9%)	1 (5.9%)	17 (7.4%)
Coumarin-induced skin ulcer	22	10 (90.9%)				1 (9.1%)	11 (4.8%)
Drug-induced skin ulcer	5	3					3 (1.3%)
Infectious ulcer	43	10 (100%)					10 (4.3%)
Nasoseptal ulcer	5	5 (100%)					5 (2.2%)
Ulcerative stomatitis	3	23 (100%)					23 (10.0%)
Recurrent labial herpes	3	24 (100%)					24 (10.4%)
Urinary bladder ulcer	9	10 (66.7%)	5 (33.3%)				15 (6.5%)
Anal fissure	7	5 (100%)					5 (2.2%)
Cervical erosion	6	12 (75.5%)	2 (12.5%)	1 (6.3%)		1 (6.3%)	16 (7.0%)
Osteomyelitis	27	2 (28.6%)	3 (42.9%)	2 (28.6%)			7 (3.0%)
Fistula	15	11 (61.1%)	4 (22.2%)	2 (11.1%)			17 (7.4%)
Total	16	184 (80.0%)	28 (12.2%)	10 (4.3%)	2 (0.9%)	6 (2.6%)	230 (100%)

laser for an average phase of 3.5 months, and one-third received argon-ion therapy for an average healing period of 6.3 months. In the cases of specially resistent or recurrent ulcers (14.4%), when the laser source was changed to another wavelength (He-Ne, argon-ion, GaAlAs, or rarely, ruby laser), the average healing term was 7.3 months.

The frequency of laser treatments was empirical in the study. Patients were ordered to receive laser therapy twice weekly (39.0%), but for people from the countryside with great traveling distances, once weekly (34.8%), others visited the center following a nonregular schedule (24.4%). Daily treatments were applied only in acute cases (1.8%). The treatment frequency of twice weekly was found most favorable; it was once weekly, the medical attendance increased with 15.4%, and following a nonregular schedule, it increased with 53.8%. Daily laser treatment was successful in acute cases only, whereas in chronic ulcer treatment it resulted in inhibition.

Discussion

The therapeutic effect of conservative therapy in leg ulcers proved to be quite successful, since 73.9% of the patients, qualified as "nonhealing" for many years, healed completely within a few months period. The fully fashioned compression stocking was effective only in the prevention of postthrombotic complications. In the treatment of active ulcers, the proper compression bandage was efficacious. The tighter the compression bandage was put on early in the morning, the less edema and pain increased during the day. The more the patient walks and moves, the faster the recovery. The beneficial effect of the compression therapy in the treatment of ulcers caused by arterial insufficiency is controversial. However, according to this study, it is highly recommended in all kinds of leg ulcers with primary or secondary edema.

Laser instruments are optical systems with the need for regular control and verification of the output, both in the visible and nonvisible wavelengths. Patient's and therapist's eyes were protected with safety goggles. None of the laser-treated patients had side effects or complications as a result of laser therapy. Lesions suspect for malignancy were investigated histologically, and the patient became a subject for laser biostimulation only after negative results.

The output of the laser determines the biological effects, while wavelength influences absorption. The indication for the laser type to be used depended mostly upon the extension of the treated area. According to previous research studies, laser biostimulation, inhibition, or coagulation are functions of the IED. The IED of 4 J/cm^2 was settled in 1971 as the most effective dose for biostimulation in wound healing, according to a series of experiments on animals and different biological systems. A more effective protocol may be possible; others reported good results in biostimulation (37-40), although using different methods and doses, experienced poor results (71).

According to the authors' observations, both in in vitro experiments and in patients, laser biostimulation of the total wound surface is not absolutely necessary because of the systemic effect; however, irradiation of the whole wound surface and, at least, the outlines was attempted. Analysis of medical attendance and the frequency of laser treatments demonstrated that the healing process dragged on when patients' visits were devoid of the plan, but the treatment of twice a week regularly made it shorter.

The average length of healing of the total laser-treated experimental group was 5.5 months, excluding the previously applied 3 months of fruitless conservative therapy. This relatively long time demonstrates that: (*a*) those qualified for the experimental group were severe cases, and (*b*) laser treatment is time-consuming. The answer to the longer healing period using the argon-ion laser rather than the He-Ne laser could be explained by the fact that larger ulcers need usually more time to recover.

The double blind test is necessary to eliminate the possibility of errors in the placebo effect. Wounds of animals originating from an inbred tribe could be excellent controls, but comparison with human nonhealing ulcers would be very difficult, considering the stage of the principal and secondary diseases, age, gender, financial and social circumstances, and the patient's attitude to the treatment. However, the main technical problem is the lack of He-Ne and argon-ion placebo lasers.

It was found that relapse of ulcer can be attributed mostly to the improper use of the compression bandage and of the bolster up in patients with chronic venous insufficiency. In this study, such recurrence in the conservative treated group was 5.3%, while in the laser treated group, it was 23.6%. Unfortunately, these data are not comparable, because the follow up of the experimental group is with retroactive from 1971, whereas, in the control group, only since 1984. Although the laser-treated patient population had much more severe problems, maybe they were more inconsistent in obeying the medical instructions, hence the high recurrence percentage. This circumstance could also be a reason why the conservative therapy did not succeed and the laser therapy became necessary. However, 97.5% of the recurrent ulcers healed, finally, with the laser therapy.

In light of the fact that these ulcers were polyresistant to the standard therapies, including skin transplantation, vascular surgery, and amputation stump reamputation, the results are more appreciable.

These experiments, which elucidate the bioregulative process of wound healing and show favorable clinical results, have convinced the authors to recommend the use of lasers to stimulate wound healing.

REFERENCES

1. Mester E, Szende B, Tota JG. Effect of laser on hair growth of mice (in Hungarian). Kiserl Orvostud 1967; 19:628-631.
2. Mester E, Ludany G, Vajda G, Tota JG, Karika G. Effect of laser on bacteria phagocytosis of the leukocytes (in Hungarian). Orv Hetil 1967; 108:1546-1550.
3. Mester E, Szende B, Gartner P. Die Wirkung der Laserstrahlen auf den Haarwuchs der Maus. Radioboil Radiother 1968; 9:621-626.
4. Mester E, Ludany G, Vajda G, Razgha A, Karika G, Tota JG. Uber die Wirkung von Laserstrahlen auf die Bakterienphagocytose der Leukocyten. Acta Biol Med Germ 1968; 21:317.

5. Mester E, Ludany G, Sellyei M, Szende B. Untersuchungen uber die Biologische Wirkung der Laser-Strahlen. Bull Soc Int Chir 1968; 26:1-6.
6. Mester E, Sellyei M, Tota GJ. Laserstrahlenwirkung auf das Wachstum des Ehrlichschen Ascitestumors. Arch Geschwulstforsch 1968; 32:201.
7. Mester E, Juhasz J, Varga P, Karika G. Lasers in Clinical Practice. Acta Chir Acad Hung 1968; 9:349-357.
8. Mester E, Juhasz J, Varga P, Karika G. Contribution a l'application clinique des lasers. Lyon Chirurgical 1969; 65:335-345.
9. Mester E, Szende B, Tota JG. Die Wirkung der uber langere Zeit wiederholt verabreichten Laserstrahlung geringer Intensitat auf die Haut und inneren Organe von Mausen. Radiobiol Radiother 1969; 10:371-377.
10. Mester E, Szende B, Tota JG. Uber die Summation fraktionert verabreichter Laserstrahlung. Radiobiol Radiother 1969; 10:379.
11. Mester E, Gyenes G, Tota JG. Experimentelle Untersuchungen uber die Wirkung der Laserstrahlen auf die Wundheilung. Z Exper Chirurgie 1969; 2:94-101.
12. Mester E, Ludany G, Vajda G, Tota JG, Karika G, Hejjas M. Untersuchungen uber die Wirkung von Laserstrahlen auf die Bakterienphagocytose von Leukocyten. Acta Biol Med Germ 1970; 25:927.
13. Mester E, Ihasz M, Kariak G, Tota JG. Effect of laser beam on the micromotility of the intestinal mucosa. Acta Biol Acad Sci Hung 1970; 21(2):171-174.
14. Mester E, Krompecher I, Kiss FA, Kalabay L, Gartner P. Laser effect on rabbit cornea treated with adrenal gland total extract of rat (in Hungarian). Kiserl Orvostud 1970; 22:308-313.
15. Mester E, Lapis K, Tota JG. Ultrastrukturelle Veranderungen in Ehrlichschen Ascites-Tumorzellen nach Laser-Behandlung. Arch Geschwulstforsch 1971; 38:210-220.
16. Mester E, Spiry T, Szende B, Tota JG. Effect of laser rays on wound healing. Am J Surg 1971; 122:532-535.
17. Mester E, Varteresz V, Doklen A, Tota JG, Hejjas M. Die Wirkung der Laserstrahlen auf die Hamoglobinsynthese in vitro. Radiobiol Radiother 1971; 5:669.
18. Mester E, Ludany G, Frenyo V, Szende B, Ihasz M, Kiss AF, Doklen A, Jaszsagi-Nagy E, Tota JG. Der Einfluss von Laser-Strahlen von geringer Energie auf biologische Systeme und die Bedeutung im Humanbereich. Arbeitsmed Sozialmed Arbeitshyg 1971; 6:13-15.
19. Mester E, Ihasz M, Doklen A, Batorfi J, Tota JG. Amino-ethylthiouronium protection on the laser radiation caused changes in the intestinal mucosa (in Hungarian). Kiserl Orvostud 1971; 23:398.
20. Mester E, Doklen A, Hejjas M, Tota JG, Ludany G, Vajda G. Effect of amino-ethylthiouronium on the laser induced phagocytosis changes in rat leukocytes (in Hungarian). Kiserl Orvostud 1972; 24:150.
21. Mester E, Szende B, Spiry T, Tota JG. Die Wirkung wiederholt angewandter Elektrokoagulation und Laser-Bestrahlung auf die Haut von Mausen. Z Exper Chirugie 1972; 5:127-131.
22. Mester E. Clinical results of wound-healing stimulation with laser and experimental studies of the action mechanism. In: Laser '75 Optoelectronics Conference Proceedings, Munich, 1975, pp. 119-125.
23. Mester E. Clinical results of wound-healing stimulation with laser and experimental studies of the action mechanism. In: In Kaplan I, Ed. Laser Surgery. Proceedings of the 1st International Symposium on Laser Surgery, Israel November 5-6, 1975 Jerusalem. New York: Academic Press, 1976, pp. 190-213.
24. Herczegh M, Mester E, Ronto G. Examination of laser-inactivation on T7 phages. Acta Biochem Biophys Acad Sci Hung 1971; 6:41-44.
25. Yew, DT, Ling Wong SL, Chan YW. Stimulating effect of low-dose laser. A new hypothesis. Acta Anat 1982; 112:131-136.
26. Tsang D, Yew DT, Hui BSW. Further studies on the effect of low-dose laser irradiation on cultured retinal pigment cells of the chick. Acta Anat 1986; 125:10-13.
27. Castro DJ, Saxton RE, Fetterman HR, Ward PH. Biostimulation of human carcinoma cells with the argon laser in vitro: a previously unreported potential iatrogenic effect of lasers. Laryngoscope 1988; 98:109-116.
28. Kiss FA, Mester E, Krompecher ST, Tota JG, Kalabay L. Laser-Strahlen und Vaskularization. Radiobiol Radiother 1972; 13:123-132.
29. Mester E, Jaszsagi-Nagy E. The effect of laser radiation on wound healing and collagene synthesis. Studia Biophysica 1973; 35:227-230.
30. Mester E, Spiry T, Szende B. Effect of laser rays on wound healing. Bull Soc Int Chir 1973; 2:169-173.
31. Mester E, Korenyi-Both A, Spiry T, Scher A, Tisza S. Stimulation of wound healing by means of laser rays. Acta Chir Acad Sci Hung 1973; 14:347-356.
32. Mester E, Mester A, Toth J. Biostimulative effect of laser beam. In Atsumi K, Ed. New Frontiers in Laser Medicine and Surgery. Amsterdam: Excerpta Medica, 1983, pp. 481-490.
33. Mester E, Mester A, Mester AF. Les effects bio-stimulants du laser - Son efficacite dans le traitment des ulceres cutanes. Lyon Chirurgical 1984; 80:457-459.
34. Mester E, Mester AF, Mester A. The biomedical effects of laser application. Lasers Surg Med 1985; 5:31-39.
35. Mester AF, Mester A. Mester's method of laser biostimulation. In: Waidelich W, Kiefhaber P, Eds. Laser Optoelectronics in Medicine 1986. Berlin: Springer, pp. 103-109.
36. Mester A, Mester AF. Data for laser biostimulation in wound-healing. In: Waidelich W, Ed. Laser Optoelectronics in Medicine. Berlin: Springer, 1988, pp. 731-735.
37. Haina D, Brunner R, Landthaler M, Braun-Falco O, Waidelich W. Animal experiments on light-induced wound healing. In: Atsumi K, Ed. Laser Tokyo '81. Tokyo: Inter Group Corp, 1981, pp. 1-3.
38. Kovacs L. The stimulatory effect of laser on the physiological healing process of portio surface. Lasers Surg Med 1981; 1:241-252.
39. Trelles MA. Soft Laser Terapia (in Spanish). Madrid: Enar Madrid Publ, 1982.
40. Trelles MA, Mayayo E, Iglesias JM. Histologic study of the action of He-Ne laser on the nasal mucosa of the

rabbit and its clinical objectives. In Waidelich W, Ed. Optoelektronik in der Medizin 1984. Berlin: Springer 1984, pp. 215-222.

41. Mester E, Neumark T, Tisza S, Mester A, Toth J, Mate L. Neuere elektronenmikroscopische Untersuchungen uber die Wirkung der Laserstrahlen auf die Wundheilung. In Waidelich W, Ed. Laser '79 Optoelectronics. IPC Science and Technology Press, 1979, pp. 330-337.
42. Mester E, Korenyi-Both A, Spiry T, Scher A, Tisza S. Neuere Untersuchungen uber die Wirkung der Laserstrahlen auf die Wundheilung. Z Exper Chirurg 1974; 7:9-17.
43. Toth M, Mester E, Vutskits Z, Ferencz G, Tisza S. Laser effect on the macromolecular synthesis if fibroblast culture (in Hungarian). Kiserl Orvostud 1975; 27:331-332.
44. Abergel RP, Meeker CA, Dwyer RM, LeSavoy MA, Uitto J. Nonthermal effects of Nd:YAG laser on biological functions of human fibroblasts in culture. Laser Surg Med 1984; 3:279-284.
45. Boulton M, Marshall J. He-Ne laser stimulation of human fibroblast proliferation and attachment in vitro. Lasers L Sces 1986; 1:125-134.
46. Saperia D, Glassberg E, Lyons RF, Abergel RP, Baneux P, Castel JC, Dwyer RM, Uitto J. Demonstration of elevated type I and type III procollagen mRNA levels in cutaneous wounds treated with He-Ne laser. Bioch Bioph Res Com 1986; 138:1123-1128.
47. Lam TS, Abergel RP, Meeker CA, Castel JC, Dwyer RM, Uitto J. Laser stimulation of collagen synthesis in human skin fibroblast cultures. Lasers L Sces 1986; 1:61-67.
48. Bacsy E, Mester E, Spiry T, Tisza S. Enzymatic-hystochemical study on stimulation of wound healing by laser. Acta Chir Acad Sci Hung 1974; 15:203.
49. Kovacs IB, Mester E, Gorog P. Laser induced stimulation of the vascularization of the healing wound. An ear chamber experiment. Experientia 1974; 30:341-343.
50. Lievens PC. Effects of laser treatment on the lymphatic system and wound healing. Laser 1988; 1:12-15.
51. Mester E, Korenyi-Both A, Spiry T, Tisza S. The effect of laser irradiation on the regeneration of muscle fibers. Z Exper Chirurg 1975; 8:258-262.
52. Trelles MA, Mayayo E. Bone fracture consolidates faster with low-power laser. Lasers Surg Med 1987; 7:36-45.
53. Vizi ES, Mester E, Tisza S, Mester A. Acetylcholine releasing effect of laser irradiation on Auerbach's plexus in guinea-pig ileum. J Neural Transmission 1977; 40:305-308.
54. Schwartz M, Doron A, Erlich M, Lavie V, Benbasat S, Belkin M, Rochkind S. Effects of low-energy He-Ne laser irradiation on posttraumatic degeneration of adult rabbit optic nerve. Lasers Surg Med 1987; 7:51-55.
55. Rochkind S, Barrnea L, Razon N, Bartal A, Schwartz M. Stimulatory effect of He-Ne low dose laser on injured sciatic nerves of rats. Neurosurg 1987; 20:843-847.
56. Mester AF, Snow JB. Effects of laser irradiation on immature olfactory neuroepithelial explants from the rat. Laryngoscope 1988; 98:743-745.
57. Kovacs IB, Mester E, Gorog P. Stimulation of wound healing with laser beam in the rat. Experientia 1974; 30:1275-1276.
58. Abergel RP, Lyons RF, Castel JC, Dwyer RM, Uitto J. Biostimulation of wound-healing by lasers: Experimental approaches in animal models and in fibroblast cultures. J Derm Surg Onc 1987; 13:127-133.
59. Namenyi J, Mester E, Foldes I, Tisza S. Effects of laser irradiation and immunosuppressive treatment on survival of mouse skin allotransplants. Acta Chir Acad Sci Hung 1975; 16:327-335.
60. Mester E, Jaszsagi-Nagy E, Hamar M. Der Einfluss von Laserstrahlung auf stimulierte menschliche Lymphocyten. Radiobiol Radiother 1974; 15:767-769.
61. Mester E, Nagylucskay S, Doklen A, Tisza S. Laser stimulation of wound healing. II. Immunological tests. Acta Chir Acad Sci Hung 1976; 17:49-55.
62. Mester E, Nagylucskay S, Tisza S, Mester A. Neuere Untersuchungen uber die Wirkung der Laserstrahlen auf die Wundheilung - Immunologische Effekte. Z Exper Chirurg 1977; 10:301-306.
63. Mester E, Nagylucskay S, Tisza S, Mester A. Stimulation of wound healing by means of laser rays. Part III. Investigation of the effect on immune competent cells. Acta Chir Acad Sci Hung 1978; 19:163-170.
64. Mester E, Nagylucskay S, Waidelich W, Tisza S, Greguss P, Haina D, Mester A. Auswirkungen direkter Laserbestrahlung auf menschliche lymphocyten. Arch Dermatol Res 1978; 263:241-245.
65. Ohta A, Abergel RP, Uitto J. Laser modulation of human immune system: Inhibition of lymphocyte proliferation by a Gallium-Arsenide laser at low energy. Lasers Surg Med 1987; 7:199-201.
66. Cseh G, K.Szabo I, Gorog P, Mester E. Changes in prostaglandine content in wounds and after laser treatment (in Hungarian). Kiserl Orvostud 1978; 30:37-41.
67. Aronoff BL, Friedman EW. Dedication Endre Mester 1903-1984. Lasers Surg Med 1985; 5:29-30.
68. Waidelich W. In memoriam Professor Dr. med. Endre Mester. In Waidelich W, Ed. Laser Optoelectronics in Medicine 1986. Berlin: Springer, 1986, p. 1.
69. Mester E, Tisza S, Csillag L, Mester A. Laser treatment of coumarin-induced skin necrosis. Acta Chir Acad Sci Hung 1977; 18:141-148.
70. Hazay L, Mester E. Laser treatment of urinary bladder ulcers (in Hungarian). Urol Nephrol Szle 1981; 9:103-105.
71. McCaughan JS, Bethel BH, Johnston T, Janssen W. Effect of low dose argon irradiation on rate of wound closure. Lasers Surg Med 1985; 5:607-614.

CHAPTER
27

Anesthesia and Operative Care

Kevin C. Moore

The establishment of surgical laser facilities in many centers has led to an increasing demand for the services of the anesthesiology department. As a prelude to this involvement, the clinical anesthesiologist should familiarize himself or herself with the basic biophysics and mode of usage of individual laser delivery systems as well as the appropriate local and national safety regulations. With this knowledge the anesthesiologist becomes a valuable member of the laser team.

Technological innovations are widening the scope of laser therapy in many specialties and this is particularly so in general surgery because of the wide variety of surgical sites and pathology. This chapter reviews the use of the CO_2 and Nd:YAG laser in general surgery from the anesthesiologist's viewpoint and discusses such aspects as preoperative patient assessment, the management of general anesthesia, intraoperative care, and postoperative analgesia.

PREOPERATIVE ASSESSMENT

The preoperative assessment of fitness for anesthesia is accepted as a fundamental requirement before surgery. The most widely used method of grading operative risk is that of the American Society of Anesthesiologists (ASA) classification of physical status that grades patients on a scale of 1–5, increasing risk incurring a higher classification. In general, the older the patient the more likely it is that he or she will have some degree of coexistent systemic disease that will increase the operative risk for surgery. Indeed, a proportion of patients are referred for laser surgery because either the extent of their disease process or their poor general physical condition precludes any form of major surgical intervention.

In reviewing 200 patients referred for Nd:YAG laser surgery, the author found that 75% were in the age group of 60–90 years (Fig. 27.1). Their ASA classification reflected their poor physical status, some 70% being graded class 3 and 4 (Fig. 27.2). Experience has shown that the surgical stress and trauma associated with laser surgery appears to be less than with conventional surgical techniques (vide infra). This allows surgery particularly of a palliative nature to be performed on patients who otherwise would be denied operative treatment. In the series referred to above, in spite of their advanced years and poor physical condition, there was no mortality directly associated with surgery or anesthesia.

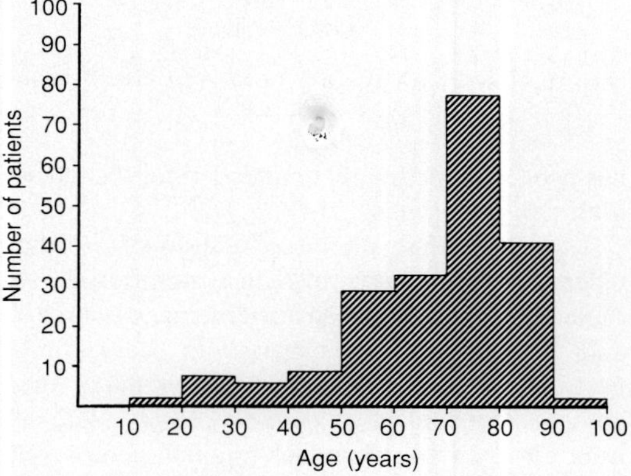

Figure 27.1. Nd:YAG laser cases: age distribution.

MANAGEMENT OF GENERAL ANESTHESIA AND INTRAOPERATIVE CARE

Endoscopy

The fiberoptic delivery system of the Nd:YAG laser is ideal for endoscopic therapy. Since 1975 its use has been widely reported for the treatment of hemorrhagic lesions of the upper gastrointestinal tract and for the palliative treatment of tumors of the esophagus, stomach, colon, and rectum. It

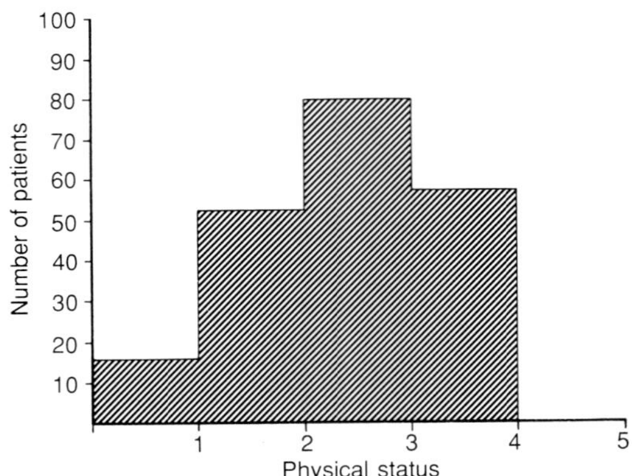

Figure 27.2. Nd:YAG laser cases: ASA classification.

has been specifically recommended for the elderly high risk patient (1).

The endoscopic photocoagulation of bleeding ulcers has been shown to reduce significantly the rebleeding rate, the need for emergency surgery, and the mortality associated with severe upper gastrointestinal hemorrhage (2). For tumor therapy, the noncontact method (NCM) of Nd:YAG laser energy application was originally employed. This involved the use of high power settings with short exposure duration and produced high tissue penetration, marked tissue charring, and troublesome smoke plume. As a consequence, episodes of treatment were often of short duration and incomplete, thus necessitating frequent initial treatments until symptoms were relieved (3, 4).

Since the introduction in 1985 of contact tips for use with the Nd:YAG laser fiber, the contact method (CM) of applying laser energy at low power has gained in popularity. The advantages of the CM over the NCM treatment of gastrointestinal lesions are the more precise application of laser energy, reduced adjacent tissue damage, no smoke plume, and, for the awake patient, less pain and discomfort (5, 6).

The choice of general anesthesia for endoscopic laser therapy seems to be mainly one of user preference. Endoscopists with no access to anesthesia services have little option. Relatively fit patients with minor lesions are ideally suited for outpatient therapy. The success of treatment without anesthesia relies on patient cooperation and the ability of the patient to cope with the unpleasant abdominal distension due to the coaxial gas flow and the discomfort and pain that is felt by some 20% of all patients (6). Frequently repeated episodes of treatment are likely to be less well accepted by the awake patient.

For patients with severe upper gastrointestinal tract hemorrhage, intubated anesthesia is recommended to avoid the danger of aspiration and to ensure adequate oxygenation. The use of general anesthesia for the endoscopic Nd:YAG laser treatment of tumors ensures patient cooperation and allows sufficient time to achieve symptomatic relief in a single treatment session. In view of the potential fire hazard of class four lasers, anesthetic gas mixtures that are explosive or inflammable should be avoided. The use of coaxial gas to cool the fiber tip can be associated with troublesome abdominal distension. In the awake patient this causes pain and discomfort, and may lead to the premature cessation of therapy. In the anesthetized spontaneously breathing patient, abdominal overdistension will embarrass respiration and impair oxygenation. Attempts to vent the excess gas by tubal drainage and suction are, in practice, not entirely successful and the situation demands strict monitoring and close cooperation between surgeon and anesthesiologist. The substitution of coaxial water for cooling purposes avoids this troublesome abdominal distension and reduces the risk of visceral perforation.

When NCM therapy is used the prospect of repeated anesthetics at 2- or 3-day intervals may persuade the endoscopist against general anesthesia. However, the combination of CM therapy and anesthesia ensures patient compliance and allows the surgeon sufficient time to perform a more complete treatment (7). As a consequence, the interval between treatments can be extended to 4 weeks for esophageal lesions and to as much as 8 weeks for rectal lesions.

Patients are frequently referred for palliative Nd:YAG laser endoscopic treatment because they are physically unfit for a major operation or because their disease process is too advanced for curative surgery. Nevertheless, general anesthesia for endoscopic procedures is safe. In the author's experience of more than 200 cases there have been no deaths directly related to anesthesia.

A further use of Nd:YAG laser energy via the endoscope is for biliary lithotripsy in patients with cholelithiasis (8). This offers a valuable alternative to early surgical intervention, which still carries a high mortality rate in elderly high-risk patients.

Open Surgery

Just as the Nd:YAG laser is the perfect endoscopic tool for photocoagulation and tumor vaporization so, for some time, the CO_2 laser has been adjudged the only laser cutting tool for general surgery and its use has been described for a wide range of body surface operations. After the introduction of contact probes for use with low-power energy in 1984, the Nd:YAG laser combined its unique coagulating properties with the cutting capabilities of the CO_2 laser. As a consequence, there has been a rapid expansion in the scope and range of operative use of the Nd:YAG laser (5).

Oral Surgery

The oral cavity, extending from the lips down to the larynx, is the territory of three surgical specialties: namely, general, orodental, and otolaryngology. The established use of the CO_2 laser in the larynx is associated with minimal operative trauma and bleeding and markedly reduced postoperative edema and pain. However, laser surgery in this site carries the greatest potential for anesthetic catastrophe due to the fire hazard associated with the use of high-power laser energy in the vicinity of combustible material (endotracheal tubes) and inflammable anesthetic gas mixtures. A simple anesthetic technique avoiding the need for endotracheal intubation and suitable for microscopic laryngeal laser surgery has been described by Spargo and colleagues (9). This involves the placement of a nasopharyngeal catheter that delivers a nonflammable anesthetic gas mixture to a spontaneously respiring patient. Careful monitoring of the airway patency is necessary. A full review of the use of the CO_2 laser in the larynx detailing the anesthetic hazards and recommended safety procedures has been given by Thode (10).

Within the oral cavity, major tongue resections are usually performed by otolaryngologists, mostly using the CO_2 laser. However, the use of low-power contact Nd:YAG laser energy within the oral cavity is increasing. General surgical usage includes resection of benign and malignant lesions of the lips, buccal mucosa, and tongue. Limited experience suggests that the low-power contact Nd:YAG laser provides the same operative and postoperative benefits as the CO_2 laser but with less danger of fire and explosion. In the author's opinion, safe anesthesia can be provided using routine nasotracheal intubation protected by a saline-moistened pharyngeal pack. Should surgery extend to the posterior oropharynx or pharyngeal region then discretion demands the use of a laser-resistant flexible metal tube for anesthesia. Figure 27.3 shows a suitable range of adult and pediatric oral and nasal endotracheal flexible metal tubes (11).

Body Surface Surgery

The surgical CO_2 laser has been used by general surgeons for a wide range of surface surgery including the resection of benign and malignant cutaneous lesions, mastectomy, axillary dissection, resection of lesions of the vulva and perineum, hemorrhoidectomy, and the desloughing of ischemic and infected ulcers. Because of its excellent cutting properties with minimal trauma to adjacent tissues its use has been associated with reduced operative blood loss, less postoperative tissue edema, and a significant reduction in the requirement for postoperative analgesia (12). This reduction in operative trauma and stress allows general anesthesia to be uneventfully performed even for the high-risk elderly patient. Routine anesthetic techniques can be used provided that they do not contravene the appropriate laser safety regulations. Where operative data are being collected for clinical research purposes the use of a standardized premedication, induction, and general anesthetic technique is vital if individual patient data are to withstand meaningful comparison. The author has reported his standard technique, which will provide safe anesthesia for the majority of surgical procedures (13). This involves premedication with lorazepam, induction of anesthesia with sodium thiopental, muscular relaxation with alcuronium (Alloferin), and analgesia with fentanyl. Ventilation is by intermittent positive pressure with a gas mixture of oxygen and nitrous oxide supplemented where necessary by a suitable nonflammable inhalational agent. Incremental doses of muscle relaxant and analgesic are given when clinically indicated. Intraoperative monitoring and recording should conform to the recommendations of the ASA (14). The meticulous keeping of records can prove valuable for research purposes and frequently stimulates interest in the evaluation of clinical anesthetic techniques. The appropriate use of regional or local anesthesia can be encouraged. Pfeffermann and his colleagues (15) have reported their use of the CO_2

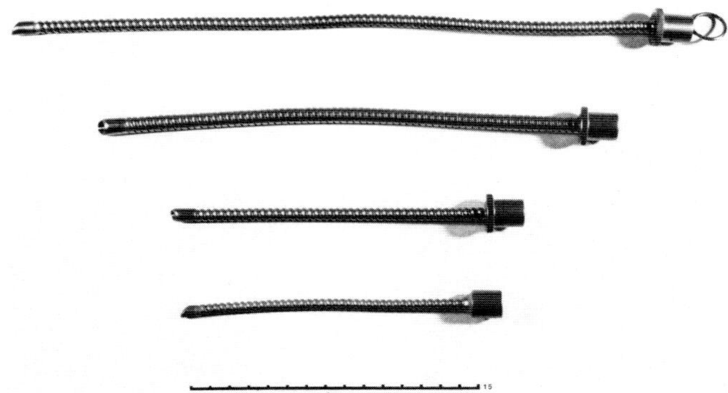

Figure 27.3. Oswal/Hunton flexible metal endotracheal tubes.

laser in rectal surgery utilizing a mixture of general, spinal, local, or no anesthesia.

With the introduction of contact tips and probes for use with low-power Nd:YAG laser energy, the surgeon now has a laser tool that can be used as a scalpel. In addition, the more precise mode of usage and reduced tissue penetration and damage make the contact Nd:YAG laser probe an excellent dissecting instrument (5). Brunner and his coworkers (16) have described its use for the treatment of benign, semimalignant, and malignant skin tumors. Comparative studies in breast surgery have shown very similar results and advantages to those for the CO_2 laser (17). In this reported study, patients undergoing Nd:YAG laser resection of primary breast carcinoma demonstrated reduced operative blood loss, a reduced need for postoperative analgesia, improved mobilization and earlier hospital discharge when compared with a similar group of patients undergoing conventional surgical excision.

The use of low-power contact Nd:YAG laser in the palliative treatment of malignant secondary cutaneous deposits that are sometimes extensive, ulcerating, and offensive has proved of particular benefit. The combination of low-power excision and photocoagulation using a focusing handpiece provides effective cleansing and toiletry, and promotes healing (N. Hira, personal communication). Even in poor-risk patients, general anesthesia can be safely undertaken because of the lack of surgical trauma and minimal biochemical and physiological upset. Overall, there would seem to be great similarity in the benefits for surface surgery using the Nd:YAG and CO_2 lasers and little difference in the techniques for anesthetic management.

Abdominal Surgery

Within the abdominal cavity, the use of the CO_2 laser is limited by its maneuverability, access to the operative site, and noncontact method of application. On the other hand, the introduction of a freely flexible contact method of applying the Nd:YAG laser has led to a marked increase in its operative use within the abdomen. Usage for a wide range of hollow viscus and solid-organ resections has been reported by several workers (5, 18). This is due, in part, to the precise nature of the dissection using contact probes with little surgical trauma to adjacent tissues. It is also due to the excellent hemostatic properties of the Nd:YAG laser, which seals small vessels. Thus, it prevents insidious capillary ooze that can be the source of troublesome blood loss, particularly in extensive tissue excision or in operations on highly vascular organs, such as the liver or the spleen.

Because of these advantages, stable anesthesia can be easily established even in those high-risk patients who might otherwise be judged unfit for major conventional operative procedures (19). Cardiovascular stability during laser surgery in the abdomen is impressive and has been shown by clinical trial to be superior to that achieved during conventional abdominal surgery. Figure 27.4 shows examples of good cardiovascular stability during major abdominal resections. In addition, the need for blood transfusion is reduced to a minimum. Reviewing some 200 Nd:YAG laser cases, the author found that only 2% required intraoperative blood transfusion.

Reports of the experimental use of both CO_2 and Nd:YAG lasers in liver and splenic resection

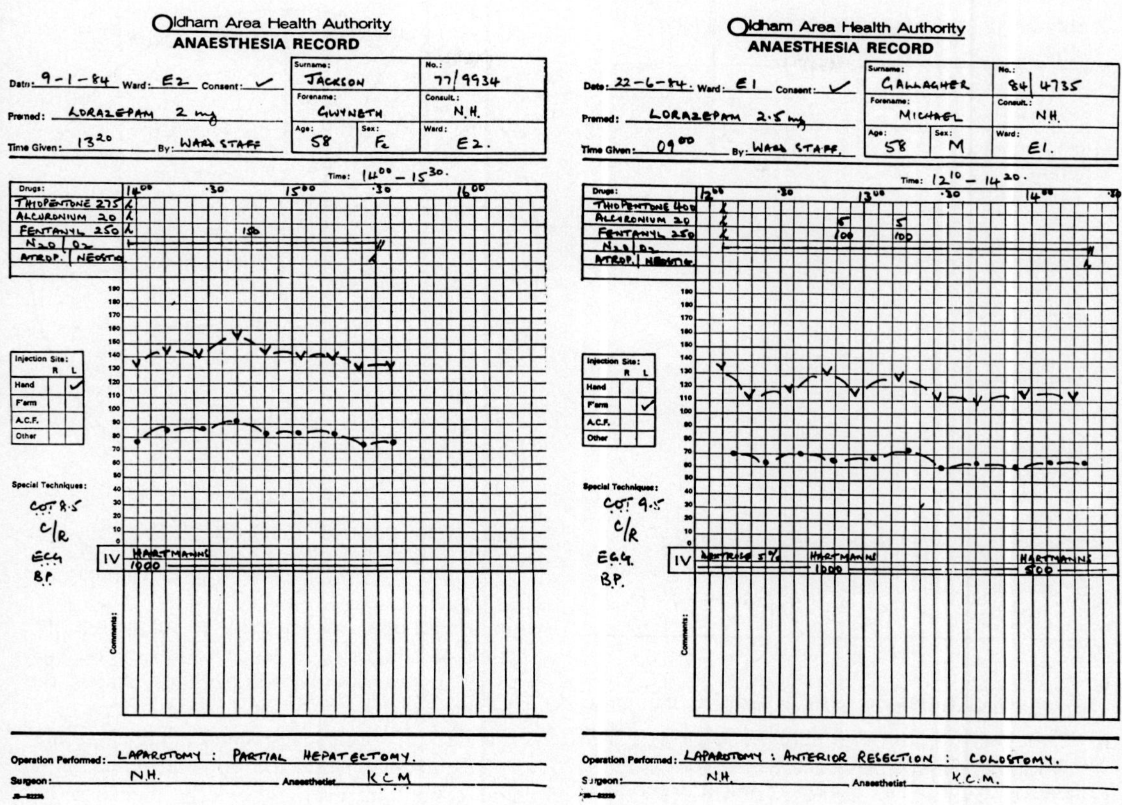

Oldham Area Health Authority
ANAESTHESIA RECORD

Date: 9-1-84 Ward: E2 Consent: ✓
Surname: JACKSON No.: 77/9934
Premed: LORAZEPAM 2 mg
Forename: GWYNETH Consult.: N.H.
Time Given: 13 20 By: WARD STAFF
Age: 58 Sex: F Ward: E2.
Time: 14 00 – 15 30.
Drugs: THIOPENTONE 275; ALCURONIUM 20; FENTANYL 250; N2O/O2; ATROP./NEOSTIG.
Injection Site: R L; Hand ✓; F'arm; A.C.F.; Other
Special Techniques: COT 8.5; C/R; ECG; BP
IV HARTMANNS 1000
Comments:
Operation Performed: LAPAROTOMY : PARTIAL HEPATECTOMY.
Surgeon: N.H. Anaesthetist K.C.M.

Oldham Area Health Authority
ANAESTHESIA RECORD

Date: 22-6-84. Ward: E1 Consent: ✓
Surname: GALLAGHER No.: 84/4735
Premed: LORAZEPAM 2.5 mg
Forename: MICHAEL Consult.: N.H.
Time Given: 09 00 By: WARD STAFF.
Age: 58 Sex: M Ward: E1.
Time: 12 10 – 14 20.
Drugs: THIOPENTONE 400; ALCURONIUM 20; FENTANYL 250; N2O/O2; ATROP./NEOSTIG.
Injection Site: R L; Hand; F'arm ✓; A.C.F.; Other
Special Techniques: COT 9.5; C/R; ECG; BP.
IV DEXTROSE 5%; HARTMANNS 1000; HARTMANNS 500
Comments:
Operation Performed: LAPAROTOMY : ANTERIOR RESECTION : COLOSTOMY.
Surgeon: N.H. Anaesthetist K.C.M.

Figure 27.4. CVS stability during contact Nd:YAG abdominal surgery.

confirm the advantages of lasers over conventional techniques (20, 22). Sultan and colleagues describe the combined use of the CO_2 and Nd:YAG lasers for resection of liver tumors (23). Circulatory disturbance is reduced during operation and, in the immediate postoperative period, the absence of incised surface ooze reduces morbidity. Hira et al. have reported a partial splenectomy after trauma in a young adult male (24). In this case the use of the Nd:YAG laser allowed the retention of a substantial portion of a badly traumatized spleen.

POSTOPERATIVE PAIN

The use of both the CO_2 and Nd:YAG lasers for breast surgery has been associated with less postoperative pain, early mobilization, and a significant reduction in hospital stay (12, 17). Other reports concerning reduced postoperative pain after laser surgery have been mainly anecdocal. Nevertheless, there appears to be a definite correlation between the use of lasers, particularly for body surface surgery, and a reduced need for postoperative analgesia.

Table 27.1 shows the author's experience of the need for analgesia after low-power contact Nd:YAG laser excision or high-power Nd:YAG photocoagulation of a wide range of benign and malignant lesions of the body surface. In the group comprising excision of discrete tumors (n = 37), 19 patients required no postoperative analgesia (51%). Those patients with ulcerating lesions (n = 35) showed even less evidence of postoperative pain with some 28 patients (80%) declining analgesia. In this latter group, because of the extensive nature of their malignant disease process, 31% (n = 11) were already established preoperatively on a regular oral dose of morphine, which was maintained unaltered postoperatively.

The absence of severe pain enables early patient mobilization after surgery and, in many cases, reduces hospital stay. Although this may

Table 27.1. Analgesia after Nd:YAG Surface Surgery

Operative Site (n)		Analgesia (n) Intramuscular	Oral	None
Primary tumor				
Breast	11	2	6	3
Cutaneous	3	0	1	2
Oral	5	0	1	4
Metastatic tumor				
Breast	6	0	4	2
Cutaneous	3	1	1	1
Oral	2	0	0	2
Benign tumor				
Perineal	7	0	2	5
Malignant ulcer				
Breast	6	0	2	4
Abdomen	5	0	1	4
Vulval	11	0	2	9
Perineal	9	0	2	7
Benign ulcer				
Ischemic	4	0	0	4

be expected for body surface surgery the same does not apply to major abdominal surgery, which is not associated with the same reduction in postoperative pain levels. Limited clinical experience suggests that there is no significant difference in analgesic requirements between Nd:YAG and conventional surgical techniques within the abdomen (13).

CONCLUSION

The indications for the use of the CO_2 laser in general surgery are well established and have proved valuable in breast surgery, axillary dissection, resection of liver tumors, tongue resection, and perineal surgery. The endoscopic application of either high-power noncontact or low-power contact Nd:YAG laser energy within the gastrointestinal tract is now a clinically accepted form of therapy. General anesthesia for all these procedures is safe provided that attention is paid to specific safeguards and laser safety regulations.

The application of low-power contact Nd:YAG laser energy is being evaluated in a wide range of general surgical procedures. Figure 27.5 shows the typical distribution of laser workload between endoscopic, body surface, and abdominal surgery. The particular benefits of the contact Nd:YAG laser are seen to best advantage in operations involving extensive tissue dissection, resection of hemorrhagic or necrotic tumors, surgery of highly vascular solid organs, and in the debridement of extensive ulcerating lesions.

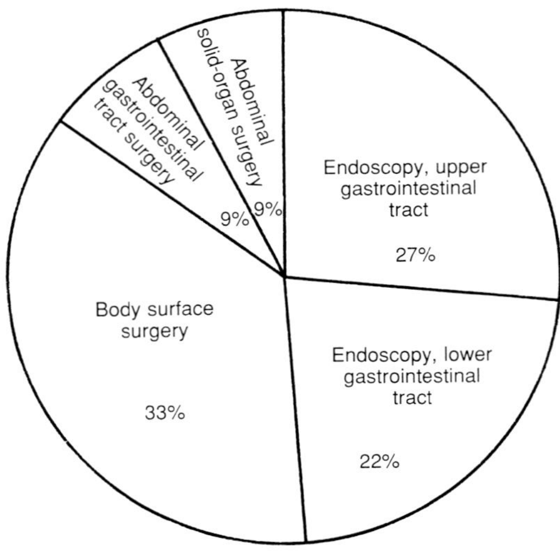

Figure 27.5. Caseload distribution for Nd:YAG laser surgery.

The lack of surgical stress and minimal circulatory disturbance helps to promote stable anesthetic conditions even in elderly high-risk patients. For body surface surgery, the reduced postoperative morbidity improves recovery and shortens hospitalization. It is hoped that this chapter will encourage anesthesiologists to participate fully in this rapidly expanding branch of surgery.

REFERENCES

1. Kuroda Y, Ichida O, Ohsato K, Koga T, Akashi Y, Tomimatsu H. Endoscopic application of Nd:YAG laser for early gastric cancer in surgically high risk patients. In Oguro Y, Atsumi K, Joffe SN, Eds. Nd:YAG Laser in Medicine and Surgery. Fundamental and Clinical Aspects. Tokyo: PPS, 1986, pp 162-167.
2. Swain CP, Kirkham JS, Salmon PR, Bown SG, Northfield TC. Controlled trial of Nd:YAG laser photocoagulation in bleeding peptic ulcers. Lancet 1986; 1:1113-1116.
3. Mathus-Vliegen EMH, Tytgat GNJ. Nd:YAG laser photocoagulation in gastroenterology: its role in palliation of colorectal cancer. Lasers Med Sci 1986; 1:75-80.
4. Brunetaud JM, Maunoury V, Ancelin JP, Cochelard D, Cortot A, Paris JC. Lasers in rectosigmoid tumors. In Oguro Y, Atsumi K, Joffee SN, Eds. Nd:YAG Laser in Medicine and Surgery. Fundamental and Clinical Aspects. Tokyo: PPS, 1986, pp. 203-209.

5. Joffe SN. Contact neodymium: YAG laser surgery in gastroenterology: A preliminary report. Lasers Surg Med 1986; 6:155-157.
6. Ell C, Hochberger J, Lux G. Clinical experience of noncontact and contact Nd:YAG laser therapy for inoperable malignant stenoses of the oesophagus and stomach. Lasers Med Sci 1986; 1:143–146.
7. Steger AC, Hira N. The palliative endoscopic treatment of inoperable oesophagogastric and rectal cancers: A low power direct contact laser technique. Ann RCSE 1987; 69:166-168.
8. Inui K, Nakazawa S, Naito Y, et al. Biliary endoscopic lithotripsy with Nd:YAG laser in patients with cholelithiasis. In Oguro Y, Atsumi K, Joffe SN, Eds. Nd:YAG Laser in Medicine and Surgery. Fundamental and Clinical Aspects. Tokyo: PPS, 1986, pp. 245-249.
9. Spargo PM, Nielsen MS, Carruth JAS. Use of a carbon dioxide laser for treatment of recurrent laryngeal papillomatosis in small children: Experiences with an anaesthetic technique. Lasers Med Sci 1986; 1:211-216.
10. Thode SA. Laryngo-tracheal laser surgery and general anesthesia. Lasers Surg Med 1986; 6:369-372.
11. Oswal/Hunton endotracheal tubes. Leyland, Preston: UK, Leyland Medical. 1987.
12. Ansanelli VW. CO_2 laser in cancer surgery of the breast: A comparative clinical study. Lasers Surg Med 1986; 6:470-472.
13. Moore KC, Steger A, Hira N. The operative care of patients for Nd:YAG contact laser surgery. In Oguro Y, Atsumi K, Joffe SN, Eds. Nd:YAG Laser in Medicine and Surgery. Fundamental and Clinical Aspects. Tokyo: PPS, 1986, pp. 124-127.
14. Standards for Basic Intra-operative Monitoring. ASA, 1986.
15. Pfeffermann R, Merhav H, Rothstein H, Simon D. The use of laser in rectal surgery. Lasers Surg Med 1986; 6:467-469.
16. Brunner R, Landthaler M, Haina D, Waidelich W, Braun-Falco O. Treatment of benign, semimalignant and malignant skin tumors with the Nd:YAG laser. Lasers Surg Med 1985; 5:105-110.
17. Moore KC. General anesthesia for Nd:YAG laser surgery. In Joffe SN, Ed. Advances in Nd:YAG Laser Surgery. New York: Springer-Verlag, 1987, p. 634.
18. Hira N, Steger AC, Moore KC. Contact low power Nd:YAG laser in general surgery. In Oguro Y, Atsumi K, Joffe SN, Eds. Nd:YAG Laser in Medicine and Surgery. Fundamental and Clinical Aspects. Tokyo: PPS, 1986, pp. 138-140.
19. Moore KC. Anesthesia for Nd:YAG laser surgery. Today's Anaesthetist 1986; 1:6-7.
20. Nims TA, McCaughan JS. Clinical experience with CO_2 laser vaporization of neoplasm. Lasers Surg Med 1983; 3:265-268.
21. Schroder T, Sankar MY, Brackett KM, Booth A, Joffe SN. Major liver resection in the pig using contact Nd:YAG laser—a new technique. Lasers Surg Med (Abstr. 83) 1987; 7:89.
22. Schroder T, Foster J, Brackett K, Joffe SN. Splenic resection with the CO_2 laser and the contact Nd:YAG laser scalpel. (Abstr.) Lasers Med Sci 1986; 1:293-294.
23. Sultan RA, Fallouh H, Lefebvre-Vilardebo M, Ladouch-Badre A. Separate and combined use of Nd:YAG and carbon dioxide lasers in liver resections: A preliminary report. Lasers Med Sci 1986; 1:101-105.
24. Hira N, Steger AC, Moore KC. Use of Nd:YAG laser in an emergency partial splenectomy. Lasers Med Sci 1987; 2:127-129.

CHAPTER
28

Postoperative Analgesia

Prithvi Raj

The present state of affairs is such that relief of postoperative pain remains largely unsolved (1). Postoperative pain is currently treated by systemic administration of non-narcotic and narcotic analgesics. Many new potent analgesic drugs have been introduced in clinical practice in the last 50 years. Their inability to provide adequate pain relief is not due to their lack of potency, but rather to improper administration (2). The reasons for inadequate analgesia are (*a*) the physicians' orders are poorly written, they are frequently inappropriate for the type and severity of pain; (*b*) they are not explicit enough and open to misinterpretation by the nursing staff; (*c*) frequently, there is a failure to understand that patients differ in their analgesic requirements.

Obviously, if parenteral drugs are to achieve their analgesic effects, an adequate plasma concentration of the drug must be attained to equilibrate with receptors specific to produce analgesia. Studies show that blood drug concentrations after intramuscular administration are totally unpredictable. This, in turn, produces a varying quality of analgesia. With the intravenous (IV) technique, some of the barriers responsible for uneven drug absorption are removed, and it is simpler to titrate a dose that will safely and quickly achieve a desired analgesic effect. An extension of this idea is the predetermined intermittent or continuous IV administration of narcotics based on a dosage schedule that can be calculated according to pharmacokinetic principles (3).

A recent innovation and an extension of the same principles governing IV administration of narcotics and analgesia is the use of mechanical devices that allow the patient to administer a predetermined dose of a particular agent (3, 4). This technique has been called "patient-controlled analgesia" and is gaining popularity in its use. The devices can be programmed to allow repetitive increments of drug to be self-administered, while limits can be set to prevent toxic amounts from being delivered (5).

Alternative techniques to systemic analgesic administration are: (*a*) various regional anesthesia procedures (infiltration, intercostal nerve blocks, epidural infusion of local anesthetics, and narcotics); and (*b*) transcutaneous electrical nerve stimulation (TENS) and cryoanalgesia.

TECHNIQUES OF ANALGESIC

Intravenous Infusion

Narcotics commonly administered by IV infusion for the control of postoperative pain are morphine, meperidine, fentanyl, burprenorphine, and methadone.

The following are examples of dosages that are suggested for morphine, meperidine, fentanyl, and methadone in patients who have undergone major abdominal surgery: morphine, 2.5–5.0 mg/hour; meperidine, 25–30 mg/hour; fentanyl, 0.045 mg/hour; and methadone, 2.5 mg/hour. Few clinical data are available for buprenorphine, although its pharmacokinetic characteristics are very similar to the other narcotics.

TRANSCUTANEOUS ELECTRICAL NERVE STIMULATION

TENS as a means of inhibiting the acute pain of injury is certainly not as effective as nerve blocks are. However, when used after abdominal surgery, it is almost as effective as parenteral narcotics and does not induce the undesirable side effects of respiratory depression, nausea, vomiting, and urinary retention. Several randomized studies have shown that analgesia provided is better than placebo effect. This was confirmed when the patients conclusively demonstrated the placebo effect with nerve stimulators that had their batteries removed. What is still lacking, however, is a good randomized controlled study of the cardiovascular effects and of the effects on stress hormones when this form of analgesia is compared with another standard for of pain relief.

Although the pain relief using TENS remains incomplete, the concurrent administration of small doses of parenteral opiates will provide the additional analgesia needed to achieve almost complete relief of pain without the side effects often associated with the exclusive use of parenteral narcotics. Some early reports of postoperative TENS claimed a reduction in the frequency of postoperative ileus and pulmonary atelectasis (6). Subsequent studies, however, have not confirmed these earlier observations. The main disadvantage of TENS is the management of the electrodes that, for their integrity and continued function, require excellent skin contact. Any movements, sweating, secretions, and disconnection of the cables, particularly to those electrodes that are included in the dressing can interfere with the continuity of analgesia; nevertheless, TENS is a practical alternative form of pain relief.

NERVE BLOCKS

Intercostal Blocks

The use of intercostal blocks for postoperative pain management has been underemphasized and, as a consequence, their application has been underutilized. Intercostal block is perhaps the easiest of all nerve blocks to perform because of the proximity of the nerve to the rib, which is its principal landmark (7, 8). Although the procedure carries the potential hazard of pneumothorax, this complication can be avoided by understanding the local anatomy and using an impeccable technique.

Most of the pain from abdominal surgery arises from the parietal peritoneum and the incision. Intercostal nerve blocks, therefore, can provide adequate analgesia and the relief from muscle spasm within the territory of innervation. In the chest, intercostal blocks can be used to provide analgesia after rib resection and thoracotomy (9, 10).

An alternative to multiple intercostal injection sites is the introduction of an intrapleural catheter and administration of 20 ml of 0.5% bupivacaine as a bolus on demand or use of 0.25% bupivacaine in a 10-ml continuous infusion (11).

Cryoanalgesia

The principal advantage of cryoanalgesia over local anesthetic intercostal blocks is the prolonged duration achieved (12). The disadvantage is that the technique is not available at every institution. In addition, it requires practice and has a long latency period to produce an effective analgesia. Where a large volume of thoracic surgery is performed, this can be a practical feasibility.

Epidural Block

Epidural analgesic agents for postoperative pain may be administered by intermittent injection or as a continuous infusion. While the intermittent method is certainly the most popular, continuous infusion technique provides a better quality of analgesia (13). For intermittent epidural analgesia to be successful, close medical and nursing monitoring is necessary to ensure immediate reinjection of the epidural catheter as soon as the patient experiences pain. Normally, however, tachyphylaxis develops rapidly.

Considerable experience has been gained in the last 20 years in the use of continuous epidural infusions (14–17). The method is comparatively safe because the solution is weak and the high resistance offered by the epidural catheter can be overcome by the use of volumetric infusion pumps. The dose can be predetermined. The dose will vary with the severity of pain and the number of dermatomes requiring analgesia. The steady-state is achieved usually after five half-lives of the drugs are attained (18). Such pumps can be set to give a bolus dose at predetermined intervals of time to prevent breakthrough pain.

DRUGS USED FOR CONTINUOUS EPIDURAL BLOCK

Only long-acting local anesthetics, e.g., bupivacaine and etidocaine hydrochloride, should be used for continuous infusion. Recently, intraspinal opiates have been used as an alternative to local anesthetics.

Spinal opiate administration does not produce an autonomic block. Loss of this modality in the postoperative period may be undersirable in patients who have undergone vascular surgery or in obese patients. Such patients are at risk for thromboembolic phenomena. This fact has prompted the combination of local anesthetics and narcotics. (19, 20). Clinicians have used combinations of bupivacaine with either morphine, meperidine, or fentanyl for continuous drip infusion. The experience shows that the combination of a local anesthetic with a narcotic provides excellent postoperative analgesia with minimal side effects.

Miscellaneous Techniques

Dextran and Local Anesthetics

Since Loder (21) used a combination of lidocaine and high molecular weight dextran (150,000) for the use of extending the duration of intercostal blocks in association with postthoracotomy analgesic treatments, investigators have tried to identify the mechanism by which such substances could prolong the action of local anesthetics. Both in vivo and in vitro studies have tended to produce conflicting data either supporting a longer duration or action or refuting such an effect. The mechanisms that have been postulated are: the pH of the solution; the absorptive effect of the dextran molecules; and the osmotic effect, a fact that is related to the size of the molecule.

Perfusion of Surgical Wounds

The perfusion of surgical wounds with local anesthetic solutions has been carried out for many years with varying degrees of success. A recent study has shown that if a wound, such as cholecystectomy, is perfused with a solution of either saline or bupivacaine over a period of 48 hours, the analgesic requirement is reduced by 70%. It seems that rather than attributing a placebo effect to the saline, it may well be that by removal of humoral substances, the genesis of postoperative pain is significantly lessened. Interestingly, no significant restoration of the vital capacity toward preoperative values occurred with either solution, results that are in agreement with other investigators who have compared similar respiratory parameters under the influence of epidural block or parenteral narcotic administration.

POSTOPERATIVE ANALGESIA IN CHILDREN

Inpatient or outpatient surgical procedures on the perineum and lower limbs in children are often associated with a stormy and combative early recovery phase. While it is normal to employ a general anesthetic technique, it is a simple matter, in addition, to perform a single-shot caudal anesthetic with 0.25% bupivacaine (22). The only potential problem with postoperative caudal analgesia is a delay in micturition in children, although this is not frequent.

The use of TENS for postoperative pain after thoracic surgery in children has recently been described (16). The impairment of respiration after operations to correct the congenital abnormality of pectus excavatum poses a challenge for adequate pain control in the postoperative period. Normally, very large doses of parenteral narcotics are required with their potential for severe respiratory depression and further hampering a return to normal pulmonary function. Intercostal blocks are difficult to do in a child. High blood levels may result from the number of intercostal spaces needing to be blocked. Thoracic epidural analgesia would be ideal, however, only a few clinicians would have the training and skill to perform this procedure.

The technique requires that two electrodes be placed parallel to the incision before a sterile dressing is applied. With the patient still under anesthesia, the electrodes are connected to an output device and the current is raised until slight muscle movement is detected. The output is then decreased until this disappears after which this setting is maintained during the postoperative period. The degree of analgesia achieved by this method can reduce the morphine requirements from as little as 3 mg during the first postoperative day to no narcotics at all during the postoperative course.

In summary, alternative techniques of providing adequate analgesia to postoperative patients is available. Regional anesthesia techniques are superior to parenteral administration of narcotics. With the introduction of spinal opiates, epidural analgesic techniques can be used with greater flexibility and reliability to provide excellent postoperative analgesia.

REFERENCES

1. Postoperative pain (editorial). Br Med J 1978; 2:517-518.
2. Mather LE. Pharmacokinetics and pharmacodynamic factors influencing the choice, dose and route of administration of opiates for acute pain. In Bullingham R, Ed. Clinics in Anaesthesiology. London: W.B. Saunders Co., 1983.
3. Hull CJ, Sibbald A. Control of postoperative pain by interactive demand analgesia. Br J Anaesth 1981; 53:385-391.
4. Tamsen A, Hartvig P, Dahlstrom B, et al. Endorphans and on-demand pain relief. Lancet 1980; 1:769-780.

5. Hull CJ. Opioid infusions for the management of postoperative pain. In Smith G, Covino BG. Eds. Acute Pain. London: Butterworth, 1985, pp. 155-279.
6. Nelson GD, Printy AL. Electrical surface stimulation for control of acute postoperative pain and prevention of ileus. Surg Forum 1973; 24:447.
7. Cronin KD, Davies MJ. Intercostal block for postoperative pain relief. Anesth Int Care 1976; 4:459-461.
8. Moore DC, Bridenbaugh LD. Intercostal nerve block in 4333 patients: Indications, technique and complications. Anaesth Analg Curr Res 1962; 41:1.
9. Faust RA, Nauss LA. Post-thoracotomy intercostal block: Comparison of its effects on pulmonary function with those of intramuscular meperidine. Anesth Analg Curr Res 1976; 55:542.
10. Galway JE, Caves PK, Dundee JW. Effect of intercostal blockade during operation on lung function and the relief of pain following thoracotomy. Br J Anesth 1975; 47:730-735.
11. Murphy DF. Continuous intercostal nerve blockade. An anatomical study to elucidate its mode of action. Br J Anaesth 1984; 56:627-30.
12. Lloyd JW, Barnard JDW, Glynn CJ. Cryoanalgesia: A new approach to pain relief. Lancet 1976; 2:932.
13. Raj PP, Denson D, Finnsson R. Prolonged epidural analgesia: Intermittent or continuous. In Meyer J, Nolte H, Eds. Die kontinuierliche Periduralanaesthesie. Stuttgart: Georg Thieme Verlag, 1983, pp. 26-37.
14. Cleland JGP. Continuous peridural and caudal analgesia in surgery and early ambulation. Northwest Med J 1948; 48:26.
15. Evans KRL, Carrie LES. Continuous epidural infusion of bupivacaine in labour: A simple method. Anesthesia 1979; 34:310-135.
16. Hinkle AJ, Koka BV. Transcutaneous electrical stimulation for pain control after thoracic surgery in children. Reg Anesthesth 1983; 8:163-165.
17. Spoerel WJ, Thomas A, Gerula GR. Continuous epidural analgesia: Experience with mechanical injection devices. Cana Anaesth Soc J 1970; 17:37.
18. Tucker GT, Mather LE. Pharmacokinetics of local anaesthetic agents. Br J Anaesth 1975; 47:213-224.
19. Muller H, Borner U, Gips H, et al. Intraoperative peridurale Opiatanalgesie. In Wust H, Stanton-Hicks M, Zindler M, Eds. Neue Aspekie in der Regional-anaesthesie, vol. 3. Anaesthesiology and Intensive Care Medicine. Heidelberg: Springer-Verlag, 1984, pp. 152-163.
20. Tucker GT, Cooper S, Littlewood D, et al. Observed and predicted accumulation of local anaesthetic agents during continuous extradural anaesthesia. Br J Anaesth 1977; 49:237-241.
21. Loder RE. A local anaesthetic solution with longer action. Lancet 1960; 2:346.
22. Schulte-Steinberg O, Rahlfs VW. Caudal anaesthesia in children and spread of 1 percent lignocaine: A statistical study. Br J Anaesth 1970; 42:1093.

CHAPTER

29

Nursing Care for Patients Having General Surgery Laser Procedures

Carolyn J. Mackety

The surgical specialty known as general surgery falls into several categories: low-risk surgery, high-risk surgery, and surgical oncology. Other surgical specialties that are in the domain of general surgery are: thoracic, vascular, colorectal, and gastroenterological. For this chapter, the perioperative care of patients who have their surgical procedures performed with lasers will be discussed. Also, because gastroenterology is a specialty that requires special nursing considerations, the nursing process will be confined to those patients who fall into the general surgical category.

Using the Nd:YAG laser with the synthetic sapphire ceramic tips on a variety of handpieces (scalpels) gives the physician tactile feedback; this mechanism was not available earlier in the development of Nd:YAG laser techniques. This method also allows the physician precision and less blood loss, contributing to quality patient care. Using this laser system suggests cost-effective care, decreasing the length of stay and, although subjective, the possibility of less postoperative discomfort to both the physician and the patient.

The low-risk patients can be those whose surgical intervention are for the following procedures: cholecystectomy; herniorrhaphy; anal procedures; lysis of adhesions; pilonidal cyst; hemorrhoidectomy; modified radical mastectomy; and exploratory laparotomies (where extensive dissection is not expected).

NURSING CONSIDERATIONS

The nursing process has the following components: assessment, planning, implementation/intervention, documentation, and evaluation. This process is a continuum in the surgical nursing environment and in collaborative practice with other team members and the patient's physician.

Preoperative *assessment* begins when the patient perceives that there is a medical problem and seeks the assistance of a physician. When the decision is made to have a surgical procedure, informed consent begins as the patient and physician discuss the risks, outcomes, and alternatives of care. Preadmission testing may be required and the patient is sent to the hospital or a certified laboratory to complete all laboratory work, x-rays and admission requirements. If the patient is having his/her procedure with the laser, an educational pamphlet (Fig. 29.1) may be available that will explain the procedure. This will be important especially if the procedure will be done as a same-day admission or as an outpatient.

If the patient is to be admitted to the hospital, the preoperative assessment begins on admission to the nursing unit or in the day of admission unit. Six areas of assessment are included.

1. current medical history
2. assessing the patient's understanding of the surgical event
3. review laboratory results to ascertain whether they fall with in normal parameters
4. assessments of physical requirements to include any handicaps, elimination patterns, nutritional and sensory needs
5. physiological assessment to assist in allaying fears related to coping with current health care needs
6. socioeconomic assessment provides information for discharge planning.

The resources for nursing assessment can be the physician, patient, family, or previous medi-

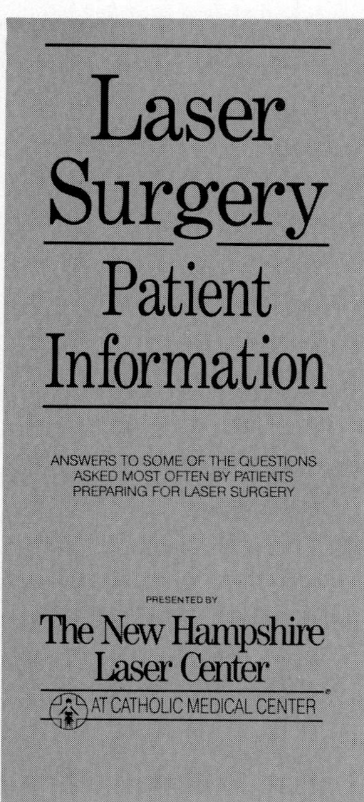

What is a laser?
The word laser stands for Light Amplification by the Stimulated Emission of Radiation. It is an intense beam of light of one single wavelength and color with a high amount of energy.

What does it do?
All matter has energy, and light energy can be absorbed, transmitted or scattered. This causes a reaction which, when a laser is used for medical purposes, allows it to cut, vaporize or coagulate tissue.

What kinds of lasers are used in medicine and surgery?
Specific lasers are named for the substance or medium used to cause the lasing and can be a gas, solid or liquid medium. Here at The New Hampshire Laser Center at Catholic Medical Center, we have the state-of-the-art in medical laser technology.

How does the laser work?
A resonator box contains the lasing medium (a solid crystal or a gas). The laser's power source pumps energy into the medium to excite the atoms and create stimulated emission. A small amount of laser light is transmitted into a delivery system. Light remaining in the resonator reflects back into the medium, "amplifying" the light by a process known as stimulated emission of radiation.

What is special about laser light?
This intense beam of light is focused in a straight line, or *collimated.* It is *coherent*–comes out all at once–and is all one color.

How does this compare with other light and power?
A regular light bulb shines incoherent light of many wavelengths. When it shines, there is no straight beam, so it shines everywhere, looks white and has no real energy. Lasers put out power ranging from .5 watts to 100 watts for medical lasers. By comparison, an electric toothbrush might be rated at 5 watts, and light bulbs put out 60 watts of unfocused energy.

What are the laser advantages in medicine and surgery?
- It can be focused to the size of a pinhead, even to a single cell.
- The tissue does not have to be touched.
- It can be used with fiber-optics to reach inaccessible places, often without incisions.
- It coagulates to reduce blood loss.
- It can be focused through body fluids.

What happens during the procedure?
If you are having laser surgery, the doctor may inject medication to numb the area of surgery. You may be asked to wear a pair of special glasses during the surgical procedure. You will probably hear the sound of the laser machine as it works and you may smell an unusual odor. Your blood pressure will be taken during the surgery, and a nurse will be with you at all times during the procedure. Please tell the doctor if you are uncomfortable at any time during the surgery.

What should I do to prepare for my surgery?
Please arrive at the Outpatient Registration area in the lobby on Level A at least one hour before your scheduled appointment.
The Outpatient Admitting Registrar will complete the necessary forms and will ask you to sign a consent form.
Also at this time, you will need to verify your medical insurance information, so please bring your cards or information with you.
If admission to the hospital is required for your procedure, arrangements will be made in advance and you will be notified.

On the day of your laser surgery, please do:
- have another adult accompany you to drive you home after your surgery
- wear casual, comfortable clothes
- bring your medical insurance card
- tell us if you have allergies

please do not:
- bring extra money or valuables
- wear a lot of jewelry or makeup
- eat or drink after midnight the night before, unless you are instructed otherwise.

You are scheduled for laser surgery at The New Hampshire Laser Center at Catholic Medical Center on:

DATE: ________________

TIME: ________________

If you have any other questions, contact your doctor, or call The New Hampshire Laser Center at Catholic Medical Center at (603) 669-5227, between 8 a.m. and 4:30 p.m., Monday through Friday.

The New Hampshire Laser Center
AT CATHOLIC MEDICAL CENTER
Enlightened Medicine.

88 McGregor Street
Manchester, New Hampshire 03102
603-669-5227

Figure 29.1. An educational information pamphlet for the laser surgery patient.

cal records. After documenting the assessment, the nursing staff can begin to plan the patient's care.

Planning the patient's care should be realistic and defined in short- and long-range goals, including discharge planning. The patient and family should be included in this planning process. Care planning may include other health care workers, such as social workers, nutritionists, pharmacists, home health care personnel, and even physical therapists, as needed.

Planning includes preparation for the surgical procedure; informing the patients how they will feel after being given their preoperative medication, what to expect during the wait in the holding area, and explaining the operating room environment. The family should be informed as to where to wait for information regarding the patient, approximately how long the procedure may take, that the physician will come and see them as soon as possible, and when or where they will be able to see the patient. The recovery room experience should also be explained. As patients emerge from anesthesia, it is difficult for them to comprehend that the tightness on their arms is from the blood pressure cuff or the IV line in their hands or arms; the calling of their names, and asking them where they are helps the recovery room personnel assess their levels of consciousness.

Planning for care during surgical intervention includes reviewing the nursing assessment to determine patient needs during the procedure. If the patient is handicapped or with some disabilities, positioning bolsters may be necessary to maintain body alignment, assuring no nerves or pressure points are compromised. Also, knowing the physician requirements for the procedure is important for the smooth administration of the case. For low-risk general surgical procedures, when done as a contact laser procedure, the following supplies and equipment may be required. This, however, is not an exhaustive list.

Implementation of the care plan requires the following supplies and equipment.

Minor instrument pan
Prep set up (area must be dry)
Sponges, dressings, tape
Light handles/suture
Nd:YAG Laser with handpiece
Scalpel tips (0.6-, 0.8-mm frosted)
Calibration ports
Back tables and Mayo stand
Laparotomy pack
Physician "specials"
Suction tubing/canisters
Drains (physician preference)
Eye protection for all
Signs on entrances to operating room
Covering for viewing windows

If a common duct exploration is done in conjunction with a cholecystectomy, a 50-ml syringe, Renografin 60, cholangiocatheter, and a t-tube will be needed. The x-ray department should be notified as soon as the gallbladder is removed, so the technician is available as soon as the cholangiocatheter is inserted into the common duct.

Kerlix super sponges with hypoallergenic tape is the best dressing for abdominal procedures. The dressings for mastectomies require pressure dressings, using fluffs, especially in the axillae preventing seroma from forming.

The major general surgical procedures include (but are not limited to):

Excision colonic tumors
Distal Pancreatectomy
Partial hepatectomy
Debulking abdominal tumor

These patients are at high risk and often are nutritionally compromised, due to the etiology of their disease. Many of these procedures often require multiple transfusions; with the use of the laser, the blood loss should be minimal.

Preoperative planning for these procedures requires organization to expedite the operative procedure, thereby reducing anesthesia time. Implementation includes setting up the room to include blood warmer or autotransfusion set-up, k-thermia blanket, positioning equipment, and suction equipment.

The following instruments, supplies, and equipment that may be needed (not an exhaustive list).

Major instrument pan
Bowel instruments
Laparotomy pack/extra sheets
Gowns/gloves
Liga-clips/applicators
Handpiece (general/oral)
Suture
Back tables and Mayo stand

Long pan extras
Self-retaining retractors
Sponges (laps/raytex) dressings
Prep set-up (area must be dry)
Suction/canisters
Probes, 0.6-, 0.8-mm frosted, chisel and flat
Kick buckets

Make sure there are enough outlets for all of the electrical equipment.

An important time for patient care in the operating room is during the anesthesia induction. The circulating nurse must be available at the bedside, if needed during this time. Organization of the room set-up will allow her/him to be free to assist the anesthesiologist during this time.

The recovery room personnel will care for patients having laser procedures with the same objectives as those having conventional procedures. They should be aware that these patients may have less postoperative discomfort and decreased wound drainage.

Postoperative care will depend on the procedure performed. Each physician have their own standard of care. There are several nursing considerations in caring for patients who must ambulate early, cough, and deep breathe. Approximately 1 hour before respiratory therapy treatments, patients should take their pain medication and support should be provided for the incision site with a folded bath blanket or pillow. It should be explained that by having respiratory therapy treatments, patients avoid fluid accumulation in the lungs, which prevents pneumonia.

Several nursing considerations should be discussed with the patient before ambulation. The patient must understand the purpose of early ambulation, i.e., to prevent venous stasis causing thrombophlebitis. It is difficult to ambulate with IV lines in the hand or arm; these are necessary because the patient will require parenteral feeding to keep up basic nutrition until a diet can be tolerated. A mobile IV pole will be necessary during ambulation.

When assisting patients to ambulate, wash and dry their legs and reapply their elastic stockings. The patients should have comfortable slippers or shoes. The bed should be moved to the lowest position, the back of the bed raised, and, using a pulley mechanism, patients should sit on the side of the bed for 1–3 min to ascertain their equilibrium. Patients should be allowed to stand for 30 sec before beginning mobilization. Short-range goals for ambulation should be planned and expanded each time the patient ambulates.

Patients who have minor operative procedures are encouraged to early ambulation and progressive care. These patients' length of stay is decreased relative to the use of the laser during their surgical intervention.

Discharge planning for patients having general surgical procedures will depend on the organ system. Low-risk patients have limited time to adjust to their hospitalization. Nurses need to be cognizant of the psychosocial effects of their disease process and provide assistance for patients to cope with their requirements. A knowledge of hospital and community resources will be helpful to meet these requirements. Successful discharge planning must define target objectives that are attainable for patients and family. The outcome of the objectives need to be evaluated and modified as patients progress toward wellness.

An example of discharge planning criteria is presented.

Hemorrhoidectomy

Objective A. Have successful bowel movements without discomfort.

1. Take stool softener as directed.
2. Dietary needs should be met to encourage regular bowel habits. Foods to include: fruit, apples, prunes, fiber, whole grain cereals, and vegetables.
    a. Avoid cheese, and chocolate as they tend to cause constipation.
3. If postoperative discomfort is anticipated, take prescribed analgesia 1/2 hour before anticipated defecation.

Objective B. Maximize wound healing.

1. Keep area clean, washing with mild soap and water after each bowel movement.
2. Sitz-bath with "ocean water" or "tea" as directed.
3. Pat dry or blow area dry with hair dryer on low heat.
4. Apply antibiotic ointment as directed.

NURSING ASSESSMENT, PLANNING, AND OUTCOME FORM

PATIENT NAME:____________________PHYSICIAN_________________

****

PART I ASSESSMENT

1. Patient understands illness and procedure that will be done? yes__no__
   If no, give patient laser pamphlet. Done? yes__no__
   a. Procedure (own words)______________________________
   b. Understands why the laser will be used? yes__no__
2. Patient understands the risks of procedure? yes__no__
   a. Risk(s) (own words)______________________________
3. Patient understands expected outcomes of procedure? yes__no__
   a. Outcomes (own words)______________________________
   b. Questions answered about laser? yes__no__
4. Other health care problems or concerns that may affect the outcome of care? (circle)
   bowel habits diet
   other diseases heart S.O.B. cancer
   hypertension vision loss
   hearing impairment diabetes
   other:______________________________
5. Family supportive and understands their role in the patients progress toward wellness? yes__no__
   Comment______________________________

===

PART II NURSING CARE PLAN

1. Patient education regarding operative procedure, risks, and outcomes explained? Completed________date. Comment______________
   ____
2. Note by O.R. Nurse: (or <u>Holding Room Nurse</u>)
   ID. band checked ___ Pre-Op meds given ____
   Consent form signed ___ Lab, x-ray reports on chart ___
   Skin integrity noted ___ Patient knows procedure yes__ no__
   Positioning problems noted?______________________________
   Patient to Operating Room at _______ a.m./p.m.
3. Patient arrived in PCAU at _________ a.m./p.m. Status____________
4. Patient to Room/Outpatient _________ a.m./p.m. Status____________

===

PART III POST PROCEDURE PLAN

Circle completed objective:
1. Ambulate, cough/deep breathe, range of motion.
2. Diet; liquid, soft, regular, special.
3. Special needs, <u>please note:</u> ______________________________

Discharge Planning:
1. Home Health Care needed? yes__no__ Contacted_______date.
2. Social Services needed? yes__no__ Contacted_______date.
   Seen yes__no__ By_________date______
3. Instructions given to patient/family? yes__no__ Date______
4. Teaching aids given? yes__no__ By_________date______
5. Problems identified that need further consultation? ____________
   ____

SIGNATURE OF DISCHARGE NURSE______________________________

===

PART IV PHYSICIAN TO COMPLETE AND RETURN TO FACILITY

1. Did your patient develop a post-op wound infection? yes__no__
2. Did you feel the patient's care plan was appropriate? yes__no__
   If no, please explain______________________________
3. What could the nursing staff do to better care for your patient?
   ____
4. What could the nursing staff do to assist you in giving better care for your patients?______________________________

Figure 29.2. Nursing assessment, planning, and outcome form.

5. Usually, on the second or third postoperative day there will be some drainage. Use a sanitary pad, this will keep the area dry and can be changed frequently.
   a. Men need to be shown how to position the sanitary pad in their underwear.

Objective C. Decrease potential recurrence of the etiology.
1. Maintain good bowel habits through good nutrition.
2. Use good body mechanics when lifting, so as not to strain.
3. See the doctor immediately if there is any change in bowel habits, rectal bleeding, or symptoms of colorectal disease.

Discharge instructions can become standard criteria, developed through collaborative practice with physicians and nursing personnel. The instructions can be printed and a copy given to the patient and family when discharged from the facility. A copy signed by the patient and nurse giving the instructions should be retained for the medical record.

Discharge planning for patients having major general surgical procedures may need flexibility and collaboration with other resources to develop a continuum of care. The objectives for developing discharge planning criteria will be to direct nursing activities in a continuous progression toward optimum health.

Patients having laser procedures for debulking of solid tumors may need to have several health care concerns identified. These nursing concerns are:

1. patient perceptions of own needs and problems;
2. patient's expectations of illness and treatment outcomes;
3. meeting the needs for activities of daily living;
4. identify the patient's ability to cope with health-related problems.

Once these concerns have been assessed, a plan can be developed, modified, and evaluated to meet the patient's and family's needs. Long-term care requirements may relate to the use of community resources, such as home health care.

Evaluation of the patient's progress toward optimum health cannot be accomplished adequately unless a feedback mechanism is built into the overall nursing care plan. Because the "minor" general surgical patient population has a decreased length of stay, the feedback mechanism would be a postdischarge phone call, about 2–3 days later, assessing the patient's progress toward wellness.

A comprehensive evaluation tool (Fig. 29.2) can be developed and completed by the physician when he/she discharges the patient. The form is returned to the health care facility and put into the patient's record. This method becomes part of the quality assurance criteria and can be reviewed by a utilization review process to measure the standard of care given at the facility.

Planning nursing care should not be bound by tradition. In today's health care environment, innovation is necessary to meet patient needs. Collaborative practice should be encouraged, awareness of hospital and community resources developed, and patient education material should be developed and readily available. Videotapes and home care for family and patients should be designed and made available to assist with the day-to-day care. Setting up a mechanism for patients to communicate with their primary caregivers if they have questions or concerns and developing discharge instructions that are easy to understand and follow are nursing's responsibility to maximize quality, cost-effective health care.

Nurses are identified as the primary caregivers and should have the knowledge and understanding of all treatment modalities available to patients. Laser therapy in the specialties of general surgery is a relatively new technique. It is nursing administration's responsibility to assure that the nurses who are giving care to these patients understand the basic tenets of laser techniques, risks, and potential outcomes when doing laser-assisted general surgical procedures.

CHAPTER
30

Laserthermia

Norio Daikuzono, Hisao Tajiri, S. Suzuki, Stephen N. Joffe

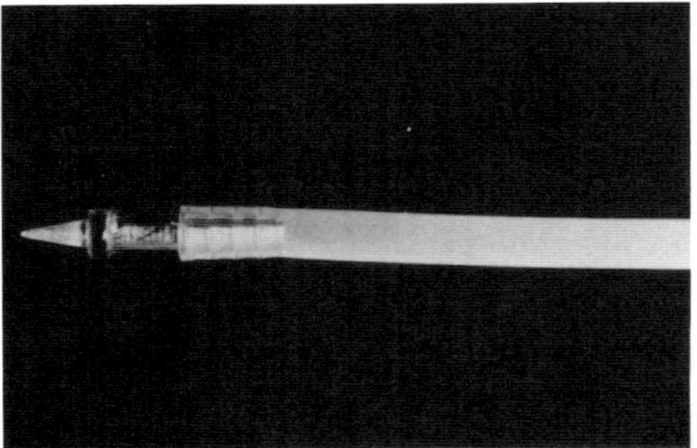

Figure 30.1. Interstitial contact probe ("frosted" on the sides) for Laserthermia.

Several kinds of energy resources have been used for hyperthermia. These include heated water, electromagnetic energy from radio frequency, microwave, sonic energy from ultrasound, scattered light from infrared light and, finally, laser energy from the Nd:YAG laser.

The contact Nd:YAG laser is assuming a greater importance in endoscopic and open surgery, allowing coagulation, cutting, and vaporization with greater precision and safety. A new contact probe allows a wider angle of irradiation and diffusion of low-power laser energy (<5 W) using the interstitial technique for local hyperthermia (Fig. 30.1). Continuous monitoring temperature sensors are placed directly into the surrounding tissue or tumor (Fig. 30.2). Using a computer program interfaced with the laser and sensors, a controlled and stable temperature (e.g., 42°C) can be produced in a known volume of tissue over a prolonged period of time (e.g., 20–40 min) (Fig. 30.3).

Requirements for hyperthermia include greater and more uniform heating with easier and more precise temperature control. A noninvasive method is desired. For certain clinical purposes, localized hyperthermia and a means of transmitting energy are important. The energy from a Nd:YAG laser, which can be transmitted by a flexible optical fiber, penetrates tissue deeper than other kinds of medical lasers.

Initially, the Nd:YAG laser for hyperthermia, using the interstitial method, required placing the bare fiber directly into a tumor (1). However, the high-power density at the distal end of the fiber caused damage to the fiber tip and vaporized the tissue. Burnt tissue, including char, absorbs laser energy and causes a very limited localized increase in temperature, which is difficult to control and is unsuitable for use in hyperthermia. Several kinds of sapphire contact probes for attachment to the Nd:YAG laser optical fiber have been introduced (2, 3). The interstitial contact probe has the ability to diffuse the laser beam on the probe surface because of its optical design. It can withstand higher temperatures and is much harder than the bare quartz fiber, which assures thermal and mechanical stability. In this chapter, local hyperthermia controlled by a computer is described, using a thermocouple as a monitor for temperature and an interstitial probe to transmit diffuse low-power Nd:YAG laser energy. This technique or interstitial hyperthermia is known as Laserthermia, which is a registered trademark of Surgical Laser Technologies, Inc. (Malvern, PA).

INTERSTITIAL PROBES

Noncontact laser irradiation can lose up to 30-40% of beam energy due to backscatter. The contact interstitial method can deliver the laser beam more effectively and quantitatively into tissue. This is very important for clinical procedures requiring a defined total dose of laser energy. The probe's conical shape facilitates mechanical pene-

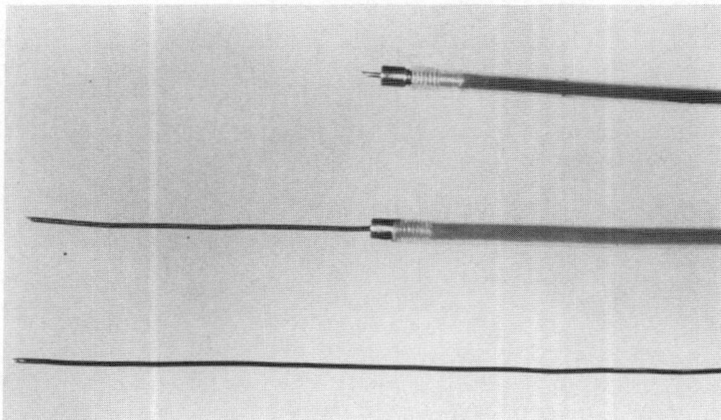

Figure 30.2. Thermocouples of various lengths are placed adjacent to the edge of the tumor.

tration of the tumor (Table 30.1). Diffused laser light on the surface of the probe has low-power density measured at less than 0.05 W/cm^2 for 1 W of total irradiation from a 3-mm long probe. In contrast, the bare fiber has a power density of 3.6 W/cm^2 for 1 W of 600-μm diameter fiber. With a longer probe, it is possible to have longer irradiation time. This means that different probe lengths can be applied based on the tumor volume. Due to low-power density on the surface and characteristics of the probe, the probe causes less local tissue damage than the bare fiber but delivers a greater amount of energy.

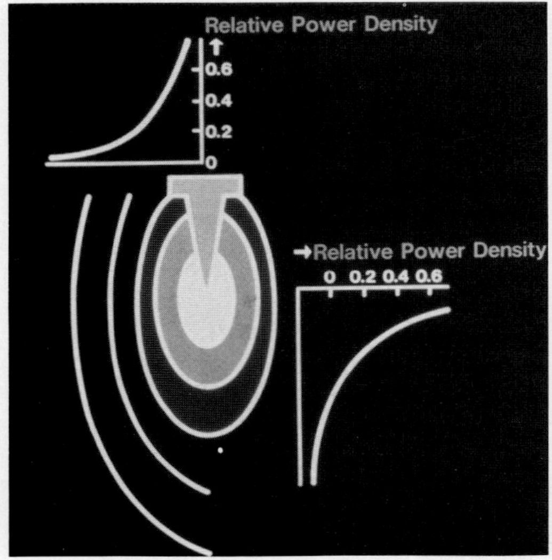

Figure 30.3. Distribution of power density from interstitial endoprobe using the Nd:YAG laser.

THERMOCOUPLE

For the practical purpose of inserting the thermocouple into the tumor, the needle-shaped stainless steel thermocouple has a stopper-like flange to control the depth of insertion. The surface of the needle is well polished for laser beam reflectence. Different length of needles are available for different clinical cases (Fig. 30.2). Comparison of temperatures measured from the thermocouple and thermograms showed there was no temperature interference from exposure of the laser beam directly onto the thermocouple during low-power laser irradiation from the probe in tissue (Fig. 30.4).

COMPUTER SYSTEM

The delivery of laser energy from the probe to increase the temperature of the tumor is computer controlled. The probe and the thermocouple are placed at fixed distances from each other.

A feedback system of measured temperature to laser energy delivery is possible, thus keeping the programmed temperature at the point where the thermocouple is located. Currently, the surgical laser requires a very stable laser generator such as the SLT Contact Laser, especially using low powers. Temperature distribution will vary with the color or the tissue, the blood flow, and the distance between the probe and the thermocouple (Fig. 30.5). The temperature on the surface of the probe has the highest temperature. To obtain a greater volume of tissue heating and controllable temperature, it is important not to obtain more than 100°C on the surface of the probe. This leads to carbonization of tissue with great energy loss leading to tissue damage of the

Table 30.1. Characteristics of Single Crystal Artificial Sapphire Compared to Quartz Fiber for Use in Laserthermia

Property	Sapphire	Quartz
Material/formula	Al_2O	S10
Melting point	2030–2050°C	1600°C
Specific heat	0.18 (25°C)	0.17 (25°C)
Thermal conductivity (g°cal. cm sec)	0.0016–0.0034 (40°C)	0.0158–0.0299 (40°C)
Coefficient of thermal expansion (10 cm/°C)	50–67	80
Elastic coefficient (10 kg/cm)	5.0	0.76
Specific gravity	4.0	2.2
Hardness (mohs)	9	7
Compressive strength (kg/cm)	28000	20000
Tensile strength	2000	900 1200
Index of refraction	1.76	1.54
Absorption degree of water	0.00	0.00
Chemical characteristic appearance	Acid- and base-proof clear	Acid- and base-proof clear
Crystal form	Hexagonal system	Hexagonal system
Transmittance for YAG laser	More 90%	More 90%

probe. A suitable low-power laser level is required, normally operating at less than 5 W, which will heat an area of 1–2 cm in diameter. A cross-sectional view of temperature distribution is almost semicircular, so that it is possible to get a known volume of tissue adequately heated easily.

METHOD OF TEMPERATURE CONTROL

At the beginning of the Laserthermia procedure, laser energy must be delivered rapidly in a continuous mode, since the tissue temperature is lower than "lower control temperature" set at 42°C. However, if the tissue temperature is within

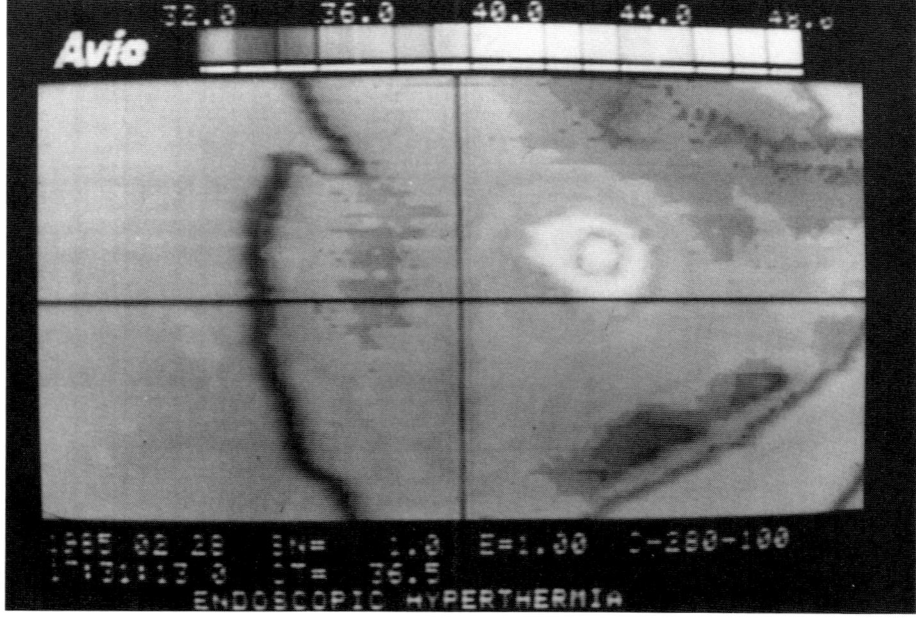

Figure 30.4. Thermogram during Laserthermia shows temperature distribution.

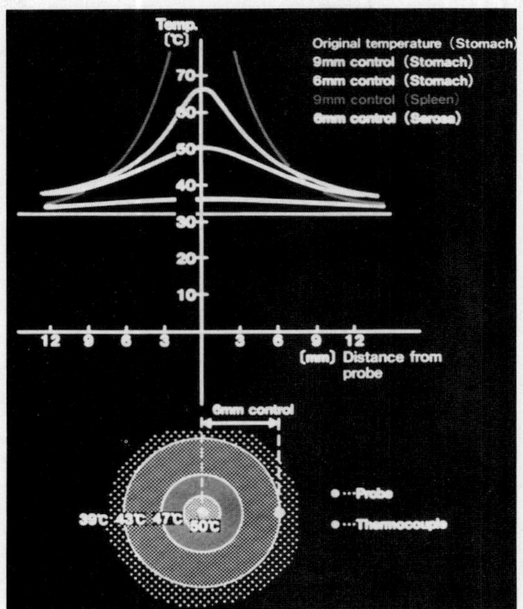

Figure 30.5. Temperature distribution in the canine stomach and spleen. Control methods for obtaining temperature control of 42–44°C using the Nd:YAG laser Laserthermia system.

the control range between the lower control temperature and the "upper control temperature," such as 44°C, the system delivers the laser energy slowly, which is possible by using the pulse mode of laser energy delivery. If the temperature is over the upper control temperature, it will stop the delivery of laser energy. For safety considerations, the system will cease delivering laser energy if the temperature is over the "abnormal upper temperature," suggesting disconnection of the thermocouple from tissue. The system allows various input ranges and conditions for controlling the system so that it has versatility for a wide variety of clinical purposes (Table 30.2).

SUITABLE POWER RANGES AND PULSE DELIVERY

From experiments in vivo, it was apparent that higher laser power caused overshooting above the upper control temperature, so the controlled range of temperature was wide and imprecise. Lower power, on the other hand, took a longer time to increase the temperature with less flexibility to response to changes in tissue conditions such as blood flow. The suitable laser power range seemed to be from 1–5 W. The laser system allows the use of continuous wave or pulse mode for laser delivery during the raising of temperature between lower and upper control temperatures. The pulse mode allows a more precise control than the continuous wave mode.

MULTIPLE LASERTHERMIA SYSTEM

The single-probe Laserthermia system heats a limited volume of tissue. To heat larger tissue volumes with a more uniform temperature eleva-

Table 30.2. Input Ranges for Laserthermia Controlling System

1. Input power	0.1–100 W
2. Total time	0.01–30 min
3. Total joules	0.1–10,000 J
4. Upper temperature (upper temperature controlled)	35.1–55.0°C
5. Lower temperature (lower temperature controlled)	35.0–49.9°C
6. Ab.-Up. temp. (abnormal upper temperature)	35.1–55.0°C
7. Ab.-Lo temp. (abnormal lower temperature)	30.0–49.9°C
8. Laser output mode (control mode)	Continuous or pulse
8–1.C (continuous)	0–30 min
8–2. P (pulse)	Programmable
8–2–1. Pulse on (pulse width)	0.1–5.0 sec
8–2–2. Pulse off (no pulse width)	0.1–5.0 sec

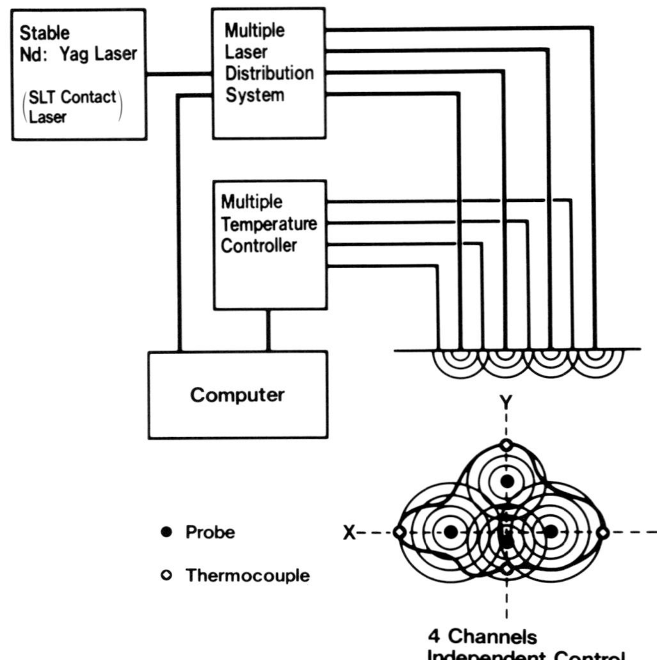

Figure 30.6. Computer-controlled, multichannel Laserthermia system.

tion, a multiple Laserthermia system was developed using a multiple laser distribution system and a computer control. Considering the rapid localized change of temperature in the tumor, each probe is independently controlled by its own thermocouple. There are no known technical problems to using more channels, which would be determined by the volume of tissue to be treated. The temperature around the probe in the tumor is higher. This is not of much concern as long as the probe does not cause tissue vaporization. The temperature should be strictly and precisely controlled at the border between normal tissue and tumor. A monitoring thermocouple should be placed at this junction and the probes should be directed to the center of the tumor. This will allow for adequate treatment at the tumor edge.

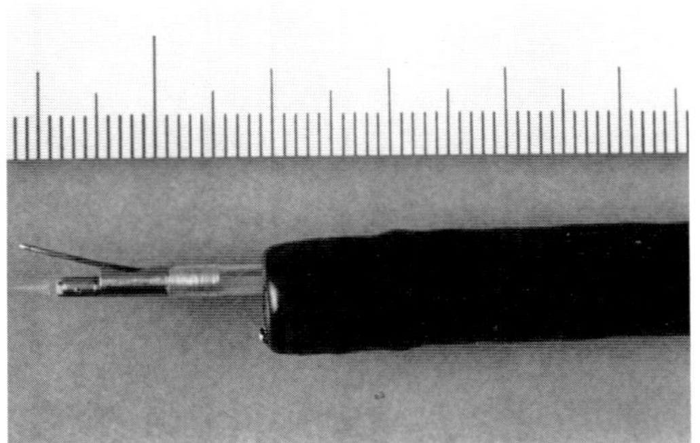

Figure 30.7. Endoscopic Laserthermia system for the endoscopic and clinical treatment of gastric and colonic carcinoma.

A single and multiple Laserthermia system has been developed that allows a precise control of temperature. These therapeutic modalities are very easy to operate, safer, and have more precise temperature control than the currently used laser system with their high power and short therapeutic durations. The single system is useful for endoscopic Laserthermia using a two-channel endoscope (Fig. 30.7). Obviously, a multiple Laserthermia system will be used for larger tumors located on an open surgical field. Recent biomedical and clinical studies of Laserthermia show that, in addition to normal efficacy of hyperthermia, it may have additional advantages based on the interaction between laser energy and cancer cells with a direct cytocidal effect with laser light on the cancer cells (4). Damage to normal tissue with Laserthermia is minimal as shown

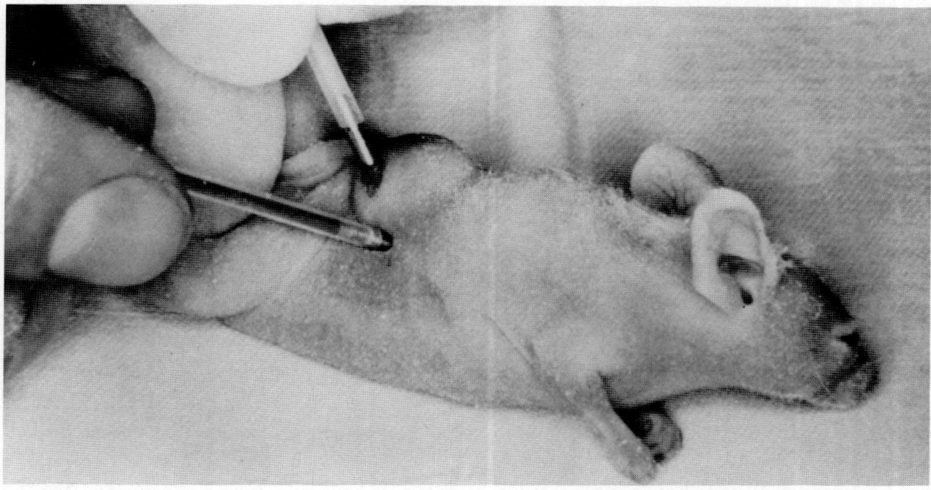

Figure 30.8. Local interstitial hyperthermia in a nude mouse with a subcutaneously transplanted human pancreatic cancer. The interstitial frosted probe is placed in the center of the tumor and the temperature sensor is positioned at the periphery of the carcinoma.

by studies measuring arachidonic acid metabolites in vivo. This method has been evaluated by different specialties (4).

EXPERIMENTAL STUDY

Human pancreatic carcinoma was transplanted subcutaneously into pathogen-free nude mice. At 5–6 weeks, these tumors were treated by Laserthermia using a frosted interstitial probe with temperature control at the margin of the tumor (Fig. 30.8). Treatment was at 10 W for 20 min at temperatures maintained at the periphery of the tumor of between 42 and 43°C. Immediately after treatment, light microscopy of the tumor showed hemorrhage, necrosis, and cell lysis surrounding the puncture point (Fig. 30.9).

At 7 days after treatment, inflammatory cell infiltration and degenerating tissues were found in

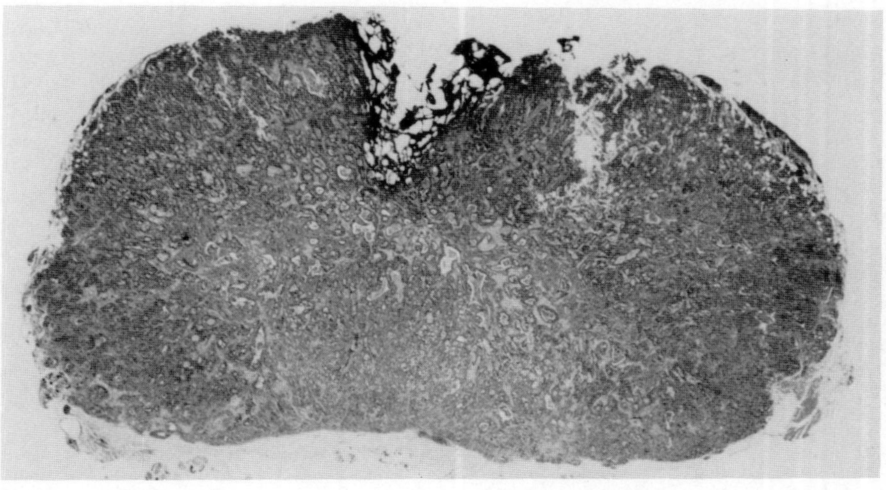

Figure 30.9. Light microscopy immediately after 20 min of Laserthermia at 42-43°C, showing bleeding and cellular destruction immediately surrounding the interstitial probe puncture site.

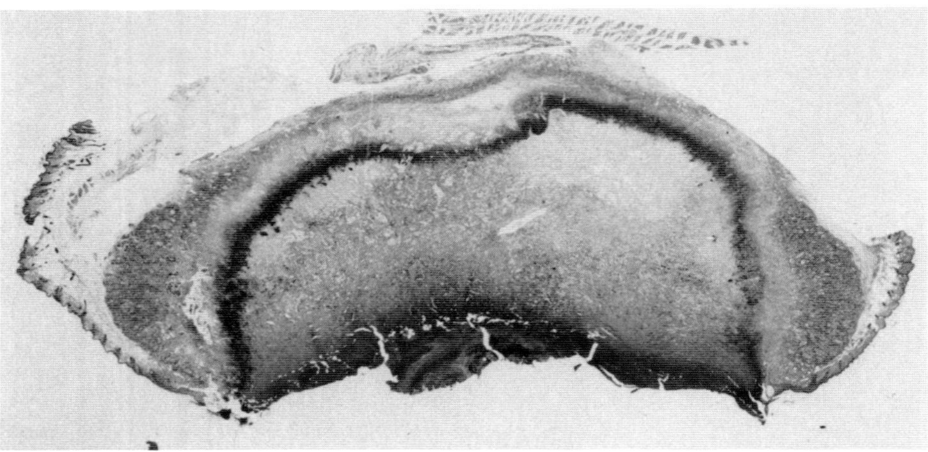

Figure 30.10. Light microscopy of a transplanted human pancreatic carcinoma 7 days after treatment by Laserthermia showing tumor necrosis clearly demarcated from the surrounding tissue.

concentric circles from the center of the punctured point accounting for 70-80% of the total volume (Fig. 30.10). Twenty minutes seemed to cause more necrosis in the tumor than 10 min of treatment. The temperature near the margin of the tumor was controlled at 42-43°C (0.5–1 cm away from the puncture point). The temperature at the center of the tumor was approximately 50°C.

Microangiography of the untreated tumor showed tumor vessel encasement with irregularity and tortuousity of the vessels. On the other hand, after local interstitial hyperthermia with the low-powered Nd:YAG laser, interruption and irregularity of blood vessels were seen near the margin of the puncture site immediately after treatment. At 7 days after therapy, the avascular area was large, corresponding to the area of necrosis. At the border of the remaining cancer tissues, the minute vessels were cut off and showed an abnormal arrangement with partial proximal dilatation (Fig. 30.11).

Initial studies on experimental pancreatic and gastric cancer and clinical applications in gastric cancer, head and neck cancer, and brain tumors

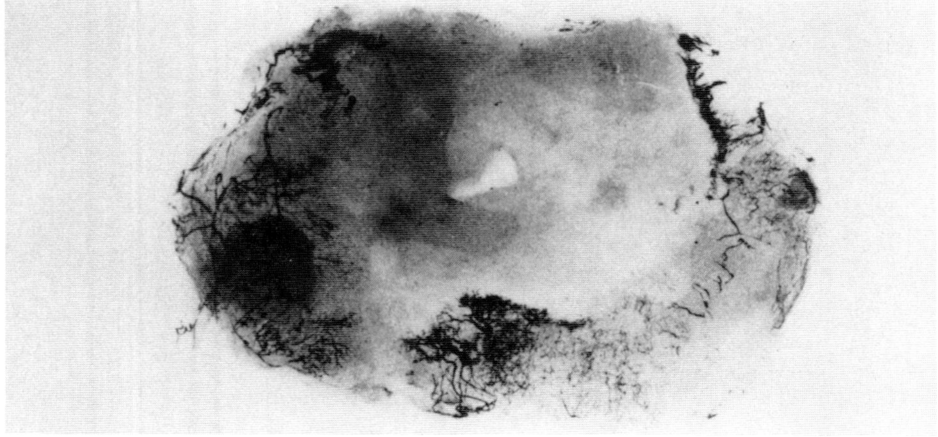

Figure 30.11. Microangiogram 7 days after Laserthermia. The avascular area corresponds very closely to the tumor necrosis seen on light microscopy.

are confirming the efficacy of Laserthermia. This new technology using a well-established principle in the treatment of cancer is expected to expand rapidly in surgical oncology as an adjuvant to other methods of treatment.

REFERENCES

1. Bown SG. Tumor therapy with the Nd:YAG laser. In Joffe SN, Muckerheide MM, Goldman L, Eds. Neodymium-YAG Laser in Medicine and Surgery. Elsevier, New York, 1983, pp. 59-70.
2. Daikuzono N, Joffe SN. Introduction of a newly developed contact ceramic probe connected to a laser optical quartz fiber for wide applications in medicine and surgery. Proceedings for 2nd International Nd:YAG Laser Conference in Munich. Springer-Verlag, 1985, pp. 302-306.
3. Daikuzono N, Joffe SN. Artificial sapphire probe for contact photocoagulation and tissue vaporization with the Nd:YAG laser. Med Instrum 1985; 19:183-178.
4. Tajiri H. Experimental studies of local hyperthermia using Nd-YAG laser. Oncologia 1986; 17:161-163.

INDEX

Page numbers in *italics* denote figures; those followed by "t" denote tables.